D1361688

QUALITY
MANAGEMENT
IN HEALTH CARE

♦

Lionel Wilson
AM, MBBS, BS, FRACGP (University of Sydney)
Managing Director, Qual-Med Pty Ltd

Peter Goldschmidt
MD, DrPH, DMS
President, World Development Group, Inc,
Bethesda, Maryland, USA
President, Medical Care Management
Corporation, Bethesda, Maryland, USA

McGRAW-HILL BOOK COMPANY Sydney
New York   San Francisco   Auckland   Bogotá
Caracas   Lisbon   London   Madrid   Mexico City
Milan   Montreal   New Delhi   San Juan
Singapore   Toronto

NOTICE
Medicine is an ever-changing science. As new research and clinical experience broaden our knowledge, changes in treatment and drug therapy are required. The editors and the publisher of this work have checked with sources believed to be reliable in their efforts to provide information that is complete and generally in accord with the standards accepted at the time of publication. However, in view of the possibility of human error or changes in medical sciences, neither the editor, nor the publisher, nor any other party who has been involved in the preparation or publication of this work warrants that the information contained herein is in every respect accurate or complete. Readers are encouraged to confirm the information contained herein with other sources. For example and in particular, readers are advised to check the product information sheet included in the package of each drug they plan to administer to be certain that the information contained in this book is accurate and that changes have not been made in the recommended dose or in the contraindications for administration. This recommendation is of particular importance in connection with new or infrequently used drugs.

Text © 1995 Lionel Wilson and Peter Goldschmidt
Illustrations and design © 1995 McGraw-Hill Book Company Australia Pty Limited

Apart from any fair dealing for the purposes of study, research, criticism or review, as permitted under the *Copyright Act*, no part may be reproduced by any process without written permission. Enquiries should be made to the publisher, marked for the attention of the Permissions Editor, at the address below.

Copying for educational purposes
Under the copying provisions of the *Copyright Act*, copies of parts of this book may be made by an educational institution. An agreement exists between the Copyright Agency Limited (CAL) and the relevant educational authority (Department of Education, university, TAFE, etc.) to pay a licence fee for such copying. It is not necessary to keep records of copying except where the relevant educational authority has undertaken to do so by arrangement with the Copyright Agency Limited.

For further information on the CAL licence agreements with educational institutions, contact the Copyright Agency Limited, Level 19, 157 Liverpool Street, Sydney NSW 2000. Where no such agreement exists, the copyright owner is entitled to claim payment in respect of any copies made.

Enquiries concerning copyright in McGraw-Hill publications should be directed to the Permissions Editor at the address below.

National Library of Australia Cataloguing-in-Publication data:

Wilson, L. L. (Lionel Leopold).
Quality management in health care.

Includes index.
ISBN 0 07 470247 5.

1. Hospital care—Australia—Quality control.
2. Hospitals—Australia—Administration. L. Goldschmidt,
Peter. II. Title.

362.110685

Published in Australia by
McGraw-Hill Book Company Australia Pty Limited
4 Barcoo Street, Roseville NSW 2069, Australia
Publisher: John Rowe
Production editors: Annabel Adair and Caroline Hunter
Designer: Asymmetric Typography Pty Limited
Illustrator: Shelley Communications

Typeset in Australia by Midland Typesetters, Victoria
Printed in Australia by McPherson's Printing Group

FOREWORD

---

1. Foreword by STEPHEN LEEDER

Lionel Wilson has led the crusade for quality assurance in medical care in Australia since the late 1970s when it was first on the medicopolitical horizon. From another perspective, that of an interest in everything that promotes the health of the community, I have admired Dr Wilson's contribution to health gain through quality health care.

Three features distinguish Dr Wilson's substantial contribution to the debate about quality: his courage, his enthusiastic persistence, and his intellectual development of the subject over the past twenty years.

I have heard him speak about quality at various points throughout those two decades. Each time my understanding about quality and its place in management has been enhanced by new ideas and developments that Dr Wilson has brought to light. Most recently I took his point to heart that quality must fundamentally be *a way* of managing, not something tacked on to conventional management. This does not diminish quality nor cast it as something lacking its own epistemology; rather, I took Dr Wilson to be saying that quality must permeate every aspect of management style.

I thus expected to be impressed with this book and I was not disappointed. Dr Wilson and Dr Goldschmidt have prepared a meticulous and instructive compendium of wise advice, beautifully laid out, easy to follow and of exemplary quality in itself.

Patient care in Australia owes Lionel Wilson a great debt for his unrelenting commitment to quality. This book puts that commitment firmly and freshly on record.

Stephen Leeder is Professor of Public Health and Community Medicine at The University of Sydney and has been based at Westmead Hospital since 1986. He is a physician with an interest in epidemiology and public health policy and has been active in Australia's development of health goals and targets and in the early phases of health gain (outcome) assessment. At Newcastle (NSW) University he was associated with the formation (in 1977) of an innovative medical school and an international centre for clinical epidemiology and biostatics and has had a longstanding interest in evaluation. He is pro-dean for medical education at the University of Sydney where a four-year graduate degree will replace the current six-year course commencing 1997. Stephen Leeder is current President of the Public Health Association of Australia and in that and other capacities is a regular contributor to the media on matters relating to health and health policy.

2. Foreword by JOHN WILLIAMSON

This foreword provides a brief history of health care quality management (QM) starting 5000 years ago. Today two philosophies compete for QM time and resources. These are the national, external 'top down regulatory micro-management' approach, versus the local, internal 'bottom up self-help strategies for QM'. Within this context, I discuss the need for this manual, and how it will enhance QM throughout the world. Implementing the QM systems this manual describes will ultimately facilitate documented improvement of modern health care, in terms of the health, economic, and satisfaction outcomes for customers, providers and payers of health care.

Doctors have long been accountable for health care outcomes. As early as 3000 BC, in the legal statutes of the Egyptians, heads of state generously rewarded physicians for exceptional medical outcomes. For example, the accomplishments of Imhoptep (2686–2613 BC), who was the physician for King Zoser, won him such acclaim that he was elevated to demi-god about 100 years after his death, and to a full deity around 525 BC. (Was this the beginning of the physician 'God complex?') A similar process took place later in the Homeric Period of Greek history, about 900 BC, with Aesculapius, to whom the caduceus, as the symbol of the medical profession, was first ascribed. Like Imhoptep, he was later made a full god, to be worshipped in the Temple of Aesculapius, along with his daughters Hygeia and Panacea.*

One of the earliest examples of what was roughly analogous to modern health outcomes management (and perhaps medical malpractice legislation) is found in the Mesopotamian Codes of Hammurabi, dating from the 18th century BC. One code states: 'If a physician should operate on a man for a severe wound with a bronze lancet and cause the man's death, or open an abscess (in the eye) . . . and destroy the eye, they shall cut off his (the physician's) fingers.' Hammurabi also addressed 'economic outcomes management', by establishing specific fees for medical care. In this early period of history it is difficult to find an example roughly analogous to what we, today, call patient satisfaction outcomes measurement. Perhaps the tried and true method of consumers 'voting with their feet'—that is, not returning to the same care provider with whom they are dissatisfied—is the universal means of consumer management of satisfaction outcomes.

Thus, throughout the span of recorded history, examples are evident of activity roughly analogous to current quality improvement functions. Such activity can be traced back in history through five streams of health care stakeholders: government, academia, health professional organisations, financing groups and consumer groups. In the past forty to fifty years, quality assurance/quality improvement (QA/QI)† has been systematised and, in many parts of the world, developed on an institutional basis, utilising formal, if not scientific, tools and methods. Currently, health care professionals are slowly learning many of the basic principles of quality management—some of which date back nearly 5000 years of recorded history.

At present, many different groups are working to improve national health care systems. Australia, for example, has been among the earliest nations to focus on a national

---

* Bettmann, OL. A pictorial history of medicine. Charles Thomas Publisher, 1972, pp 16–17.
† In the United States this term was established by the Institute of Medicine of the National Academy of Science (a private and highly respected organisation) to encompass all of the quality or 'Q' words, including utilisation review and risk management as required by the US Congress for the one third of patients who are federally funded.

program of QA.†† In the early 1980s, this activity utilised many of the concepts and resources of the National Organization for Quality Assurance in Hospitals (known often by its Dutch abbreviation, CBO) in the Netherlands. (Subsequently CBO would organise and operate the 'World Health Organization's Collaboration Centre for Quality Assurance in Health Care', based in Utrecht, the Netherlands.)

'New, revised and repackaged' QI technologies are increasing at an exponential rate. Unfortunately, their application has had rather mixed results in terms of QI cost-effectiveness, especially when assessed in terms of the impact on final outcomes (health, economic and satisfaction outcomes of care rendered). The 'top down regulatory, micro-management approach' has a particularly dismal track record. Studies by the Institute of Medicine in the USA have shown that this regulatory QI policy has had little positive— and likely serious negative—effect on the US health care system (or non-system).

This regulatory approach leaves health care professionals with the impossible task of trying to keep up with constantly changing and expanding regulations. Many caregivers have all but given up hope that these regulations will do anything more than waste their time with increasing paperwork, at the expense of time with patients.

Within this historical context, as well as the continuing QI technology explosion, the contribution of this manual will be of universal value. The authors, Lionel Wilson and Peter Goldschmidt, are important pioneers of the current QA/QI field. Their knowledge, insights and experience make them well qualified to produce this important volume which is truly a magnum opus for these authors. This manual's target readers are appropriately as broad as the field of health care itself—direct and ancillary clinical professionals, administrative and management personnel, to name a few. It provides readers with both ideas and resources to develop a solid foundation for designing, implementing and evaluating QM programs.

This publication provides a comprehensive overview of the field of QM. It is truly an encyclopedia of recent QA/QI technology encompassing most, if not all, current QI theory, principles and methods. Further, it is also an invaluable means for identifying other QA/QI resources. For example, it provides a useful means for keeping up with the rapidly expanding QI field. It stresses what, in the future, will likely be among the most important resources for QA/QI—namely medical informatics and computerised 'Decision Support Technology' (DSTs). This manual's listing of the major serial publications and newsletters in the QI field facilitates retrieving other important published resources. This contribution alone will prove of major benefit to QA/QI professionals trying to keep up with, and applying ongoing developments in, health care quality assessment and improvement technology.

The material in this volume applies to a range of health care facilities and systems, beyond its main focus on hospital care in Australia. For example, information in this work is equally applicable to quality management in ambulatory care, long-term care and nursing home care. Its wider application internationally will also be very important. American readers may have difficulty accommodating to traditional spelling of common English words, such as 'centre'. However, this is a minor consideration when weighed against the substantial value this book will have for improving QA/QI activity in the USA, Canada, and elsewhere.

---

†† Organised around Australia's AMA/ACHS Peer Review Resource Centre. This resource centre model was espoused by CBO in The Netherlands, whose philosophy was that QI must be a 'bottom-up' voluntary effort, in contrast to most QI systems that stressed a 'top-down' regulatory approach. Each hospital group must design their own approach, to be facilitated by information, tools, consultation and training by the QI resource centre for any given region. (See Quality assurance in The Netherlands: Parts I and II, Australian Clinical Review, December 1985 (pp 160–167) and March 1986 (pp 4–8).)

In any event, QA/QI, if not all health care professionals throughout the world, will find this encyclopedic volume of major importance. Its use as a means of obtaining a familiarity and understanding of the overall field of 'QA/QI' will be of as much value as that for solving specific QI problems or designing and implementing specific QI programs. The authors are to be congratulated for their enormous effort to produce a book that will make such an important contribution to the field of health care and that of quality improvement.

Salt Lake City, Utah
November 1994

Dr John Williamson is the Director of the Salt Lake Regional Medical Education Center, in the US Department of Veterans Affairs. He is a Professor in the Departments of Medicine and Medical Informatics at the University of Utah. For thirty-five years he has focused on quality improvement (QI) technology, particularly health science information management, the foundation for QI. He is internationally recognised as a pioneer in these fields. He has written ten books and monographs and over 100 articles on these subjects.

Dr Williamson's early emphasis on health care outcomes as the key to health care improvement was the topic of his 1978 book Assessing and Improving Health Care Outcomes, the Health Accounting Approach to Quality Assurance. *The principles embodied in this approach are now recognised as fundamental to effective QI. Since the early 1960s, Dr Williamson has written extensively on structured group judgment for quality assurance priority setting, as well as on the vital importance of an outcomes based approach to quality improvement. He designed the concept of a Quality Improvement Resource Center to facilitate voluntary participation of both providers and consumers in developing QI systems. The WHO International QA Collaborating Center, in the Netherlands, has promulgated this innovation—regarded as standard today—in 46 centres throughout the world. In the US, his early research influenced the provisions of the quality assurance section of the Bennett Amendment to the Social Security Act, and later of the National Health Maintenance Act, which is still in force today.*

Among his many awards and honors, Dr Williamson was the 1993 Recipient of the prestigious John P. Hubbard Award, given by the National Board of Medical Examiners in recognition of an individual who has made a significant contribution to the pursuit of excellence in the field of evaluation in medicine. He was the recipient of the first US Department of Veterans Affairs Career Quality Achievement Award in 1992. The award citation recognised his unique contribution to the Department's mission and his numerous and significant contributions to the health care field. The plaque that Dr Williamson received in 1990 for the Utah Medical Association Distinguished Service Award reads: 'In recognition of pioneering research in medical quality assurance and its application to the patient.' The citation recognised him as someone who has 'made a difference in medicine'. In 1986, he received the American College of Medical Quality's Founder's Award for his outstanding contribution to the field of medical quality assurance and utilisation review through his teaching and writing.

3. Foreword by ANGUS MACIVER

Anybody who has sat at a dinner table when the conversation has turned to the experience of hospital care will know how many people in our community are dissatisfied with the treatment that they receive in our hospitals.

FAI Insurances Limited is the insurer of many private hospitals and health care institutions throughout Australia and was for many years the owner of a major private hospital group. Through its experiences in those areas FAI has become aware of the reasons why so many people have become disgruntled with the quality of care that they have experienced in hospitals. As a major insurer in the areas of medical malpractice and professional liability, for a number of reasons we felt it was incumbent upon us to take steps to promote quality management—that is, the systematic improvement in the quality of care and reduction in risk to patients, staff and the hospital. Firstly, we are concerned about the quality of care received by patients and want to promote improvements in the quality of that care. Secondly, we want to help contain the rising cost of care attributable to inappropriate utilisation. Thirdly, we want to make sure that such professionals as doctors remain insurable, by encouraging them to adopt prudent risk management procedures. Finally, we want to promote a safe and productive environment for patients and staff.

Sponsoring this manual is an important response to our concerns. The manual applies to all types of health care while focusing on hospitals. The manual has been written to increase the awareness among administrators, managers, doctors, nurses and other health professionals that they must continue to strive in all areas of hospital activity to promote two things—excellence of their own performance particularly with respect to improving patients' health outcomes, and overall quality of the service of which they are a part. We hope that the manual will encourage and assist hospital managers, doctors and nurses to achieve those aims.

Sydney, Australia
November 1994

Angus Maciver joined FAI Insurances Limited in 1974 and founded its Professional Indemnity Division. He is the general manager of that division and is also a director of FAI. He has developed a keen interest in medical malpractice insurance and is very much involved in risk management and claims prevention techniques.

Maciver delivered a paper at the first Medico-Legal Seminar held in Sydney in 1988 sponsored by the New South Wales Medical Defence Union and the Law Society of New South Wales. He is constantly sought after to present papers on risk management to various professional groups around Australia. He was educated at Fettes College, Edinburgh, Scotland, and afterwards received his Bachelor of Law degree from the internationally renowned London School of Economics.

FAI's Professional Indemnity Division is now the largest malpractice underwriter operating in Australia. It underwrites policies for professionals in South East Asia, North America and the United Kingdom, as well as in Australia. The company underwrites the insurance program for the seven thousand members of the New South Wales Medical Defence Union, and was the first Australian underwriter to back the Victorian and West Australian Medical Defence Associations. The company insures many private hospitals and nursing homes in Australia and overseas. FAI is Australia's third largest general insurance company, with a premium income of A$540 million and assets in excess of A$2.4 billion (1993).

Our quality guarantee

Improving the quality of medical care is an activity of an order of magnitude more difficult than improving the quality of manufactures. Many doctors, hospital managers and politicians are puzzled by how to improve the quality of the nation's hospitals. This manual provides the picture needed to solve the quality management jigsaw. It contains everything you need to know to get started on, and a map to guide, the long journey toward quality maturity. Any hospital that successfully implements the complete, comprehensive quality management program that we describe in this manual will improve its quality of care. Guaranteed!

PREFACE

The past fifty years have witnessed an explosion in medical technology and in government programs designed to give everyone access to medical care. The result is a paradox: despite large expenditures, there has been modest improvement in the nation's health, and most of that improvement may have resulted from factors other than medical care. Rising costs, frustration with government programs, and disappointment with both hospitals and the doctors who work in them have diminished the optimism and excitement of dazzling technological developments. Seemingly uncontrollable demands for health care resources and rapid medical care cost inflation are propelling us toward an unprecedented examination of the production of health improvement or, stated more familiarly, health care quality and accountability for results. The era of quality management has arrived.

Essentially, health care quality management involves deciding what interventions will maximise a patient's health status improvement, measuring the extent to which such interventions are being implemented properly, closing any gaps between what should and is being done, and searching for better interventions and ways to assure and improve health care quality and its management. Providers should strive to improve health status at least cost and with greatest patient satisfaction. If maximal attainment of all three aspects of quality is not feasible, the trade-offs should be as acceptable as possible to patients, providers, payers and the general public.

Quality is as central to health care as it is to the production of other goods and services. Yet the conceptual and practical aspects of quality—quality assurance and quality improvement—are virtually unknown to most doctors, hospital managers, and board members, and the civil servants who run and the politicians who are responsible for health care programs. We have written this manual to fill this gaping void.

The context of this manual

This manual is about quality management—the management of quality. Management of organisations involves setting objectives and policies—including what to produce and how to produce it—and getting these things done through other people. Quality is customers' perception of the value of an organisation's products and services. Recently it has become fashionable to talk about TQM (total quality management) and CQI (continuous quality improvement), or both as a single concept—TQM/CQI—without much understanding about what these terms mean, especially in health care. TQM/CQI are concepts that industry developed in the search for market share and profits in an increasingly competitive world of rising customer expectations. In health care, there is a tendency to think of TQM/CQI as a package that a hospital, for example, can purchase, give to employees, and expect quality to improve. Nothing could be further from the truth, as many industrial organisations have found already to their cost.

In this manual we eschew use of the term TQM (except where describing its evolution in industry) because quality management in hospitals encompasses more than traditional (industrial) TQM. Nevertheless, the idea that TQM/CQI can somehow be grafted onto or incorporated into an existing organisation is bound to disappoint and may be a recipe for failure. Quality management requires reorganisation for total quality. Failure to grasp this fundamental reality will doom from the outset efforts to achieve quality maturity—the state and reality of continuous quality improvement.

Quality management applies to everything that goes on within hospitals, including clinical and patient care, clinical support services such as imaging and laboratory services, operational services such as laundry and housekeeping, and administration. To date, quality management in hospitals—where it has applied at all—has been limited generally to such operational services as the laundry because they are simple situations and most resemble industrial operations. However, hospitals' core business is clinical care. Accordingly, this manual focuses on clinical care—a subject that hospitals have either ignored completely or addressed inadequately. Nevertheless, the same quality management principles that we describe in this manual in relation to clinical care apply to everything else that goes on in hospitals.

Readers will find that many of the philosophical principles of industrial TQM coincide with those we enunciate in this manual. Indeed, to comprehend fully the concepts and issues involved in quality management in hospitals, readers must become familiar with some of the theory and concepts of quality that have evolved over many years in industry. Most importantly hospital professionals need to know how to manage quality, organise a quality management program, implement such a program, and institutionalise quality management processes particularly those relating to clinical care. This basic platform for implementation is so critical to success that it is this manual's primary focus.

Problems and opportunities

We wrote this manual in response to some of the major problems facing health care today and the great opportunities to improve the quality of hospital care. It intends to offer a practical guide for discussing and improving care in Australian hospitals. The manual provides a language and context for rational discussion, and describes specific steps any hospital can take toward quality maturity. While written expressly for the Australian environment, readers in all countries, including Canada, the United Kingdom, and the United States, may find the manual's contents useful in their quest to improve the quality of care.

In managing health care quality, we face the following principal problems:

- Lack of knowledge: we have little idea about the effectiveness of most medical interventions, a problem exacerbated by the inadequacy of quality measures.
- Lack of accountability: we currently have no way of knowing whether or not hospitals are producing high quality care, or any real measure of the variability in care either between hospitals, or among providers of care within hospitals.
- Increasing cost pressures: liability costs are rising and, although costs in the Australian public sector have been capped, the pressure on costs of care is considerable, raising concerns about value-for-money and our ability to afford the level of care we demand.
- Rationing: as health care expenditures consume ever larger fractions of government and personal budgets, the reality of rationing care takes many forms including hospital waiting lists and waiting for appointments with some types of specialists.

- Quality management is no panacea: much confusion surrounds the pursuit of quality management, and quality assurance and improvement, as if they were a panacea; a quixotic (if not chaotic) pursuit of the 'holy grail'.
- Potential for waste: the potential exists to waste vast sums on inappropriate and ineffective initiatives, while giving rise, on the one hand, to false expectations about what can be accomplished, and, on the other, to such damaging effects as increased cynicism that nothing really works.

This manual describes the following principal opportunities:

- Health improvement: effective quality management would meet expectations of health improvement for less money.
- Diminution of litigation: full implementation of quality management, including credentialling of medical staff, can be expected to reduce the level of litigation against hospitals and doctors.
- Greater patient satisfaction: quality management takes seriously patient satisfaction, which is an important element of the quality of care.
- Better value for money: improving quality is seen as a way of increasing efficiency, getting the same or greater effectiveness for less cost, and staving off unpleasant rationing (while improving value-for-money and patient health status).
- Greater employee safety and health: occupational health and safety programs are an integral part of quality management; to improve the health and welfare of staff is to improve the greatest asset of any hospital.
- Elevation of staff satisfaction and morale: to be part of an institution whose entire focus is on quality of service is a great stimulus and source of pride to any professional group. Health professionals have been educated to strive for high quality care. Quality management enables hospital professionals to practise in an environment which actually strives for excellence rather than in one which pays lip-service to quality.

Benefits and costs

In the present environment of diminishing budgets, hospital managers may question the cost of a quality management program. How can such a program be justified at a time of financial austerity?

The expectation—or at least the hope—is that quality management will save money in the long run (although it may require additional expenditure in the short run) because it will reduce such things as waste, inappropriate use of equipment and unnecessary interventions. Doubtless, this is true in some, if not all, circumstances. Even if it turned out that quality management cost more than it saves, the resultant better value for money is itself worthwhile. There is even value in knowing that the care one receives is effective and meets standards with low variability, and is not hit-or-miss. Fundamentally, quality management is part of management and is, or should be, an inescapable cost of doing business, in the same way that accounting for the use of finances is a part of doing business. The question is not whether or not to conduct quality management, but rather how it should be done and how much time and money should be applied.

What assurance does Ms Smith, who is about to undergo surgery, have about Dr Jones' performance in meeting standards? Who knows what Dr Jones' performance really is? What are the personal and social costs if Dr Jones' performance or that of the hospital in which he works is substandard? Performance can be improved only if it is first measured. Then we can investigate reasons for variations in performance and eliminate substandard care and focus on strategies to improve care. We need a system to improve care, because quality is the product of the system of care and not that of individual doctors working in isolation. Australian hospitals should measure the costs and benefits of their quality management initiatives to know which ones are the most cost-effective. We believe that summative assessments of costs and benefits will show that benefits far outweigh costs.

The challenge

When we decided to write this manual, we realised that the undertaking was a large one. However, it was only during the course of the project that we fully realised the width and breadth of the canvas on which this picture had to be drawn. Quality management encompasses all of the various activities which together ensure quality of care and services, and the process of co-ordinating and organising such activities. Quality management embraces all the multiple and various functions and activities which together are required to ensure quality maturity. It includes quality assurance, quality improvement, utilisation review and risk management. Quality assurance is conformance to performance specifications and, by extension, the improvement of these specifications. Utilisation review monitors the way in which resources are used in the hospital. Risk management is the minimisation of financial loss to the hospital, the single largest factor currently being malpractice litigation. The scope of this range of material is very great.

The audience

While directed primarily to hospital professionals, the concepts and indeed many of the manual's practical aspects apply to the much wider health care community. The manual intends to assist health professionals and others who are responsible for health care—and in particular hospital care—to improve the quality of care, particularly patients' health outcomes. Hospital boards and managers are responsible for quality management and hence the quality of care—a point we emphasise repeatedly. We also direct this manual to all health professionals, and doctors in particular, who may find for the first time a detailed account of the subject in a manner that is easy to understand and substitutes facts for myths. For this reason we deal with medical staffs' principal concerns about their legal risk. We draw doctors' attention to the fact that quality management intends to facilitate provision of high quality care and is inherently neither condemnatory nor judgmental of medical or any other staff, and that medical staff in particular have a vital part to play in quality management.

We are the first to acknowledge the interest and the involvement of nurses and many other health professionals in various aspects of quality management in Australian hospitals. Indeed, their interest has in general far exceeded that of medical staff. Accordingly, at first glance many nurses and other health professionals may feel that we make far too little reference to nursing and other special hospital services. Quality management is about improving patients' health status and in that context, doctors are usually the key decision makers, even though nurses and other allied health professionals also will be involved in the care process. It is not of much benefit to the patient if nursing care was of the highest standard when the surgeon performed the wrong operation. This logic prompts us to reject the concept of 'QA for nurses', 'QA for physiotherapists' and so on. In our view quality management and quality assurance are for patients.

To this day in Australia, hospital medical staff have seen an unbridgeable gap between what they consider to be 'clinical' and what is 'management'. Dealing effectively with what has become an increasingly legally hazardous environment, and improving the quality of care, involves bridging this gap. Quality management represents such a bridge.

The problem of jargon

Health care quality management is a new and rapidly evolving field. The borrowing of terminology from related basic disciplines, often with altered meaning, and the invention of new terminology, often characterises this stage of development. Considerable confusion results, hampering communications and retarding implementation of concepts. In this manual we confront this problem and provide readers with a coherent framework with which to understand the basic concepts underlying quality management. We hope that by giving readers a language with which to communicate about quality management it will be possible to speed implementation of useful concepts and avoid implementation of useless ones that sound good but are flawed. Necessarily, our efforts are imperfect; we have avoided writing in the kind of language that would require readers to acquire an entirely new and unfamiliar vocabulary. Thus, by restricting our efforts to more precise definitions of familiar words and concepts, we have not removed all of the ambiguities that an entirely new vocabulary would have allowed.

Sticking to the familiar, we may be seen incorrectly as emphasising the negative rather than accentuating the positive, which is our—and should be readers'—goal. Lately, for example, it has become fashionable to avoid the use of words such as 'problem', or 'deficiency' or 'inadequacy', substituting instead such phrases as 'improvement opportunity'. Unfortunately, new-speak terms such as improvement opportunity are applied ambiguously and have lost any precise meaning they may have once had. Everything is capable of being 'improved', but, for quality management purposes, the term has no meaning devoid of a proper term of reference. For this reason we continue to prefer simple words such as problem, defined meaningfully, in preference to more politically acceptable phrases such as improvement opportunity, defined ambiguously; even while we recognise the value of positive thinking and the importance of word forms in emotionally-laden communications.

Variability of content

We have quite consciously indulged in a degree of variability in the detail of different sections of the manual. We have written some sections, such as those dealing with credentialling of medical staff, in considerable detail, while to some readers other sections may appear to be somewhat superficial. This variability represents our perspective of the emphasis required presently and reflects our experience of hospitals' current interest in and understanding of quality management's various elements. In drafting this manual we conducted an extensive review of worldwide activity in quality management, including what one might refer to as 'state-of-the-art' technologies. However, the manual has been written primarily for Australian hospitals and we have chosen to include only those elements and material that we regard as the most suitable for present Australian conditions.

Structure of the manual

Quality management in all its aspects is so extensive a topic that a professional's greatest problem is gaining an oversight and some perspective of the subject matter. This manual intends to meet this need. Nevertheless, because of its length this manual will no doubt appear somewhat daunting to some readers. Consequently we have prepared two brief, but differently focused, summaries of the entire manual. 'The 18 Cs of quality management' provides a thumbnail sketch of the vital elements of a quality management program. The 'Executive Summary' provides readers with an overview of the manual's entire subject matter and provides the most complete summary of essential material. Readers will find both summaries useful to gain perspective on a vast subject.

We divided this manual into seven self-contained but related parts. Each part contains a number of chapters. Summaries and lists of chapters at the beginning of each part and lists of sections at the beginning of each chapter enable readers to move quickly and easily through a large volume of text. The chapters, sections and paragraphs follow, as far as possible, a logical sequence with frequent subheadings to permit easy use and reference. At the conclusion of each chapter is a list of references that have been noted in the text.

We oriented much of the manual's subject matter towards the practical implementation of systems, programs or projects; hence the use of the word 'manual' throughout the text. Nevertheless, we realise that most people do not want to read a manual of this size from cover-to-cover, and sporadic reading exposes them to the risk of becoming lost or at least deprives them of a full perspective of the subject. We designed the manual's structure and content to minimise this risk. Consequently, anyone who reads the manual cover-to-cover in one or more consecutive sittings may be struck by a certain amount of constructive redundancy.

At one time or another we have been faced with requests for some authoritative, complete and coherent text on quality management in hospitals. As far as we are aware, there is no such text available. Most material on the subject that is available is in journals and concentrates—in a way suitable for journal articles—on some small aspect of the subject or on a particular project. None of the material attempts to provide an overall view and perspective of what constitutes a quality management program and the context in which it must operate. In Australia, a few monographs have tried to describe a range of methodologies but there is no written material which adequately provides readers with the context, the purpose, or the approach necessary for quality management implementation. In addition, in Australia it has not been easy to access the large amount of North American reference material dealing with the theoretical concepts of quality of care. For these reasons we believe this manual represents a unique contribution at the present time.

The future

Throughout the manual we constantly make reference to the current situation in Australian hospitals. Our comments and suggestions are made with a deep understanding of the difficult environment in which doctors, nurses, hospital managers and others sometimes work. For quality management to become a reality in Australia, there are a number of essential factors:

- Incentives must be put in place for the hospital industry collectively to do better. The manual supplies the rationale for these incentives, describing the value of quality management and why good intentions and noble motives alone are insufficient for success. Hospital boards and, given the preponderance of public hospitals, governments, both state and federal, must provide the necessary incentives.
- To be effective, quality management programs that hospitals implement should meet certain guidelines or standards and an outside body should check that they do.
- Regulators, including government can, and perhaps should, mandate that quality be measured and results published, and provide the incentives and sanctions to improve quality. However, they do not deliver the care. Only providers can improve the quality of care.
- Also important is the knowledge about what to do and how to do it; the manual makes a start. Vital to success is adequate resources which take the form of:

—Money. Like any other hospital activity, a quality management program requires allocation of budgeted resources.

—Staff. Training programs will be required to provide skilled and properly trained quality managers.

—Expert consultants. Experts in the area are very limited and hence some form of resource centres (regional or otherwise) will be required to provide to hospital staff the level of knowledge consistent with success.

• Needed above all else is the will to succeed. Hopefully the manual will spur some people to action. Demonstrating what can be done should inspire the less inspired to a commitment.

Today the accreditation of hospitals in Australia is an accepted part of quality management. This change in the health care delivery system took thirty years to be accepted fully; from the early 1960s—when a knowledgeable group of practitioners first formally accepted the idea—to 1990—when the state of Queensland finally acceded to join the program. We anticipate that it may take another thirty years until quality management, as defined in this manual, is working well in all, or almost all, Australian hospitals. We hope this manual fulfils its purpose of being a stimulus for and offering a guide to the implementation of effective quality management programs.

Special thanks

We would like to record our thanks and appreciation to FAI Insurances Limited and Mr Angus Maciver whose original idea it was to write this manual and who accepted the burden of underwriting a significant part of the cost of this extensive undertaking and wrote a Foreword to the manual. If this manual fulfils its purpose, the hospital industry in Australia will need to acknowledge the important initiative taken by FAI Insurances.

We would also like to express our thanks and appreciation to Dr John Williamson and Dr Stephen Leeder for writing Forewords to this manual, and to the many contributors and facilitators mentioned in the Acknowledgments, which details their contributions to this challenging undertaking. We trust that readers find our and their efforts to have been worthwhile.

LIONEL L. WILSON
PETER G. GOLDSCHMIDT
Sydney, Australia
September 1995

ACKNOWLEDGMENTS

The breadth of quality management and the required range of expertise is so extensive that we have sought contributors, experts in several special fields, to complement our knowledge and experience, and facilitators to assist us accomplish tasks or review and comment on drafts of chapters. We acknowledge their contributions with appreciation. However, the views expressed in the manual are entirely our own.

Contributors

Emeritus Professor David Ferguson

David Ferguson's contribution to the chapters on occupational health and safety reflects his extensive experience and distinguished career.

David Ferguson was the first professor of occupational health in Australia. He played a major role in the development of the disciplines of occupational medicine and ergonomics and served as president of the professional bodies in both these disciplines. He was on the board of the International Commission on Occupational Health for six years, and of the Asian Association of Occupational Health, and was a consultant to the World Health Organization. He is now a consultant occupational physician. His qualifications include a Doctorate in Medicine; Fellowship of the Australasian College of Physicians; Fellowship of the London and Edinburgh Royal College of Physicians; and Fellowship of the Australian College of Occupational Medicine. He was awarded the Order of Australia (AM) in 1986.

Mr John Pavlakis

John Pavlakis' contribution towards the chapters dealing with quality management and the law and his general advice and guidance to the authors in this area has been invaluable.

John Pavlakis is a partner in Blake Dawson Waldron, Solicitors. He practises in the area of professional indemnity, in particular the defence of claims against medical practitioners. He has represented providers in many cases of alleged medical negligence against hospitals, as well as acting in disciplinary matters.

Mr Robert Todd

Robert Todd's contribution deals with the chapter on defamation and his valuable advice and help in this area is acknowledged.

Robert Todd is a partner at Blake Dawson Waldron, Solicitors, who practises predominantly in the areas of defamation and commercial litigation. He advises national, metropolitan and local newspapers, publishers and broadcasters on all aspects of their publishing activities as well as acting for individuals in defamation actions.

Facilitators

A number of individuals and organisations provided invaluable assistance in this manual's preparation. We gratefully acknowledge their contributions. They are, in alphabetical order: Ms Yosephine Allies who freely wordprocessed the manuscript for Part II, as well as many other individual sections of the manual; the American Hospital Association Resource Center, specifically Ms Eloise Foster and Ms Anne Kiger for their assistance in describing the HEALTH file; Interwest Quality of Care, Inc, specifically Dr John Williamson and Ms Charlene Weir, for their assistance in analysing the contents of the HEALTH file, and the US National Library of Medicine, specifically Mr Sheldon Kotzin, who gave permission for the use of HEALTH file contents; Ms Caroline Marsh, previously of the New South Wales Department of Health, Legal Section, and now of Blake Dawson Waldron, Solicitors, for bringing us up to date with recent legislative amendments in the Australian states and the Commonwealth relating to provisions for qualified privilege. Finally, we thank the following American reviewers for their contribution to this manual. They are (in alphabetical order): Dr Dennis Bertram (State University of New York at Buffalo, New York); Patricia Schroeder (Nursing Quality Connection, Thiensville, Wisconsin).

To test the applicability to the Australian scene of some of our ideas we sought the help of a number of persons in different areas of the health industry who were prepared to read and comment on sections of the manual. We have taken their views and comments into account and are grateful for their efforts. The experts who read one or more draft sections are, in alphabetical order: Mrs Barbara Anderson, formerly Manager Education and Resource Unit, ACHS; Mr Geoff Cornwell, formerly Manager, Western Suburbs Hospital, Sydney; Professor C J Eastman, Professor & Chairman Division of Laboratory Medicine, Westmead Hospital, Sydney; Mr Roy Harvey, Head of Health Services Division, Australian Institute of Health & Welfare, Canberra; Associate Professor Helen Owens, formerly NHMRC National Centre for Health Program Evaluation, Melbourne; Emeritus Professor T. S. Reeve CBE, Royal North Shore Hospital, Sydney; Dr Sidney Sax CBE, Visiting Fellow, Australian Institute of Health, Canberra.

We acknowledge with gratitude the willingness of those who reviewed the full manuscript for our publisher. Their names in alphabetical order are as follows: Dr Frances Cunningham, formerly Senior Policy Adviser to Minister for Health NSW, presently Senior Research Manager Medical Benefits Fund of Australia; Dr John Duggan, Editor, Journal of Quality in Clinical Practice, Hamilton NSW; Ms Anne Harrison, Australian Physiotherapy Association; Mr Roy Harvey, Head of Health Services Division, Australian Institute of Health & Welfare; Mr Peter O'Connor, Executive Director, NZ Council on Healthcare Standards, Wellington, New Zealand; Mrs Joy Packer, Quality Manager, St George Hospital, Sydney; Mr John Rasa, Rasa Management Services, Thirroul NSW; Ms Joanna Westbrook, School of Health Information Management, Cumberland College of Health Sciences; Dr John Williamson, Professor of Medicine and Professor of Medical Informatics in the University of Utah School of Medicine.

ABOUT THE AUTHORS

Dr Lionel L. Wilson

Lionel Wilson is a key figure in the development of quality management in Australia, in all its manifestations. He is generally acknowledged as being a driving force and seminal influence in the introduction and development of quality management to Australia's health services from the mid 1960s until the present time. He played key roles in the introduction to Australia of hospital accreditation, the delineation of clinical privileges (credentialling of medical staff), and the use of formal quality assurance methods. He is adviser to the Commonwealth Department of Human Services and Health on matters related to quality management and quality assurance in hospitals.

Dr Wilson's many accomplishments include: Federal President of the Australian Medical Association, Chairman of the Australian Council on Healthcare Standards, Chairman of the World Medical Association, and Life Governor of the Australian Medical Postgraduate Federation. He has had a long and varied association with both public and private hospitals, including membership of the board of Sutherland Hospital, a large Sydney Metropolitan hospital, for ten years. His consultancy, Qual-med Pty Ltd, offers specialty services on all matters relating to the implementation of hospital quality management programs.

In 1993 he was invited to lecture on quality management and quality assurance in the first postgraduate diploma course in these subjects in Australia by La Trobe University's School of Health Systems Sciences in Victoria.

Lionel Wilson is a graduate of Sydney University Medical School and a Fellow of the Royal Australian College of General Practitioners. He is a member of the Order of Australia, a Fellow of the Australian Medical Association, a recipient of the Gold Medal of the Australian Medical Association, the first recipient of the Medal of Achievement of the Australian Council on Healthcare Standards, and a Life Governor of the Australian Postgraduate Medical Foundation.

Dr Peter G. Goldschmidt

Peter Goldschmidt is President of World Development Group, Inc, a business development consultancy that specialises in quality management, medical technology assessment and integrated clinical information systems. He was formerly Director of the Health Services Research and Development Service, US Department of Veteran Affairs (VA), Washington, DC. The VA operates the world's largest unified health care system, with current expenditures of over US$15 billion annually.

For the US Department of Defence, he designed the Civilian External Peer Review Program which, since 1986, has been in use worldwide. This computerised structured

xviii

quality review system permitted for the first time the routine assessment of the quality of care. Beginning in 1992, the VA adopted this same design to monitor its quality of care. In 1987, he designed QSM, a product that permitted for the first time the routine measurement of the quality of care. His activities for the US Congress Office of Technology Assessment have included writing a background paper on quality of care indicators and serving on the advisory panel for its study of VA Decentralised Hospital Computer Systems.

Dr Goldschmidt was principal consultant to the Quality Management Workgroup of (Hillary Clinton's) Interagency Task Force for Health Care Reform. As a consultant to the (US) Institute of Medicine, he designed the *Medical Technology Assessment Directory*. For the World Health Organization in Geneva, he conducted a worldwide survey of health manpower development. He has also conducted international missions for the World Bank, the US Agency for International Development, and the US Trade and Development Agency. He was a member of the special Pan-American Health Organisation expert committee on health information systems.

Dr Goldschmidt's most important studies include the *Medical Practice Information Demonstration Project* for the US Department of Health and Human Services, and a *Comprehensive Study of the Ethical, Legal, and Social Implications of Biomedical and Behavioral Research and Technology*, a study mandated by the US Congress.

Peter Goldschmidt is a graduate of University College Hospital Medical School (London), the University of Westminster School of Management Studies (London), and the Johns Hopkins University School of Hygiene and Public Health (Baltimore, USA).

OVERVIEW OF CONTENTS

The manual consists of seven parts that cover all the components necessary for a full understanding of quality management. It describes what it means and what is required to become a 'quality-mature' hospital. However, the subject of quality management is so vast that we claim only to provide a coherent overview of its essential elements. The manual does not, and cannot, provide all of the information necessary to implement every facet of a quality management program in all types of hospitals. A textbook of medicine, no matter how comprehensive, cannot equip its reader to become a competent practitioner. Similarly, the successful implementation of a quality management program requires more than reading this manual. However, it provides a good start.

Part I: Background

Part I explores the historical, legal and attitudinal background to and context for the introduction of quality management in Australian hospitals

An understanding of where we have come from provides perspective about where we currently stand, and where we should be going in the future. According, Part I describes the historical and cultural context of the current drive for quality management, quality assurance, and especially quality improvement. This part also voices the insurance industry's concerns regarding the issue of legal liability.

Part II: Concepts in quality management

Part II describes the concepts that underlie quality management and improvement and provides the key to a deeper understanding of this large body of knowledge—some understanding of which is essential if hospitals are to approach quality management rationally and seriously. This part gathers together relevant samples of this discrete body of knowlege which has developed over the past twenty to thirty years. It includes such recent directions as practice policies, practice guidelines, clinical indicators and severity of illness.

To date, Australian hospitals have been deprived of any significant theoretical and conceptual input into discussions on quality management and quality assurance. In recent years some of them have become enamoured with industrial quality management concepts and have even attempted to graft them onto their existing structures. What does total quality management (TQM) mean and what is quality improvement? What is meant by quality assessment and quality improvement? What is the difference between quality assessment and quality measurement? This part explores these issues and relates quality management activities in hospitals to their counterparts in industry to demonstrate their essential similarities and differences and to permit the reader to see quality management in hospitals in a wider context.

This part also lifts the curtain on the concepts subsumed under, and those necessary to operationalise, quality management. These include such concepts as: the production of health, practice policies, the quality improvement spiral and utilisation review, providing a theoretical basis for what are, in general, poorly understood concepts. Finally, it examines the question of managing quality assessment, quality assurance and quality improvement.

Part III: An effective quality management program

Part III describes the structure and organisation of a quality management program and practical implications for the implementation of these essential elements.

One puzzling factor of Australian initiatives in quality management is why so few hospitals have established effective programs. The reasons for the lack of success are multiple, but essentially lie in the undue emphasis on so-called 'methodologies', and almost no attention to the organisational and administrative framework necessary to use them effectively in the broader context of quality management. Accordingly, this part seeks to redress this imbalance by providing considerable detail on such organisational and administrative elements which, in most Australian hospitals, are assumed to be unimportant, and which, even when present, are often functionally deficient.

Part IV: Quality management methodologies

Part IV describes three essential methodologies that every hospital must implement as part of an effective quality management program. None of these techniques has any precedence over any other. Hospitals will need to use all of them at the appropriate stage of their journey toward quality maturity. These methodologies are:

- the process of credentialling and appointing medical staff;
- patient satisfaction surveys;
- structured quality review.

In most Australian public hospitals an appointment system for medical staff has long been in existence. In few hospitals, however, is there an effective formal system of credentialling of medical staff. Credentialling of medical staff (deciding what any doctor can or cannot do in the hospital at any one time) is a crucial part of quality management, and in today's highly litigious environment is an effective form of risk management. Credentialling of medical staff by their peers must have a rigorous formality if legal exposure is to be minimised.

The conduct of properly structured and organised patient satisfaction surveys is an important mechanism for measuring the interpersonal aspects of the quality of care.

The concept of structured quality review is a potent tool for assessing and improving the quality of care. It provides a highly structured process which pays due recognition to the implications of the law of natural justice.

Part V: Risk management

Part V deals with risk management; specifically professional liability and occupational health and safety. Effective quality management programs have consequential benefits for hospitals and doctors by minimising the risk of legal actions and costs associated with medical and hospital malpractice, and for patients in terms of more health status improvement, cost containment and greater satisfaction.

Risk management, or the management of financial exposure, is becoming a much broader issue than that traditionally perceived in Australia. In an acute care hospital, risk management refers not only to the traditional occupational health and safety of employees, but also to the management of financial exposure to hospital and medical malpractice costs. To be effective, risk management requires not only the introduction of specific systems, but also in many instances an attitudinal change on the part of hospital managers and the health professionals who work in the hospital.

Part VI: Quality management and the law
Part VI looks at current concerns among some members of the medical profession about the legal implications of quality management activity.

Part VII: Newsletters and journals
Part VII lists alphabetically and chronologically newsletters and journals that focus exclusively or principally on one or more aspects of health care quality management, and provides a one-page description of each publication.

CONTENTS

————

PART I Background and context of quality management in Australia

PART II Concepts in quality management

PART III Building an effective quality management program

PART IV Quality management methodologies

PART V Risk management

PART VI Quality management and the law

PART VII Quality management resources

LIST OF FIGURES

———

Chapter 6 Quality management, assurance and improvement

Chapter 7 Practice policies and criteria

Chapter 8 Structured quality improvement

Part III: Building an effective quality management program

Chapter 1 Introduction to and purpose of Part III

Chapter 3 The quality management committee and an effective committee system

LIST OF TABLES

Part V: Risk management

Chapter 3 Occupational health and safety

Part VII: Quality management resources

Chapter 1 Introduction to and purpose of Part VII

Chapter 2 Quality management periodicals

LIST OF ABBREVIATIONS

ACHS	Australian Council on Healthcare Standards	HIC	Health Insurance Commission
ACR	Australian Clinical Review	HIV	Human Immune-deficiency Virus
AHA	Australian Hospital Association	HMO	Health maintenance organisation
AHS	Australian Hearing Service	ICU	Intensive care unit
AIDS	Acquired Immune-Deficiency Syndrome	IMS	Indicator-based performance monitoring system
AMA/USA	American Medical Association	IQC	Interwest Quality of Care (Salt Lake City, Utah, USA)
AMA	Australian Medical Association	IR	Infra red
CABG	Coronary artery bypass graft	JCAHO	(US) Joint Commission on Accreditation of Healthcare Organizations
CEO	Chief executive officer	JIT	Just-In-Time (inventory system)
CI	Conformance improvement		
CQI	Continuous quality improvement	MAAC	(Hospital) Medical Appointments Advisory Committee
CRI	Continuous R&D improvement	MDU	Medical Defence Union
CT	Computerised tomography	MMA	Medical management analysis
CTI	Continuous technology improvement	MeSH	Medical Subject Headings (of the US National Library of Medicine)
DOD	(US) Department of Defense		
DRG	Diagnosis related group	MQIS	(US) Medical Quality Indicator System
DST	Decision support technology		
ECG	Electrocardiogram	MRSA	Methicillin Resistant Staphylococcus Aureus
ENT	Ear nose and throat		
GDP	Gross domestic product	NAL	(Australian) National Acoustics Laboratory
GIO	Government Insurance Office (of NSW)		
GNP	Gross national product	NHS	National Health Service (of the UK)
GP	General practitioner		
GPS	Group problem solving	NSW	New South Wales
HCFA	(US) Health Care Financing Administration	NSW-MDU	New South Wales Medical Defence Union

NLM	(US) National Library of Medicine	RMO	Resident medical officer
OH&S	Occupational Health and Safety	SCI	Structured conformance improvement
OPA	Outcome/process assessment	SI	Specifications improvement
ORA	Outcome risk adjustment	SMR	Structured medical record review
PDCA	Plan-Do-Check-Act (Quality improvement cycle)	SOM	Structured outcome measurement
PRO	(US) Peer Review Organization	SPC	Statistical process control
PSRO	(US) Professional Standards Review Organization (Predecessor of PRO)	SPI	Structured problem identification
QA	Quality assurance	SPR	Structured problem resolution
QAHC	Quality assurance, health care	SQC	Statistical quality control
QAS	Quality assessment system	SQI	Structured quality improvement
QC	Quality circle	SQR	Structured quality review
QCA	Quality of care assessment	SSI	Structured specifications improvement
QFD	Quality functional deployment	TB	Tuberculosis
QI	Quality improvement	TQM	Total quality management
QM	Quality management	TQC	Total quality control
QMC	Quality management committee	UCDS	(US) Uniform clinical data set (derived by HCFA for use by PROs)
QMD	Quality management department	UK	United Kingdom
QPM	Quality performance measurement	UM	Utilisation management
QSM	Quality Standards in Medicine (Boston, Massachusetts, USA)	UR	Utilisation review
		US	United States (of America)
		USA	United States of America
		VA	(US) Veterans Administration (now this same abbreviation is used by its successor, the US Department of Veteran Affairs)
R&D	Research and development		
RF	Radio frequency		
RM	Risk management	VMO	Visiting medical officer

GLOSSARY

Readers who want to discern the meaning of an abbreviation (for example, 'QM') should first find the full term in 'List of abbreviations' (that is, 'quality management', in the case of the example), and then find the term in this glossary. Definitions of terms are consistent with their use in this manual, and may vary (often for reasons described in the manual) from those with which readers are familiar. Readers who are generally unfamiliar with health terms may also wish to consult a medical dictionary for terms that are not defined here. Readers in the US may also wish to consult Lexikon: Dictionary of health care terms, organisations, and acronyms for the era of health care reform. Oakbrook Terrace, Illinois: Joint Commission on Accreditation of Healthcare Organisations, 1994.

abdominal swab a piece of gauze or towelling used during the course of an abdominal operation

acceptable quality of care clinical care that has met all explicit and/or implicit criteria that medical peers, or others, consider necessary for care to be considered acceptable and/or that has not violated any such criteria that would cause them to consider care unacceptable

accessibility (the extent of) an individual or population's ability to obtain health care services. This concept often includes knowledge of when it is appropriate to seek health care, the ability to travel to, and the means to pay for, health care. Compare to **availability**. Availability and accessibility affect the effective demand for health services (the extent to which individuals or populations use health care services). Latent demand expresses the extent to which individuals or populations want to use health services but cannot do so because they are unavailable or inaccessible.

accountable health plan (scheme) a health financing and delivery concept whereby a single organisation is responsible for both collecting payments from, and delivering comprehensive health care services to, contributors (sometimes referred to as subscribers or members), often through a vertically integrated health care system. The plan may contract with providers for the delivery of health care services, for example, but remains responsible, and accountable to contributors, for services' quality, including quality improvement

accreditation *see* **hospital accreditation**

acquired immunodeficiency syndrome (AIDS) a disease first recognised in the US in 1981, caused principally by the human immunodeficiency virus (HIV) that destroys cell-mediated immunity

Agency for Health Care Policy and Research (AHCPR) an arm of the US Department of Health and Human Services, concerned principally with enhancing the quality (effectiveness and appropriateness) of health care services and the accessibility of such services through scientific research and the promotion of quality improvement

appropriate care *see* **appropriate intervention.** *See also* **acceptable quality of care**

appropriate intervention an intervention that can reasonably be expected to benefit a particular patient, because he/she fits the profile of patients for whom the intervention is known or assumed to be effective. *See also* **indicated intervention**

appropriateness the quality of being appropriate. In health care, the extent to which an intervention is suitable for a particular person (patient) time and place. *See* **appropriate intervention**

Australasian College of Obstetricians and Gynaecologists a learned college whose members are obstetricians and/or gynaecologists. Membership is gained by examination

Australian Council on Healthcare Standards (ACHS) an organisation established in 1974 in order to conduct the process of accrediting hospitals in Australia

Australian Medical Council a national body consisting of the presidents of the state medical boards and various medical school representatives; it now accredits Australian medical schools

Australian Quality Award an award for which Australian companies can compete that is based on concepts and procedures similar to those of the Baldridge Award in the US

availability the existence (supply) of relevant health care services in a defined geographic area. Services' availability does not mean that they are accessible to all who may benefit from them *See* **accessibility**

Baldridge Award in the US, the Malcolm Baldridge National Quality Award, named for a former Secretary of the US Department of Commerce, exemplifies current TQM/CQI specifications

benchmarking involves searching for, comparing oneself to, and learning from, the best. Often used mistakenly to mean merely comparing one's performance with that of others

bylaws a hospital's bylaws constitute its internal legislation—self-imposed rules to regulate conduct. They provide the legal and administrative framework by which the hospital intends to achieve its objectives

case-based based on individual cases—for example, an assessment of the quality of care based on judgments regarding individual episodes or continua of care. Contrast to **population-based**

case-mix the proportion of patients of different diagnostic categories that are treated by providers

clinical indicators population-based screens to detect malprocesses that do, or could likely, give rise to maloutcomes of clinical care. They do not measure hospitals' quality of care; they are not quality indicators

complication an adverse patient event related to medical intervention, especially an event that is an expected consequence of, or that sometimes occurs in relation to, the patient's disease or its treatment. *See also* **incident, maloccurrence** and **maloutcome**

continuous quality improvement the process of continually improving the quality of care, by improved conformance to practice policies or standards, and/or by their redesign. Same as **kaizen**

contra-indicated (contraindication) refers to an intervention that is inappropriate or improper for a patient because of the patient's state; often refers specifically to such an intervention that would otherwise be appropriate. For example, a patient's physiology might be such that he is unlikely to survive a surgical operation that, if he were in better shape, would produce health benefits. In such circumstances, the operation would be contraindicated

corporate reengineering the process of continually redesigning and rebuilding an organisation based on the efficient production of its goods and services

cost-benefits analysis an analysis that weighs all an intervention's costs against all its benefits, usually measured in monetary terms, from society's perspective

cost-effectiveness analysis an analysis that produces data about alternative interventions' discounted streams of effects and the direct costs of producing them

cost of care the monetary cost of (inputs required for) delivering specified health care services to an individual. Contrast to **price (of health care services)**

cost-worth analysis an analysis that determines whether an intervention's (monetised) effects are worth its costs

credentialling the process of matching the hospital's resources and the desired activities of individuals on the medical staff with their qualifications, experience, and competence to determine what any member of the medical staff is permitted to do in the hospital at any point in time. Also referred to as delineation of (clinical) privileges

criteria (practice criteria) the basis for quality assurance, guidance or instructions to quality assurance personnel about judging how patients should have been managed. These provide indirect guidance or instruction to providers about how patients should be managed. They can be derived from practice policies, if they exist or, if not, must be formulated de novo

customer a person who buys a good or service using their own money (or other resource) or that to which he/she is entitled, for example, through a government health care financing scheme. By extension, a customer may be viewed as the recipient of a good or service within an organisation in which the person is employed. For example, an employee may be the personnel department's 'customer'. A person beyond the organisation affected by a good or service, should only be termed a customer if he/she buys, that is, willingly enters into a transaction for, a good or service. Other persons affected by goods or services may be beneficiaries or victims, certainly *not* customers

decision support technology (DST) any systematic aid to help individuals make decisions; primarily computerised expert systems to aid many processes of medical care including diagnosis, treatment and quality assurance

deep sleep popularised in the 1970s, a therapy as a treatment for a range of psychiatric conditions

defamation the holding of a person up to hatred, ridicule or contempt or a statement that tends to lower the person in the estimation of a right thinking, ordinary, decent Australian

delineation of clinical privileges the determination of what any medical practitioner is permitted to do in the hospital at any one time. *See* **credentialling**

Deming Method method for improving quality developed by the American quality guru Edwards Deming, based on his 14 point 'message to management', including the use of statistical process control

Deming Prize prize established in 1951 in honour of the American quality guru Edwards Deming and administered by the Japanese Union of Scientists and Engineers. Japanese companies compete for the prize which awards quality improvement prowess; the prize is the forerunner of the US Baldridge Award

diagnosis the process of categorising a patient or deciding the nature of a disease based on the patient's characteristics, symptoms, signs and signals (results of laboratory tests or other diagnostic interventions)

diagnosis related groups (DRGs) groupings of diagnoses (or procedures) in a hospital that have the same propensity to consume resources. In 1983, the US Health Care Financing Administration developed a prospective payment system based on DRGs as means of paying hospitals for services to Medicare beneficiaries in order to contain costs and promote efficiencies in care delivery. *See also* **case-mix**

diagnostic accuracy indicates the proportion of people that a test classifies correctly as having or not having a particular disease or other characteristic of interest

diagnostic intervention an intervention conducted for the purpose of establishing a diagnosis or categorising a patient for a particular purpose, usually treatment selection

disability adjusted life years (DALYs) variant of **Quality Adjusted Life Years (QALYs)**

domains of clinical practice specific areas of clinical practice established for a particular purpose (specifically credentialling) that may or may not coincide with commonly recognised specialities in medicine

dysfunction a failure of, or abnormal, function

effective producing a desired result or outcome. *See* **effectiveness**

effectiveness the quality of being effective. In health care, interventions' effectiveness is a statistical concept. An effective intervention improves the health status of a specified patient population beyond that of doing nothing or that which is obtainable with supportive care (the placebo effect), even if some patients' health status is unchanged or worsened by the intervention. The manifest variation in the extent of individuals' health status improvement describes the intervention's risk. Because, at least in principle, an intervention's effectiveness (which is defined by and therefore depends in part on provider characteristics) can be measured, the term effectiveness is preferable to the term **efficacy**

efficacious possessing the potential to produce a desired result or outcome. *See* **efficacy** and **effectiveness**

efficacy the power to produce desired results or outcomes; generally synonymous with **effectiveness**, but in health care often erroneously considered to be different from effectiveness, based on the fallacious concept that an intervention's efficacy is its effectiveness under ideal conditions of use and the equally fallacious idea that the difference between an intervention's efficacy and its so-called effectiveness represents improvement potential

encounter *see* **health care encounter**

false negative a false negative results when a diagnostic test indicates that a patient does not have a disease (or other characteristic of interest) when, in fact, he/she does

false positive a false positive results when a diagnostic test indicates that a patient has a disease (or other characteristic of interest) when, in fact, he/she does not

gross domestic product (GDP) a monetary measure of the totality of goods and services produced in a community, usually a country

hazard an object or situation that is potentially harmful

health *see* **health status**

health care encounter a person's contact with the health care system, for example, a telephone conversation with a public health nurse, a visit to the doctor, admission to the hospital; sometimes limited to the face-to-face provision of a service by a health care professional

Health Care Financing Administration the US government entity responsible for federally funded health schemes, principally **Medicare** and **Medicaid**

health care system a conceptual (or in some situations a concrete) system that consists of the totality of entities (and their interrelationships) that intend to maintain or improve people's health through the delivery of personal health services. The term 'health system' is broader and includes all entities, not just those that deliver personal health services, such as medical doctors and hospitals

health care technology *see* **medical technology**

health maintenance organisation an organisation that agrees to provide a defined (often comprehensive) range of health services to an individual (or group) for a specified period (usually a year) in exchange for a prospective (usually monthly) per capita (or sometimes per family) subscription (payment)

health outcome an outcome that affects a patient's health status. *See also* **outcome**

health state the state of a person's health at a given moment in time, often measured in functional terms, for example, able to do usual activities but in principle, also encompassing mental and emotional well-being—for example, able to engage in meaningful personal or social relationships

health state discount the extent to which a health state's value is reduced in the present because that state occurs at some future time. Discounts are usually calculated as an annual percentage reduction in a health state's value. For example, people often ignore (discount heavily) present risks (such as those from smoking) that result in future, especially long-term, health problems (such as lung cancer or circulatory disease). In health status measurement, discounting health states permits the comparisons of interventions that produce markedly different effectiveness (health benefits) streams (and risks)

health state weight the relative value that a person or population puts on different health states that are exhaustive and mutually exclusive (so that the resultant weights sum to one)

health status an integrated measure of health, or the health quality of life, that encompasses mortality, institutionalised morbidity, ability to carry out activities and, in principle, mental and emotional well-being, over a defined period (for example, the patient's lifetime, ten years after the beginning of treatment). Operationally, health status is the product of summing each health state (an expression of an individual's functional ability) multiplied by its weight (an expression of a health state's value relative to alternative states) and by its discount (an expression of value relative to the present)

health status improvement the improvement of a patient's health status (over what it would otherwise have been)—the desired outcome of medical intervention. Health status improvement may result from an intervention even if the patient's health status is worse after the treatment than before it because, without the intervention, the patient would have been even worse off

health system a conceptual system that consists of the totality of entities (and their interrelationships) that intend to maintain or improve people's health

hospital accreditation the formal process of surveying a hospital against predetermined criteria and standards to determine whether or not it complies with applicable standards; such standards believed to be related to the hospital's ability to provide services of acceptable quality

Hospitals and Health Services Commission in Australia, the defunct Commonwealth Government initiative in the early 1970s, established to engage in health services research

hospital malpractice literally, bad practice on the part of a hospital; those interventions and actions that take place in a hospital (or fail to take place when indicated) that a court of law considers (or, in the case of potential malpractice, might consider) negligent

human immunodeficiency virus (HIV) the aetiological agent responsible for AIDS **(acquired immunodeficiency syndrome)**

inappropriate (intervention) an intervention that cannot reasonably be expected to benefit a particular patient because he/she does not fit the profile of patients for whom the intervention is known or assumed to be effective

incident an event that occurs in connection with patient care that merits reporting or is reported because of a deviation from expected or standard practice that could have resulted in patient health status loss, putative malprocesses that actually resulted in patient health status loss, or an actual or potential injury to a staff member or visitor

incident report a written report of an event that occurred in connection with patient care including, for example, a deviation from expected or standard practice that could have resulted in patient health status loss, putative malprocesses that actually resulted in patient health status loss, or an actual or potential injury to a staff member or visitor

incident reporting a system for identifying, processing, analysing and reporting incidents with a view to preventing their recurrence

indicated intervention an intervention for a particular patient who can be expected to benefit from it because he/she fits the profile of patients for whom the intervention is known or assumed to be effective, and for whom no contra-indication exists

intervention an action that intends to change the course of events (to achieve a desired, or to avoid an undesirable, outcome). In health care, a process (or an action that is part of a process) that intends to improve a patient's health status. Health care interventions may be classified as preventative, diagnostic, therapeutic or rehabilitative. They comprise a technology and its delivery mechanism

Joint Commission on Accreditation of Healthcare Organisations founded in 1951, the private, non-profit organisation that accredits hospitals in the US; until 1987, the Joint Commission on Accreditation of Hospitals

just-in-time (JIT) the process of manufacturing (and delivering or receiving) small batches of products and using them right away to minimise in-process and finished product inventories. This has the added benefit of allowing defective parts to be identified early, thereby avoiding production of large numbers of defectives. Same as **kanban**

kaizen *see* **continuous quality improvement**

kanban *see* **just-in-time**

Kellogg Foundation a private foundation in the US. Its objectives are directed to funding projects in agriculture, education and health

maloccurrence literally bad occurrence; any untoward event related to medical care. Sometimes adverse event or adverse patient occurrence, especially if the event is not an anticipated or natural consequence of the patient's disease or treatment. *See also* **complication, incident** and **maloutcome**

maloutcome literally, wrong outcome; deviation from expected or required outcome. In health care, the occurrence of an outcome contrary to expectations, especially one that more likely than not arose from malprocess

malpractice literally, bad practice on the part of a doctor or hospital. *See* **hospital malpractice**

malprocess literally, wrong process; deviation from expected or required process. In health care, includes use of inappropriate interventions, use of appropriate interventions that were implemented improperly, mismanagement of complications, and any other action that should not have been but was applied, that should have been but was not applied, and that was applied improperly whether or not it should have been applied—whether or not the patient suffered a maloutcome. The concept of malprocess does not usually extend to inefficient care—for example, use of a brand name instead of a generic antibiotic or poor scheduling of tasks—if the only difference was one of cost and the inefficient care did not adversely affect the patient's health status

management the process of setting an organisation's objectives and policies, allocating resources and directing people toward achievement of objectives, including measurement of results to improve performance. Also the group of people (managers) who are responsible for running an organisation, especially its central (top) managers

management information system a system comprising mechanisms to collect, process, store, transmit, analyse and report data that is designed to monitor an organisation's performance or that of its constituent elements or provide other information for management decision making, especially, but not necessarily exclusively, on the part of managers

manufacturing quality control a system encompassing product design and manufacturing that intends to produce a product to specifications with as little variance as possible

Medibank established in 1974, the Australian federal funding mechanism for medical and hospital services, renamed Medicare in 1984

Medicaid the US federal-state funding mechanism, administered at a state level, that enables the medically indigent (people who cannot finance their own medical care) to obtain health care

medical technology drugs, devices, medical and surgical procedures, etc. that comprise interventions, and their organisational and support systems (interventions' delivery mechansims); sometimes health care technology. *See also* **product technology** and **process technology**

medical technology assessment the assessment (evaluation) of medical technology in terms of its effectiveness and cost, and sometimes also its ethical, legal, social and other implications

Medicare (in Australia) the national tax funded financing mechanism that meets both medical and hospital costs

Medicare (in the US) the federal mechanism administered by the Health Care Financing Administration that funds medical and hospital services for defined populations, predominantly the aged and disabled

Natural Justice rules that have been developed over time to ensure that individuals' rights and interests are protected in decision making processes; in the US comparable to the right to due process

needle stick injury injury from hypodermic needles. *See* the broader term, **sharps**

negative predictive value the probability that people whom a test suggests do not have a given characteristic, truly do not have it

occupational health and safety that branch of health science and practice relating to the identification, control and elimination of health hazards in the workplace, and the prevention and treatment of accidents and diseases related to work and the work environment

organisation an entity consisting of individuals with assigned roles and responsibilities who are working to achieve a common purpose

orthogonal arrays an analytic tool used in manufacturing to approach rather than guarantee the attainment of an ideal design, especially for a product that consists of multiple parts whose interactions affect its quality or performance

outcome the results of production processes which precede them in space-time, acting on inputs in a given environment. In health care, the term 'outcome' usually refers to post-intervention results or measurements—the observed outcomes of an intervention—whether or not one can confidently attribute those results to the preceding intervention (process)

outcome/process assessment a case-based method for quality assessment and/or measurement that relies on comparing what was done (process) and achieved (outcome) in a particular case to what should have been done and achieved for that type of case

outcome risk adjustment a population-based method for quality measurement that relies on statistical adjustment of one or more outcome measures—for example, mortality rates—for factors that affect patient outcomes and are beyond the provider's control in order to produce a relative quality score; whatever differences exist after such adjustments are attributed to the providers' performance

paradigm shift a fundamental change of mind-set (new model of reality) that permits one to look at the same set of facts but draw substantially different inferences than one did previously (with the old model of reality)

Pareto effect (sometimes, principle) named after the Italian economist (1848–1923) who showed that most effects (often taken to be 80%)—for example, quality defects—result from few causes (often taken to be 20%)—for example, quality problems

patient outcome the result for the patient after health care (intervention), especially patient health status—whether or not care process produced it. *See also* **outcome**

patient satisfaction the subjective sense of quality, particularly regarding the interpersonal aspect of care, that patients experience after one or more health care interventions or encounters

pattern analysis the statistical analysis of data related to medical practice—for example, screening data and/or structured medical record review findings—in order to reveal patterns of or variation in practice or care (for example, quality problems)

peer review in North America, health care peer review refers traditionally to the process of retrospective review of a practitioner's medical records by colleagues to determine whether or not care was delivered within boundaries set by acceptable standards of practice. In Australia, the term is used ambiguously to cover any review of patient activities, and rarely in the North American sense. Because of ambiguities associated with the term, this manual avoids its use in favour of such terms as 'structured medical record review' and 'structured quality review' for retrospective assessment of the quality of care involving review of practitioners' medical records

Peer Review Organisations (PROs) organisations established in the US to review the quality of care and the appropriateness of settings (use of resources) for care provided to Medicare patients in hospitals. PROs are under contract to the US Department of Health and Human Services which administers the Medicare program. PROs replaced PSROs with passage of the *Tax Equity and Fiscal Responsibility Act* of 1982

Peer Review Resource Centre an organisational unit, established by the Australian Medical Association in 1979, to provide resources, training and support for quality assurance activities

personal health services the delivery of health care to individuals at primary and higher levels by doctors, nurses and other health workers and the organisation, financing and management of such care

placebo effect is manifest when an intervention (which may be no more than supportive care and attention) improves a patient's health status (usually temporarily) without having a known specific effect on the health problem or its manifestations

Plan-Do-Check-Act (PDCA) cycle describes a process for assuring that products conform to specifications, thereby assuring, and hence improving, product quality; sometimes referred to as the Deming cycle, or the Shewhart cycle. Specifically, the PDCA cycle refers to establishing product and production specifications (sometimes referred to as quality planning), producing products, checking that products meet specifications (sometimes referred to as quality measurement) and, if not, determining why not, and acting to eliminate quality problems' root cause (sometimes referred to as quality improvement)

policy management setting objectives and formulating policies for the health system, its components and their interrelationships; obtaining resources for the health system and allocating them among its components; monitoring health conditions and outcomes; evaluating system performance and economic, ethical and social impacts; and assessing prospects

population-based based on populations—for example, an assessment of the quality of care that depends on the statistical manipulation of parameters derived from observations of individuals in a defined population. Compare to **case-based**

positive predictive value the probability that the people whom a test suggests have a disease or other characteristic, truly have it

practice policies pre-established clinical decision rules for treating individual patients that take into account their preferences regarding ends and means, and that are the starting point for defining these processes and their expected resultant outcomes

practice standard refers to a performance relative to a care process, either the outcome of a specific care process (for example, the time from the induction of anaesthesia to the beginning of the surgical operation must be 30 minutes or less) or a patient outcome of one or more or all care processes (for example, the patient died during the admission). As used in this context, standard pertains to individual cases; not to populations of cases. *See also* **standard**

price (of health care services) the amount a provider charges an individual or his/her health care scheme (or which he/she/it must pay) for specified health care services. Contrast to **cost of care**

primary care basic health care services provided by a health care professional—for example, doctor or nurse—to a patient, especially the treatment of ordinary health problems or initial assistance on entering the health care system. In Australia and other industrialised countries the term often applies to care provided by general practitioners as opposed to specialists. In the US increasingly, and in developing countries especially, nurse practitioners and other non-medical graduates may delivery some primary care services

procedure any medical or health care intervention, especially one that involves manipulations or a series of steps to accomplish, such as a surgical operation

process a particular method of doing something, generally involving a number of steps or operations, that results in an outcome or produces an output

process reengineering the redesign of a process, often from square one, to improve the quality of its output and/or production efficiency, especially in light of new technology to achieve competitive advantage; often associated with reduction in personnel which may be its objective

process technology know-how pertaining to production processes. In health care, knowledge about how to deliver interventions or implement practice policies (product technology) most cost-effectively. *See also* **product technology**

product technology know-how pertaining to the design of products, especially in relation to their manufacture or production. In health care, knowledge about disease processes and interventions to alter their course. *See also* **process technology**

Professional Standards Review Organisations (PSROs) predecessors of PROs

provider in health care, an organisation or individual that provides health care services—for example, a hospital, doctor or nurse

provider performance a measure of a provider's achievement of an important function, such as improving patients' health status

provider profile the result of a statistical analysis of a provider's performance, especially in relation to others

public health programs activities to protect the health of a population or community including, for example, health education, product safety, consumer protection, sanitation, occupational health and safety, recycling and environmental programs

quality the totality of a product's or service's characteristics that bear on its ability to satisfy customers' desires. *See also* **quality of care**

quality adjusted life years (QALYs) sometimes referred to as disability adjusted life years (DALYs), a measure or estimate of the number of years lived that is weighted by (adjusted for) the quality of life of those years (for example, the extent of disability or functional ability). *See also* **health status**

quality assessment the process of examining a single episode or continuum of care, a unit of a provider's performance, to determine whether or not care was appropriate

quality assurance assurance of a product's quality. In health care, the process of ensuring that clinical care conforms to criteria or standards; a subset of quality management. The term implies quality assessment and corrective action if and when quality problems are detected

quality circle a mechanism whereby a small group of employees meet, usually voluntarily, to identify and solve work-related problems, especially those related to product quality or the cost of production

quality control refers to mechanisms, usually in industry, that intend to assure products meet specifications by, for example, measuring product quality in comparison with specifications and taking corrective action and, by extension, mechanisms that intend to prevent production of defects by, for example, controlling inputs to processes

quality control circle the original (Japanese) name for a quality circle. Shopfloor workers would voluntarily meet as a small group to look for ways to improve the production processes on which they worked

quality cost the cost of producing products that do not meet specifications including, for example, the value of inputs (materials, labor, etc.) in scrapped products, the cost of repairing or reworking defective products in the factory or those returned by customers, and the intangible costs of loss of reputation, etc.

quality functional deployment (QFD) a set of planning and communication routines that focuses and coordinates an organisation's skills to design and produce products that customers desire. It offers a systematic way of listening to customers to determine exactly what they want and of determining how best to translate customers' desires into products and services at a price customers are willing to pay

quality improvement generally, results from more perfect conformance to product specifications and/or their improvement so that specifications more perfectly meet customers' desires, including improvements to production processes that, for example, result in lower costs and, hence, lower product prices. In health care, results from more perfect conformance to practice policies that are known or assumed to produce maximum health status improvement within patient's preferences and society's resources. Alternatively, results from refashioning those policies, including the introduction of new interventions or technologies that are known or assumed to produce greater patient health status improvement than previous policies, and/or changes to health care processes that reduce the cost of care, increase patient satisfaction with, or perfect value trade-offs relevant to the implementation of existing or refashioned practice policies and/or the delivery of care. *See also* **quality** and **quality of care**

quality indicator a measure of quality; specifically, a variable that measures the quality of care

quality of care has the following four dimensions: technical quality (sometimes referred to simply as the quality of care), cost of care, patient satisfaction, and value trade-offs among the preceding three dimensions. Widely (and inadequately), the degree to which health services for individuals and populations increase the likelihood of desired health outcomes and are consistent with current professional knowledge—*see* **technical quality of care.** *See also* **quality cost**

quality management the aspect of management concerned with quality policy and an organisation's production function from this perspective including, for example, mechanisms for producing products to specifications, designing products that customers desire, and producing the technologies that expand what can be produced (product technology) and how well it can be produced (process technology), and mechanisms for improving quality management. Quality management's goal is quality maturity; its product, quality improvement

quality management program a set of coherent activities intended to implement quality management within an organisation and thereby enable it to achieve quality maturity

quality maturity the end result of implementing quality management. A quality mature hospital continuously improves its quality of care and services, as well as the mechanisms that produce such continuous improvement

quality measurement the process of quantifying the quality of a provider's entire output, expressed, for example, as the proportion of cases treated appropriately (the summation of individual case quality assessments)

quality problem a deviation from expected or specified process that if avoided would improve product quality; deviation from expected or required product quality presumed to arise from malprocess. *See also* **malprocess** and **maloutcome**

Quality Standards in Medicine (QSM) a Boston-based company that markets a commercial product of the same name to assess the technical quality of care through structured quality review. The QSM product includes diagnosis and procedure-specific automated outcome/process assessment screens; it also supports structured medical record review of cases failing screens, and produces reports of screening and review results, including those for profiling hospital departments and individual medical practitioners. QSM's international database permits users to compare their performance with respect to detailed screening criteria

reengineering *see* **corporate reengineering** and **process reengineering**

research and development the generation of new knowledge; development of technology; assessment of existing and new health policies, practices and programs; transfer of technology; dissemination of information; and development of methods and mechanisms for these purposes

resource development the provision of health system inputs, encompassing, for example, production of health workers, construction of health facilities, and manufacture and distribution of health care products

risk the chance of harm—a measure of the extent to which a person is exposed to potential harm

risk management the aspect of management concerned with minimisation of financial loss to an organisation, commensurate with the achievement of its purpose. In health care, designing and implementing a program of activities to identify and avoid or minimise risks to patients, employees, visitors and the institution, to minimise financial losses (including legal liability) that might arise consequentially, and to transfer risk to others through payment of premiums (insurance); a subset of **quality management**

sensitivity a measure of how well a test detects people who have a given characteristic, that is, the extent to which people who truly manifest a characteristic are so classified

separation in Australia, a patient discharged from hospital

severity of illness a conceptual measure of a patient's probability of death without treatment; a term that often refers to the collection of data about a patient's disease as a means of adjusting risk for a particular outcome such as death.

sharps hypodermic needles, scalpels, or similar devices

Shewhart cycle *see* **Plan-Do-Check-Act (PDCA) cycle**

specificity a measure of how well a test detects people who do not have a given characteristic and, hence, does not label them as having a disease that they do not have

standard the expected or required level of attainment on a criterion variable. *See also* **standard of care**

standard of care the level of conduct used to assess health care, particularly, medical practitioners' conduct for purposes of determining its adequacy or, especially, liability in negligence law or malpractice cases

statistical process control measuring all or samples of products and suspending production when products outside pre-set tolerances appear, permitting the cause of problems to be investigated and remedied, and assuring products meet specifications

statistical quality control *see* **statistical process control**

structure conceptual or physical elements or components arranged in a particular way so that they constitute and operationalize a process. For example, the facilities and members organised to deliver health care services

structured medical record review a systematic process whereby expert clinicians examine medical records to confirm quality problems identified by outcome/ process assessment screens or to identify quality problems if outcome/assessment screens are not used

structured outcome measurement the strategy of measuring the long-term outcomes (end results) of health care interventions. It examines the extent to which conformance to specifications actually improves patient health status in comparison to expectations (expressed in practice policies), and produces information to improve them

structured performance benchmarking the strategy of measuring competitors' (colleagues') performance to identify the best performers; to discern what processes, patient flows and organisation seems to produce this performance; and to establish where one's own performance stands in relation to the best with a view to improving it

structured problem resolution evaluation of and selection among alternative improvement action to remedy quality problems and eliminate their root causes

structured quality improvement a hospital-wide strategy to systematically identify quality problems, discover their root causes and eliminate routinely these causes

structured quality review a method of identifying quality of care problems. It involves steps necessary for identifying, confirming, and illuminating quality of care problems and for revealing patterns of care. The term refers specifically to a process involving automated outcome/process assessment screens, structured medical record review of cases failing screens, and pattern analysis of screening and medical record review findings

system a set of elements and their interrelationships that may be conceptual (the system's purpose is in the mind of the beholder) or managed (the system is designed to achieve a particular purpose). The system's purpose is a function of the whole and cannot be accomplished by any of its constituent elements

technical quality of care the central measure of provider performance—the extent to which a provider improves patients' health status, especially in comparison to what is achievable

technique the formal or practical method or procedure of carrying out a task or an operation

technology the application of knowledge and science to achieve a practical purpose; know-how. It is a method for accomplishing a desired end, and represents a way of doing something. *See also* **medical technology**

therapeutic intervention an intervention for the purposes of treatment; specifically, one intended to improve a patient's health status

total quality management (TQM) a management philosophy that is customer centred, product focused, measurement oriented, improvement driven and all pervasive

trade-off *see* **value trade-off**

treatment the management of illness; the application of remedies to disease; the use of interventions to improve patient health status

unindicated (intervention) an intervention which is not indicated and, therefore, inappropriate. *See also* **indicated intervention** and **appropriate intervention**

utilisation review the process of reviewing the appropriateness (including necessity, intensity, timing, place) of the use of resources (including procedures, services, facilities) involved in patient care, particularly interventions, investigations, length of stay, etc.; a subset of quality management. The term does not usually encompass the efficiency with which services are provided (such as the cost of diagnostic test); rather it is limited to the use of services (for example, the appropriateness of the number of times a diagnostic test was performed on a patient). Operationally, medical necessity and other judgments about the appropriateness of care are often subsumed under quality assurance

value trade-offs giving up the attainment of one objective in order to attain another; or accepting a lower level of accomplishment of one objective in order to be able to attain greater levels of accomplishment of others; specifically, trade-offs among quality of care, the cost of care, and patient satisfaction with care

vertically integrated health care system a system under a single management structure that provides care to individuals at two or more levels; especially, a health care system comprising primary care providers, hospitals, tertiary care centres and other health care facilities (for example, nursing homes) and services (for example, home care). *See also* **accountable health plan (scheme)**

World Health Organisation (WHO) the technical agency of the United Nations (established by treaty in 1948 and headquartered in Geneva, Switzerland) that is concerned with people's health

THE EIGHTEEN Cs OF QUALITY MANAGEMENT

Quality happens when quality counts

This section outlines how hospital managers must think and what they must do to develop an effective quality management program to achieve operational quality maturity—the perpetual state of striving ceaselessly for excellence and the reality of improving continuously the quality of care.

Centrality: Quality is the heart of the job

Hospitals are health-producing facilities. Quality involves improving people's health status, not merely providing health services. Quality is the hospital's main purpose, not something to be considered as a side issue at the end of the day. Hospital directors' and managers' policies and decisions must put quality at the core of everything that the hospital does. Doctors have a vital role to play. However, quality is the product of the care system, not of doctors alone. Quality management involves a hospital-wide program for achieving operational quality maturity.

Commitment: Actions speak louder than words

Directors and managers must commit to quality if quality management is to succeed. This commitment must be manifest in policies, budgets and actions. Hospital directors and managers must delegate responsibility to quality managers to establish and run effective quality management programs. They must insist on accountability for results, with both appropriate incentives and sanctions. Managers must communicate their commitment to quality to the entire hospital by words and, most importantly, deeds.

Consistency: Always hold steadfastly to the same principles

Both commitment and action must be consistent with the hospital's policy and its plan for achieving quality maturity. Not only must there be a policy on quality management, but managers must also adhere to the policy and institute incentives and sanctions to promote this end. Providing incentives to do what needs to be done is perhaps even more important than devising sanctions for the occasional person who does not want to co-operate.

Continuity: Stay the course; avoid stop–go

Quality management demands a continuous commitment to action. A stop–go approach will achieve nothing. Hospital directors in particular must realise that there will be resistance, difficulties and problems, but they must persist. In particular, budgets must be adequate and maintained. Even though the quality management budget cannot be sacrosanct, if resources run short, cutting the QM budget in line with across the board cuts is short-sighted and self-defeating.

Coherence: Clarity and harmony among ideas and actions

An effective quality management program is coherent and is managed to ensure that its many complex aspects are functioning according to a predetermined plan in the most cost-effective manner. The various parts of the program must all be based on a common, articulated set of principles, and work in harmony. The effect of the whole can only be realised if all of the parts exist, work at sufficient performance levels, and are integrated. Isolated use of methodologies, for example, may achieve little if anything; and may be counter-productive.

Comprehensiveness: Cover all aspects in relevant detail

Managers must direct their efforts to all areas of the hospital with equal vigour; not just to cleaning and nursing services, for example. Further, the program must cover in detail every relevant aspect of technical quality (quality assurance and improvement), cost (utilisation review and risk management), patient satisfaction and value trade-offs among these three competing aspects of quality. To pay lip-service to quality management, to emphasise form over substance, or to implement a program that focuses on selected projects results neither in an effective quality management program nor much quality improvement.

Competence: Everyone must be trained and perform properly

Quality demands that everyone is trained sufficiently and works competently. Managers must be trained in management; quality managers, in quality management. Hospital managers and staff must accept that the introduction of new technology must automatically involve training in its use, if quality is to be assured. Learning on the job by trial and error is no longer acceptable. Hospitals and their medical staffs who are serious about the quality of patient care must establish a formally structured credentialling mechanism for medical staff to determine what any doctor is permitted to undertake in the hospital at any one time. Where needed, hospitals must put in place similar mechanisms to judge the training and performance of other technical staff, for example, critical care nurses.

Conformance: Adhere to, and improve, care policies and processes

Quality improvement results from conformance to practice policies (that describe how patients should be managed and who should manage them) and from better practice policies that provide more health status improvement, lower costs, and/or greater patient satisfaction. Quality managers must:

- compare what is being done and achieved with what should be done and achieved;
- establish priorities to ensure cost-effective use of quality management resources;
- investigate root causes of variation in processes and outcomes, if not obvious;

- develop and implement plans to resolve quality problems and eliminate their root causes in order to improve the match between what patients need and desire and what they receive, and to reduce variability in processes and to improve outcomes.

Quality managers must also facilitate the acquisition of new knowledge and information to improve practice policies and production processes through benchmarking, outcomes measurement, and research and development.

Computation: Measure, provide feedback, monitor improvement

Quality management involves measurement, feedback, and the use of data to improve care. At present, the quality of care is largely unassessed; there is no feedback and, consequently, there can be no systematic improvement. Hospitals must:

- specify and assess the quality of their care; feedback information to improve care processes;
- monitor processes and outcomes to identify and resolve quality of care problems;
- support and maintain well-documented clinical records and good clinical information systems in order to aggregate and analyse clinical data, which is essential to good care and to quality management.

Comparison: Judge your performance against what colleagues and competitors are achieving

Quality management involves relevant, valid comparisons among doctors and departments and, where possible, hospitals. Comparison is important as a spur to the continuous search for improvement. Without knowing how others are doing, one does not know what is possible, and hence how one is really doing—even if one's performance is improving.

Credibility: Success must appear likely

The quality management program must be credible to all participants but, because they are so integral to its success, particularly so to the hospital's medical staff. It must be based on sound concepts and successful experience—evidence derived from scientific assessment. Its mechanisms must be plausible. The key to credibility is communication: Why is quality management necessary? What must be done? This manual intends to provide credible answers to these questions.

Communication: Tell everyone why quality matters and how to improve it

Instituting quality management in a hospital demands attitudinal and behavioural change. Communication and education:

- is perhaps the most demanding of its requirements;
- must start on day one and continue indefinitely for all hospital staff, clinical and non-clinical, to ensure that they understand the meaning of quality management and to enable them to become the instruments of improvement;
- must be a two-way process to establish a meaningful dialogue.

Hospitals must enlist employees in the quest for quality. They must encourage them to suggest improvements, thus becoming part of the improvement process. Successful quality management requires shared concepts and common terminology. This manual intends to meet this pressing need.

Co-ordination: The left hand must know what the right hand is doing

Co-ordination of the various activities that comprise a quality management program is essential to ensure its effective functioning, the smooth integration of a series of complex activities, and to avoid wasting time and effort. Such co-ordination is the responsibility of the quality management committee, the hospital's most important committee. The quality management department, headed by a qualified quality manager, is the principal resource for implementing the hospital's quality management program including quality assurance, utilisation review and risk management.

Collaboration: One for all and all for one

Hospitals are production systems. Quality depends on the proper functioning of system elements and the co-ordination of their individual purposes to achieve those of the whole. Such co-ordination requires collaboration between departments and among their members. Quality improvement is the central goal; quality management, the process for its achievement and the structure for collaboration. Interdepartmental, interdisciplinary teams must collaborate to identify and resolve quality of care problems, and to improve production processes. A well-articulated system of committees is the appropriate mechanism for such collaboration, but must be a substitute for existing—and not merely another layer of—bureaucracy.

Co-operation: The hospital is part of a larger system

Hospitals must co-operate with community groups, regulators, suppliers and everyone else who affects the quality of what they do and how they do it. They must find out what customers—patients and communities—expect of them and organise to deliver it. Quality management is the delivery vehicle. Everyone's efforts must be guided by an understanding of what is required and the system organised to produce it. Individual goals must be harnessed for and subordinate to this common goal. Failure to satisfy customers and other stakeholders makes achievement of both individual and organisational goals difficult, if not impossible.

Celebration: Success is not always its own reward

Successes should be recognised and rewarded. Hospitals should honour and reward suggestions which improve quality or save costs. They should celebrate outstanding performers and performances. Pay and promotion should depend on measured performance.

Change: People like to change, when not being forced to change

Quality improvement requires planned change. People may want to change, but may not want to be told to change. Managers must provide the environment, including incentives, that engenders a willingness to change and facilitates improvement. Hospitals must manage change. It must not be haphazard and unco-ordinated, the latter resulting only in chaos. All change is painful, and education and incentives are necessary to make it understandable and acceptable. Quality management involves establishing mechanisms to ensure that if and when quality problems are revealed, they can be resolved by a process of relatively painless but effective change.

Cost: Quality management is a cost of doing business

The only relevant issue is deciding which quality management program best suits the hospital's circumstances. Quality management strives to improve value for money. Its principal benefit is giving patients health status improvement with greater certainty. Quality management can also reduce costs. Effective quality management requires bringing rewards in line with value added.

EXECUTIVE SUMMARY

E11 | Quality management can improve quality—but only if action replaces talk

See Part II, Chapter 1 and Part III for details.

Quality management (QM) portends a revolution in health care's production function: what health care is provided and the way that services are delivered. It promises a paradigm shift: from an emphasis on providing services to one of improving outcomes.

Most hospital managers, doctors and other health care professionals are quite unfamiliar with quality management and the revolution it portends in health care. They can either shape the revolution or allow it to shape their work. Health care quality management promises to fulfil a cherished dream: knowing realistically what one can expect from medical intervention and being sure of getting it. Quality management can be as liberating for hospitals and doctors as it is reassuring for patients.

In the late 1980s hospitals and other health care facilities began to notice quality management's success in industry. Industry's motivation is clear: increasing profits, by avoiding the cost of reworking or fixing defective products, and by delighting customers. Hospitals' interest in quality stems from regulatory requirements and a desire to follow fashion, to market themselves as high quality providers, to reduce malpractice and other risks, to counter external quality assurance initiatives and cost containment pressures, and, at least in some cases, to improve practices.

To date, hospitals' renewed interest in quality has resulted in more talk than action, especially at the clinical level where it matters the most. The current quest for quality, inspired by industrial example, is only one of a number of historical forces driving health care toward quality management. Others include: payment strategies, utilisation management, risk management, quality assurance, medical technology assessment and, most recently and perhaps most importantly, the ability to quantify quality. The quality management activity that has occurred in Australian hospitals to date has been patchy, fragmented, and lacking any integration within an individual hospital.

E12 | Health care in trouble

See Part II, Chapters 1 and 3 for details.

E12.01 | *Health care is (one of) the largest economic sectors*

Government's guarantee that all citizens should have access to health care, and the concomitant growth in the health care system, is one of this century's most important social changes. In all industrialised countries, health care has become one of the largest

1

economic sectors. Countries continue to devote more of their resources to health care, although in Australia the Commonwealth government has capped it at about 8% of GDP (gross domestic product). Growth in health care expenditures provides the means to develop and deliver medical technology, which in turn stimulates demand for more health care services. This spiral is stressing the health care system and threatens to propel expenditures out of control. Despite the supposed miracles of modern medicine, people are increasingly dissatisfied with the health care system.

E12.02   *The health system is a conceptual entity*

The health system represents the totality of interventions that intend to maintain or to improve the population's health (which is the summation of individuals' health). The health system and its component systems are conceptual entities that consist of myriads of interrelationships among their various elements, including government, each under the control or influence of different groups and with its own sociopolitical traditions. The health system is not the result of rational design efforts to achieve some predetermined purpose; it is not managed. It has no identifiable clients (or customers); merely everyone collectively regardless of such things as philosophy, purpose or desires. The health system consists of the following five principal components:

- personal health services;
- public health programs;
- research and development;
- resource development; and
- system policy management.

Personal health services (referred to collectively as the health care system) respond to individuals who seek help. They account for the largest share of total health care expenditures; hospital care accounts for a substantial fraction of these expenditures. Public health programs target populations and some, particularly health education, may impact on personal health services. This manual focuses on personal health services.

E12.03   *Health care is one, perhaps minor, determinant of health*

A person's health status is the result of four sets of interrelated factors and their interactions. They are: biology and our genetic programming; behaviour; the prenatal and postnatal environments, encompassing such physical factors as climate and pollution, biological factors such as viruses and bacteria, economic factors such as food, shelter and clothing, and social factors such as population aggregation, workplace and support systems; and the health system.

Increasing wealth, better nutrition and public health measures are often credited with improving life expectancy because, until recently, effective medical interventions are thought to have been lacking. The age of modern medicine is less than fifty years old. Modern medicine's contribution to health is controversial. This controversy stems from the failure to assess adequately medical technology and to measure meaningfully health care outcomes in relation to health care processes. Each day, worldwide, we spend billions of dollars on health care interventions on the presumption that they are effective.

E12.04   *Large increases in expenditures; modest gains in health status*

In the past decade, substantial increases in per capita health care expenditures have been accompanied by relatively modest gains in health status, measured inadequately by life expectancy at birth (an established way of measuring the population's health that tells us nothing of the health quality of life). Health status (the preferred measure) quantifies a person's health throughout life (or for a defined period) and includes the number of years lived and the health quality of life, taking into consideration morbidity, institutionalisation and functional ability. It provides the common metric necessary to evaluate all of the health effects of alternative, disparate interventions. However, to date, health status has not been measured routinely—in fact, it has hardly been measured at all.

E12.05 | *Medical care may not be as effective as presumed*

Questioning the effectiveness of medical care is a relatively new phenomenon. For far too long people have simply assumed that health care services result in health status improvement, the ability to palliate translates into the ability to cure, and advances in medical science result in more effective interventions. Two principal perspectives cast doubt on the effectiveness of modern medical interventions: large increases in health care expenditures have produced modest gains in life expectancy (and perhaps even less health status improvement); and inadequately designed research studies show medical interventions to be effective, whereas well-designed research studies show that most medical interventions are ineffective.

E12.06 | *Little is spent on science; little is known scientifically*

Too little useful research is being done, too few research results are useable, and information that is relevant and valid is too hard to find. Most interventions are introduced in practice without scientific assessment of their effectiveness, let alone their cost-effectiveness. Knowledge of cost-effectiveness of medical interventions is essential for meaningful quality management. For example, in an era of increasing scarcity, cheaper treatments that are as effective as those that exist now may be more valuable socially than marginally more effective treatments whose cost is so high that few people or health financing schemes can afford them.

E13 | Problems in Australian hospitals

See Part I, Chapter 1 for details.

Like most of the industrialised world, Australia is experiencing problems in its hospitals. Many of the difficulties relate to the great expansion of medical technology and the consequent increasing rate of specialisation.

The hospital industry in Australia, as in any industrialised society, is large and complex. While common wisdom suggests that Australia enjoys hospital services which are soundly based, hospitals and society cannot ignore the rising rate of hospital and medical litigation over recent years, and the rising tide of complaints and dissatisfaction with hospitals. Rising health care costs coupled with the community's expectations for better value for money from hospital services is adding a further dimension to the problem.

There has been an insidious emphasis on how many patients individual facilities treat, rather than on the extent to which hospital episodes improved patients' health status, the cost of services provided, and patients' satisfaction with the care they received. Certainly, anecdotal accounts and insurance company experience suggest that the quality of care and services in hospitals has suffered. There is insufficient evidence to know if the apparent linkage between the number of patient complaints and the level of litigation and the quality of care and services is real or whether it merely reflects a greater community awareness and a greater propensity to complain.

Few if any hospitals can guarantee patients that they monitor routinely their quality of care, let alone inform them of the quality of care they can expect to receive. There are few if any hospitals in Australia that can demonstrate an effective quality management program. This situation persists despite historical initiatives pertaining to hospital accreditation, credentialling of medical staff and, more recently, quality assurance in the context of quality management.

The reasons for this failure are many and varied, but boil down to the lack of incentives for hospitals to introduce quality management programs and no sanctions if they do not. Moreover, doctors, not unlike their counterparts in many comparable industrial settings, find quality management threatening and, in the case of doctors, quite foreign to their culture and traditions. Put very simply, doctors tend to believe, incorrectly, that their efforts alone reflect the quality of care and hence quality assurance efforts must be about finding fault with doctors. However, quite unlike their counterparts in industry, doctors' failure to embrace quality management does not lead to the demise of their organisation with consequential loss of employment.

E14 | Quality really matters: industry leads, hospitals follow

See Part II, Chapters 1 and 2 for details.

Worldwide, industry has recognised that it is 'quality or else'. In the West, many people attribute Japanese manufacturers' success to their relentless pursuit of quality. The idea that quality is the key to success has spawned a series of movements with various names, such as TQM (total quality management), CQI (continuous quality improvement), the Deming method, and a host of management techniques such as QCs (quality circles), SPC (statistical process control), and QFD (quality functional deployment).

Companies are devoting considerable time, attention and resources to quality management; not for competitive advantage, but for their survival. Some have succeeded. But in many companies the quality revolution is on paper rather than on the shop floor; lip-service to quality management cannot improve quality. In others, quality management programs have simply ground to a halt because they have failed to produce expected results. Often they focused on the structure of quality management processes, rather than on their outcome or effectiveness, and failed to focus on what matters most to customers: the quality of goods and services.

Hospitals have yet to come to grips with the quality revolution. Quality management is, or should be, an essential component of hospital management. It provides the information to reassure patients about the hospital's quality of care and to improve continuously the quality of that care. Hospitals, and everyone who works in them, must gear everything that they do to improving patients' health status. In this decade and beyond, quality management will be one of the hospital's most significant challenges.

E15 | Quality management is a production-level tool

See Part II, Chapters 2 and 3 for details.

E15.01 | *Quality maturity is the goal; quality improvement, the product; quality management, the process*

Quality management (QM) is customer centred, product focused, measurement oriented, improvement driven and all pervasive. Its goal is quality maturity—the state of striving ceaselessly to continuously improve quality (and its inseparable twin, productivity) to produce greater value for money. (See Figure E-1 on page liv). Quality management encompasses all of the forms and functions necessary to achieve quality maturity.

A quality-mature hospital increases patients' health status maximally, at least cost, with greatest patient satisfaction, and perfects trade-offs among these objectives if they cannot all be met simultaneously. Quality is measured explicitly; results used continuously to review and, if necessary, revise practice and process policies and change care systems and processes to improve quality. Changes in culture, organisation, incentives and the hospital's operating environment are needed to facilitate progress toward this end.

Quality management is a production-level tool, useful to manufacturers in the production of goods and to hospitals in caring for patients. Viewing a hospital as a

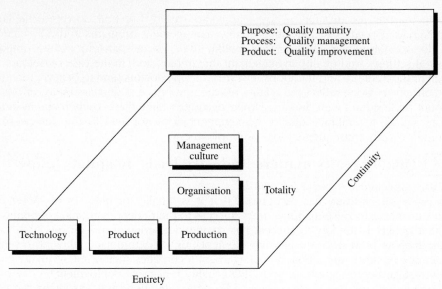

Figure E-1 *Dimensions of quality management*

complex production system is difficult for many health professionals, but necessary if they are to really understand quality management. Key concepts include the following:

- Quality and costs are so intertwined that one cannot be managed without regard to the other.
- The quality of goods (produced by manufacturers) or services (health improvement produced by hospitals) results from production systems, not the efforts of individuals working in isolation (e.g. production workers or doctors).
- Quality management is synonymous with, and required for, good management: achieving an organisation's purpose by improving its product and production system.
- Quality management is an integral part of production or service delivery, not something separate.
- Quality management can, and should, be subjected to the same scrutiny and continuous improvement to which it subjects an organisation's production function.
- Concepts and techniques needed to implement quality management exist already but, as with all aspects of production, can be improved continuously.

E15.02   Quality management means meaningful measurement

Measurement is essential for quality management, which involves considerable use of statistics. Health care has been devoid of meaningful feedback to improve its quality. Actions may be hit-or-miss, and without feedback no one will know that anything has really improved. Feedback of results to improve practice policies, care processes and quality control elements is the principal missing link to integrate systems and improve the quality of care.

E15.03   Health care is a far greater quality management challenge than manufacturing

Virtually all quality management experience stems from manufacturing, necessitating constant reference to industry and industrial analogies. Health care, however, represents a more complex quality management challenge, even though the same basic principles apply. Industrial quality management techniques cannot be applied uncritically, and have limited applicability, to clinical care. Health care quality management requires use of more sophisticated techniques (outlined in this manual) than those used in industry; however, industrial techniques can play a part in improving operational efficiency.

E15.04   *Variance reduction: as important in health care as in manufacturing*

The greatest difference between manufacturing and health care is what constitutes quality and how to achieve it. Manufacturing quality gurus often define quality simply as meeting specifications; zero defects is a quality absolute to be achieved through zero variation in inputs and of manufacturing processes. Since hospital patients often exhibit large variation in factors affecting outcomes, simple statistical analyses can exhibit large, but quite appropriate, variation in the processes applied to patients. Achieving zero defects in health care requires perfecting the fit between what patients need and desire and what they receive. Achieving a perfect patient–process fit and ensuring that specified processes are implemented properly, thereby ensuring zero production defects, is far more difficult than achieving zero defects in manufacturing. Variance reduction must strive toward improving poor performance (and, secondarily, eliminating poor performers) to protect patients while encouraging good performers to do even better, to improve the average, and reduce variation in, quality of care.

E15.05   *Technology, product design and production determine quality*

The quality revolution began in production (making the product to specifications) and spread to product design—first to enhance products' 'manufacturability' (thereby improving production quality) and then to produce designs that delighted customers at value-for-money prices. Now the quality revolution is spreading to the generation of the technology that improves production processes and product designs.

Quality is determined ultimately by technology (which usually limits product designs and production processes); mostly by product and process specifications; immediately by conformance to specifications; and additionally by operational efficiencies that reduce production costs. In health care, product technology is knowledge about disease processes and interventions to alter their course; process technology is knowledge about how to deliver interventions most cost-effectively. Product specifications are manifest in practice policies (standing rules on how to treat types of patients and what to expect as a result) and process or procedural policies (process specifications or step-by-step procedures, for example for conducting specific surgical operations).

Today, most if not all hospitals lack, and for the foreseeable future will continue to lack, the means to develop technology, and to formulate *de novo* practice and process policies. Consequently they must usually limit their quality management efforts to adopting or adapting practice and process policies developed, for example, by professional societies (that are based on knowledge and technology developed, for example, by government-funded research) and to improving conformance to these policies. By measuring outcomes in relation to processes, hospitals can contribute significantly to improving knowledge, as well as the quality of their care. This manual focuses on practice policies and their use to define and, through structured quality improvement, to assure and improve hospitals' quality of care.

E15.06   *Quality management is more than traditional quality assurance*

Traditionally, at least in the United States, the term quality assurance (QA) has been associated with postproduction (retrospective) review of care, sometimes called medical audit. In North America, medical audit has been confined largely to episodic, sporadic or haphazard retrospective case-by-case review of medical records and, if deficiencies were found in care or its documentation, feedback to the doctor—who was as likely to argue about the so-called deficiencies as to reflect on or change his or her practices to prevent their recurrence. Almost certainly there was no follow-up to see if problems recurred or not. Three factors virtually precluded meaningful efforts to change practice and improve the quality of care: limiting QA to doctors' activities, with its implicit, erroneous assumptions that doctors alone produce patients' health status improvement and that they are the cause of, or their (re)education would resolve, all problems; lack of pattern analysis to identify problems and investigate their underlying causes; and absence of systems to rectify any problems for which causes could be elucidated. In Australia, the term quality assurance has been used loosely to embrace almost any activity intended to review clinical or non-clinical services. Most of such activity has been unstructured and rarely associated with review of patients' medical records by colleagues.

E15.07 | *Assuring quality requires attention to all production phases*

The idea that health care is a production function and that quality management is a production-level tool for its improvement suggests classifying quality control mechanisms by their temporal relationship to production processes: preproduction, intraproduction and postproduction. Health care quality control mechanisms include the following:

- Preproduction—to control the inputs to production processes, for example:
  —Admission policies: to control the types of patients the hospital treats.
  —Credentialling: to control who treats patients.
  —Practice policies: to control how patients are treated.
- Intraproduction—to assure conformance to practice policies (product specifications) during the process of care delivery, for example:
  —Decision support technologies, to help providers make the right decisions at the right time, will be increasingly common in the next thirty years.
  —Robotics, to help implement procedures flawlessly—here today, more tomorrow.
- Postproduction—to measure and monitor performance toward its improvement, by comparing what is being done and achieved to what should be being done and achieved, and making necessary changes in the production system to close any gaps, for example using:
  —Structured quality review (SQR), which involves automated screening of medical records to identify, and structured medical record review to confirm, quality of care problems, and statistical analysis of findings to describe patterns of care, and illuminate quality problems, toward improving conformance with practice policies.
  —Structured outcome measurement (SOM), to examine long-term outcomes (end results) of care and their relationship to practices, to improve practice policies and care processes.

Hospital accreditation, relying as it has until quite recently on preproduction surveillance of structures, is insufficient to assure quality. Hospitals must develop and deploy a complete quality management system that encompasses mechanisms to assure and improve quality at all three production phases.

E15.08 | *Quality management encompasses all quality improvement activities*

Quality management embraces all the multiple and various functions and activities which together are required to ensure quality maturity. (See Figure E-2 on page lvii.) In hospitals, quality management includes:

- Quality assurance/quality improvement (QA/QI)—to ensure that care conforms to practice policies (pre-established process and outcome criteria and standards); to

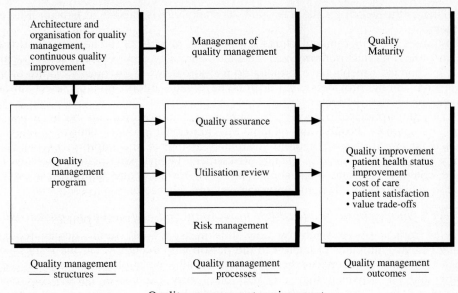

Quality management environment

Figure E-2 *The dynamic of quality management and quality improvement*

provide information to validate and improve practice policies; and to correct identified deficiencies in performance, thereby improving the quality of care.
- Utilisation review (UR)—to ensure patients receive only needed (but all necessary) interventions (procedures, days of care etc.), in the least expensive setting, for the shortest possible duration. In practice, UR is best subsumed within QA.
- Risk management (RM)—to reduce the hospital's exposure to financial loss consequent to providing care. Such exposure is reduced inherently by effective QA/QI.

E16 | Quality: foremost in customers' minds

See Part II, Chapters 3 and 5 for details.

E16.01 | System quality differs from production quality

At the health system level, access to care is clearly an important quality consideration and may obviously influence a population's health. However, it is irrelevant at the production level, which involves patient–provider interactions. Maximising providers' performance for individual patients does not necessarily maximise system performance, although it may contribute to improving it. Moreover, the last units of achievable health status improvement may be gained at considerable cost, and if some of these resources were used elsewhere, they may yield more population health improvement per dollar. This manual focuses on production-level quality, that is, patient health status improvement by individual hospitals.

E16.02 | Quality defines a product or service; it is not an aspect

Quality is good; high quality is very good; low quality is, well, to say the least, not good. 'Quality' evokes a powerful and positive image that somehow encompasses the ideals of truth, beauty, and abundance; the quest for it is eternal, a crusade that sometimes is as compelling as the search for the holy grail. Its attainment is elusive; its accomplishment ephemeral.

Customers can gauge manufactures' quality by a number of dimensions, apart from price, including: product performance, reliability, durability, serviceability, aesthetics and image. In contrast, patients have virtually no measurements of the quality of care to use in selecting among providers and doctors have little information to select among interventions for their patients.

Health care's principal purpose is to maintain and improve patients' health status. To assure and improve health care quality, this functional product definition must be translated into product specifications. All quality assurance and improvement activities begin with quality assessment. Quality assessment begins with practice policies (or practice criteria) that state what should be done for particular types of patients to maximise achievable health status improvement and what to expect consequently.

E16.03 *Quality must be measured to be improved; defined to be measured*

Quality is defined operationally by how it is measured. Measuring quality requires defining essential attributes of interest to the person who intends to use the results—the customer. Products and services that rank high on all aspects of quality, the very best, are few and far between; they are also often very expensive. Quality has many characteristics; trade-offs among them must usually be made. Quality and costs are so intertwined that one cannot be managed without regard to the other.

E16.04 *Provider performance is paramount*

Health care quality (provider performance) has the following four essential dimensions:
* technical quality—measured by health status improvement;
* resource consumption—measured by the cost of care;
* patient satisfaction—measured by patients' perceptions of the subjective or interpersonal aspects of care;
* values—measured by the acceptability of any trade-offs that must be made among the three previous outcomes.

Practically, hospitals must measure provider performance with reference to conformance to practice policies and their expected patient outcomes. Today, interventions' effect on health status must usually be assumed because it is not—but ought to be—known scientifically. Today, hospitals do not measure, and patients do not know, providers' quality of care. Consequently hospitals cannot improve the quality of their care and neither hospitals nor patients can select rationally among providers.

E16.05 *After 5000 years, a breakthrough in the quest for quality*

Patients and providers have long been concerned about the quality of their health care. However, lack of technology has precluded its meaningful measurement. In this century, and particularly in the last decade, great strides have been made in measuring the quality of health care. They are principally advances in: health care quality concepts, knowledge engineering and computer technology. The last few years have seen the emergence of the first practical methods for routinely assessing and measuring health care quality.

E16.06 *Quality measurement is more than quality assessment*

Quality measurement is necessary to quantify quality and to conclude that improvement has occurred. Quality (performance) measurement quantifies a hospital's or a doctor's performance in diagnosing and treating patients. It provides an actual measure of a hospital's performance; patients or payers can choose among hospitals based on their quality scores. Quality (of care) assessment determines whether or not care provided to an individual case met specified standards of medical practice. It provides a judgment about the quality (appropriateness or acceptability) of an episode or continuum of health care; hospitals can use these assessments to improve the technical quality of their care. If these assessments involve all aspects of the quality of care and appropriate probability samples of or all cases, hospitals can aggregate them into a quality score in order to measure quality and to monitor quality improvement.

E16.07 | *Measuring quality: outcome/process assessment is better than outcome risk adjustment*

Two approaches are emerging to measure quality:

- Outcome risk adjustment systems adjust statistically a hospital's patient health outcomes (e.g. deaths) for factors affecting the outcome that are beyond the hospital's control in order to obtain a measure of its performance.
- Outcome/process assessment relies on specifying the processes that if implemented properly would result in the maximum achievable patient health status improvement (given the patient's preferences for ends and means and society's resources), and case-by-case assessment to see if a provider followed specified processes and achieved expected outcomes. Outcome/process assessment reveals what quality problems exist and may illuminate their causes; outcome risk adjustment does not.

E17 | Health care is a production function

See Part II, Chapters 1, 4, and 6 for details.

E17.01 | *Health care's purpose is to improve patients' health status*

Health care's purpose is to improve patients' health status to the maximum extent possible, using specific interventions consistent with patients' preferences and constrained only by patients' means, providers' circumstances, and society's resources and mores. Hospitals exist to manufacture health. The idea that health can be 'manufactured' or that hospitals are health-producing 'factories' is a perspective on health care that is rarely articulated, and foreign to most doctors. Quality management requires viewing hospitals as health-producing facilities—organisations designed to 'produce' health. However, hospitals are not industrial factories and the production of health in hospitals differs markedly from the production of manufactures in factories. Consequently, industrial quality management methods may not be, and often are not, useful for improving the production of health.

E17.02 | *Care processes, patient characteristics, the environment—and their interactions—produce outcomes*

Health care production systems consist of a series of processes (shaped by structures), each of which may be a production subsystem with its own process elements. (See Figure E-3 on page lx. The output of one process is an input to a subsequent process. Three sets of variables—and their interactions—produce patient outcomes: health care production processes (producer); patient's characteristics at the time of entering the process, including his or her health problems; and the environment in which production processes take place (coproducers). Interactions among variables may be the greatest determinant of patient outcomes. An effective medical intervention (process) transforms patients (input): patients' postprocess health status (outcome) is greater than it would have been at that point in time without the process. Knowing the determinants of health does not mean that we can alter them favourably; knowing health status does not tell us what produced it.

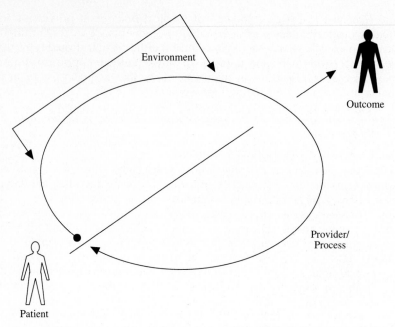

Figure E-3 *The production of outcome: Health care process (intended producer), patient, environment (coproducers), and their interactions*

E17.03 *It is easier to measure outcomes than to attribute them to interventions*

Attribution of patient outcomes to care processes is the key to quality improvement. Measuring a postprocess outcome tells nothing about whether or not the process produced the outcome. A patient's recovery or death may have everything, nothing, or something to do with care processes. It is one thing to observe an effect and quite another to confidently attribute that effect to the preceding intervention.

Attribution of outcomes to processes must either be assumed or inferred. The strength of the inference depends on the strength of the evidence. Attribution may be based on judgment, examination of interventions and events preceding outcomes, or, preferably, on research results. Plausible mechanisms are not necessarily valid chains of cause and effect. The greater the period between intervention and measurement, the more uncertain becomes attribution of outcomes to processes because of the increasing opportunity for occurrence of postprocess outcome-influencing events.

E17.04 *Quality management requires that outcomes be assessed, not assumed*

Outcomes measurement provides information on the end results of care in relation to the processes that preceded them and other coproducers, for example patient characteristics. This information can improve the design and content of practice policies, confirm or cast doubt on interventions' effectiveness, point to the need for better interventions, and help set research priorities. However, outcomes measurement cannot provide incontrovertible evidence about interventions' effectiveness and can never be a substitute for clinical trials or other experimental research. Patients select doctors and doctors select interventions; substantial patient–provider selection bias may exist.

E17.05 *Design of health production systems requires scientific evaluation*

Research studies, especially randomised controlled clinical trials (which can overcome patient–provider selection bias), provide the best information for designing practice policies and production processes. Only through scientific evaluation can one produce the certain knowledge necessary to (re)design health production systems to realise achievable health status improvement and to raise the level that is achievable. Today we spend far too little on such research; it is too narrowly focused to be useful for quality management and often too poorly done for its results to be useable.

E17.06 Hospitals must strive to establish a complete quality management system

Hospitals are health care's principal production facilities—organisations designed to 'produce' health. They must put in place a complete quality management system—the structures and processes necessary to improve continuously the quality of their products and production processes. (See Figure E-4 below.) An effective quality management system assures and improves continuously the appropriate treatment of individual patients and treatments' effectiveness. It encompasses mechanisms to:

- control or assure product quality at each of production's three phases: preproduction, intraproduction and postproduction;
- generate the information needed to validate and improve practice policies and their constituent product and process technologies;
- manage and improve quality management.

Quality control takes places at two levels: the organisation and the workface. Organisations design production systems to produce products to specifications. What occurs at the workface determines products' quality. Ideally, organisational quality control mechanisms promote workface quality and workface experience shapes organisational quality control mechanisms.

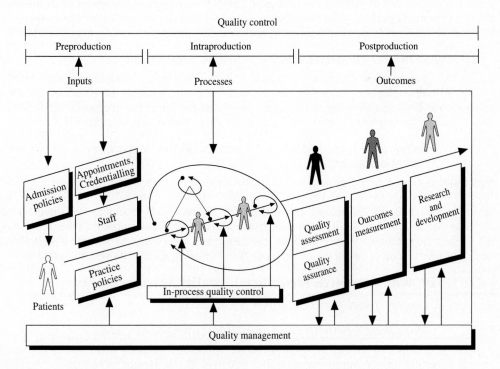

Figure E-4 *Health care quality management system*

E17.07 | *Analyse variation in processes, outcomes to identify improvement opportunities*

Quality management's central goal is to improve product quality and to reduce production variance. Variation in patient outcomes or deviations from specified processes or expected outcomes may signify a quality problem. Hospitals' goal is to reduce the variation in the fit between what patients need and want, and what they receive. They must implement interventions, for example a surgical operation, as uniformly as practical. Uniformity of process facilitates assessment of variation in outcome by eliminating the obvious factor—variation in process. Variation in outcomes detracts from quality because it represents risk to patients. Quality managers must reduce variance in outcomes while simultaneously increasing average patient health status improvement. In some circumstances they may face trading-off increased average health status improvement and reduced variation in such improvement.

All strategies for improving the quality of care depend ultimately on analysing variation in production performance and resultant outcomes. They are principally:

- structured performance benchmarking;
- structured quality improvement;
- structured outcome measurement.

E17.08 | *Identify the best performers; find the difference that makes the difference*

Structured performance benchmarking refers to the strategy of measuring competitors' (colleagues') performance to identify the best performers, to discern what processes, patient flows, and organisation seem to produce this performance, and to establish where one's performance stands in relation to the best. Consequently, one can align one's production system with that of the best performers toward improving one's performance. Today, structured performance benchmarking is beyond the means of all but large-scale hospital systems or those that engage in collaborative arrangements for this purpose.

E17.09 | *Find and eliminate quality problems' root causes*

Structured quality improvement refers to a hospital-wide strategy to systematically identify quality problems, discover their root causes, and routinely eliminate these causes. Quality-focused hospitals must design and deploy mechanisms for these purposes. This is the basic strategy for improving hospitals' quality of care, and it is now practical.

E17.10 | *Relate long-term outcomes to care processes to validate and improve practice policies*

Structured outcome measurement refers to the strategy of measuring the long-term (end results) of health care interventions. It examines the extent to which conformance to specifications actually improves patient health status, and produces information to improve them. It is not a substitute for, but may help prioritise, needed research. Only the largest hospitals are likely to have the resources necessary to launch a structured outcome measurement program or conduct the clinical trials that its results suggest.

E18 | The way forward: structured quality improvement

See Part II, Chapter 8 and Part IV, Chapter 4 for details.

E18.01 | *More health benefits than pursuing cures for diseases*

Structured quality improvement (SQI) is likely to be the greatest advance in the next twenty years. If implemented successfully, SQI has likely greater potential to improve health care's cost-effectiveness in the next twenty years than any other technology—even 'cures' for such specific diseases as cancer. It operationalises the quality improvement spiral. Structured quality improvement pertains mostly to conformance improvement (getting done what needs to be done in the way it should be done each and every time) but also informs specifications improvement. Structured performance benchmarking and structured outcome measurement provide information mostly for specifications improvement (what to do and how to do it).

| E18.02 | *Quality improvement results from conformance to, and better, specifications*

The quality improvement spiral is the combined continuous operationalisation of two interlocking cycles: the conformance improvement (CI) and specifications improvement (SI) cycles. Practice policies are their common point of origin. (See Figure E-5 below.) The CI cycle refers to the process of perfecting conformance to specifications. The SI cycle refers to that of reviewing and revising product specifications (practice policies that are the basis for QA activities). The CI and SI cycles must be repeated endlessly to assure and improve quality continuously. For all practical purposes, the conformance improvement cycle is synonymous with the quality assurance cycle.

| E18.03 | *Quality assurance cycle: repeat endlessly to improve quality continuously*

The term quality assurance denotes a cyclical process involving retrospective quality assessment—retrospective review of care outcomes and processes based on

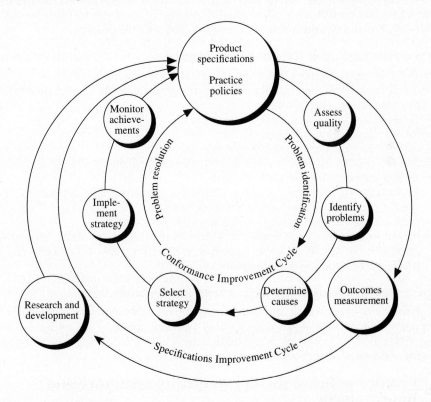

Figure E-5 *Continuous quality improvement through conformance and specifications improvement cycles*

documentation in the patient's medical record—and subsequent steps to improve care processes to close any performance gaps. Quality assurance (QA) and quality improvement (QI) are important but distinct aspects of production and product quality; continuous quality improvement (CQI) is performing QA/QI on a continuous basis. Quality is improved both by better conformance to specifications, and by better specifications (those that produce more health status improvement, or the same improvement at less cost or with greater patient satisfaction, and/or less variation in outcomes).

E18.04 | *Specifications improvement: knowing right things to do*

The specifications improvement cycle intends to improve quality through better product specifications—the practice policies that are the starting point for the conformance improvement cycle; ideally, those that if implemented properly would result in maximal patient health status improvement within patients' preferences and society's resources. Quality managers can derive information to formulate or revise practice policies from their or others' clinical experience, structured quality improvement, structured performance benchmarking, structured outcome measurement and research reports.

E18.05 | *Conformance improvement: doing right things right*

The conformance improvement (or QA) cycle intends to improve quality through conformance to product specifications and thus to reduce variability in health care processes and outcomes. It starts with specifying what should be done and achieved, continues with assessing the extent to which it was done and achieved, and ends with efforts to close any performance gaps. Quality managers must put in place mechanisms to identify systematically and resolve routinely quality of care problems.

E18.06 | *First find, then fix, quality problems*

Structured quality improvement involves a hospital-wide system for:
- structured problem identification—to identify systematically quality problems, and their root causes. This involves:
  —defining and measuring or assessing quality;
  —identifying quality problems;
  —determining quality problems' root causes.
- structured problem resolution—to resolve routinely quality problems and eliminate their root causes. This involves:
  —evaluating and selecting among alternative improvement actions to remedy quality problems and eliminate their root causes;
  —planning and implementing chosen improvement actions;
  —measuring quality to ascertain if it has improved, to attribute any observed improvement (or its lack) to improvement actions, and to identify any other problems that they may have created.

E18.07 | *Quality improvement begins with quality assessment*

Quality assessment—measuring and monitoring provider performance—is presently the key to quality improvement in hospitals. Quality assessment results can inform admissions policies, credentialling decisions and practice policies—the starting point for quality assessment and hence of the quality assurance cycle.

E19 | Practice policies: the key to quality assurance and improvement

See Part II, Chapter 7 for details.

E19.01 *Effectiveness is a statistical concept; providers' performance depends on interventions' appropriate use*

One must distinguish between an intervention's effectiveness and providers' performance—the extent to which providers use an intervention appropriately and implement it properly. Effectiveness is a statistical concept. An effective intervention improves a population of patients' health status. Measuring an intervention's true effectiveness depends on determining the difference in health status between intervention, doing nothing, and a disease's natural history in such a way that one can confidently attribute the difference to the intervention, for example through a well-designed, well-controlled randomised clinical trial. An appropriate intervention can reasonably be expected to benefit a particular patient because he or she fits the profile of patients for whom it is known or assumed widely to be effective.

E19.02 *Specifications are the heart of quality*

Only by specifying a product can its quality be assured (by producing it to specifications) and improved (by specifying a product that meets customers' desires better). Health care's product is defined by practice specifications: what providers should do for patients (care processes) and what to expect as a result (outcomes). They may take the form of practice policies—standing rules for treating patients—(referred to sometimes as guidelines or parameters) or practice criteria (referred to sometimes as criteria and standards)—rules for judging whether or not patients were treated appropriately.

E19.03 *Process specifications define health care's product; an individual patient's outcome cannot be attributed to care process*

Process specifications define health care's product because it is impractical to measure routinely patients' health status improvement and virtually impossible to attribute reliably any measured improvement to specific interventions. Practice policies—pre-established clinical decision rules for treating individual patients that take into account their preferences regarding ends and means—are the starting point for defining these processes and their expected resultant outcomes. For all practical purposes, in the immediate future, quality management relevant to clinical care will be limited in most hospitals to adopting and adhering to practice and procedural policies, and to ensuring conformance to these policies.

E19.04 *Practice policies express how to achieve achievable patient health status improvement*

Practice policies:
- are the basis for practice, providing direct guidance or instructions to providers about how patients should be managed, including who should manage them and where they should be managed;
- represent the best way to manage individual patients;
- make explicit assumptions between health care processes (specific medical interventions) and stated patient outcomes;
- must take into account:
  —hospitals' facilities and other resources (and doctors' and other providers' skills) for treating patients;
  —patients' preferences regarding ends to be achieved and means to achieve them;
- may encompass socioeconomic considerations.

One must clearly distinguish synthesising knowledge to determine best practices (which involves only technical issues) from formulating policies—what should be done in specific circumstances (which involves such social issues as judging an intervention's cost-benefit). Practice policies must be highly specific to be useful. Their complexity virtually requires that they be computerised at the point of service delivery, in decision support technology. Nevertheless, even simple practice policies, if formulated and used consistently, can improve the quality of care.

If available, which usually they are not, fully-elaborated practice policies can be translated easily into practice criteria, to assess retrospectively the quality of care. If not available, practice criteria serve this latter purpose. Practice criteria are the basis for quality assurance, guidance or instructions to QA personnel, including medical record reviewers, about judging how patients should have been managed. They provide indirect guidance or instruction to providers about how patients should be managed.

E19.05 | *Technology limits achievable patient health status improvement*

Conformance to practice policies will only improve patients' health status if they embody effective interventions. Conformance to valid practice policies will improve quality, but only to the limits of the underlying technologies. Additional health status improvement requires better technologies. Nevertheless, conformance to valid practice policies—doing what is known or assumed to be effective—may provide greater additional health status improvement than the introduction of new treatments under development or that could plausibly be developed in the near future.

E20 | Quality problems: search systematically, resolve routinely

See Part II, Chapter 8 for details.

E20.01 | *Systematic surveillance is essential to find quality problems*

For effective quality management, hospitals must have in place systems to identify systematically and resolve routinely quality problems—deficiencies that if resolved would improve the quality of care. Hospitals can employ the following problem identification mechanisms:

- systematic review of care or cases (patient records that document care processes and outcomes);
- systematic surveys of people's perceptions and suggestions;
- incident reports, including patient complaints and allegations of malpractice, and compliments;
- quality assurance studies;
- group problem-solving techniques, for example quality circles.

At a minimum, hospitals must perform hospital-wide systematic surveillance of care or cases, using either, or preferably both, of the following methods:

- structured quality assessment—reviewing care case-by-case—for example structured quality review or unaided structured medical record review to identify and characterise quality problems;
- structured quality monitoring—population-based screening—watching rates of events in populations of cases to trigger review of providers' care if rates exceed pre-established limits.

Structured quality review (see below) is the most cost-effective way to identify quality of care problems. The careful tracking and reporting of hospital incidents, and patients' complaints and compliments, is an important supplemental mechanism for identifying potential or actual problems. An incident is something that happened as a result of or in connection with patient care, especially something that merits reporting. Hospitals should track all incident reports, including patients' complaints, investigate individually all serious incidents, and analyse statistically incident reports and investigations' results in order to identify patterns with a view to reducing incidents. Patient satisfaction surveys help to assess the interpersonal aspects of quality of care and are an important tool in overall quality management and quality assurance (see below).

E20.02 | Screening can be a cost-effective way to identify quality of care problems

Screening's central purpose is to focus expert clinician reviewers' attention on cases likely to exhibit quality problems, thereby reducing their workloads to manageable levels and improving their productivity. It substitutes data analysis or less expensive medical abstracter or nurse reviewer personnel for expensive expert clinician reviewers. Case-based screens identify cases that exhibit potential quality of care problems and their nature. Population-based screens identify providers whose cases exhibit specified events at a higher or lower rate than that specified (threshold) or whose performance lies at the extremes of statistical distributions (cut-off). Ultimately, quality assessment depends on expert clinician review of medical records—either those failing case-based screens or those of providers identified by population-based screens. Case-based screens are more useful than population-based screens for identifying potential quality of care problems.

Structured quality assessment intends to identify quality problems by employing mechanisms to look either for a given problem (e.g. nosocomial infection) in all cases or for all problems in a given case, or, preferably, both (all problems in all or relevant statistically significant samples of cases). It may involve use of case-based screens to identify quality of care problems. These screens divide cases into those that can be presumed acceptable because they met screening criteria and those that require further review by expert clinicians to confirm or deny quality problems. Their utility depends on the extent to which they can accurately classify cases as containing an important quality problem or not. Ideally, case-based screens must identify all cases with important quality of care problems (sensitivity) while rejecting those with no quality problems (specificity). The sensitivity and specificity of emerging computerised quality assessment screens is now sufficiently high to make their use worthwhile.

Structured quality monitoring may involve the use of population-based quality of care screens (referred to often as rate-based or clinical indicators). Such screening may trigger the further investigation of a provider's cases to confirm (or deny) a quality problem's existence and to identify problem processes, including those that might have produced observed maloutcomes. Clinical indicators are rate-based screens that depend on thresholds or cut-offs to trigger further review. Sentinel events are indicators with zero thresholds. Population-based screening can only identify providers who seem to be experiencing quality problems and may miss those who are delivering substandard care but who do not exceed screening thresholds or cut-offs. Population-based screens'—clinical indicators'—sensitivity and specificity is largely unknown.

E20.03 | Determine problems' root, not only their apparent, causes

To fix problems and ensure they remain fixed, hospitals must establish problems' root causes, those that if eliminated would prevent the problem's recurrence, not only their apparent causes, which are merely the problem's antecedent manifestations.

E20.04 | Problems are fixed only if they remain fixed

Hospitals must put in place a system for fixing quality problems and checking that they stay fixed. Hospitals that attempt to identify quality problems without institutionalising the means to resolve them are wasting their resources.

Structured problem resolution involves: selecting among potential improvement actions (solutions to problems); implementing chosen solutions; and assessing quality to ascertain if it has improved. Problems are resolved only if they stay resolved and do not reappear after so-called improvement activities end. Resources and other constraints are likely to mean that not all problems can be resolved immediately; priorities must be set. Some problems are likely to be more important than others and therefore should be resolved first. For some potential improvements, the cost of their attainment may not be commensurate with their benefits and therefore they should be deferred.

Resolving quality problems may require changes in one or more of the following three areas:

- care processes—how doctors and other health care providers treat or manage patients;
- patient flows—how patients are routed into and from clinical processes, how the hospital manages care delivery, and the interrelationships among care processes;
- organisational management—how the hospital structures the production system or enterprise, and how it manages people and processes.

E21 | Quality: the challenge of history

See Part I, Chapter 2 and Part II, Chapter 1 for details.

E21.01 | *The challenge of measuring providers' performance*

Interest in formal quality assurance activities has waxed and waned throughout history. In recent times—1858—the English founder of modern nursing, Florence Nightingale, was concerned about the outcomes of hospital care, and thought of statistical adjustment of mortality data to permit proper comparisons, although she lacked the technology to make the necessary measurements. Early this century in the United States, a Boston surgeon, A. E. Codman, wanted to tally patient outcomes (the end results of care) to give credit for success and to fix responsibility for failure, although he too lacked the necessary technology. His efforts led ultimately to the formal accreditation of hospitals with the creation, in 1952, of the Joint Commission for the Accreditation of Hospitals (now the Joint Commission for the Accreditation of Healthcare Organisations). Now, after 5000 years, the technology is emerging to meaningfully measure health care providers' performance. It represents the key to quality management and promises to unlock untold improvements in the quality of care.

E21.02 | *Meeting the quality management challenge in Australia*

To look at the current Australian quality management scene with the benefit of historical perspective is to add a logic and understanding to three developments on the road to quality management that many medical practitioners see as threatening intrusions into their professional lives: hospital accreditation, credentialling of medical staff and quality assurance.

In the late 1950s and early 1960s concerns about the standard of care in public hospitals in New South Wales led to efforts to introduce hospital accreditation. In retrospect, these efforts could be seen as the first steps toward quality management in Australian hospitals. After more than a decade of effort, the concern about the standard of hospital care resulted, in 1974, in the establishment of the Australian Council on Healthcare Standards (ACHS). It took some thirty years for accreditation to be accepted throughout Australia.

In the early 1970s two serious incidents in New South Wales hospitals brought the issue of what doctors do in hospitals to the public agenda and resulted in the development of the concept of credentialling of medical staff, which had the effect of easing the widespread government and community concern. The first of these episodes involved the death of a young woman during an operation for thyroidectomy. The surgeon was a qualified anaesthetist and the anaesthetic was provided by a series of three general practitioners. The second episode involved a solo GP in a small country hospital conducting a total hindquarter amputation with the Director of Nursing giving an open ether anaesthetic. Unfortunately, once the concerns had subsided, credentialling remained purely conceptual and has never been effectively implemented in Australia, although it is the norm in the United States.

The formal introduction of quality assurance into Australia commenced in 1977 following a challenge by the Commonwealth government to the medical profession. Attitudes to quality management and its subset—quality assurance—have changed for the better since the late 1970s and early 1980s, and considerable activity is occurring in a number of areas. For example, in 1991 the ACHS introduced its clinical indicator project and revised its standards to introduce quality management as a requirement for hospital accreditation. Nevertheless, the fact remains that today there is no Australian hospital that can boast an effective quality management program, and one has to question the effectiveness of many QA projects in improving the quality of care for patients.

E21.03 *Hospital accreditation challenges governments and providers*

The development of hospital accreditation in Australia provides a good illustration of the difficulties encountered when attempting to introduce change into an extremely conservative industry. The greatest resistance in Australia, where public hospitals dominate the industry, was initially from state government hospital authorities which saw hospital accreditation as an intrusion into their area of responsibility.

Members of the medical profession, with some notable individual exceptions, have never felt comfortable with hospital accreditation. Accreditation's focus on structure, and to a lesser extent on process, while ignoring outcome, has added to doctors' dissatisfaction because they have a subjective view of quality which relates almost entirely to the value of the medical care that individual doctors provide. In fairness to doctors' concerns, while accreditation may help to expose organisational deficiencies, it neither ensures that patients receive quality care nor documents that care improves patients' health status.

Hospital accreditation is still evolving in Australia. While it has played the major role in upgrading the quality of Australian hospitals, there is no doubt that it has not met its founders' expectations in all respects. Until quite recently, one could criticise accreditation for not raising standards of medical records to the level necessary for quality management and case-based payment, and not explicating those pertaining to quality management and quality assurance. Now the ACHS is applying considerable efforts to address these issues. The ACHS has revised its standards on medical records and quality management and, if implemented with vigour, they should have far-reaching effects on the industry. However, the ACHS must still face the widely-held view that accreditation is a paper tiger: many forms but little substance. Whether true or not, such perceptions provide the ACHS with a continuous challenge to its role and credibility.

E21.04 *Technology challenges doctors' competence*

Concerns about the quality of services in Australian hospitals emerged in the late 1950s for which, in retrospect, it is difficult to pinpoint clear reasons. Most importantly, hospitals were not able to adjust to the enormous changes brought about by the technological explosion following World War II. With the technology came a concomitant elevation of expectations, a factor fuelled to some extent by the enthusiasm of the medical profession. In the late 1960s, problems associated with medical staff undertaking procedures for which they were inadequately trained or experienced was a manifestation of this failure to adjust to a rapidly changing hospital environment.

Until quite recently, the Australian hospital and medical cultures have been derivatives of those of the United Kingdom. Attitudes of medical staff, training of doctors and nurses, and hospital staffing arrangements bore the unmistakable stamp 'made in the UK', in part because many specialists had trained there. However, the geographic, political and medical environment of Australia is very different from that in the United Kingdom and consequently problems began to appear in the early 1960s. Instinctively, answers were sought from a more comparable environment—that of the United States. Hospital accreditation in Australia was deliberately fashioned on the US model developed by the Joint Commission on Accreditation of Healthcare Organisations. A system of credentialling of medical staff (delineation of clinical privileges) was developed in the first instance without any knowledge of the US model. Significantly, a blueprint for a system ultimately emerged that was identical with that pertaining in North America.

Unfortunately, formal credentialling of medical staff has posed too big a threat to long-established traditional attitudes derived from the United Kingdom. In Australia, as in the United Kingdom, quality of care in hospitals has been seen to equate with the postgraduate qualifications of medical staff and there has been a failure to implement effective credentialling. This failure has meant that one of the most important elements of quality management and the minimisation of the risk of medical and hospital malpractice litigation is missing in the overwhelming majority of Australian hospitals. The Royal Australian College of Obstetricians and Gynaecologists was the first of several colleges to acknowledge problems inherent in granting good-for-life qualifications by demanding recertification at periodic intervals. Credentialling is not only about the training of doctors but also about the link between their training and the hospital's resources. Postgraduate qualifications may certainly indicate a general competence at a point in time. However, credentialling is about specific, often procedural, competence, and the hospital's ability to provide the resources needed to conduct procedures to standards.

E21.05   *The government challenges the medical profession*

The third phase in the historical development of quality management activity in Australia commenced in 1976 when the Commonwealth government challenged the medical profession to engage in what was referred to as 'peer review'. Significantly, issuing this challenge to doctors and not to hospital managers reflected a lack of systems thinking which still exists to the present day. The Australian Medical Association took up the challenge and effectively engaged in technology transfer following a study tour of the United States, Canada and (West) Germany. The AMA embarked on a massive educational program that resulted in a considerable lessening of apprehension as doctors for the first time began to hear something of the techniques and principles of assuring quality of care. Nevertheless, there is no doubt that a degree of concern remains among doctors who have conceptual difficulty moving past the individuality of clinical care to the systems approach required for quality management.

E22   Hospitals must focus on, commit to and organise for quality

See Part I, Chapter 1, Part II, Chapters 6 and 9, and Part III for details.

E22.01   *Quality pertains to everything hospitals do*

Everything that hospitals do must be geared to improving patients' health status, reducing the cost of its attainment, and increasing patient satisfaction with the interpersonal aspects of care. Quality management applies to everything that goes on within hospitals, including clinical and patient care such as doctors' decisions, nursing and physiotherapy. It also includes clinical support services such as clinical laboratory and imaging services, and operational services such as laundry and housekeeping, and administration. However, this manual focuses sharply on clinical care—the core business of hospitals' production function—and, because they play such a vital role in its provision, on doctors' performance. To date, quality improvement in hospitals, where it has been attempted at all, has been limited generally to such operational services as the laundry because they are simple situations and most resemble industrial operations. While useful, such isolated efforts can achieve little quality improvement.

Quality management is about improving patients' outcomes and hence providers' performance. It is not about the condemnation or judgment in isolation of doctors, nurses or anyone else in hospitals. Quality management is primarily about continuous improvement in the quality of care, solving problems in a complex production system, and only rarely about weeding out 'bad apples' (poor performers resistant to or incapable of improving their practices through encouragement and education).

E22.02 | *Quality improvement requires a quality management program to improve quality*

An effective quality management program is the hallmark of a quality-mature hospital. It institutionalises the structures and processes necessary to assure and improve quality, and the mechanisms to administer, control, and evaluate them to permit their adaptation to changing circumstances and to ensure that they continue to produce these outcomes.

The quality of a hospital's product defines the reason for its existence. Quality management is the process for assuring and improving quality. It involves interlocking structures and processes and outcome-based feedback to manage the production of health. Quality management is, or should be, a hospital's primary business, not an incidental activity to be thought of only after the daily pressures of caring for patients have ceased. To achieve quality maturity, a hospital's quality management program must institutionalise:

- the hospital board's and management's commitment to quality, manifest, for example, in the existence of appropriate hospital by-laws and adequate budgets;
- a systems view of product and production quality, to develop a complete quality management program;
- an organisational structure to operationalise the program.

E22.03 | *A proper organisational structure is essential for success*

An effective quality management program includes the following organisational elements:

- a well-constituted quality management committee and an effective committee system;
- a quality manager with the knowledge and management skills to guide and control the program successfully;
- a quality management department, with appropriate staff, to focus, co-ordinate and support quality management activities;
- clinical information systems to ensure the adequacy of data in medical records and to provide the necessary technology to aggregate, manage and use such data.

The absence of all or a number of these key elements of an adequate organisational framework is the major reason for failure to implement quality management in Australian hospitals. Methodologies for assessing the quality of care, and for identifying and resolving quality problems, have been a focus of interest for many health professionals. However, this focus on methodologies has occurred to the exclusion of the organisational structure necessary to effect quality improvement. A quality management program's structure and organisation are this manual's central themes, because most Australian hospitals frequently do not consider these critical elements sufficiently, and sometimes they ignore them completely.

Small hospitals (100 beds or less) face additional difficulties in implementing quality management. However, there are a number of strategies to maximise the use of their limited resources and to allow a small hospital to embark meaningfully on quality management and, eventually, to achieve quality maturity. Such strategies include: making use of resources and services from a common network of hospitals or developing an association with a larger nearby hospital; and organising such functions as credentialling of medical staff on an area or regional basis and reducing the number of committees by combining them.

E23 | Hospitals' policy and resource allocations manifest commitment to an effective quality management program

See Part III, Chapters 2, 4, 5 and 6 for details.

E23.01 | *Directors and managers must commit to quality*

The initiation of quality assurance in Australia in 1977 saw the burden for this activity placed on the shoulders of the medical profession. In the ensuing years, the medical and nursing professions were criticised for failing to undertake effective quality management activity. While doctors and other health professionals must play a key role in any quality management program, the prime decision makers in the process are hospitals' directors and managers. Quality management is a subset of management. A hospital's board of directors has the main responsibility. Without the board's and manager's commitment and involvement, very little will happen.

E23.02 | *Commit totally to total quality*

The most important impression that the hospital's board and its manager must convey to the rest of the hospital is a total commitment to the concept of quality. Directors on hospital boards show great concern about building a new car park or running the hospital canteen and, unfortunately, have a limited understanding or concern for their primary responsibility—the quality of care and services they provide to patients. Hospital managers likewise have seen quality of patient care as something to be left to health professionals. Directors' and managers' total and continuous commitment to quality is essential to quality management's successful implementation.

E23.03 | *Boards must direct, managers lead the quest for quality*

A hospital's board must first develop and approve a quality management policy and then insist that the manager implements its policy decisions and provide the day-to-day leadership to drive quality. The board must ensure that the hospital manager establishes a quality management committee to guide hospital-wide quality management and a quality management department to support the hospital's quality management program. It must monitor reports to ensure that the hospital manager is properly conducting the program that embodies the board's policy.

To a large extent directors and managers generally have failed to accept or even understand their responsibilities for the quality of care and hence for quality management. Included in their responsibilities is the development and approval of appropriate hospital by-laws that clearly spell out everyone's quality management responsibilities and obligations. Further, quality management and all its attendant activities requires resources. Such resources include a quality manager and staff, a quality management department, external consultants when necessary, and the funds to meet these costs. The allocation of resources in a hospital is the responsibility of its directors, not doctors or nurses. Quality management deserves a separate line item in the hospital budget.

Mercedes-Benz spends 8% of its operating expenditure on quality control. Most Australian hospitals spend little or nothing. While no one would suggest that Australian hospitals should (or would know how to) begin spending immediately this proportion of their operating expenses on quality management, without a specific allocation of resources to a quality management program Australian hospitals will never be in a position to achieve excellence, and the quality of patient care will continue to be compromised. Clinical information systems in particular are an essential ingredient of quality management and should be seen as a top resource priority for any hospital board.

E23.04 | *Educate to change attitudes, maintain commitment*

A quality-mature hospital implies attitudes and behaviour on the part of everyone in the hospital that will realistically require major change from those that pertain in most Australian hospitals today. Changing attitudes and behaviour is a large undertaking and cannot be achieved easily overnight. Hospital boards of directors, managers, medical and nursing staffs, and the entire range of professionals and workers who constitute a modern hospital must adopt appropriate attitudes towards health care quality. The educational effort required is extensive and continuous and is perhaps the main reason why it may take five to ten years or longer to achieve quality maturity. Further, while attitudinal and behavioural change justifies a large educational commitment, technical education also plays an important role. Hospitals are responsible for ensuring that nurses who require continuing technical education, or medical staff who have been shown to be unaware of certain technical aspects of care for which they bear responsibility, actually receive such education or training.

E24 | **Hospitals must (re)organise for success**

See Part III, Chapter 3 for details.

E24.01 | *An effective committee system is the hospital's central nervous system*

Quality management requires an organisation geared to improve quality. A hospital cannot succeed by creating another committee and grafting it onto an ineffective organisational structure. It must organise for quality and ensure that all of its committees function effectively as a coherent whole and, if they do not, reorganise them to achieve this end. The failure of hospital committees is a critical element in the failure of their quality management and quality assurance activity. Instituting a well-functioning system of multidisciplinary committees is an important, albeit difficult, task in any hospital.

The quality management committee is a policy decision-making body that sits at the apex of an extensive, integrated system of committees. These committees are a hospital's nervous system. What committees exist, and how they interrelate, to whom they report, and the presence of properly prepared terms of reference for individual committees, bear greatly on their effectiveness as part of a quality management program. Committees are a necessary forum for discussion and decision making, a critical element in democratic or participatory management, a mechanism to permit the orderly generation and transfer of information, and the means to bring together diverse expertise and perspectives.

E24.02 | *The quality management committee is the hospital's most important committee*

The quality management committee (QMC) plays a central role in quality management. It is the hospital's instrument for developing and co-ordinating policy on quality management throughout the hospital. It sets reporting requirements and reviews and acts on reports from subcommittees, departments and divisions, and it advises the hospital manager and board. The QMC should be multidisciplinary and comprise members from most, if not all, of the hospital's major clinical and non-clinical departments. However, this committee should not comprise more than ten to fifteen persons.

E24.03 | *The quality management committee is the apex of a complete committee system; all other committees must relate to it*

The number and types of committees reporting to the quality management committee will vary from hospital to hospital. Such factors as a hospital's size will obviously influence the number of and interrelationships among committees. A range of committees is needed because a single committee, namely the quality management committee, cannot do everything. Essential committees include the following, for example: medical appointments advisory committee; credentials committee; quality of care committees; practice policies committee; medical records committee; infection control committee; various clinical support committees; housekeeping and administration committees; and occupational health and safety committee. (See Figure E-6 on page lxxv.) In many, if not most hospitals, many of these committees already exist. However, their existence is not enough: they must be efficient and integrated to be effective.

E24.04 | *Committees must function effectively and efficiently*

Far too little attention is paid to hospital committees and how they function, and in many instances members of hospital committees function in isolation, unaware of the greater purpose and role of their committee. All too often a new standing committee is formed when an ad hoc working party would have sufficed, resulting in simply too many committees, with a consequential waste of valuable professional time.

From a clinical viewpoint, most hospitals to date have functioned almost in spite of their committees. Quality management, and the more circumscribed quality assurance, cannot function effectively unless the committee system, on which its implementation relies, is both effective and efficient. Achieving this end poses a significant challenge.

Doctors in particular hate committees. Presently, most hospital committees are indeed a waste of busy medical practitioners' time. Agendas are poorly prepared, minutes follow no set pattern and are sometimes even legally suspect. The standard of chairmanship more often than not is poor, and committee members themselves have little understanding of how they should effectively conduct themselves in a committee. In this environment, busy doctors tend to vote with their feet, which renders the committee even less effective. While readers may think this situation only applies to their hospital, experience suggests that unsatisfactory committee functioning is the rule rather than the exception. A group of well-intentioned people sitting down around a table and talking about a problem does not automatically produce an effective committee. In most committees, in most hospitals, an attitude prevails which sees discussion of an issue or a problem as being all that is required of committee members. Not only must committees serve as vehicles for exchanging information, but they must also be effective decision-making bodies that can initiate action.

E24.05 | *Chairpersons must know how to run committees*

Of all problems probably none represents a greater hurdle to a committee's effectiveness than the standard and capacity of the chairperson. Nurses, medical academics or senior members of the visiting medical staff are not born with the understanding needed to chair a committee. Chairmanship is a skill which has to be learnt and, hopefully, can be taught. Hospital managers must provide committee chairpersons with the training necessary to acquire this skill.

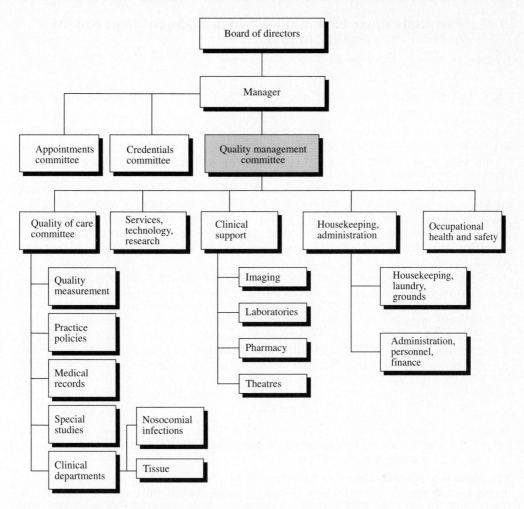

Figure E-6 *Quality management committee structure*

E24.06 | *Multidisciplinary committees are essential*

Patients receive hospital care from a complex matrix of providers from a variety of disciplines. Assuring the quality of care similarly requires a multidisciplinary approach. It is a misnomer to talk of quality assurance for doctors, for nurses, or for allied health personnel, as if there was some quarantined arrangement for the care conducted by these different disciplines. The only form of quality assurance or quality management that hospital staff should discuss is that for patients. All committees, therefore, should be multidisciplinary. The only exceptions should be the medical appointments advisory committee and the credentials committee which should consist solely of medical practitioners (and, if they exist, the equivalent committees for nurses or for other providers should be composed only of those types of practitioners). Frequently, however, a covert hesitancy on the part of hospital professionals to expose themselves to what they mistakenly anticipate will be a critical environment in multidisciplinary committees places additional barriers in the way of implementing effective committee structures.

E25 | Hospitals must have a quality management department headed by a quality manager

See Part III, Chapter 4 for details.

E25.01 | Hospitals need resources to support quality management and to improve quality

For over fifteen years Australian hospitals and health professionals have been attempting to introduce meaningful quality assurance activity, with remarkably little success. Reasons for this lack of success include a lack of commitment from hospital managers, a lack of structure, and the inadequacy of resources that have been made available to them to carry out this complex task. In the complex service environment of any hospital it is simply insufficient to initiate a quality management program, or any part of it, and assume it will automatically be carried through successfully and without difficulties. This reality is no reflection on health professionals, but rather a realistic posture for activities that are new and, because of the complexity of hospital services, are subject to a variety of obstacles and difficulties.

A quality management department and a quality manager are new concepts for Australian hospitals. They are integral elements of the organisational structure necessary for quality management. The collection into one functional unit of all those hospital professionals involved in quality management is an important ingredient in the management of a very extensive program. A properly resourced quality management department is essential for successful implementation of a hospital-wide, integrated quality management program that embraces the necessary range of activities. Medical staff often greet this suggestion with apprehension and believe it is merely another management stratagem to control them. Similarly, the suggestion is likely to provoke fear in hospital administrators that it is just another cost burden for the hospital.

E25.02 | The quality management department: the key resource for quality management

The quality management department is responsible for implementing the hospital's quality management program. Busy doctors and nurses will not have the time or authority to conduct the range of requisite activities, even if they have the expertise and inclination. They need competent professional support. The quality management department exists to teach, support and assist doctors, nurses, and others in the hospital to operationalise mechanisms and implement techniques that can assure and improve the quality of their care and services. It is not a mechanism for interfering with the clinical work of doctors, nurses, or anyone else.

Certainly, quality management bears a cost; but administrators must weigh this cost against the cost of needless deaths, iatrogenic illness, extra days in hospital, and defending and paying malpractice claims. No administrator would deny the need for a finance or accounting department, for example, merely because there is an intrinsic cost. Moreover, the cost of establishing a department of quality management is not as great as might seem at first glance. Rather it can be seen as a rationalisation and better use of staff, most of whom will already be employed in the hospital.

In many hospitals such staff as quality assurance 'co-ordinators', medical record personnel, infection control nurses, occupational health and safety officers, and staff involved in the hospital's preparation for accreditation exist already. Bringing them together under the umbrella of a quality management department adds a cohesion and co-ordination to their activities that is frequently absent now. Being part of the establishment of the quality management department, under the quality manager's competent professional leadership, would help to improve their productivity and to focus their effort on the principal goal of improving patient care.

The functional relationship between the quality management committee and the quality management department is often a cause of confusion. Figure E-7 below sets out the functional interrelationships between the quality management committee and the quality management department.

E25.03 | *The quality management department facilitates and supports quality management*

The quality manager, who heads the quality management department, is responsible for implementing the hospital's quality management policy and program. As depicted in Figure E-8 on page lxxviii, the department's responsibilities include:

- Planning: producing plans to implement the board's policy—both a five to ten year strategic plan and an annual implementation plan.
- Supporting: staffing the quality management committee and supporting the quality management program.
- Implementing: maintaining the structures and operating the systems necessary to conduct and/or support conduct of quality management activities, for example credentialling, risk management, quality assessment, and improving care processes and hence the quality of care.
- Informing: operating clinical information systems and keeping medical records.
- Controlling the program: matching plans against progress.
- Managing quality management: evaluating the benefits of solved quality problems against the cost of solving them.
- Monitoring progress: reporting to the quality management committee, hospital manager and board of directors in relation to all aspects of the program.

Key functions of the quality management department include:

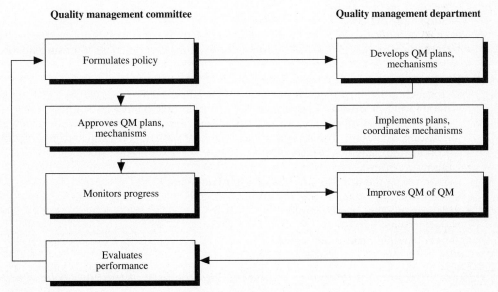

Figure E-7 *Functional relationships between quality management committee and quality management department*

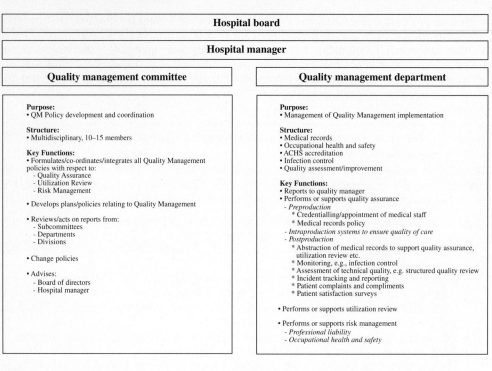

Figure E-8 *Comparison of role and functions of quality management committee and quality management department*

- Preproduction quality control, for example:
  —ACHS accreditation;
  —credentialling/appointment of medical staff;
  —medical records policy;
  —admission policies;
  —practice policies.
- Intraproduction quality control—production systems and practices to ensure quality of care.
- Postproduction quality control, for example:
  —abstracting medical records to support QA, UR, etc.;
  —monitoring process and outcomes, for example nosocomial infections;
  —assessing technical quality, for example by means of structured quality review;
  —tracking, analysing, and reporting incidents and patient complaints/compliments;
  —conducting patient satisfaction surveys.
- Utilisation review:
  —monitoring the appropriateness of use of services;
  —measuring the cost of care.
- Risk management, for example:
  —professional liability;
  —occupational health and safety.

E25.04 | *The greatest barrier to improving quality: lack of trained professionals*

No quality management program can succeed in the absence of a quality manager who has the knowledge and experience necessary to guide its implementation. In most states of Australia, over the past five years or so the number of quality assurance 'co-ordinators' has increased markedly. However, many of these professionals lack either the motivation, the knowledge or the management skills—or sometimes all three—to enable them to run an effective program. The present dilemma for Australian hospitals is that very few health professionals exist with adequate education, knowledge and management skills to adequately match this role.

Perhaps one of the greatest barriers to improving the quality of care in Australia at the present time is the lack of an adequately trained pool of quality managers. The course in quality management that La Trobe University in Victoria established in 1993 through its Lincoln School of Health Systems Sciences is a welcome beginning and should be replicated around Australia. However, for some time to come hospitals themselves will need to make arrangements to identify and train appropriate professionals for this new role.

E25.05 | *The quality manager must be a highly trained professional*

Hospitals need a quality manager whose job is to implement the hospital's quality management policy and to direct its quality management department. The quality manager should be second only to the hospital manager. He or she must:
- be a health professional who has a deep understanding of hospitals;
- have a sound knowledge of quality management and quality assurance theory, technology and application;
- know how to manage;
- report directly to the hospital manager like any senior manager, and unlike most quality assurance (QA) 'co-ordinators', even if a nurse, must not be part of the nursing establishment reporting to the director of nursing.

Up to the present, the majority of QA co-ordinators in Australia have been nurses. Indeed, nurses perceived the need for quality management before most other health professionals. Many nurses possess all the qualifications and other criteria to fulfil the role of quality manager. However, hospitals have often selected QA co-ordinators on the most haphazard of criteria; consequently they often possess little or no background knowledge and certainly have a minimum of management expertise. In many hospitals QA co-ordinators are part of the nursing staff establishment rather than part of the hospital's central management team. From the medical staff's perspective, this position does not allow the nurse QA co-ordinator to institute programs that may involve major changes in clinical care.

Quality management is a central management function; the quality manager cannot be part of the nursing establishment, even when he or she is a nurse. Instituting a program of quality management needs a senior professional (who may well be a nurse) who is in a position to affect policy decisions and have some standing and authority.

E26 | Clinical information is the basis of high quality practice and of quality management

See Part II, Chapter 9 and Part III, Chapter 5 for details.

Quality management and the assessment and improvement of clinical performance (QA/QI) are primarily about statistics. Aggregating and analysing clinical data enables staff to identify and analyse patterns of care. In the absence of good clinical information systems, including a disease index and the capacity to manipulate the data into a range of reports, quality assurance and improvement is simply not possible. Good clinical information starts with the raw clinical data entered into patients' medical records. What data clinicians and others record, and how well they record such data, determines a quality management program's effectiveness. Quality relates not only to what is done and how well it is done, but also to how well it is documented. High quality care is also care that is well documented. Quality management programs must target—and they result in—improved recordkeeping, which improves care directly and makes possible further quality improvement through data analysis and use of resultant information.

The quality of medical records in many instances is simply not good enough to meet the demands of quality management. This unfortunate state of affairs exemplifies the poor quality (risk) management that exists in almost all Australian hospitals: inadequate medical records are common additive factors in instances of hospital and medical litigation. In many cases even where no negligence has occurred a hospital or doctor cannot defend a charge of negligence because supporting evidence is absent from the medical record. So important are medical records to quality management that medical records personnel should form part of the quality management department.

E27 | Methodologies must not stand in isolation but must be integrated with other elements of the quality management program

See Part II and Part IV for details.

E27.01 | Separate wheat from chaff

Pundits advocate that hospitals use this or that technique to manage or improve quality. Few of these techniques have universal application and even fewer are suitable for use in Australian hospitals presently, because of the current stage of their development or the current sophistication of Australia's hospitals. Most importantly, use of isolated techniques will likely achieve little quality improvement. Hospitals must articulate a complete quality management system, implement it through an effective quality management program, and use suitable techniques that will lead to documented quality improvement.

It was not so long ago that a genuine claim could be made that assessing quality of care simply could not be done, or was only possible by researchers. That excuse no longer exists. The technology is now available to assess and assure the quality of clinical care. This manual describes in some detail those techniques that are most appropriate for use in Australian hospitals, in their present stage of quality maturity, and that are generally not being conducted or are not understood. Other techniques, such as infection control and incident monitoring, that Australian hospitals commonly perform, attract only a passing reference. The following three techniques receive special emphasis. Their implementation would bring immediate, substantial and substantiated improvements in the quality of care if hospitals were to act upon their results:

- credentialling and formal appointment of medical staff—which are vital components of a quality management program;
- structured quality review (SQR), which involves retrospective assessment of the quality of care by examining patients' medical records to compare what was done and achieved to what should have been done and achieved;
- patient satisfaction surveys to assess the interpersonal dimension of quality.

E27.02 | Credentialling medical staff is critical for quality management

While most public hospitals in Australia have formal appointment and reappointment procedures, very few hospitals have effective credentialling procedures. Credentialling, or the delineation of clinical privileges, is the mechanism by which the board, acting through the medical staff, determines precisely what each member of the staff is permitted to do in that hospital at any one time. There is probably no more vital aspect of quality management than ensuring that doctors undertake only those activities for which their training, experience and competence has prepared them, and the hospital has adequate resources to support.

At present, most hospitals consider higher qualifications to be the only requirement indicative of competence. Moreover, once appointed to a hospital a doctor is permitted to continue to practise based on this qualification until his or her retirement, regardless of lack of efforts to keep up with advances in medicine, illness, infirmity, or differing standards of moral behaviour which is part and parcel of the human condition. It were as if the only guarantee of the quality of an automobile manufacturer's products were its engineers' qualifications on joining the company. Qualifications are important but not sufficient. Manufacturers emphasise the quality of their products, not their workers' qualifications, regardless of their products' quality. Hospitals must do the same.

The existence of an effective credentialling process is one manifestation of the hospital board's commitment to quality management, and it is also an important component of the hospital's risk management activity. To be effective, credentialling must be annual and must be specific, each doctor applying for the precise practices he or she wishes to carry out. It is the one part of a quality management program that the medical staff alone must conduct. However, if credentialling is to function smoothly, the quality management department must provide proper administrative support. The credentialling process requires hospitals to:

- constitute a credentials committee, composed of five to nine medical practitioners from the hospital's principal specialties;
- prepare carefully and observe strictly the credentials committee's terms of reference;
- prepare carefully and check rigorously the credentials committee's minutes, to avoid any chance of them being legally vulnerable;
- ensure that committee members adhere absolutely to confidentiality requirements;
- observe strictly the rules of 'natural justice';
- conduct the entire credentialling process with a proper degree of formality;
- subject all medical staff (visiting and hospital staff) to the same process;
- obtain information concerning individual doctors' performance from a number of sources including the medical staff association, the hospital manager, and the results of such quality assessment activities as structured quality review.

E27.03   *Structured quality review: an effective and efficient way to find quality of care problems*

Assessing quality is the first step toward its improvement. This seemingly obvious fact is often one that hospital staff either do not recognise or choose to ignore. Quality assurance implies a mechanism to identify quality problems and a mechanism—and the will—to fix problems and eliminate their root causes. Only when a hospital has investigated and eliminated problems' root causes, and evaluated improvement actions' effectiveness can it state that it has improved the quality of care.

The process of structured quality review (SQR) is probably the most effective method that is available presently to assess the quality of care. It is a practical, and the most potent, way to identify technical quality of care problems. Because it can be implemented easily with a minimal commitment of resources, SQR is likely to be the initial method for, and remain the mainstay of, problem identification in hospitals for some time to come. Problem identification is the first step toward problem resolution and should be seen primarily as an educational process. Since SQR is the first step towards problem resolution, hospitals must commit to changing their care processes and institutionalise mechanisms to plan and implement change before attempting structured quality review.

Structured quality review is a postproduction (retrospective) technique for assessing the quality of care, based on an examination of patients' medical records. It involves the following three steps necessary to identify, confirm and illuminate quality of care problems, and to reveal patterns of care:

- screening—use of automated outcome/process assessment screens (described in this manual) to identify cases that harbour potential quality problems and thus that require further review;
- review—use of structured medical record review, a structured process for examining medical records, to assess the quality of care (of cases failing screens) and to characterise quality problems;
- analysis—use of statistical (pattern) analysis of screening information and medical record review results to reveal patterns of care (the nature and distribution of quality problems) to illuminate their causes and to guide subsequent investigations.

Medical staff play an important part in the process of assessing quality of care. However, because of the time and skills required to support quality assessment, hospitals should rely on automation or support staff to do as much as possible, thus preserving doctors' time for what only doctors can do. The quality management department is responsible for managing the structured quality review process, including:

- selecting or assisting clinical departments in their selection of cases to review;
- tracking review cases;
- ensuring reviews are conducted in a timely fashion;
- assuring the quality of reviews; and
- processing review results.

Decisions need to be taken on which medical records to review and which medical staff are to review them. Setting up the review process is likely to require expert assistance and training medical staff in the review process.

Structured quality review should result in:

- a judgment about the appropriateness (acceptability) of care that encompasses all aspects (by all providers) of clinical care (including support services) and its documentation;
- a list of process problems, deviations from practice policies or criteria (standards), that if resolved would improve the quality of care, and who is responsible for them, for example individual doctor, nursing service, pharmacy or the system of care;
- a list of maloutcomes with a judgment as to whether or not each more likely than not resulted from malprocess (for subsequent analysis) and their putative antecedent malprocesses;
- statistical analyses of patterns of care (processes and outcomes) found in these case-by-case reviews, to examine the distribution of problems and to identify the nature and magnitude of improvement opportunities.

E27.04 | Interpersonal aspects of quality are important

Properly conducted patient satisfaction surveys represent an important instrument for assessing quality of care. They assess principally the interpersonal aspects of quality, but may also shed light on such other aspects as the effects on patients of changing service arrangements. Conducting patient satisfaction surveys requires a good deal more than asking a convenient handful of patients a few off-the-cuff questions relating to the quality of hospital food. Such surveys are intended to collect systematically patients' opinions about the quality of care they received. In particular, clinical care should be a prime target of such a survey.

Conducting patient satisfaction surveys requires a structured approach to sampling and questionnaire design and administration if their results are to be credible. Hospitals should appoint a subcommittee of the quality management committee to act as a survey users group. Its functions include: setting priorities among questions; reviewing and approving protocols (including samples, questionnaires and data analysis plans); and assisting in the evaluation of survey results and their implications for changing care processes. Once again, it is essential to have mechanisms in place to assure that any changes demonstrated as necessary by the survey actually take place.

E28   Utilisation review: the greater the demands on resources, the more efficiently they must be used

See Part II, Chapter 6 for details.

As the twin spotlights of efficiency and economic reality focus on hospitals, their use of resources becomes increasingly important. Given the increasingly fierce competition for resources in today's hospitals, their unnecessary or inappropriate use for one patient means less resources for others whose need may be more genuine. The appropriateness of admissions, the length of hospital stays, and the justification for such things as investigations, treatments, and the use of drugs are some components of utilisation review. In practice, hospitals can best subsume most utilisation review activities within the processes of quality assessment and improvement.

E29   Risk management: minimising financial loss benefits everyone

See Part V for details.

E29.01 | *Hospitals must evaluate and reduce risks*

Risk management as a distinct activity is almost unknown in Australian hospitals. Any hospital faces many risks of financial loss. Such risks can be arranged in four categories: professional liability, occupational health and safety, environmental hazards, and commercial risks (the latter two being beyond this manual's scope).

Every hospital should periodically evaluate the risks it faces and plan accordingly. This plan must include, for all types of relevant risks: prevention (avoiding risks or controlling hazards); damage control (minimising damage when a hazard has not been avoided); and risk transfer (getting someone else to pay for any damage that occurs in exchange for a fixed insurance payment). Such a plan must include common risks and the very infrequent risks that, if they were to occur, would be disastrous or materially affect operations. Prudent risk management requires assessment of risks that cannot be prevented entirely, and the purchase of appropriate insurance. Some risks are not insurable, emphasising the need for preventive risk management. An effective quality management program can minimise risks; one by-product of improved quality is effective risk management.

E29.02 | *Ultimately, quality management can reduce malpractice litigation and financial loss*

Risk of professional liability, where hospital and doctor are so frequently involved in joint legal action, is of greatest interest to medical staff. An effective quality management program results in a diminished level of malpractice litigation or in the total amount of awards, and is a potent element in risk management. Surprisingly, this link between professional liability and quality management does not seem to have been adequately made in Australia. Credentialling is a very important aspect of risk management, as is incident reporting and the handling of patient complaints. Patient satisfaction surveys may also minimise risk, as well as improve quality. A satisfied patient rarely becomes a litigant.

Eliminating malpractice may reduce but not eliminate malpractice suits. Not all bad outcomes result from malpractice. Medical care involves risks that cannot always be prevented. However, bad outcomes which were once seen as acts of God increasingly are seen as evidence that something went wrong and someone was at fault. Nevertheless, an effective quality management program can reduce the risk of a suit and improve the chances for defending oneself against allegations of malpractice if one is brought. Inevitably, a few patients will suffer serious adverse outcomes, and some may have involved malpractice. The hospital can control the losses resulting from such outcomes by having a well-formulated management strategy, prepared well in advance, for handling such incidents when they occur.

E29.03 | Hospitals are potentially dangerous worksites: occupational health and safety is an important part of quality management

Hospitals are potentially dangerous places in which to work and staff must be constantly alert to these dangers. The range of hazards encountered in hospitals is greater than that of almost any other type of workplace. Incidence rates for compensatable injury and illness are about double the average rates of all combined service industries and equal to those of manufacturing industry. Despite high incidence rates of work-related disease and injury, most hospital workers are poorly served by health and safety programs. It is an ironic paradox that hospitals bristling with health professionals whose whole ethic is caring for patients on many occasions give the appearance of either failing to recognise worker health and safety as deserving attention, or, at least, giving it low priority.

Hospitals should strive to prevent occupational injuries and diseases if at all possible, since in many cases there are no satisfactory treatments for, by way of example, degenerative back disease (from inadvisable patient lifting), AIDS (from needle sticks), or mesothelioma (from exposure to asbestos). Hazard control results in risk reduction. Management, through the hospital's quality management program, has an obligation to minimise occupational health and safety hazards, and to diminish the risks that employees face. It may need to correct the traditional attitudes that occupational health and safety is a benefit bestowed by an industrial award and is therefore separate from hospitals' health culture.

An effective occupational health and safety program should be an integral part of the hospital's quality management program. In the broadest sense, it encompasses such functions as hazard control (its core business), health promotion, stress management, employee health services and employee management. It can contribute to product (health care) quality in the following ways: prevent injury to patients; prevent direct injury to staff; and improve the work environment and worker morale, thereby contributing to improvements in both health care quality and productivity.

The hospital's occupational health and safety (OH&S) committee should be a subcommittee of the hospital's quality management committee. It carries out the QMC's responsibilities pertaining to OH&S. Principally, it recommends policy to the quality management committee, develops the program, and evaluates efforts to improve occupational health and safety and the OH&S program. The OH&S director should chair the hospital's OH&S committee, and be a member of its quality management committee. The quality management department should generally be responsible for all OH&S activity, and the OH&S director should report to the quality manager. In large referral (especially teaching) hospitals, there may be a separate OH&S department. Its director would report to the hospital manager (as would the quality manager). Such an OH&S department may engage in consulting, teaching and research.

E30 Getting started is the greatest hurdle

See Part III, Chapter 6 for details.

E30.01 *Commitment is the key to success*

One of the greatest hurdles hospitals face in establishing an effective quality management program is how to get started. No three words sum up the requirement better than: commitment, commitment, commitment. The commitment must exist with the directors, the management, and medical, nursing and other staffs. (See Table E-1 below.)

Table E-1 *Getting started*

The time frame for completion of these activities will vary greatly from hospital to hospital depending on individual circumstances. The three-year implementation suggested here may be reasonable for some hospitals and overly optimistic for others. Achieving quality maturity may take 10–12 years.

When	What	Who
To start	obtain board commitment	hospital manager
after commitment	establish QM planning group	medical nursing staff/hospital manager, outside consultant
next	appoint quality manager	hospital manager, outside consultant
next, or at same time	assessment of QM activities with report	outside consultant
next	develop QM policy, QM plan	quality manager, planning group
next, or at same time	begin hospital-wide education for QM	quality manager, planning group
next	form QMC from planning group; terms of reference	quality manager, chair planning group
next	commence committee restructuring; agenda, minutes, chairmanship	quality manager, consultant
at end of 1st year	review progress and revise plans	QMC, quality manager
next	consolidate 'QA' activities, functions in separate QMD	quality manager, MRA, OH&S officer etc.
with committee restructuring completed	establish mechanisms to effect changes identified by assessment, monitoring activities	QMC, QMD
next	begin to implement QM plan	QMC, quality manager
at same time	plan and initiate patient satisfaction survey	quality manager, outside experts
at same time	review and co-ordinate system for recording & tracking incidents, complaints, compliments	quality manager, DON, OH&S officer
at same time	reinforce education, communication program to hospital staff	quality manager
next	review needs to focus attitudinal, behavioural change program	QMC, quality manager
next	commence upgrade of medical record dept. if necessary	quality manager, MRA

continues

Table E-1 *continued*

When	What	Who
next	initiate simple projects e.g. study blood products' usage	relevant clinical, support depts., quality manager, QMC
at same time	review and upgrade infection control	quality manager, infection control sister, clinical & support depts.
at end of 2nd year	review progress and revise plans	quality manager
QMC, QMD functioning well	formalise risk management, including OH&S, programs	quality manager, OH&S officer, chair QMC, HM
12 months before reappointment triennium	commence discussions with medical staff about credentialling	quality manager, HM, medical staff, consultant
next	review need for additional QM staff	quality manager
next	form additional committees if necessary	quality manager
QM program established and a core of supportive medical staff	commence quality assessment using SQR	quality manager, medical staff, MRA, consultant
next	review needs to focus contents of education program	quality manager, QMC
next	begin process of charting progress in improving care	QMD
at same time	expand studies, extend quality assessment, extend monitoring	QMC, quality manager, clinical, other staff
at end of 3rd year	review progress and revise plans	quality manager
at end of 5th, 10th, 15th years	evaluate QM program, revise policies, structures, activities etc.	quality manager, QMC, HM, board, medical and other staffs
on continuing basis	assess, improve, and continue hospital-wide education program	quality manager, QMC
on continuing basis	manage QM implementation	quality manager
on continuing basis	monitor QM program's cost-effectiveness	quality manager, HM, board

List of abbreviations:

DON	director of nursing	QM	quality management
HM	hospital manager	QMC	quality management committee
MRA	medical records administrator	QMD	quality management department
OH&S	occupational health and safety	SQR	structured quality review
QA	quality assurance		

E30.02 | *Align attitudes to commit to quality*

Commitment and a mind-set which sees quality of care and services as the hospital's prime purpose, are both the most important and, at the same time, the most difficult aspects of a quality management program to achieve. Commitment is essential for action. Attitudes, which are inherent and which act as barriers to effective implementation, also inhibit commitment if people believe that one cannot change them. Attitudinal barriers include the following:

- Quality of care is something only for health professionals.
- Doctors are responsible for quality.
- Quality can be assured through training and qualifications.

- If a problem occurs, the doctor's qualifications or his or her education are at fault.

This set of assumptions and attitudes is an unfortunate misrepresentation of the problem and leads to the concept of 'weeding out bad apples' or to seeking solutions for unacceptable care in the continuing education of doctors. Correct attitudes and a useful formulation of the problem include the following:

- Quality is a subset of management.
- The hospital produces quality.
- Quality can only be assured through appropriate processes implemented properly.
- If problems occur (maloutcomes attributable to malprocess), they can only be corrected by improving the system of care or care processes.

This formulation of the problem obviously predicates a very different solution, which this manual describes. Quality-focused organisations emphasise education to rectify attitudes, ensure a productive, quality-producing climate and facilitate learning. Employee education is an important aspect of introducing a quality management program into any hospital. Obviously, where appropriate hospitals shoudl also focus education efforts and training to rectify any performance deficiencies and to improve doctors', nurses' and others' skills. An effective quality management program permits such focused education and training.

E30.03 | Communication, education must begin early, continue indefinitely

A hospital cannot expect to impose a quality management program on hospital professionals who have no real understanding about its aims and objectives and who are told little if anything about the ways and means. Communication and education must commence on day one and must continue indefinitely. Hospitals must employ all appropriate methods of communication for different staff members, including, for example, meetings, seminars, workshops, videos, audio-tapes, newsletters and articles.

E30.04 | Achieving quality maturity requires a long-term commitment

The time frame for implementing an effective quality management program will obviously vary from hospital to hospital. However, as a guide, we suggest:

- Board education, establishing the quality management committee and the quality management department could take one to two years.
- Getting activities underway to produce meaningful results could take two to five years.
- Refinements to the program could take an additional two to five years.
- Achieving quality maturity will take five to twelve years.

While every hospital will have differing needs and will probably be at different stages of commitment, knowledge and implementation of the various aspects of quality management, the following activities require attention.

E30.05 | First establish a quality management planning group

The biggest problem most hospitals and hospital staff face is where to start and what to do. Every hospital must have the resources to provide the structures and processes necessary to conduct meaningful quality management and to assist and support its individual departments, divisions and professional groups to plan projects, explain the correct methodologies, assist with decisions about priorities and generally guide them through what initially will be strange territory.

For the hospital that is starting from scratch, the first step is to establish a quality management planning group. This group will eventually become the nucleus of the quality management committee and hence its membership should go some way toward reflecting this fact. Everyone involved in starting quality management, including board directors and managers, should read this manual, in whole or in part. For the quality manager, reading the manual from cover to cover is essential. The hospital manager, heads or directors of divisions and others should read the front matter and such other parts of the manual as either interest them or affect their work. For a hospital board member, such detailed reading is probably not necessary; reading the Preface, the Eighteen Cs of quality management, and this Executive summary will suffice. The hospital manager's task is to gain an understanding of what quality means, and what questions he or she needs to ask to ensure that it is being achieved in his or her hospital, and how to evaluate answers. The quality manager must be capable of instituting and running a program that results in documented improvement in the quality of care.

E30.06 | *Appoint the quality manager early: select the right person*

The appointment of a quality manager is the next step. A hospital should take it early so that it can involve the quality manager in the program's development. Most hospitals would be well advised to seek outside consultant advice to delineate the quality manager's role, develop a proper job description and assist with personnel selection. The right appointment to this position is crucial to ultimate success. The identification of suitably qualified quality managers is not an easy task at this time. The appointee needs management skills, technical knowledge, and, ideally, should understand and have experienced hospital culture.

The newly-appointed quality manager should develop a quality management implementation strategy. It consists of an initial assessment, a resultant plan, and such decisions as those regarding the appropriate form of and timing for the establishment of an organisational structure, education and communication, and specific quality management activities.

E30.07 | *The quality management plan must be flexible and dynamic*

A hospital must:

- decide where it is going and where it wants to be;
- assess where it is in relation to where it wants to go;
- develop a strategic plan to close any gap;
- develop a year-by-year implementation plan to implement the strategy;
- annually review progress against the plan and determine why it has been better or worse than expected, and plan the following year accordingly. At the same time, the strategy should be reviewed for appropriateness and, if necessary, so should quality management objectives and policies.

Hospitals must first—or preferably retain a consultant to—assess whatever quality management activities are under way. The quality management plan is the blueprint for action and its contents will vary according to the results of each hospital's assessment.

E30.08 | *Claims about existing quality management activities often do not match reality*

The current understanding of quality management in Australia, and the focus to date in hospitals on isolated quality assurance projects, means that most hospitals will have little conceptual understanding about where they are, let alone where they should be going. Further, most hospital managers when asked about quality assurance respond in a manner which completely belies the reality of the situation when assessed by an independent observer. The assessment should include the organisational structure for quality management, including committees and their effectiveness; the attitudes of directors, manager and staff; clinical information systems; and factual evidence of what existing quality management efforts have achieved. This assessment's timing will vary from hospital to hospital. For some, it will trigger the hospital's journey toward quality maturity. For others, it will occur after the quality manager's appointment.

E30.09 | Change requires planning and implementation mechanisms

Effective change requires planning and appropriate implementation mechanisms. Existing organisational units and mechanisms should be able to resolve most quality problems. The quality management department is responsible for co-ordinating changes that cross organisational lines and, when necessary, establishing task forces to investigate, plan and co-ordinate implementation of planned changes. Implementation plans should describe what is to be done, how it is to be done, who is responsible for doing it according to what timetable, with what resources etc., and must specify expected results, expected implementation and operational costs (or savings), and the means to measure results and costs (or savings) and to attribute them to the chosen strategy (or other factors).

E30.10 | Directors must persist, managers must insist on a proper quality management structure

Establishing the quality management program's organisational structure must be one of a hospital's earliest initiatives and, after gaining commitment, is perhaps the most difficult step of all. Medical staff are likely to resist creation of the quality management department on the grounds that it is merely another management instrument to 'control' them. Most hospitals will need to restructure and revise their committee system. Modifying or revamping committees is also likely to provoke further resistance, as entrenched members attempt to preserve what they see as their rightful prerogatives. Hospitals must approach this aspect of getting started with patience, and good communication and negotiation skills. Above all, the board must persist and the manager must insist that a proper quality management organisational structure exist.

E30.11 | Integrate committee functions

The review of existing committees' functions should now occur. Pay attention to terms of reference, interrelationships, lines of reporting of the entire committee system, and the means to service and support the committee system. Where appropriate, disband or merge unneeded committees and add vitally-needed committees—such as quality management committees—in individual departments.

E30.12 | Improve clinical information systems to improve care

Quality management depends on good clinical data and the capacity to aggregate and analyse that data. Hospitals should give the quality manager responsibility for medical records and clinical information systems. The hospital manager should transfer existing staff who carry out these activities to the quality management department at the earliest possible opportunity. One of the quality manager's first tasks (after establishing the QMC and the QMD) is to ensure that medical records (which contain vital raw data) are of an acceptable standard, and that the department has the resources and the appropriate technology to use these data effectively.

E30.13 | Quality management must include occupational health and safety

Occupational health and safety is an important aspect of risk management and the hospital should integrate such activities into its quality management program. Transferring responsibility for occupational health and safety (OH&S) to the quality management department is an important step toward this integration. At an appropriate stage, most likely within the first twelve to eighteen months, the hospital should pay attention to its OH&S program. Appropriate actions will flow from an initial assessment of OH&S activities.

E30.14 | *Credentialling medical staff requires long lead times*

The credentialling of medical staff cannot be implemented overnight. A long lead time of discussions with and explanations for the medical staff will be essential. In this area, in particular, most hospitals will require outside assistance. A hospital should have an effective credentialling program in place within the first two years.

E30.15 | *Early on, be content with modest achievements*

Once the quality management committee and the quality management department headed by the quality manager are in place—and not before—is the appropriate time to commence some specific quality management activity. The usual tendency is to try to do too much initially. Most medical staff, in their initial enthusiasm, will claim to be able to undertake quality management without the need for a quality management department. We cannot overemphasise that they cannot, because they do not know what they do not know. In the absence of the quality management committee, quality management department and quality manager, medical or nursing staff's initial enthusiasm will only end in failure and frustration.

The quality manager's expertise and guidance, the QMD's support, the QMC's active participation, and the hospital board's commitment and authority, are all necessary to contemplate and complete the long and complicated journey toward quality maturity. Once they are in place, the hospital and/or its individual departments can begin to undertake productive projects that fit into its overall quality management plan. The hospital should attempt only one or two projects in the first instance. One example might be a patient satisfaction survey. Activities should emphasise end results. If we do so-and-so, what can we improve subsequently? Are we committed to make such improvements, if results warrant? Unless the answer to this latter question is a resounding 'yes', the hospital is only wasting the time and effort it is about to put into quality management activities. Simultaneously, the quality management department should assess what resources are available to conduct these activities, determine what additional staff and consultant resources may be required, and plan to obtain them.

E30.16 | *Progress toward quality maturity requires evaluation of progress*

Periodic evaluation is the only effective method of ensuring that quality management activity is achieving its intended goal and is really worthwhile, and that the hospital is productively using its quality management resources. It is very easy to create the impression of extensive quality management activity without in fact achieving very much. It is therefore essential, particularly in this day and age of fiscal responsibility in hospitals, to ensure that a great deal of time and money is not being wasted on projects that do not achieve their stated aims.

The hospital must assess and evaluate its quality management activity on an ongoing basis. It must subject it to the same degree of scrutiny to which quality management subjects clinical care to improve processes and outcomes. Evaluation is necessary to find the most cost-effective way to conduct quality management. Monitoring the extent to which problems are resolved, determining the extent to which observed changes are attributable to chosen improvement actions, and evaluating their cost-effectiveness provides vital information for improving future quality improvement efforts. The quality management department should systematically record this information, for example in a project completion report, and store it in a computerised database for subsequent analysis.

Presently, such quality management activity that does exist is largely unevaluated, precluding efforts to improve its cost-effectiveness. These issues highlight the need for effective information systems in hospitals that can track quality management activity's costs and benefits.

Each year the hospital's quality manager should compare what the quality management program achieved and spent with what it planned to achieve and spend. This evaluation focuses on the program's ability to identify and resolve quality of care problems.

E31 | Quality management and the law: much of the apprehension is unwarranted

See Part VI for details.

There is a widespread concern among medical staff about their legal exposure if and when they engage in quality management activities. This concern, while genuine, is largely unwarranted and doctors' fears are exaggerated. The legal risks incurred in quality management programs, particularly by doctors, are risks of legal liability for negligence, defamation and denial of natural justice. By structuring quality management programs with a proper degree of formality, as described in this manual, hospitals and doctors can certainly minimise any risks that might exist, particularly with respect to activities such as the credentialling of medical staff. Further, an effective quality management program is the best way of minimising the risk of malpractice litigation, and the mechanisms described in the manual are the answer to doctors' concerns relating to defamation.

E32 | Quality maturity demands patience and persistence; there are no quick fixes

See Part II, Chapter 9 and Part III for details; Part VII for printed resources to help keep current.

E32.01 | *Quality management must include—and focus on—all clinical activities*

Quality improvement depends on describing through data, understanding through analysis and improving through action. Quality management is useful for improving the quality of hospitals' care. It must include all of the hospital's activities, especially clinical care, the core of its production function. Improving catering or the laundry, while useful, will make very little difference if the quality of clinical care remains unaltered.

Health care system policy decision makers and hospital managers must provide the will, the means, and the incentives to measure care processes and outcomes, and to use the resultant information to improve quality. There are no quick fix solutions. Managers must stay the course and avoid sounding the retreat at the first sign of resistance. Managers must also back demands with deeds. They must recognise excellence and reward success. Managers' failure to change can doom quality management efforts every bit as much as their lack of commitment to the structures and processes necessary to implement quality management.

Managing quality costs money. But the lack of quality (quality-cost) can be, and almost invariably is, even more costly. Initially, quality management may increase costs because the hospital must pay for the quality management program and, in some cases, doctors may be undertreating patients now (in comparison to best practices). But in principle a quality-mature hospital can expect lower costs from:

- reduced liability insurance premiums, malpractice claims and monetary damages;
- reduced iatrogenesis, specifically preventable errors and clinical complications;
- reduced unnecessary tests and treatments;

- improved clinical efficiency resulting from quicker diagnosis, better treatment selection etc.;
- improved operational efficiency, with resultant better use of resources;
- improved productivity through enhanced employee protection, job satisfaction and morale.

Quality management's main benefit is improving the quality of care and reducing variability, giving patients more health status improvement with greater certainty. If quality-focused care costs less than present care, that is an added benefit. Certainly it provides better value for money.

E32.02 | *Toward quality maturity: the longest journey starts with the first step*

For many years, manufacturers have recognised quality as the key to success and sustained commercial profitability. Because hospitals' success has never been—but should be—measured in terms of successful outcomes of care, cost-effectiveness in care processes, and patient satisfaction, very little if anything has ever been done to manage quality. In health care, the intention to do good (improving patients' health status), manifest in the processes of health care services, has been confused with doing good (measured improvement). The hesitancy to recognise the link between the level of litigation—which is too high—with this failure to introduce effective quality management programs is surprising, to say the least. Perhaps it has all been too hard. Attitudes in any professional group are difficult to change—and the hospital and medical professions are no exception. In Australia, governments, hospitals and the health professions must recognise the importance of health care quality management, and the considerable shift in intellectual paradigms and individual attitudes and behaviour that must take place to implement it. The establishment of model pilot programs in each of the Australian states would be a useful first step. These pilots will demonstrate that once a program has commenced it must be continued indefinitely with the objectives of improving quality and reducing costs. It will not be easy—but the time to start is now.

E32.03 | *This manual offers a vision of the destination—and a map*

The journey to quality maturity is long and difficult. The traveller needs a clear vision of the ultimate destination, and the will to get started and the commitment to keep going. Also essential is a map to find the way, and a preparedness to learn from the journey to correct one's course from time to time. This manual intends to create the vision, prepare readers to undertake this arduous journey toward quality maturity, and provide the necessary map.

BACKGROUND AND CONTEXT OF QUALITY MANAGEMENT IN AUSTRALIA

SUMMARY

Part I provides the context in which quality management in health care has developed in Australia and the forces that will influence its future development. With any new idea it is just as important to know where we have come from as it is to know where we are and where we are going. Part I provides an historical and contemporary context of the introduction of quality management into Australian hospitals and their associated services. It explores rising hospital and medical malpractice costs, one of the important elements driving quality management. This part also analyses the explosion of medical technology and its associated costs which have combined to change dramatically the world of the acute care hospital. Armed with such an insight, health professionals will better understand the forces driving quality management and come to accept that it will inevitably become an intrinsic part of their professional activities.

This part also defines what is meant by quality management and how it differs from what hospitals have been doing. It includes some of the key historical milestones of the development of quality management—such as hospital accreditation and the early attempts to introduce effective systems for the delineation of clinical privileges (credentialling) for hospital medical staff—and examines two critical questions: Why quality management has not yet been effectively introduced and why it should be introduced now.

Chapter 1   *Introduction to and purpose of Part I*—provides an introduction to and a context for this part.

Chapter 2   *History of quality management in Australia*—summarises the key features in the various stages of the history of quality management, including hospital accreditation, credentialling of medical staff and quality assurance. It also looks at the changing face of hospitals and the hospital and medical culture.

Chapter 3	*Hospitals—a changed and changing environment—* examines the issues relating to the technological explosion, questions of costs and appropriateness of hospital care and problems associated with medical staffing patterns.
Chapter 4	*Hospital and professional liability—*explores hospital and medical malpractice litigation and the medical defence organisations. Comparison is drawn between hospitals and other professional groups and some illustrative cases and comments are provided.
Chapter 5	*Why we need quality management—*explains why quality management is not only desirable but also essential. Definitions of quality of care and quality assurance are provided and the prevailing attitudes of doctors explored, together with issues of continuing medical education, risk management and utilisation review.

Chapter 1

INTRODUCTION TO AND PURPOSE OF PART I

---

110   Contents

The general failure to implement effective quality management programs in Australian hospitals has to be seen against the politics, financing and organisation of what are perhaps the most complex of all organisations in a modern industrialised society. This chapter provides an introduction to the manual's subject matter and describes:

- **111.** Purpose of this part
- **112.** Contents of this part
- **113.** Purpose of this chapter
- **114.** Hospitals and the health agenda
- **115.** Quality management
- **116.** Why this manual

111   Purpose of this part

This part provides readers with the historical and contextural elements essential to gaining an accurate perspective about quality management in Australia. Apart from the historical account we have identified those issues that are driving hospitals and health care generally inexorably towards quality management. At the same time, because health professionals tend to believe that they are unique, we have drawn attention to the situation of a number of different professional groups to compare the circumstances. In discussing malpractice litigation, we have been at pains to present valid data. As others have found, obtaining such data in Australia is extremely difficult. While the data presented is far from adequate, unfortunately, it was the best available to us.

112   Contents of this part

This part presents developments in a manner designed to provide readers with sufficient material to gain perspective of a range of events that span over thirty years. In the interest of readability, it describes briefly only the most important historical events. Author Lionel

Wilson participated in most, if not all, of them, permitting him to add the insight of his personal experience. Readers of this part will obtain a greater perspective and a deeper understanding of the remainder of the material in the manual through the following five chapters in this part:

- Introduction to and purpose of Part I
- History of quality management in Australia
- Hospitals—a changed and changing environment
- Hospital and professional liability
- Why we need quality management

113 Purpose of this chapter

This chapter is an introduction to Part I and intends to describe the context of past and present efforts to introduce quality management into Australian hospitals. The chapter provides a brief background about hospitals and the health agenda and changed community perceptions which are influencing them and the health professionals who work in them. It also explores briefly the efforts to implement quality management to date and some of the inherent difficulties to be faced in such a task. Finally, there is an answer to the reader's question 'Why this manual?'

114 Hospitals and the health agenda

114.1 Rising costs and the drive for quality management

The problems of hospitals dominated the health agenda in Australia in the 1980s and all evidence suggests that the 1990s will be no different. In this regard, Australia does not differ substantially from most other industrialised societies, with the exception, perhaps, that in Australia the various vested interest groups in the health industry tend to be more vigorous and vocal. Hospitals—how they are managed, how they are funded, who gains admission to them and above all what services are conducted in them—will continue to be on the national health agenda well into the future.

Budgetary pressures and the ever-increasing force of malpractice litigation will demand programs and technologies which will enable us to answer questions such as:

- Can we quantify the clinical activities in our hospitals?
- How well are we conducting those clinical activities?
- How appropriate are they?
- How does one hospital compare with another in these matters?
- How do medical providers match up to professional standards?
- How does one provider compare with his or her colleagues?

To a large extent the medical and hospital malpractice experience in the 1980s, which has carried through into the 1990s, is a manifestation of the hospital industry's inability to cope satisfactorily with the widening complexity and expanding technology of hospital care, and the increasing tendency of the community to resort to legal solutions for dissatisfaction with medical and hospital services.

114.2 Changed community perceptions

The community's perceptions, attitudes and expectations about health services have had a considerable impact on the level of hospital and medical malpractice litigation. The idea that sick people and, in particular, small premature babies actually die is no longer accepted as inevitable. The community expects that all babies born will not only survive but will be perfect in all respects, and if a baby is born with a mental deficit, for example, it must be the result of someone's error or fault. Increasingly that someone is seen as the doctor or the health care system. Moreover, people see the proper avenue for retribution to be the legal system.

115 | Quality management

115.1 | *The implementation failure*

Quality management programs are about continuously improving patient care and, most importantly, patient outcomes, on a hospital-wide basis. Occupational health and safety (OH&S) of employees is also an integral part of quality management because attention to OH&S improves the quality of patient care and the work environment. Quality assurance is about product quality and hospitals' product is patients' health status improvement. Quality of care is principally the degree to which the hospital's services improve patients' health status consistent with their values.

As Joyce Craddock points out: 'It is one thing to be interested in quality of patient care, as all health professionals are, and another to introduce programs which will ensure quality.[1]

Throughout the hospital industry, both in the private and public sectors, health professionals generally acknowledge the desirability of improving patient care and understand the need for better occupational health and safety programs. However, in spite of the increasing risks—legal and otherwise—in the hospital environment, there has been a universal failure to implement programs which would be effective in achieving those goals. The number of malpractice claims and the rising awards, together with the continuance of preventable incidents, are surely manifestations of the inadequacies of current quality management approaches and illustrate the room for improvement.

There are a number of factors which can be adduced to explain this implementation failure, namely:

- lack of adequate understanding about quality management;
- a general failure to provide specific budget allocations to this area of hospital activity;
- inadequate organisational frameworks essential for quality management activity in most hospitals;
- poor clinical information systems;
- a general shortage of health professionals with the necessary skills and training required to administer quality management programs;
- a widespread disbelief that quality of care needs improvement, or can be improved within existing technological and sociopolitical constraints.

There is continuing confusion in the minds of medical staff and hospital management alike, concerning the nature of quality management. Its subset—quality assurance—is still widely seen erroneously as inherently an inspectorial exercise with punitive overtones, essentially for the purpose of 'weeding out the bad apples'. While hospitals do have a responsibility to limit the activity of that small percentage of unsafe doctors, far greater improvement can be realised by assisting every doctor improve his or her care and generating the information and knowledge that make such improvement possible.

Improving quality of care and preventing maloccurrences demands sound information. At the present time we have no measures of the number of patients misdiagnosed, treated inadequately or improperly managed. In short, we have no measures of the health status improvement which is possible now but not being realised. We have no measure of the number of unnecessary tests or treatments, or those performed inaccurately or improperly. This lack of information about what is being achieved and what present achievements cost is the central problem that a quality management program is designed to solve.

Perhaps the greatest barrier to effective quality management implementation in Australia is the shortage of skilled manpower to assist, manage and implement such programs. Another reason for the poor implementation of quality management programs is the belief that measuring the quality of care (required to know if one is improving it) is impossible or, if possible, difficult and expensive. In other words measurement, and hence improvement, is either impossible or impractical. While this may have been the case, it is no longer so. In addition, there has been a worldview that the introduction of new, more advanced technology has improved the quality of care and hence removed the need to measure it. The fear of finding inadequacies or less than expected gains may have retarded quality assurance efforts even further, whereas in reality more, and more perfect technology, demands greater attention to quality management. The invisible nature of poor quality care (because quality is not yet measured routinely) is one reason for the difficulty in persuading professionals and, for that matter, the larger community of the importance of effective quality management.

For the most part, reference to quality management in Australia has largely been focused on individual studies and projects both of a clinical and operational nature. While individual studies are important, even more important, as this manual emphasises throughout, are those organisational and structural features without which a quality management program (and individual projects) cannot hope to succeed. At the present time, deficiencies in these areas remain among the greatest barriers to effective quality management and quality assurance activities in Australia.

115.2 The quality management jigsaw

Quality management's jigsaw puzzle nature is another barrier to effective implementation in Australia. While many of the pieces of the jigsaw are familiar to hospital professionals, most are not. In addition, unlike any ordinary jigsaw, this one has no picture on the front of the box to tell us what it is all supposed to look like when it is completed. Unfortunately, at the present time there are few, if any, hospitals in Australia where it is possible to picture the successful implementation of an integrated hospital-wide program in a complete form. The failure to implement effective quality management programs is at least partly due to this inability to conceptualise the totality of such a program and to know what steps to take to ensure its successful introduction.

This manual describes the essential elements of the quality management jigsaw, supplies the reader with the all-important picture of how the pieces fit together to form the essential structure of an effective quality management program, describes the organisational framework which is essential if an integrated quality management program is to become a coherent entity, and provides a guide to achieving that end.

115.3 Inadequate academic interest

While quality assurance has been much talked about in Australian hospitals since 1977, there has been little awareness of the body of theory or discussion of quality assurance concepts which have developed over the past twenty-five years in the United States of America. To date in Australia, with few exceptions, there has been little academic focus of interest in quality management, and scientific medical publications have in general paid scant attention to the topic. Accordingly, while this publication has a practical direction, Part II explores quality management's theoretical underpinnings, a subject that is receiving increasing attention worldwide.

| 115.4 | *The plus and minus of quality management* |

No pretence is made that the actions suggested throughout this book are easy to implement or that they represent a panacea for all the problems of hospital care. Nevertheless, the approach to quality management that this manual advocates will lead to:

- better patient care;
- more effective use of resources;
- greater professional satisfaction and improved morale;
- diminished patient complaints;
- diminished malpractice;
- the means by which hospitals, boards and management can best meet the demands of community accountability.

However, implementing a quality management program will:

- not eliminate malpractice litigation, although it will likely diminish it and provide better defence against such actions;
- not solve all of the hospital's problems, because as medical care improves expectations also rise;
- not meet community's and funders' perceptions of how health resources should be allocated.

116 Why this manual

In spite of nearly twenty years of effort in Australia to introduce effective quality management programs, there is still widespread confusion about goals and objectives. This confusion abounds throughout all sections of the health industry from politicians to professionals at the workface. Quality assurance is still widely seen as some part-time activity of doctors and nurses and, to date, directors on hospital boards and hospital managers have not seen quality of care as part of their particular responsibility. There has been little discernible evidence that the hospital industry has recognised the enormous organisational change required if quality management is to be effectively implemented.

Adding to these difficulties is the absence of easy access to texts which could shed light on this subject. Indeed, we are not aware of a text anywhere that adequately describes what has to be done and how to do it. Accordingly this manual is largely about what has to be done and how to do it in an Australian context. Further, while busy hospital professionals may not be so interested in obscure theory, it is important for all to realise that a body of theory underlies the practice of quality management and that some understanding of this theory certainly assists in the difficult task of implementing a quality management program and improving the quality of patient care and related outcomes.

References

1 Comments made during the course of a lecture by Dr Joyce Craddock at Royal North Shore Hospital, Sydney 1989.

Chapter 2

THE HISTORY OF QUALITY MANAGEMENT IN AUSTRALIA

---

120 Contents

This chapter deals briefly with the history of quality management in Australia including:

- **121.** Purpose of this chapter
- **122.** Australian hospital culture
- **123.** The medical culture
- **124.** The changing environment
- **125.** Quality of care concepts
- **126.** Three strands of activity
- **127.** Doctors' characteristics

121 Purpose of this chapter

Some account of the story of the Australian development of systems aimed at improving quality of patient care in hospitals is helpful in achieving a perspective about its progress and will serve to highlight both implementation successes and failures. This chapter intends to orient readers to the Australian situation.

The development of quality management is an interesting and evolving story that is far from complete. It reflects a maturing process on the part of the Australian hospital industry as it moves away from traditional cultural links and attempts to find more appropriate solutions to challenging contemporary problems. This story also reveals the inevitable evolution of Australia's health care system.

122 Australian hospital culture

Many of the difficulties to which this manual alludes have their basic roots in the health and hospital culture which Australia, starting as a British colony a little over 200 years ago, inherited from the United Kingdom. Many of the anomalies in the Australian health care system in general are due to the adoption or adaptation of systems which may have worked well enough in the United Kingdom, but which we have found and continue to find to an increasing degree are inappropriate to Australia with its differences of geography, organisation and political structure. The United Kingdom continues to evolve along its own course while we in Australia are trying new approaches that fit with our evolving society.

The development of quality management, therefore, can also be seen as an attempt to look for more appropriate mechanisms in a changing Australian hospital and medical environment. Right from the very beginning of European settlement in Australia hospitals and doctors, like many other aspects of Australian society, were based on the English or Scottish model. Hospitals, seen essentially as charitable institutions for the indigent sick, were supported by charity or government finance. Such institutions and the doctors working in them were seen as performing 'good works', and the idea of making anyone accountable, either financially or medically, would have been seen as offensive to many public-spirited individuals and quite out of keeping with the nature of the services provided.

As Australia moved towards the end of the nineteenth century this predominantly public sector hospital industry came under the control of powerful state government hospital authorities which, understandably, saw these public hospitals as part of their fiefdom and responsibility.

While there has been some variation between the Australian states, private hospitals developed later in the scene and initially were small units of what was essentially a cottage industry. Indeed, in the state of New South Wales where the public hospital system has always predominated, it has only been within the past twenty years or so that private hospitals have begun the change from small units with individual owner–operators to larger hospitals and chains of hospitals, organised and managed with the sophistication expected in today's hospital environment.

123 The medical culture

As with hospitals, since the beginning of European settlement the Australian medical profession has been an image of its English and Scottish counterparts. The socialisation of the medical student and the fostering of what may be called the health culture both occur in university medical schools that are essentially still models of English or Scottish medical schools, with the exception of the University of Newcastle in New South Wales (founded in 1975, with first admitted students in 1978). This medical school, while retaining the English/Scottish model at the bedside, has diminished the influence of self-contained academic departments and introduces the student to clinical care in the first year (while traditional schools reserve the first year, at least, for teaching basic science subjects). Based on clinical problems, the student is then exposed to both clinical and basic science subjects in tandem.

However, while this relatively new medical school has a good deal to say about self-evaluation and self-audit, there is no area of this medical course specifically devoted to the topic of quality management and quality assurance. It is likely that other medical schools reflect this barren situation. Thus medical students, early in their careers when they are exposed to those basic principles which should be guiding them throughout their professional careers, never address the central issues of what are the outcomes (end results) of care, and how we know what they are and how to improve them. It remains to be seen if planned changes to the structure of the medical courses, due to occur in a number of medical schools before the end of this decade, will significantly address these deficiencies.

The Royal College system in the United Kingdom was initially used to obtain postgraduate qualifications. With the advent of increasing specialisation there was a perceived need to have Australian training and Australian qualifications, and counterparts of these colleges were eventually established in Australia. It is only relatively recently that the majority of specialists in Australia have ceased to obtain their postgraduate training in the United Kingdom.

The majority of doctors practising in Australia's hospitals are visiting medical staff, who have private practices as well as hospital obligations. Teaching hospitals and major metropolitan and country base hospitals employ a small number of full-time staff specialists. Historically, visiting medical staff provided their services to public (i.e. non-insured, indigent) patients in public hospitals on an honorary basis. The 'honorary system' was not only an extension of the concept of charity to the indigent sick, but was also an enormous saving to governments in providing these hospital services. In the 1960s pressure from specialist physicians (internists) and surgeons led eventually to payment for services to public patients on a part-time salaried sessional basis. In some states privately insured patients were accommodated in public hospitals and were charged on a fee-for-service basis. In the last decade of the twentieth century the extent of this saving is becoming painfully obvious as state governments struggle to find the funds for medical staff now remunerated for their services to public (now no longer necessarily indigent or non-insured) patients in these hospitals.

Since the early 1960s visiting medical staff have been remunerated for service to public patients in public hospitals, with a variety of rates of sessional payment and a variety of conditions attached to such payments in different states. However, the historic attitude that doctors are providing charity to these patients still persists with some medical staff and there is no doubt that attention to public patients, on some occasions at least, is on a less personalised basis than is the case for 'private' patients, who, whether privately insured for the doctor's fee or not, are responsible for paying the doctor directly. Doctors do not have automatic admitting rights to either public or private hospitals, and increasingly over the past twenty-five years general practitioners have been excluded from having any access to most metropolitan hospitals and have played a diminishing role in even the larger country hospitals.

Australian medical care is provided in a two-step process. General practitioners provide primary, first contact care. When necessary, the primary care doctor refers a patient to a specialist; most specialists apply for and obtain admitting rights to hospitals. The reimbursement system embodies this referral arrangement to ensure that patients' access to specialist services results only from a general practitioner or another specialist practitioner. The system is designed to limit patients' direct access to specialist services and is approximately 80% effective.

Limiting patients' access to specialist services can save money and improve quality (by limiting both inappropriate self-referral and care delivered by specialists that could be better and less expensively delivered by general practitioners). However, patients may be irritated by the need to see a general practitioner when their problem 'obviously' needs a specialist's attention. Further, general practitioners may inappropriately refer to specialists or fail to refer to them when advisable, especially if there are incentives to save money by not referring patients. Measures to monitor practitioners' quality of care, including the appropriateness of referrals, are essential.

Post-hospital care, in theory at least, is once again the responsibility of general practitioners. In practice this does not occur as regularly as it should and many postdischarge patients are being followed up by their hospital specialist in the hospital's outpatient department or in the specialist's private rooms. Traditional hospital outpatient clinics have declined in recent years, more so in some states than others. There are a number of reasons for this trend, including the financial drivers in the doctors' payment system whereby, for some specialist services, a fee can be raised in the specialist's rooms but not in the hospital's outpatient department. Another reason is a deliberate attempt by surgeons to diminish the use of public hospital outpatient departments. Those that have survived now cater mainly to welfare recipients or provide technically sophisticated services that cannot be easily provided outside of a hospital environment.

124 | The changing environment

By the late 1950s it had become clear to some leaders of the medical profession that many of the problems in the hospital system were arising in an environment which had become closer to that of the United States of America than that of the United Kingdom. In retrospect it is hardly surprising that organisational arrangements which suited the small densely populated United Kingdom, with its centralised government, would sooner or later run into difficulty in a country the size of the United States, organised as a federation and with a geographically dispersed population no bigger than that of the Los Angeles metropolitan area.

Further, while a British health culture existed in Australia, the country had adopted only part of the United Kingdom system. For example, while in Britain hospitals are mainly staffed by employed specialist practitioners ('consultants' on salaried contracts most of whom engage in little or no private practice), in Australia the staffing arrangement was closer to the US model of visiting staff, with each specialist mostly engaged in their own private practice.

In the late 1950s efforts commenced to investigate the United States and its hospitals, and the way medical staff related to them, to a degree that had not occurred previously. It was not long before attempts were made to adapt some of these US systems to Australian conditions. Hospital accreditation, credentialling of medical staff and the move to introduce quality assurance were tangible evidence of this trend.

125 | Quality of care concepts

Quality of care, particularly from the point of medical practitioners and copied for the most part by other health professionals, has depended on:

- medical education;
- registration with its attendant disciplinary and complaints mechanisms;
- the Royal College system for specialist training;
- medical malpractice litigation (which some might see as a quality management tool) to right wrongs and prevent their occurrence (or at least recurrence), although it has many imperfections including the potential for abuse and costly defensive medicine. It needs to be emphasised that only a fraction of the poor care that occurs is ever brought to the courts' attention and many cases that appear in courts do not involve poor care.

Until the late 1950s and early 1960s quality of care in hospitals was seen to be covered by the registration of doctors and nurses and the idea that if doctors in particular were adequately educated and trained, quality would take care of itself. The idea, passed down to us from the British Royal College system, that qualifications equate with quality was never true, but erected a significant barrier to understanding the need for quality management, both within the medical profession and the community at large.

As recently as 1992 a prominent leader of the Australian medical profession while commenting about quality management asserted that in his view: ' . . . if we choose our doctors well, educate them in such a way that we give them an inquiring . . . mind and examine them thoroughly, that is the best we can do.'[1] This approach might have worked quite well in the low technology environment which endured until after World War II;

however, the technological explosion which started to make itself felt in the 1950s and which we are still experiencing also exploded this rather self-satisfying and highly subjective view of quality.

126 Three strands of activity

The movement to provide formal systems for managing quality in Australia's hospitals has had three quite distinct and separate streams of activity which are only now slowly converging into one comprehensive concept—quality management. Those three streams are: hospital accreditation; credentialling of medical staff; and the quest for assuring and improving the quality of care and services.

126.1 Hospital accreditation

Towards the end of the 1950s a small group of clinicians who happened to be officers of the New South Wales Branch of the Australian Medical Association (AMA) saw that serious deficiencies existed throughout the public hospital system in that state. Their concerns included: the inadequacy of medical records, particularly in relation to the use of blood; the poor and variable quality of medical staff organisation in New South Wales public hospitals; and a vague worry about the issue of how doctors' activities should be controlled and who should do it. The wholistic notion of quality of care simply did not exist.

On 7 July 1959, following an address on hospital accreditation in the United States by Dr Ed Crosby of the American Hospital Association, the New South Wales Branch Council of the AMA determined to establish ' . . . a Conjoint Board to draw up a scheme of accreditation of hospitals based on the accreditation scheme in the United States of America . . . '[2] Thirty years were to pass before hospital accreditation became acccepted by all state governments in Australia. The story of hospital accreditation illustrates the difficulties inherent in the introduction of change to the health industry.

Those thirty years were characterised by: indifference followed by opposition and frank hostility from state governments; continuing frustration as seeding funds were denied both in Australia and in the United States; and the establishment and ultimate disbandment of three joint committees. Those years also saw the dogged perseverance and persistence of a small group of individuals who, without realising it, were pioneering the concept of quality of hospital services in this country.

Eventually, in 1970 what had been a state activity by the AMA in New South Wales and subsequently the Australian Hospital Association in Victoria became a national activity under a federal joint committee, recognised by both parent bodies.

In 1972 the federal joint committee of the AMA and AHA became the Australian Council on Hospital Standards. There were still no resources, no funds and no staff. Then in 1973 the newly-elected federal Labor government established the Hospitals and Health Services Commission. A seeding grant of A$25 000 was made from the Commonwealth government to the Australian Council on Hospital Standards and this enabled the appointment of its first executive director. Once established, in 1974 the ACHS (now the Australian Council on Healthcare Standards) successfully applied for a three-year grant from the Kellogg Foundation in the United States and, it was thought, after fifteen years of effort, it was simply a matter of getting on with the job. In reality the struggle had only just begun.

Another three years were to pass (1977) before continuing discussions and pressure persuaded the New South Wales Health Commission (which was responsible for the state's public hospitals) to participate in the program. In the meanwhile, in Victoria's less centralised environment, in 1975 Geelong Hospital became the first hospital to be accredited in Australia. Queensland was the last state to agree to participate in the program in 1990.

The greater part of the 1980s was taken up with refining the hospital accreditation program. Refinements included the training of surveyors, rewriting standards, and accommodating some of the key stakeholder groups who did not have a seat on the Council. The end of the decade also saw some interesting initiatives including the clinical indicators project, expansion of the Education Unit, and assisting organisations in New Zealand and the United Kingdom to establish hospital accreditation programs.

The 1990s have witnessed an extensive and sincere appraisal by the ACHS of its approach and methodology in assessing a facility's capacity to deliver quality care. That appraisal is still in progress.

126.2 | *Credentialling of medical staff (delineation of clinical privileges)*

The second strand of activity in the history of quality management related to what doctors did in hospitals. The period from 1965 through 1970 produced a number of quite horrendous incidents involving doctors undertaking hospital procedures which were beyond their training, experience and competence in totally unsuitable conditions. These incidents were seen as the tip of an iceberg. They led to a public outcry and subsequently to the development, once again by the New South Wales Branch of the AMA, of a system for credentialling medical staff—a system to determine what any doctor can do in the hospital at any one time. Some of these incidents, following complaints against the doctors under the *Medical Practitioners Act*, were subject to in camera inquiries resulting in legal action for damages. One incident that occurred at this time resulted in twenty years of media controversy and finally was subjected to a Royal Commission.[3] As far as the authors are aware, an effective credentialling program has never been implemented effectively in any hospital in Australia, largely due to entrenched resistance by doctors.

126.3 | *Quality assurance*

Even while initiatives in hospital accreditation and the credentialling of medical staff were underway at least in New South Wales, pressures were mounting on hospitals and health professionals at a federal level.

Following an inquiry into health insurance in 1976, the minister for health in the Fraser government, Mr Ralph Hunt, challenged the medical profession to engage in 'peer review' in hospitals within three years or the government would do it for them. Looking back from the 1990s it was an extraordinary challenge. The Australian Medical Association (federally) took up this challenge and an AMA/Commonwealth government fact finding group went to Canada, the United States and (West) Germany to find out what 'peer review' meant and how one was supposed to implement it. The AMA's acceptance of this challenge represented the beginning of the third strand of activity in the development of quality management in Australia.

The next four years witnessed an enormous effort by the AMA to educate the health community about what was at first referred to as peer review, then medical audit, then clinical review, then quality assurance, and now quality improvement. Throughout the 1980s a great deal of effort was expended in hospitals particularly by nurses and other health professionals—now quite independently of the AMA—to chase this holy grail. Indeed, nurses and allied health professionals have been more involved and shown more interest in quality management than have most doctors.

127 | Doctors' characteristics

Doctors are trained to be independent, self reliant and individualistic—and quite rightly so. They are taught to rely on their own judgment and in general are not accustomed to sharing their decision-making processes with others, except perhaps in a non-judgmental way with colleagues. The idea of being formally accountable, other than to their own professional ideals, is totally foreign to them. Generally doctors have difficulty accepting that it is possible to measure, in any meaningful way, either the processes or outcomes of patient care.[4]

As a general rule, when asked to consider 'problems' associated with patient care, doctors tend to think only about the rare and unusual rather than about commonly encountered conditions. They are also more accustomed to thinking about individual cases rather than either patterns or systems of care. Doctors, like many action oriented people, hate committees. They tend to relate, in general, to one-on-one situations, and the way hospitals conduct business reflects this preference. Doctors prefer corridor conversations to what they see as the protracted time wasting of committees.

While there is great variation in medical staff organisation throughout Australia, in larger hospitals there is usually a series of departments or divisions reflecting the traditional clinical specialties. Many of the difficulties associated with the involvement of medical staff in quality management issues are due to the unwillingness or inability of busy doctors in private practice to spend time on staff organisational meetings and the reluctance of heads of departments to exert anything like clinical or administrative control over their colleagues.

Medical staff association meetings have a tendency to become a forum for medico-political—or what the nurses might call industrial—discussions. It is perhaps not surprising that trying to involve medical staff in anything other than clinical care has always been a frustrating exercise. While the situation is slowly changing, to most clinicians the word 'management' carries with it the spectre of alien and mindless control over them.

References

1 Australian Medicine. From the President vol. 4, no. 21 16 November 1992.
2 Minutes of the NSW Branch of the Australian Medical Association, July 1959.
3 Report of The Royal Commission into Deep Sleep Therapy vol. I-b, Sydney, 17 July, 1990.
4 NSW Parliament Public Accounts Special Committee. Funding Infrastructure and Services in New South Wales. Minutes of Evidence. Arnold P, p. 210. Report No. 72. June 1993.

Chapter 3

HOSPITALS—A CHANGED AND CHANGING ENVIRONMENT

---

130 Contents

Within the practising lifetime of most medical practitioners, hospitals have changed and are still changing at a rate which has produced considerable discomfort to the health professionals who work in them. In this chapter we explore these changes:

- **131.** The technology explosion
- **132.** Costs of hospital care
- **133.** Appropriateness of hospital care
- **134.** Accountability
- **135.** Medical staffing patterns
- **136.** Fragmentation of care

---

131 Purpose of this chapter

This chapter looks at the changes that have occurred in hospitals, largely from the perspective of the technological explosion. It is an attempt to provide some logical explanations for the enormous changes that hospital professionals, particularly doctors, find so disturbing, and which impinge on the day-to-day activities of all hospital professionals.

132 The technology explosion

The rising tide of medical and hospital malpractice litigation is the outward manifestation of changes that have occurred in our hospitals and the society in which they function over the past thirty years. Medical technology exploded in the years following World War II and continues at an increasing rate. It is one of the root causes of our current difficulties in hospitals. Australia is not alone; this phenomenon is common to all developed, industrialised societies.

There is an argument that all technology is good and the more of it there is the better. However, medical technology poses a number of problems. In Australia and elsewhere

15

the effectiveness of much medical technology in improving health status has not been adequately assessed. Clearly, not all medical technology is useless. Innovation has provided a wider choice of investigations and therapies; however, it has also led to the inappropriate use of a number of devices and other interventions, with the attendant risk of damaging effects. Further, there is no doubt that it has added considerably to hospital costs. Increases in costs are measured annually in budgets; the effectiveness of care has simply been assumed. Certainly, the increase in life expectancy that has occurred in this same period is not commensurate with the rise in costs, even if one attributes all of the gain to medical care, which is a very unlikely circumstance.

Australia has already begun to encounter a number of problems with medical and hospital technology quite apart from its cost-effectiveness. They include, for example:

* the training of practitioners to use the technology;
* the continued competence of practitioners, which is important in Australia's small scattered population. Such matters as the volume of throughput per year has a critical bearing on continued competence;
* the siting and control over technology;
* how the technology is to be financed;
* who should receive the technology and under what circumstances.

While medical technology has provided some of the most amazing progress in hospital care, many medical practitioners are only too well aware of the difficulties in keeping pace with this growing development. The question arises about the controls necessary to be applied to medical staff who wish to carry out new technology and the requirements for training in such circumstances.

In spite of the difficulties that result from new medical technology, we do not suggest turning the clock back, even if it were remotely possible to do so, because technology has produced significant advances in care. The difficulties to which we refer can be summarised as follows:

* not everything is effective and we do not know what is and what is not;
* some effective technologies cost more than they are worth (at least to society, if not to the patient);
* effective technology is not always used appropriately or implemented properly;
* the potential for harm (iatrogenesis) with more sophisticated technology is increasing;
* advances in technology manifest ethical and sociopolitical dilemmas, including those concerned with its distribution, such as who should receive it, under what circumstances and who should pay.

The demand for the assumed benefit of these technological advances as a right of every member of the community has led to a profound change in the character of hospital care, which has brought with it a difficult adjustment problem for the health professions and an environment which has left many patients overawed by technological marvels, yet still increasingly dissatisfied with the quality of the care they have received.

133 | Costs of hospital care

Until relatively recently, governments have been willing participants in encouraging the community to partake to the full of all the benefits which modern sophisticated hospital care can provide. The underlying assumption has been that modern hospital medicine only has benefits; 'more is better'.

As in other comparable societies, the health agenda for the 1990s appears to have changed. Whereas until recent years patients' demands for services was the main consideration, there is now recognition that resources are finite and the quantity and range of services to be provided have to fit within a budgetary constraint. Doctors and other health professionals are increasingly being forced to make decisions relating to the 'rationing' of services. For hospital medical staff nurtured on the 'more is better' approach this has been, in many cases, a very painful adjustment.

A diminished flow of funds to, and the increased demands on, public hospitals, has meant that the appropriateness of all aspects of hospital care now becomes a major consideration. If the totality of the provision of hospital services is limited by resources, the need for doctors and hospitals to have more information on the effectiveness and costs of medical interventions becomes imperative. Inappropriate care, whether in the form of unnecessary investigations, unnecessary procedures or even unnecessary hospital admissions, means that there is less money to carry out those activities which are appropriate, necessary and effective.

134 Appropriateness of hospital care

The appropriateness of care provided in hospitals is one facet of quality care. While unnecessary and excessive investigations carry a cost burden, they may also indicate a less than adequate quality of care. Some investigations, such as radiology, also carry with them the risk of patient harm. Unnecessary surgical interventions not only lead to avoidable costs (often hidden in the hospital's total budget), but also expose the patient to unnecessary risk. Care that is maximally effective and that avoids superfluous interventions equates with high quality.

135 Accountability

Another portion of the health agenda that has changed and is still changing is the question of the independence of medical practitioners and the degree of accountability expected of them. The idea of a trained medical professional, skilled in his or her work, conditioned to the idea of adherence to a detailed code of professional behaviour, and accountable to no one but his or her own professional ideals for the quality of care he or she provides, also has fallen victim to the changed environment in which medicine is now practised.

The very technology which has handed such power and prestige to an extensive range of medical specialties has led to doctors as a group being perceived as mere technicians and, in the eyes of many, expensive ones at that. Where previously doctors were seen as dispensing a very personalised form of care and support, they are now seen as dispensers of high-powered technology which, while capable of miracles, is nevertheless seen as very impersonal. This transference of therapeutic agent—from doctor to machine—has meant a transfer of mythical powers, once held by the doctor, to the healing machine. This depersonalisation of the medical profession has resulted in the community's diminished willingness to accept medical practitioners' fallacies, errors and omissions.

Ironically, a much better educated community is much less prepared to accept the inadequacies of purveyors of modern medical technology than were their parents and grandparents who accepted with loving affection the inadequacies of their medical practitioners. Compared with today's hospital doctor, yesterday's practitioner, armed merely with a stethoscope, was in relative and absolute terms therapeutically impotent. The public's expectations concerning the miracles of modern medicine have grown faster than the reality of medical technology. In part these expectations are fuelled by the medical profession who, ironically, often stand in the way of measuring its effectiveness and improving the quality of care.

This change in attitudes towards doctors is manifested in the demands of the community and governments which represent it, for increasing degrees of accountability by doctors for the appropriateness and quality of the services they provide. For the medical profession to deny this desire for accountability is the surest way for its practitioners to lose even more of their independence, in terms of clinical freedom and financial independence, than has already occurred.

Effective quality management programs fulfil the requirement of medical staff, other hospital staff, and of the hospital itself to be accountable to the community. At the same time, however, such programs meet the genuine need of hospital professionals to understand what is happening in their hospital and, where problems are found to exist, to provide a mechanism to resolve them.

136 │ Medical staffing patterns

In capital cities, metropolitan areas and major country regions, Australian hospitals have followed the UK specialist model of medical staffing, in contrast to the generalist model adopted by most Canadian hospitals. There are, of course, many small rural hospitals where general practitioners are the only practitioners available. These hospitals, however, represent a minority of total hospital beds.

The 'specialist' model of hospital staffing is characterised by all medical staff being specialist medical practitioners in one or other specialty or subspecialty. All patients are admitted under the care of an appropriately designated specialist. When taken to its logical conclusion, the 'specialist' model results in no general practitioners having hospital access and eventually, as in some teaching hospitals in Australia, there are even no general medical or surgical beds, all beds being allocated to one or other subspecialty.

In the 'generalist' model, general practitioners access rights to hospital beds and are encouraged to continue to tend their patients, even though the care may be transferred temporarily to one or more specialists or specialist teams. While able to attend to their own patients within their granted privileges, general practitioners are expected to call on specialist medical advice when required.

137 │ Fragmentation of care

While both systems of staffing have their advocates, their advantages and disadvantages, the problem with the specialist model which we are now witnessing in Australia is the potentially high level of fragmentation of patient care. In addition, specialists tend to focus more on specific health problems rather than on the patient and his or her capacity to cope with life. Specialists also tend to favour more, and more expensive, interventions.

At the extreme, in tertiary referral hospitals such as teaching hospitals it is not uncommon for four or more teams of specialty services to care for the one patient at the same time, each specialist team responsible for a different range of medical problems. In such circumstances it is difficult at times even for hospital staff, let alone the patient, to know which particular doctor or team has primary responsibility for the patient's care. In addition, in large complex hospitals there is the usual number of nursing and allied health staff, all of whom play a large part in the totality of care provided to any one patient. How, in our efforts to assure quality of care, can we integrate these many and disparate providers?

In this at times overwhelming conglomeration of service providers, it is surprising that some medical practitioners can still assert that the quality of care provided to the patient equates solely with the medical care which they themselves provide. Part of the answer to this serious fragmentation of care may be to develop a meaningful role for the general practitioner. Not all general practitioners will desire such a role but those who do, particularly in the major teaching hospitals, could play an important co-ordinating and bridging function.

Chapter 4

HOSPITAL AND PROFESSIONAL LIABILITY

---

141 | Purpose of this chapter

This chapter underscores the problems that occur all too frequently in hospitals of all sizes and in all locations, whether they be major teaching institutions or hospitals of a humbler nature. We have attempted to paint a balanced picture in perspective and to avoid dramatising or exaggerating the current situation in Australian hospitals. The availability of hard data is very limited. The facts presented here are far from ideal, but we obtained even this material with great difficulty. Even this limited data demonstrates there is a problem.

Anyone who keeps a file from the daily press over several consecutive months would find that reported hospital maloccurrences represent a much larger issue than hospitals or doctors recognise. Doctors and hospitals feel very threatened by such media reports and often respond by accusations of 'doctor bashing' or claims that the reports are one-sided and biased. Nevertheless, the fact is that some patients do die as a direct result of hospital mishaps and others suffer significant pain and disability—and better quality management might well have prevented some of these tragedies.

To put the concerns expressed in this chapter into perspective, we believe that Australia has a solid, admirable base of good quality health care. In spite of the millions of medical services rendered in any one year which are satisfactory by any standard, the likely volume of services which are not satisfactory cannot be ignored. Moreover, an effective quality management program would improve services which are now considered satisfactory. Indeed, quality management emphasises continually improving products and services, not merely correcting problems in the production of existing products and services.

The case studies we describe are merely the tip of an iceberg, the full extent of which can only be surmised. All these case studies, in one aspect or another, reflect a lack of the attitude (or its extension into action) that says quality of care is the most important aspect of our work in this hospital, and by their very nature they indicate the absence of effective quality management programs.

142 | Hospital and medical maloccurrences

Every profession in Australia over the past decade has faced ever-increasing problems in relation to professional indemnity claims and, consequently, rising professional indemnity premiums. The medical profession has been no exception and does not stand out among other professional groups. Most of the professions have responded to these problems by instituting schemes for their members that intend to cut losses in the long term and thereby achieve more stable premiums.

Since the late 1960s in the state of New South Wales—and we have no reason to believe other states are different—there has been a succession of incidents that have produced media and community reaction relating to care provided in hospitals both public and private. These incidents merely represent the tip of a large iceberg. They manifest the failure of our hospitals to adjust to fundamental changes, related to a great extent, if not predominantly, to the explosion in hospital and medical technology. They represent the inevitability of the impact of technology in the absence of effective quality management systems.

143 | Forces driving hospital malpractice claims: how to counter them

143.1 | Four forces affect claims' rates

In spite of the apparent downward trend in the number of claims in one state for public hospitals, claims for malpractice and dissatisfaction with the health care industry will likely increase, and the factors responsible will be with us for years to come. Four forces principally drive hospital claims. They are:

- a better informed community;
- the legal profession;
- media hype;
- hospital indifference.

143.2 | A better informed community

The Australian community has become much more aware of its rights to sue hospitals and doctors and many people no longer look upon hospitals and medical practitioners as being somehow divine. Society has accepted the supposed benefits of medical technology to such an extent that there is a commonly prevailing attitude that if something went wrong someone must have been at fault. Not only have the community's expectations been increasing, but so too has its understanding of the use of legal avenues for redress.

143.3   *The legal profession*

There are an increasing number of legal practitioners in our society who are encouraging clients to bring claims because they see such clients as an ongoing source of revenue for their practice. The disappearance or diminution of the third party or workers' compensation areas of legal practice added to the pool of legal practitioners looking to benefit from hospital and medical malpractice litigation. It is by no means fanciful to claim that the day of the US style ambulance-chasing lawyer has already arrived in Australia.

143.4   *Media hype*

The media has focused its attention increasingly on stories of hospital and medical malpractice. A scan of the popular press over an eighteen-month period commencing in 1992 produced a list of 142 stories of hospital and medical misadventure and reports of problems related to the hospital industry and its associated professional groups—mainly doctors.

143.5   *The price of indifference*

Hospitals in Australia cannot continue to ignore the reality of today's litigious environment if they wish to preserve their and their medical staff's financial integrity. For medical practitioners, their professional autonomy is also at stake. Indifference to the issue will result in the doubling of insurance premiums and a continued doubling until underwriters start to drop out of the hospital indemnity business altogether. When the insurers start to avoid the business, hospitals will find themselves in a situation similar to that in the United States in the 1970s when for a time hospitals could not obtain indemnity cover at any price. At present, in the United States the price of indemnity continues to rise. Indemnity insurance for an obstetrician currently stands at over US$50 000 per annum. A practitioner must deliver a substantial number of infants just to generate the income to pay this premium. Consequently, obstetrical care is becoming scarce or unavailable in some areas of the United States. A similar trend is becoming apparent in Australia.

143.6   *The solution to counter rising claims*

Hospitals in Australia must start to take an increasing interest in quality management and risk management techniques, not merely to satisfy the insurance industry and avoid an uninsurable environment, but even more importantly for the benefit of their patients. Many hospitals and their medical and nursing staff have taken significant steps in this direction. Hopefully, some thoughts and ideas in this manual will help to guide them further down this difficult path.

144   The medical defence organisations

144.1   *Nature of medical defence organisations*

In Australia indemnity against medical negligence is carried by a number of organisations in the various states. Most of these organisations are mutual societies. The New South Wales Medical Defence Union, characteristic of most of these organisations in Australia, faced a growing crisis in the mid 1980s associated with a rapidly escalating claims experience.

Due to the number of organisations and their reluctance to release data, obtaining detailed claims experience is very difficult. However, the Review of Professional Indemnity Arrangements for Health Care Professionals conducted by the Department of Human Services and Health has recently published an interim report. We are grateful to the chairman of that Review, Ms Fiona Tito, for permission to use material from the report. (See Tables I-4-2 and I-4-3 on pages 25 and 26.)

144.2 │ Corrective actions taken

Action taken by the various medical defence organisations to reduce severity of claims includes:

- employing full-time staff with medical and legal qualifications;
- working closely with insurers;
- educating members in claim prevention and risk management by circular and by seminar;
- encouraging members to report possible claims incidents so that problems can be resolved quickly;
- encouraging members to ensure that dissatisfied patients are sent away in a happier state of mind and are thus less likely to resort to litigation.

144.3 │ Hospitals and health insurers

While doctors and hospitals are feeling the financial consequences of hospital and medical malpractice, vital players in this scene are the organisations that play an important intermediate role. They comprise:

- the commercial insurance industry, which insures hospitals against these risks;
- the medical defence organisations, which are mainly mutual benefit societies and which provide indemnity for medical practitioners against negligence actions; and
- the health insurance industry consisting mainly of non-profit registered health benefit funds, which reimburse privately insured patients for the costs of occupying private beds in public hospitals and for the costs of private hospital bed days.

All three groups of insurers have a large vested interest on behalf of their client populations to diminish negligence, hospital maloccurrences and episodes of poor quality care in hospitals. To date, the interest in effective hospital quality management programs on the part of any of these groups has been almost non-existent. We find this difficult to understand and we would hope that, in patients' and in their own interests, this situation will change.

145 │ Comparison with other professional groups

145.1 │ Property valuers

Property valuers were hard hit in the 1980s in legal actions for negligence. Their institute (the professional association) has produced a handbook on valuers' liability and risk management, written by leading lawyers who practise in the area. There is no doubt that this initiative had a considerable effect on valuers' actions and on the incidence of claims.

145.2 │ Insurance brokers

The National Insurance Brokers' Association, whose members were being crippled in the early 1980s by massive rises in professional indemnity premiums caused by lack of professionalism and the inevitable high incidence of claims, has spent considerable time and money on improving the quality of service provided by its members. The Association has also produced videos which have been sent to all members. In addition, it has sent senior brokers specialising in risk prevention for professionals, to members' offices all over Australia to run loss prevention seminars. The Association has put together a well-run professional liability insurance scheme for its members. Through the Association's educational efforts, premiums have declined.

145.3 │ Lawyers

The legal profession has made professional indemnity insurance compulsory for its members. This provision allows them to compile their own claims statistics and to advise members where and why claims are recurring in certain parts of legal practices. Such a scheme enables the profession to educate its members in loss prevention, the provision of better service and to negotiate better terms with insurers or reinsurers.

145.4 | *Other professions*

In the case of some professional groups, insurers have exerted strong pressures to ensure radical steps were instituted to improve professional standards. For example, some firms of engineers have been unable to buy a professional indemnity policy unless they have a system of checking all of the drawings produced by members of staff, organised at their head office. In the case of architects, firms have been made to take better site notes and to confirm oral conversations with clients in writing. Insurers have insisted that financial planners' staff members and licensed dealers attend regular seminars and are only allowed to recommend investments which are approved in writing by the firm's principal.

145.5 | *The hospital industry*

In the area of legal risk minimisation, the hospital industry stands out for the following reasons:

- it has done little if anything to put its own house in order;
- whether in the private or public sector there is no planned approach to reduce claims and the costs of either premiums or damages;
- there is no compulsory insurance for operators of private hospitals;
- there is no readily accessible set of statistics providing an adequate claims profile;
- neither the public nor the private sector has even commenced to advise its constituent parts about the problem either in written or other form.

The hospital industry in Australia has still not taken adequate steps to introduce effective quality management, nor have hospitals seen fit to engage in effective risk minimisation policies. It is almost as if, in the face of a significant level of claims, the hospital industry does not believe there is a real problem. It would appear that as an industry, hospitals:

- do not perceive that there is a problem, or;
- while seeing the problem, believe that the cost of fixing it is greater than allowing it to continue, or;
- perceive the problem, but do not know how to set about fixing it, or;
- perceive the political costs of fixing the problem to be too high.

Until hospitals instal currently available clinical information systems to demonstrate the nature and extent of problems in hospitals and introduce effective quality management programs, doctors and administrators will continue to face media attacks, and the level of litigation directed at doctors and hospitals will continue to increase.

146 | **Hospital and medical claims statistics**

146.1 | *Trends in medical 'claims'*

One of the biggest problems in the interpretation of data available from medical defence organisations in Australia is that there is little or no uniformity in the definition of terms used. 'Claims' have different meanings, sometimes referring to notification of incidents and sometimes only being recorded as such when a payment has been made. Table I-4-1 (see page 24) shows the number of 'claims' made for one major medical defence organisation.

Table I-4-1 *Claims experienced by one medical defence organisation against doctors*

Year	Number of claims
1984	146
1985	249
1986	365
1987	382
1988	416
1989	773

Note: Data are the latest available.
Source: Private communication with FAI Insurances Pty Ltd.

The membership of the organisation from which these claims statistics have been obtained represents approximately 20% of the total indemnity organisations' combined membership in Australia. Due to the unreliability of the data from medical defence organisations generally, and the variable use of terms, we consider it to be unwise to draw definitive conclusions. Certainly, regardless of absolute numbers, Table I-4-1 reveals that the number of 'claims' rose significantly over a six year period.

The interim report of a review of professional indemnity arrangements contains aggregated claims data from an Australia-wide survey of medical defence organisations. These data, reproduced in Table I-4-2 (see page 25), demonstrate a much smaller incidence of 'claims' than that suggested in Table I-4-1, which pertains to data from a single medical defence union. They do not distinguish between doctors involved in hospital incidents and doctors involved in incidents in their own practices. While the number of claims in Australia seems to have doubled between 1985 and 1988, they seem to have reached an uneven plateau. Table I-4-3 (see page 26) shows that over a quarter of finalised claims did not involve a monetary settlement, and that almost one half of finalisations were delayed for five or more years.

Obtaining data on hospital legal liability claims has been even more difficult than for medical practitioners. However, it has been possible through the New South Wales Health Department to obtain the number of legal liability claims made against New South Wales public hospitals in each financial year from 1981 to 1993/94. In order to put this data into better perspective, Table I-4-4 (on page 27) combines it with the number of separations (discharges) from New South Wales public hospitals (acute) for the same years and the approximate number of claims per 100 000 separations.

These data on hospitals' claims represent the situation in one state of Australia—New South Wales—and only relate to public hospitals. While the number of claims is probably not so high in the smaller states, and proportionally may well be less, such observations, in the absence of data, can only be conjecture. Certainly, from media reports there would be no reason to believe that the number of maloccurrences in hospitals and the resulting litigation were not matters for serious concern. In New South Wales, the number of claims suggests that there is a trend of diminishing incidence since 1985/86. Nevertheless, 335 claims in 1993/94 still represent an increase of 500% from 1981/82. Since there were 203 public hospitals in New South Wales in 1991/92 (the latest year for which we have published data on the number of public hospitals in New South Wales), 316 claims in that year were equivalent to more than one claim for every public hospital in the state during that year.

The number of claims, however, is only part of the picture. Unfortunately it was not possible to obtain the dollar amounts that these claims represent nor actual settlements.

Table I-4-2 *The number of claims filed against Australian medical defence organisations by year of report and year of occurrence* [a]

Year of occurrence	Year of claim report								
	1991	*1990*	*1989*	*1988*	*1987*	*1986*	*< 1985*	*1985*	*Total*
1991	552	0	0	0	0	0	0	0	552
1990	391	492	0	0	0	0	0	0	883
1989	190	340	580	0	0	0	0	0	1110
1988	136	164	334	528	0	0	0	0	1162
1987	82	112	185	406	513	0	0	0	1298
1986	69	69	100	191	354	380	0	0	1163
1985	72	45	74	120	150	298	321	0	1080
1980-1984	240	255	506	591	369	391	443	1588	4383
1975-1979	24	17	15	16	20	33	48	817	990
before 1975	5	3	4	6	7	8	3	104	140
Total	1761	1497	1798	1858	1413	1110	815	2509	12761

[a] This table covers 4 medical defence organisations representing 78.5% of all members in responding medical defence organisations (MDOs). The response from one MDO was completely inconsistent and excluded from this table. The response from another MDO was edited to make logically consistent.

Source: Department of Health, Housing & Community Services, Survey of medical defence organisations. Prepared by statistical consultancy, Australian Bureau of Statistics. Unpublished material, April 1993: Table 14.1.

However, we suspect that if extrapolated to the rest of Australia, these claims and the costs of defending and settling them would probably amount to many thousands, if not millions, of dollars of wasted funds in a public hospital system very hard pressed for finances.

146.2 Private hospital claim statistics

Statistics on private hospitals are not easy to come by, but access to one insurer, FAI Insurances Ltd, provides some revealing information. In 1989 FAI, one of Australia's largest insurers, insured over 100 private hospitals and it was handling 150 possible malpractice claims against those hospitals.

FAI divides claims into two groups. There are 'definite claims', that is, a writ has been served on a hospital. In addition there are 'possible claims', where a hospital receives a letter from a disgruntled patient raising the possibility of a claim at a future date. Insurers treat both types in the same fashion in that they open a claim file and place a reserve on the claim.

146.3 Cost of defending claims

In New South Wales claims against hospitals are commonly brought to the New South Wales Supreme Court, resulting in a sequential chain of costs. Insurers will brief the best available Queen's Counsel, who in New South Wales charges from $3000 to $6000 per day. Junior Counsel charge up to one-half that fee, to which must be added the fees of solicitors and the costs of expert witnesses. With only two parties involved, legal costs can soon add up to $12 000 per day in court and this does not include the costs of preparation of the case. In New South Wales, Legal Aid has largely been discontinued for civil actions.

However, existing grants of Legal Aid have been continued and in certain special circumstances litigants may still apply for government aid in the running of a case. Such litigants can only qualify where they demonstrate that they have a genuine case and do

Table I-4-3 *Analysis of claims finalised by Australian medical defence organisations during the reporting period ended in 1991*[a]

| Year | Delay | Amount of finalisation ($) | | | | | Summary | | |
		0	1-100 000	100 001- 1 000 000	over 1 000 000	Total	Per cent of total	Cumulative number	per cent
1991	0	36	46	0	0	82	9.02	82	9.02
1990	1	55	66	1	0	122	13.42	204	22.44
1989	2	55	62	0	0	117	12.87	321	35.31
1988	3	11	50	2	0	63	6.93	384	42.24
1987	4	21	82	2	0	105	11.55	489	53.80
1986	5	17	75	4	1	97	10.67	586	64.47
1985	6	12	57	3	0	72	7.92	658	72.39
1980–84	7–11	45	145	13	2	205	22.55	863	94.94
1975–79	12–16	10	22	4	0	36	3.96	899	98.90
before 1975	>16	5	5	0	0	10	1.10	909	100.00
TOTAL		267	610	29	3	909	100.00	909	100.00

[a] One medical defence organisation did not respond to this question, hence the table represents 75.2% of all responding MDO members.
Source: Department of Health, Housing & Community Services. Review of Professional Indemnity Arrangements for Health Care Professionals. Survey of medical defence organisations: prepared by Statistical Consultancy, Australian Bureau of Statistics. Unpublished material, April 1993: Table 11.2.

not have sufficient funds to prosecute it to a proper conclusion and/or where the case is of public interest. If a plaintiff with Legal Aid loses the case, Legal Aid does not pay all the defendant's costs, which would normally be the losing side's responsibility. One successful defence of a claim in the Supreme Court by the New South Wales Medical Defence Union cost the Union $120 000, because the plaintiff had Legal Aid.

146.4 *Quality of care—the human factor*

We have laid considerable emphasis in this chapter on the tangible effects of the costs of litigation both for doctors and hospitals. However, our emphasis on risk minimisation, litigation costs and the insurance costs, as important as they may be, should not overshadow the other consequences of poor quality care. One of the medical profession's main ethical directives is *primum non nocere* (first do no harm). Patients would rather avoid pain and suffering than receive monetary damages which, while intended to compensate, can never make them whole.

For example, a young man who had his leg amputated because of failed or non-existent infection control, the lady who died following a medication error in which she received a fatal dose of morphine, the mother who has an unnecessary caesarian section, the baby born prematurely with an intellectual deficit due to an inappropriately induced labour, all represent human suffering and anguish which should be—and in these cases could have been—avoided. (See case commentaries later in this chapter.) The fact that some compensation has resulted through the legal system is, in our opinion, important but of secondary importance. Moreover, only a small fraction of cases in which patients are harmed ever get to court. The patient does not recognise the harm or the doctor's or hospital's liability, or fails to pursue an action.

Table I-4-4 *Number of legal liability claims filed against NSW hospitals, 1981–94, and their rate per 100 000 separations*

Financial year	Number of claims	Number of separations	Number of claims per 100 000 separations
1981	63	885 615	7.1
1982	206	(no data)	(no data)
1983	66	890 676	18.6
1984	152	799 967	19.0
1985	362	761 224	47.6
1986	348	845 885	41.1
1987/88	345	867 146	39.8
1988/89	310	900 810	34.4
1989/90	273	948 738	28.8
1990/91	310	1 004 002	31.0
1991/92	316	1 027 369	30.8
1992/93	427	1 074 842	39.9
1993/94	335	1 215 943	27.7

Footnotes:
(a) It should be noted that data was collected before 1987 in calendar years and after 1987 in financial years. No data re number of separations or number of claims per 100 000 separations was collected for the year 1982 (calendar) in NSW nor for the first half of 1987. Sampling factors were used in all years and the figures given are for weighted untrimmed separations. The 1984–85 figures are attributed to the doctor dispute in NSW. (Personal communication. Ryan S. NSW Health Services Research Group, Department of Statistics, University of Newcastle, Shortland NSW.)
(b) There is generally a time difference from the year a claim is lodged or registered with the insurer and the year in which the claim is acted upon. For example, in 1993/94, 27.7 claims per 100 000 separations refers to the number of claims lodged. The actual number of claims acted upon, proceeding to a court action or settled in 1993/94 could have been more than or less than 27.7.
Source: Private Communication with NSW Health Department.

147   Illustrative cases and comments

147.1   *Sources of cases*

This section provides examples of common problems which arise in hospitals and become the matter of litigation either for the hospital or the doctor or both. Following each set of examples is a commentary that describes how the maloccurrence might have been prevented. We believe that the case studies presented here provide a realism for hospital professionals beyond descriptions of rising malpractice costs and exhortations to implement quality management programs. In addition, they serve to illustrate the dimensions of the problems described previously.

A hospital administrator might—although we would like to hope they would not—dismiss these illustrations as isolated incidents that might have happened to anyone. To the contrary, we believe that neither hospitals nor doctors become embroiled in these types of incidents in an isolated fashion. Rather, when an incident occurs it usually represents the end of a long line of mishaps that either were not noticed, or were noticed, but as the patient took no action, no corrective action on the part of the hospital followed. Many of the incidents which follow represent a system failure which an effective quality management or risk management program would have averted, or at least alerted the hospital to the likelihood of a recurring problem.

The following case studies derive from the case files of FAI Insurances and The Medical Defence Union and are described with their kind permission. The majority of the studies relate to Australian hospitals; however, some are from the United Kingdom. None are from the United States or other countries. Nevertheless, the comparability is universal and the lessons to be derived are global. Both the description of and the comments that follow these studies are those of the authors, not those of FAI Insurances or The Medical Defence Union.

The summaries presented are of necessity only summaries of complex accounts of events and as such some readers may feel that there is insufficient detail to enable them to make their own judgment. The summaries have been selected because in each case litigation did proceed and because they illustrate quality management issues. They also provide readers with examples of what we see as failed quality management programs, or more likely the absence of any quality management program at all. In selecting actual case studies, we have attempted to avoid the bizarre and unusual and have concentrated, for the most part, on commonly recurring situations. They are everyday situations or routines which are more often than not elementary in nature. The incidents generally took place either in the hospital ward or operating theatre and most involved some element of medical malpractice.

147.2 | *Patient Falls*

CASE 2.1

The patient in this case was in the ward and required assistance in having to be moved temporarily from her bed. In the process of being lifted and moved by nursing staff she fell and broke her left leg.

A claim was brought against the hospital with the allegation being that the hospital failed to provide sufficient or competent staff to move the patient safely.

CASE 2.2

In this case the patient was being prepared for surgery and was taken for a preoperative shower. He mentioned that he was feeling light-headed and giddy. He was left alone in the shower and fell, suffering concussion and injuring his arm.

An action was taken against the hospital for failing to properly attend the patient to and from and during the shower.

CASE 2.3

The patient was admitted to hospital for a curettage and cancer check, which was performed successfully. Soon after returning to her bed after surgery, the patient got out of bed and, in a disorientated state, fell and injured herself. She was knocked unconscious and suffered concussion. The bed had not been fitted with safety rails.

A successful action was brought against the hospital for negligence as a result of this episode.

CASE 2.4

A 62-year-old housewife was admitted to hospital for a sinus washout and laryngoscopy under general anaesthetic. After an uneventful operation she was placed in the left lateral position prior to extubation. During extubation she coughed, rolled on to her back and, although the anaesthetist was holding her shoulder, he could not prevent her falling off the table onto the operating theatre floor. She sustained a laceration and haematoma of the right temporal region and bruising around the right shoulder. There was no bone injury but she remained in hospital four days longer than expected. She complained subsequently of episodes of light-headedness, headaches and a sensation of drumming in her ear, but neurological examination revealed no abnormality.

The Union considered the claim which followed to be indefensible. An anaesthetised patient should not be allowed to fall off an operating table. Since no member of the theatre staff had been available to assist the anaesthetist, the health authority was invited to share in the settlement. The claim was concluded on these terms for a modest sum.

COMMENTS

- Patient falls in hospitals, whether in the wards or elsewhere, are the commonest incidents that occur. A hospital with an effective quality management program ensures that all incidents including falls are formally recorded and, even more importantly, tracked. An incident tracking system helps to identify trends and patterns of maloccurrences and even demonstrates, in the case of falls, individual areas of risk, such as a particular ward, corridor, shower or bathroom.
- Frequently, as in these cases, there is not only harm done to a patient, with resulting legal costs to hospital and doctor, but also additional days of stay which renders the episode a very costly one indeed in a hospital environment hard-pressed for funds.
- Once the problem has been identified its probable causes can be tackled and corrective action, such as an educative program for nursing staff or installation of additional support arrangements in showers, can be undertaken.
- We discuss incidents and incident reporting in a later section of this chapter and again refer to the subject in Part II, Chapter 8 and Part III, Chapter 4.

147.3 *Poor documentation/inadequate medical records*

CASE 3.1

This patient had surgery to remove varicose veins. The operation itself was performed without incident. Despite the fact that the patient had advised of an allergy to rubber on the Admission Form, postoperative rubber bandages were applied to her legs. The patient suffered a severe rash resulting in extreme pain and further treatment.

An action was brought against the hospital alleging that the hospital had failed to properly and reasonably act upon her medical history of allergy.

CASE 3.2

A 29-year-old woman was admitted to hospital by a specialist obstetrician for elective caesarian section, her third.

After delivering a healthy baby, the surgeon noted the patient had a minor degree of placenta praevia. The placenta was removed without difficulty but as the surgeon was closing the abdomen the anaesthetist expressed concern about the patient's falling blood pressure. The surgeon completed the operation.

When the drapes were removed he noticed that the patient was bleeding heavily per vaginam—and she was returned to the operating table where hysterectomy was performed to stop the bleeding. While being transfused with 7.5 litres of blood and 4 litres of volume expander, the patient's heart arrested. She was resuscitated successfully but was found ultimately to have suffered hypoxic cerebral damage. Histopathology revealed that the patient had placenta praevia accreta.

A claim for damages was instituted on her behalf. The Union's experts acknowledged the difficulties faced by the surgeon but were concerned about the poor quality of the medical records, the inconsistencies of the medical reports and the surgeon's delay in recognising the excessive blood loss.

The patient suffered severe injuries; she was virtually blind and quadriplegic but despite only limited intellectual abilities, she was aware of her disabilities. The Union and the member agreed that the claim was indefensible and it was settled out of court for A$1 000 000.

COMMENTS
- The problem of poor documentation by hospital medical staff is a constant and recurring problem. Both in and out of hospital inadequate medical records result in more medico-legal angst than any maloccurrence on the part of the doctor.
- Obstetricians as a group are currently extremely concerned about their exposure to legal claims and the cost to them of indemnity insurance and yet, in the course of our encounters, they of all hospital medical staff seem to be least mindful of the need for good, detailed documentation of clinical activity. As we record elsewhere, a tendency by some obstetricians to make no medical notes in the circumstances of a normal confinement led on one occasion to a very heavy settlement for a legal action against an obstetrician and the hospital.
- We discuss the problems and issues related to medical records and clinical information in Part III, Chapter 5.

147.4 Absence of practice policies
CASE 4.1

A 31-year-old mine official was referred to an orthopaedic surgeon because of continuing problems with his left knee following an injury sustained some years before. The surgeon advised physiotherapy but as that was unsuccessful the patient was admitted for surgery. After the patient had returned to the ward it was discovered that the surgeon had operated on the right knee instead of the left. A series of omissions had led to the mistake: he had not checked the consent form, he did not look at the patient's wristband nor the theatre list, he did not take his notes to the theatre and he had failed to mark the limb which was to be operated on. The claim which followed could not be defended and was settled out of court.

COMMENTS
- The behaviour of this surgeon, to say the least, was sloppy and careless, and in keeping with the general assumption that this type of behaviour is rarely an isolated instance, we would believe that this or similar occurrences had happened on previous occasions.
- However, as we discuss in Part II, practice policy committees should determine the type of procedures necessary to avoid situations similar to the above. Practice policies should be documented.

147.5 Absence of adequate infection control
CASE 5.1

This patient had surgery performed to a leg. The operation was without incident or complication. After the operation, bandages were applied over the wound but were not changed for five days. The wound became infected and the patient required pain killers and had to stay in hospital for a further three weeks.

A successful action was brought against the hospital for pain and suffering.

CASE 5.2

The patient, a young male, was admitted to hospital for reconstructive knee surgery. The operation was performed by a staff surgeon. The knee became badly infected and resulted in subsequent amputation of the leg. A study and review of hospital records indicated that sterilisation procedures in force had not been properly adhered to by staff. It was also possible that some of the equipment used in the operation had not been suitably cleaned for the purpose of the surgery.

As might be imagined, the hospital was found liable and a judgment of very heavy damages was made.

CASE 5.3

The patient had surgery performed successfully, but a few days after discharge she developed staphylococci sores around her mouth and nose. She was advised that she had 'dirty mask syndrome'. The incident resulted in a series of outbreaks, with resulting anguish and scarring.

A settlement was made to the advantage of the patient and involved the insurer and the hospital in significant financial cost.

COMMENTS

- These cases of failed or non-existent infection control programs demonstrate the risk to hospital and doctor, not to mention the patient, of inadequate attention to this essential element of a quality management program.
- These instances suggest that nursing practices and protocols either did not exist or supervision of staff was such that they were not routinely followed. These case studies also clearly demonstrate the added cost to the patient, the hospital, the health insurance fund and the entire system by poor quality care.
- As with previous problems, it is impossible to believe that theatre staff had adopted an attitude to sterilisation and sepsis on these occasions which were different from all other occasions. Good infection control is an example of monitoring on a continuing basis which is integral to an effective quality management program. The fact that the records, in one case, revealed inadequacies in the infection control procedures would confirm our suspicion that this incident was not isolated.
- Hospitals that have large proportions of surgical cases sometimes use the monitoring of infection control as their major quality management activity. A good infection control program, with an experienced infection control nurse, would have identified the problems in these hospitals; would have determined whether the problem was one of nursing or medical origin; and would have looked at the technique of sterilisation and determined the need for further training for nursing staff. Such an infection control nurse would have more than paid for his or her salary with the amount of any one of these claims.
- The prevention of these claims and the trauma to the hospitals, including the effect on morale, adds real meaning to the term 'risk management'. The ultimate proof of the adequacy of infection control procedures is the absence of nosocomial infections. Their occurrence should be a signal for action in order to analyse the causes and improve procedures.
- We refer to such monitoring as part of the role of the QM Committee and the QM Department in Part III, Chapters 4 and 6.

| 147.6 | *Medication errors*

CASE 6.1

- This patient was an elderly woman who was admitted to hospital for investigation of cellulitis of her left foot. On the night of admission the patient was given three times the prescribed dose of morphine. The error arose through the misreading by the nurse of the doctor's order. In spite of countermeasures and although the patient apparently returned to normal, after five to six days she developed septicaemia and died. Not surprisingly, legal action resulted in heavy damages.

COMMENTS

- Medication errors are still very common in most hospitals. Doctors on their part constantly fail to associate their illegible handwriting with the reason for their precise orders not being accurately executed. Poor medication protocols and delivery systems in many hospitals, and human error, are the reason why nurses have the major involvement in medication errors. All medication errors should be treated as incidents and all should be formally recorded. It is part of a quality management program to track all incidents including medication errors. By a system of tracking it may be possible to understand why medication errors are occurring and institute effective preventive measures. They may include, for example, an education program for nursing staff, a review of nursing practices and procedures, or some action to discipline a medical practitioner who repeatedly fails to write legibly.
- A quality management program, by insisting on good incident reporting and tracking, will provide the information to determine why errors are occurring and data from which action may be taken to diminish this problem. We make reference to incidents and incident reporting later in this chapter and again in Part II, Chapter 8 and Part III, Chapter 4.

| 147.7 | *Retained abdominal swabs*

CASE 7.1

This patient was admitted for abdominal surgery and was operated on by a visiting surgeon. Subsequently, the wound became infected. The patient suffered respiratory problems and severe nausea for approximately two years. An X-ray eventually revealed a retained abdominal swab as the cause of the problems. Subsequent abdominal surgery resulted in cessation of all symptoms.

Here both the surgeon and the hospital were liable for the claim.

COMMENTS

- A retained abdominal swab is a hazard in any abdominal surgery. However, were the procedures and protocols for theatre activity adequate? Did the hospital have any information as to whether or not that surgeon had had a similar incident previously and, if so, on how many occasions? Did the hospital know how many other incidents of a similar nature had occurred in its own theatres with other surgeons? An effective quality management program would be monitoring all such incidents and tracking the record of its surgeons in the hospital. We do not know whether or not this patient's symptoms over a period of two years resulted in readmissions, but the tracking of all readmissions, something rarely done in Australian hospitals, would probably have picked up this patient sooner than otherwise occurred. Reference to incident reporting and tracking is made later in this chapter and again in Part III, Chapter 4.

147.8 | Retained sutures

CASE 8.1

In this case a patient was admitted to hospital for removal of her gall bladder. The operation, for some reason, was conducted in the obstetric ward. While the procedure is said to have been carried out without problems, there was a failure postoperatively to remove the sutures from the wound. Despite pain and discomfort, and only after several postoperative visits to the doctor, was the problem identified and the sutures removed.

A successful legal action against both doctor and hospital was the result.

COMMENTS

- It is difficult to imagine a situation more calculated to trigger litigation than a hospital which permits a surgeon to conduct a major procedure in an obstetric ward. In addition, the quality of nursing care is also subject to question. It would appear that a quality environment had not been created in this hospital. The very existence of a quality management program which can be seen as effective is a useful deterrent to the occasional member of the medical staff or nurse who thinks it might be easier to cut corners. Preventing the surgeon operating on this patient under the circumstances described would have been a good example of risk management. We discuss risk management in Part V.

147.9 | Informed consent

CASE 9.1

In this case the patient entered hospital for the purpose of having varicose veins removed from her right leg. During the course of the procedure, the surgeon noticed a lump in the region of the patient's groin and that the right thigh was swollen. Faced with the alternative of abandoning the procedure, he elected to continue the removal of veins and explored the lump for diagnosis. The removal of tissue in the groin resulted in considerable scarring.

The surgeon was sued on the grounds of not having adequately examined and diagnosed the condition beforehand and for the unauthorised removal of tissue.

COMMENTS

- The question of informed consent is becoming an important issue. The action of the surgeon in this instance could be said to have occurred to anyone. However, it is up to the hospital to create a climate in which any surgeon would think very carefully before conducting a procedure without consent. It has been said that just as eating in company tends to lead to better table manners, so does the mere existence of a quality management program generate greater care on the part of all hospital professional staff.
- Few surgeons can still be unaware of the legal consequences of failing to obtain informed consent. In addition, in this case inadequate preoperative assessment of the patient occurred. An important part of any quality management program is the development by medical staff of practice policies which are helpful guidelines for clinical staff. While many practice policies have been implicit up to the present time, the responsibility of a surgeon under circumstances which occurred in this case perhaps should be spelled out in explicit practice policies. We discuss the question of practice policies in Part II, Chapter 7.

147.10   *Accident and Emergency departments*

CASE 10.1

This case involved the death of a 20-month-old infant. The parents of the child had taken the sick infant to the hospital in the early hours of the morning suffering from diarrhoea and vomiting. Upon arrival at the hospital the parents received what they described as a very cool and rude reception by the doctor, who at first simply inquired as to why they would bring a child to the hospital at such an hour. The child was obviously distressed and demanding fluids and the parents continually asked why the child was blue and whether it was dehydrated. The child was sent home and died two hours later from dehydration.

Both the hospital and the medical officer concerned had heavy damages awarded against them.

CASE 10.2

While playing cricket a solicitor was hit on the tip of his little finger by the ball. In the local casualty department a medical student observed that the finger was swollen and that there was splitting of the pulp tissues. The student recommended an X-ray of the finger. However, the casualty medical officer deemed it unnecessary and arranged only for the wound to be cleaned and sutured. The finger later became infected and an X-ray revealed that a dislocation of the distal inter-phalangeal joint had been missed.

The solicitor immediately made a claim against the casualty officer who was, fortunately, in benefit with the Medical Defence Union. The MDU advised that resisting the claim would be difficult and settled the matter accordingly.

CASE 10.3

A 31-year-old man had just 'put his shoulder out' and was seen by a casualty officer who found a full range of shoulder movement. An X-ray revealed, to the treating doctor's eye, no fracture or dislocation. However, a radiologist reported subluxation of the right acromio-clavicular joint. Five weeks later, this dislocation was diagnosed at another hospital.

A claim resulted alleging that the casualty officer had denied the patient the opportunity to undergo surgical repair by failing to diagnose the injury. Examination of the patient for medico-legal purposes revealed loss of power at the shoulder but, as the surgeon put it, 'no practical disability'. Nevertheless, the Union's expert adviser felt that it would be difficult to defend the failure to diagnose the injury and to bring the patient back for review. He doubted, however, that early surgical repair of the injury would have improved the patient's condition. Much discussion occurred in committee at the Union and reference was made to the frequency of the injury in rugby football and to the success rate of conservative treatment which enables some players to continue to play. Because the patient had been 'deprived of a chance', successful defence seemed unlikely and settlement was made.

COMMENTS

- There is no one area of hospital activity where, from the point of view of the doctor or the hospital, risk management assumes greater importance than the department of accident and emergency.
- There are a number of lessons to be derived from these cases. The first is that any hospital offering an accident and emergency service must understand that the 'emergency' exists in the patient's mind and ensure that the skill and experience of the medical and nursing staff is consistent with the demands of such a service. All

too often, such accident and emergency services are staffed by the most junior and inexperienced of medical staff.

- The second lesson is that the art and skill of oral and, when indicated, written communication with the patient is a vital and integral part of the care provided. The rude and intolerant professional will often convert a concerned and dissatisfied patient into a litigant, at great cost to both the professional and the hospital. Of equal importance is good documentation about what was found, what inferences were made, and what was communicated to the patient and how it was communicated.
- The accident and emergency department must strive to keep a constant balance between the need to train junior staff and the imperative of having experienced staff constantly present. An active quality management program which, for example, monitors the accuracy of X-ray reporting of junior staff and instructs junior staff in the importance of good documentation, as well as monitoring that it is being observed, is vital, as is the need for well-documented practice policies.
- The level of interpersonal care can be assessed by well-constructed patient satisfaction surveys. Patient satisfaction surveys are described in Part IV.
- The instances cited above represent the few which ended in legal action. From the point of view of quality of care provided, there is no way to account for all those similar circumstances where without any legal action there would be little or no awareness of less than ideal clinical care.

147.11 │ Inadequate facilities and resources

CASE 11.1

A 46-year-old solicitor was referred to an ENT surgeon privately because of a firm swelling between the hyoid bone and the upper border of the larynx. A diagnosis of thyroglossal cyst was made and the patient was admitted for its excision. At operation the anaesthetist found the patient difficult to intubate and two doses of suxamethonium were necessary. The operation was uneventful and the patient returned to the ward. There was some bleeding into the dressing and suction bottle and the wound was tender. Two hours postoperatively the patient began to complain of severe pain and he became very distressed. The bleeding increased and a pressure bandage was applied.

The resident medical officer (RMO) was called but ten minutes later the patient complained of difficulty in breathing and he became cyanosed. The RMO noticed that the patient's neck was swollen. The staples were removed but there was little blood clot in the wound. The patient then arrested and resuscitation was commenced. The RMO was unable to intubate the trachea and an attempted tracheostomy was also unsuccessful. Thirty minutes after the arrest the consultant ENT surgeon arrived and performed tracheostomy. Sinus rhythm was re-established and the patient was transferred to the intensive care unit. Over a period of time he remained unresponsive to all stimuli; his pupils were fixed and a CT scan revealed multiple brain infarcts. As there was no evidence of brain stem function the patient was certified dead and the ventilator was switched off.

The Union's expert advisers noted that the emergency arrangements at the private hospital were deficient. The RMO was responsible for all emergency work but he was relatively inexperienced. The ward had been inadequately equipped to cope with emergencies and there was no tracheostomy set readily available. The subsequent settlement was shared by the Union and the private hospital.

COMMENTS

- The facilities and staffing of any hospital must match the level of procedural activity undertaken by the medical staff. If the hospital is unwilling or unable to provide a level of facilities and staffing, it should have a credentialling mechanism which denies medical staff the right to undertake procedures which cannot be adequately serviced.

- An effective quality management program must include a structured credentialling program for all medical practitioners who work in the hospital. We do not know, for example, whether the anaesthetist was experienced or not. In a hospital with a credentialling program, we would not have to wonder. We discuss credentialling in some detail in Part IV.
- In addition, a quality management program entails the development of documented practice policies by the medical staff that should lay down the course of action to be taken in a range of circumstances including emergencies.

147.12 *Inadequate credentialling of medical staff*

CASE 12.1

A 24-year-old man complained of pain and developed neuropraxia following the excision of an osteochondroma from the upper end of the fibula. Two days later a junior doctor evacuated a haematoma but the patient continued to complain of pain and became pyrexial. The consultant orthopaedic surgeon re-explored the leg nine days later and found dead muscle in the lateral and anterior fascial compartments. Despite skin grafting the patient was left with severe disfigurement, deformed toes and the possibility of premature degenerative changes in his knee joint. He eventually had a below-knee amputation.

The man's claim was settled by the Union because the first exploratory operation after an excision of an osteochondroma should not have been delegated to an inexperienced doctor and because there had been unacceptable delays.

COMMENTS

- Deciding what individual doctors are permitted to do in any hospital should be a decision by a properly constituted credentialling process, about which we have more to say in Part IV. A credentialling mechanism which is formal and detailed is an integral part of any quality management program.
- In the case of junior medical staff, well-documented practice policies should be available in a hospital giving clear guidelines concerning what can and what cannot be undertaken by doctors in training.
- The responsibility for actions of junior medical staff rests with their senior visiting medical staff and with the hospital.

148 Incident reporting

Our comments about the case studies reported above show the importance of an effective system of incident reporting and tracking as part of an overall quality management program. In many Australian hospitals, still, 'incidents' are seen merely as mishaps which occur to either patients or staff as a result of physical accidents. Incidents are really much wider than this traditional perspective. The purpose of recording incidents is to identify patterns of care or circumstances which expose the hospital or its staff to unnecessary risk, or which represent opportunities for improving the quality of care. Incidents can be grouped into the following categories:

- staff/patient/visitor accidents (e.g. patient slips in shower);
- staff–patient mishaps (e.g. staff hits patient);
- staff mistakes (e.g. swab left in abdomen; nurse drops patient);
- patient–patient incidents (e.g. patient hits patient);
- patient–staff mishaps (e.g. patient rapes staff member);
- visitor–staff, visitor–patient incidents (e.g. visitor kills patient).

While incident reporting does occur in many Australian hospitals, in most hospitals they are directed to either nursing administration, medical administration or the hospital manager. In some hospitals that is about as far as they go. In addition, we frequently find that many incidents are not reported for a variety of reasons. Nurses fail to report medication errors for fear of retribution. Doctors react very strongly when requested to report medical incidents, seeing it as unwarranted criticism. We have also experienced heads of departments who simply did not understand the meaning of an 'incident' as used in the hospital context. However, the main problem is that these reports frequently are not collated and tracked in a way which enables the detection of patterns of behaviour or events which could lead to effective preventative action and hence improved quality of care.

It is important to know that a surgeon left a swab in an abdomen. It is much more important to know how many times this particular surgeon or this particular theatre team have left swabs in an abdomen. In other words, is it a person failure or the failure of the hospital's operating room procedures? The quality management department should be tasked to collect and to analyse and present the results of such analyses in a form which is meaningful to clinicians and administrators. Proper analysis of incident data may lead to better reporting, promoting a virtuous quality improvement spiral.

Chapter 5

WHY WE NEED QUALITY MANAGEMENT

| 150 | Contents |

It is still necessary to justify quality management to most Australian hospitals. This chapter explains why we need quality management and deals with:

151. Purpose of this chapter
152. Definition of quality of care
153. QM in hospitals: misnomers and lack of integration
154. The missing ingredients—parallels with industry
155. Attitudes of medical staff
156. Quality of care and qualifications
157. Continuing medical education
158. Little utilisation review, even less risk management

| 151 | Purpose of this chapter |

This chapter argues the necessity of and justification for quality management (QM) and quality assurance (QA). In spite of a good deal of talk within hospitals and the medical and nursing professions, lasting now for almost twenty years, such arguments are still required and have not yet been convincing enough to overcome barriers to action. Medical technology, changes in the hospital environment and general expectations about quality and accountability are propelling hospitals towards quality management, often still without their conscious awareness. How hospitals respond to the need for quality management will affect not only the destination but, more importantly, the journey itself.

| 152 | Definition of quality of care |

Once we start to talk about the quality of care we are immediately faced with the need to define what we are talking about. The quality of care literature is beset with jargon and semantics and, like all abstract concepts, quality of care is extraordinarily difficult to define and even more difficult to operationalise. (Part II explores quality dimensions and how it can be measured.) The result is that there are as many definitions of quality of care and quality assurance as there are people prepared to write about the topic.

According to the Institute of Medicine in the United States, for example:

Quality of care is the degree to which health services for individuals and populations increase the likelihood of desired health outcomes and are consistent with current professional knowledge.[1]

To begin to translate the abstract idea of quality to the practical realities in hospitals, we have found the following four short statements of Dr Paul Sanazaro in the United States to be helpful:

The prime purpose of quality assurance activities is to be continually improving the quality and appropriateness of care and services received by all patients.[2]

This is a deceptively simple statement, as we will show, but one which clearly focuses on improvement in patient care and not on catching aberrant practitioners. By implication, it also means that QA is not only about medical care—a point that one needs to emphasise constantly to doctors—but is rather about the totality of patient care. Similarly, it is not directed at any particular practitioner or group of practitioners, nursing, medical or other, but rather about all care delivered to all patients in any one facility.

Quality assurance itself can best be defined as adherence to standards and criteria that are based on current knowledge and sound experience.[2]

The only standards which apply to medical and hospital care in Australia at the present time are organisational standards for health care facilities developed by the Australian Council on Healthcare Standards. These standards make no reference whatsoever to the processes or outcomes of patient care. Recently, the ACHS has begun an initiative to develop so-called clinical indicators in an attempt to develop some measure of clinical outcomes. While commendable, this initiative is still in its early stages.

Clinical indicators represent a series of coarse screens for populations of patients that may or may not indicate a quality of care problem. (Part II, Chapter 8 discusses clinical indicators.) Criteria serve to assess either the process or outcome of care. The development of explicit criteria for the retrospective evaluation of medical care is costly in terms of money and human resources. (Part II, Chapter 7 explains their use.) It is possible, however, and a good deal more practical to make use of explicit criteria developed at great cost elsewhere and, if necessary, to modify them to suit Australian conditions.

Care and services can be considered appropriate when they are indicated by the patient's condition and when they are neither excessive nor deficient.[2]

While there is a good deal of anecdotal evidence to suggest that many services in Australian hospitals are inappropriate, there is little in the way of objective evidence (because no one has made the requisite measurements). Certainly, when considering the level of pathology and radiology investigations there is a widespread perception by both administrators and medical staff that many of them are inappropriate and unnecessary.[3] The question of accuracy of reporting of X-rays and pathology tests is also important. Without formal systems of review there is no way of determining whether these problems exist or not. More importantly, without a formal and structured quality management program, there will be no way to correct problems even if or when they are found to exist.

Assurance under the term quality assurance may be defined as maintaining and formally accounting for the quality and appropriateness of care.[2]

The last of Sanazaro's four statements has particular relevance for Australian hospitals and the traditional Australian hospital culture. If anything is characteristic of the Australian hospital scene, it is the almost complete absence of the formal accounting of quality. In most Australian hospitals, particularly teaching hospitals, there is a great deal of activity, including meetings of medical staff, case presentations and individual supervision of activity, all of which claim to have an impact on the quality of care. However, rarely are quality of care problems or the way in which such problems were resolved ever documented formally. This formal accounting, in a useful way, is the nub of any effective quality management program.

153 | QM in hospitals: misnomers and lack of integration

While hospitals, which jointly represent a multibillion dollar industry faced with potentially crippling legal and financial consequences of malpractice litigation, are still asking why they need a quality management program, no one in the wider industrial world would think to question the need for quality control programs. For almost twenty years doctors in hospitals in Australia have been encouraged by such bodies as governments and the ACHS to involve themselves in what was confusingly referred to initially as peer review, then clinical review, and more recently as quality assurance, quality improvement and quality management. The rapid development of interest, knowledge and techniques in this area has produced, in the space of a few years, a bewildering array of new terms.

In Australia lack of familiarity with concepts underpinning quality management and a failure to understand basic principles has resulted in the use of the terms 'peer review', 'clinical review', 'quality assurance' and 'quality improvement' almost interchangeably with little regard for their real meanings. As a result communication has been seriously impeded and it becomes impossible to have meaningful discussions about, for example, quality improvement if it means something different to everyone taking part. The absence of a common understanding of the terms used has only served to heighten the latent concerns of medical staff and reinforce many of the existing barriers to implementation.

Hospitals have made little effort to institute quality management. In major teaching hospitals and small country hospitals, whether public or private, hospital professionals' efforts have been piecemeal, fragmented, and totally lacking in cohesion and integration. We are not aware of any hospital in Australia where a patient can be admitted, confident that the quality of care he or she will receive will be subject to a formally structured process of scrutiny. Why is this so? If so much discussion about quality assurance, including seminars, workshops and meetings, has taken place, and so many health professionals have tried to become involved, why have the results been so poor? What have been the missing ingredients necessary for success?

154 | The missing ingredients—parallels with industry

154.1 | Industrial quality control

We believe some of the missing factors can be identified by looking at the wider industrial world and thereby assisting health professionals to see the hospital world, to which they are perhaps a little too close, in a somewhat better perspective. If we take as an analogy a high quality motor car, such as the Mercedes Benz, we will see that the factory manufacturing this product has its board of directors, management, a range of highly skilled and qualified professionals and a host of other workers. Comparison of the analogy with the hospital 'factory', whose product is health status improvement, is instructive. It helps to illuminate why we have not been more successful in our struggle to introduce quality management programs into Australian hospitals.

Our Mercedes factory takes quality control very seriously indeed. Management allocates 8% of the total operating expenditure to the quality control program and, unlike the current situation in our hospitals, the quality control program involves the entire factory and everyone working in it [Personal communication with Mercedes Benz (Australia).] This quality control program is not something left to the whim of the professional engineers, and we certainly do not find the fragmented arrangements so common in hospitals, where one group of professionals may be engaged in some quality management activity but not the remainder. The idea that key professionals, such as the medical staff, could opt out of a total quality control program, when translated to the environment of our Mercedes factory, would be seen as ludicrous. In industry the quality control program is a policy issue for the directors and the management; not one left to originate from professional staff. Nevertheless, even in general industry, both management and professional staff have to be committed to and participate in the program if it is to succeed.

It is worth reminding ourselves about the respective roles of board and management. The board is concerned about the company's wellbeing. The company's prosperity (and board members' wellbeing) depends mostly on the quality of its end products and the board wants to assure it. The management is concerned with the mechanisms necessary to achieve desired product quality. If the quality of the end product is not adequate, it is the responsibility of the board to bring in more effective management. The board does not concern itself directly with finding out why the product is unsatisfactory or with trying to fix inadequate quality management mechanisms.

The Australian hospital industry has tried, with varying degrees of enthusiasm, to introduce quality management programs into a complex environment with little more than minimal resources. Looking to health professionals to initiate such programs without the commitment, involvement or support of the governing body or management and without specific allocation of resources for this purpose was a fundamental error. Unlike industry, boards of directors and management of hospitals have been very slow to appreciate their pivotal role in the introduction of quality management programs. Without a commitment by a board of directors to a quality control program, whether the facility be a Mercedes factory or an acute care hospital, no policy will be developed, no resources will be allocated and the end result will be that very little will be achieved.

No one in the car industry would believe for one moment that the quality of their product should rest solely on the qualifications of their engineers, and yet the hospital industry continues to do just that. In the matter of qualifications of staff and its relationship with quality, patient care in hospitals is no different in principle from the Mercedes car. Analogous with car production, patient care in a hospital is a multidisciplinary affair, and systems relying on the qualifications or ad hoc efforts of medical, nursing or other staff alone will never be sufficient to assure the quality of care, especially since improving health status is far more complex than manufacturing products. Implementing a QM program in a hospital is infinitely more difficult than one for manufacturing. It is not possible to simply copy the approach of the manufacturer and expect it to work in a hospital environment. However, what the hospital industry does need to copy from industry is the commitment to quality, entailing as it does the measurement of performance and the seeking of ways to improve.

154.2 *Hospital-wide and integrated quality management*

Industry uses such terms as total quality management (TQM), total quality control (TQC) and continuous quality improvement (CQI) to describe the environment we have alluded to by way of our Mercedes analogy. These terms imply an involvement by the entire facility and everyone working in it. These concepts are aimed at ensuring continuing efforts to improve the quality of all goods or services produced. In similar fashion, the quality management program of a hospital involves the entire hospital and all staff who work in it. A QM program purview is much wider than clinical services and the performance of doctors or nurses. It embraces management, outdoor staff, telephonists and all the spectrum of staff that goes to make up the workforce of a modern hospital. The integration of the search for quality by all these staff is part of a QM program because they are part of the production process and their performance shapes product quality. Integration means communication. The fragmentation of care and the isolation of units and departments, and the professionals who work in them, renders communication a constant and common problem.

When it comes to quality management activity the integration between different professionals such as nurses and medical staff, the integration between different specialties such as physicians and surgeons, the integration even within the subspecialties of the major specialties, and the integration between the different service areas of a hospital, presents a challenge that cannot be solved without special organisational arrangements. The primary structure for this hospital-wide integration is the quality management mechanism itself, because quality management focuses on the hospital's main product—namely, the improvement of patients' health status. How to achieve a program which involves the entire hospital and everyone working in it on a continuing basis is a major challenge yet to be faced in Australia.

155 | Attitudes of medical staff

There is still a widespread feeling among some medical staff and many hospital managements that this whole question of quality management is really a potentially expensive whim of a few enthusiasts and that in reality the standard of care in Australian hospitals is high and may even be improving. This attitude is largely explained by attitudes which equate quality with qualifications and confuse quality (excellence) with sophisticated technology. As a result, quality management as a systematic activity is not perceived as an important part of their hospital activity and holds a low level of interest for many hospital medical staff.

While the lack of effective quality management can only be partially attributed to medical staff, as we have emphasised, it has to be recognised that doctors' attitudes can be summed up as follows:

* some doctors think QM is unnecessary;
* some think it necessary but not achievable;
* some think it is achievable but not cost-effective or not worthwhile;
* some think it is worthwhile but impractical because some doctors think it unnecessary.

Common wisdom suggests that overall quality of hospital care in Australia has a sound basis. That does not mean, of course, that there is no room for improvement, and in some areas more than others. However, even if hospital care were perfect, it needs to be demonstrated that no improvement is needed or, if needed, such improvement is not possible. Why do we need to demonstrate or document quality of care? Apart from having a fiduciary responsibility, unless one looks for inadequacies or improvement opportunities they will not be found. Further, publishing data about performance spurs competition and extends our ideas about what is achievable. Demonstrating how good hospital care is, or identifying areas needing improvement, is part and parcel of a quality management program.

156 | Quality of care and qualifications

156.1 | Undue reliance on 'qualifications' to assure quality

Astonishingly, most medical staff and directors on hospital boards, particularly those in teaching hospitals, ask, 'But don't we already have high quality patient care in our hospital because we have well-trained and highly-qualified specialist medical staff?' The linkage of quality to higher specialist qualifications is repeatedly invoked.

The answer is that for the great majority of our hospitals we really do not know whether we have high quality care or not. As we do not routinely measure any aspect of quality including the process or the outcome of hospital care in Australia, how can we judge quality? Even if some patients do receive high quality care, we have no way of knowing how variable the quality of care to all patients is. One feature of high quality care is low variability of quality from patient to patient. For a given patient, low variability is an assurance of what to expect.

If we were to measure the quality of care indirectly by the number of patient complaints or the number or size of legal actions taken against medical staff and hospitals, we might have an indirect measure about the quality of hospital care. Unfortunately, even these data are difficult to come by. One thing, however, is certain: while well-qualified and experienced medical staff are an important ingredient of quality care, they in no way guarantee it.

Medical staff in Australia tend to have difficulty when faced with such an assertion, because they are trained to think only in terms of medical care, and because the concept of higher medical qualifications equating with quality of care is embedded in the hospital and medical culture. This attitude of medical staff conveniently ignores situations where, for example, a specialist anaesthetist conducts thyroid surgery; where a general surgeon engages in major urology; where a general surgeon undertakes gynaecological procedures and vice versa; and where hospital staff undertake new (experimental) procedures as if they were simply routine, sometimes with disastrous results.

The incidence of medical and hospital malpractice litigation does not fall only on practitioners who lack higher qualifications. Indeed, recent case studies include academics, staff specialists and visiting specialists, as well as general practitioners.

156.2 *Not doing rather than not knowing*

The basis of most quality of care problems can be traced to deficiencies within the system of care, not the individual performance of providers (doctor, nurse or other staff member). Nevertheless, occasionally, poor performance is a cause of poor quality care. In these cases it is only rarely that poor quality care is due to actual lack of knowledge on the part of the health professional. Rather, most quality of care problems due to poor performance are due to lack of skills and are the result of attitudinal problems such as lack of motivation, lack of interest and extremes of personality. Where quality management demonstrates lack of knowledge or skills on the part of a medical practitioner, some form of medical education is indicated. However, unfocused continuing medical education will not improve quality of care. Quality management is a valuable tool to improve the efficiency and effectiveness of continuing medical education.

157 Continuing medical education

157.1 *Lack of problem identification mechanisms*

Hospital medical staff are always quick to point out there are many meetings and discussions and 'other forms of review' in their hospital. Closer inspection will usually reveal that what medical staff are referring to are meetings structured on the medical education model. These and similar meetings are often incorrectly designated 'peer review'. This medical educational model, involving case presentations and discussions, is usually heavily orientated towards 'interesting cases' and is important intellectually for medical staff as well as beneficial in improving diagnosis and management—but it is not effective quality assurance. It cannot systematically identify problems in caring for patients, since it traditionally focuses only on single cases.

In addition, for a variety of reasons such meetings will usually ignore patient care problems relating to an individual practitioner, even if they do surface, and generally are directed solely at vigorously examining issues of diagnosis or management in unusual or rare and interesting clinical situations. Moreover, such meetings are rarely multidisciplinary and hence will never hear about aspects of care other than medical care, thus avoiding critical aspects of the total quality of care picture. Educational meetings in the form of lectures, or case presentations and discussions, are an important part of the care process but are not a mechanism to assess and document the quality of care.

There are two links between educational meetings and quality assurance. Firstly, problems of care which do surface in the course of a clinical meeting should be referred to a quality management committee which is geared to explore the issues and take corrective action. Secondly, educational meetings should represent the consequence of effective quality management to ensure that they focus on problems of inadequate knowledge, skills or attitudes highlighted by the quality management activity.

157.2 | Lack of problem resolution mechanisms

One of the main weaknesses of medical educational meetings being used or mistaken for a mechanism for assuring quality of care is such a meeting's inability to resolve identified problems because of the lack of an effective problem resolution mechanism and the absence of any feedback loop. This lack of action is due to the absence of organisational structure and lack of integration of such activities which alone renders effective action possible.

We have witnessed such a meeting where a real issue of inappropriate medical services did arise. Services which had been conducted on a number of patients were clearly regarded by the meeting as unnecessary. After considerable discussion and increasing frustration those present came to the conclusion that they could do nothing further because there was no mechanism by which they could resolve the problem that they had identified. Instances like this merely serve to emphasise the need for formally structured quality management programs that are able to provide a mechanism for problem resolution.

The universal absence of an organisational structure to convert identified problems into action which leads to problem resolution is the key weakness throughout hospitals in Australia. Furthermore, where elements of quality management do exist they are characterised by a lack of integration and coherence, which renders useless any value they may have otherwise had.

158 | Little utilisation review, even less risk management

158.1 | Clinical care

Most hospitals when asked about quality management or quality assurance will seriously assert that such activity does exist in their hospital. Doubtless, sporadic instances of review do occur but are usually limited to one or two individuals in a particular department, and because there is an almost universal lack of an organisational structure to enable it to happen, there is rarely any action as a result of such studies. Utilisation review in the form of data relating to the use of investigations is often presented to directors at board meetings. Rarely if ever is such data available to medical staff. Even more rarely is any effort undertaken to determine why the utilisation of a particular modality of investigation has risen, let alone any effort to apply corrective action should that be necessary. Risk management, other than in a very limited sense as it applies to vehicles and workers' compensation, is an unknown entity in Australian hospitals and the level of hospital and medical litigation is testimony to that.

158.2   *The work environment*

Too little attention is paid, and not only in Australia, to the relationship between the performance of medical staff and workload. Even the greatest surgeon is likely to make mistakes when confronted with an unbearable case load. The workload and intolerable hours of work for many junior medical staff has been highlighted recently in several states in Australia. As the day-to-day care of patients in teaching and metropolitan hospitals frequently falls to these trainee medical staff, it would be instructive to see some objective data concerning the quality of care that their patients are receiving. The work environment does not consist solely of hours of work. Satisfactory facilities for visiting obstetricians to rest—and even sleep—while supervising a confinement; adequate space and facilities for medical staff to write and complete documentation, and other comforts which enable very busy and often stressed professionals to perform under ideal circumstances, may all make a significant contribution to ultimate quality of patient care.

References

1 Institute of Medicine. Medicare: A strategy for quality assurance. Lohr KN, ed. Washington DC: National Academy Press, 1990.
2 Sanazaro P. Unpublished paper presented to a meeting of International Quality Assurance. Orlando, Florida, USA. 1986.
3 McLean RG. Diagnostic imaging: reversing the focus. Leading article. Medical Journal of Australia. Vol. 161, 17 October 1994.

Part II

Concepts in Quality Management

SUMMARY

Over the past 100 years or more, manufacturing has developed and progressed the concepts of quality management, quality assurance and quality improvement. The same principles of quality management apply to any organisation, be it a factory or a hospital. The difficulty is to translate the well-developed concepts from industry to an idiom that is understandable and makes sense to hospital professionals. Using industrial analogies, Part II does just that.

For many health professionals, some of these concepts may seem strange and unnecessarily complex. However, as in any other area of activity in health care, practical application is always assisted by a theoretical framework and, to aid understanding, this part deliberately repeats relevant basic concepts in each of its nine chapters. As a result they can stand alone while at the same time they provide a coherent whole. The nine chapters, each of which focuses on a particular aspect of quality management, are:

Chapter 1 *Introduction*—provides a brief overview of the material in the remaining eight chapters.

Chapter 2 *Total quality management*—describes this management philosophy in some detail and how the reality differs from the popular perception of many industrial organisations and hospitals.

Chapter 3 *The health system*—describes the health system and its parts and emphasises the importance of distinguishing between quality of the health system and quality of health care provided at the workface or production level.

Chapter 4 *Health as a production function*—introduces health care as a production system, involving a major paradigm shift, and demonstrates how this approach aids in a fuller understanding of requirements for quality management.

Chapter 5 *Quality and its measurement*—describes the assessment and measurement of clinical quality of care and the various methods by which this can be approached.

Chapter 6 *Quality management, assurance and improvement*—provides a framework for understanding the real meaning of these terms and introduces concepts such as conformance to standards and problem identification and resolution.

Chapter 7 *Practice policies and criteria*—practice policies provide guidance or instruction to providers about how patients should be managed, including who should manage them and where. This relatively recent development is explored together with associated concepts of criteria.

Chapter 8 *Structured quality improvement*—elaborates on the mechanisms to improve quality by identifying problems and resolving them in a structured fashion.

Chapter 9 *Management of quality management*—describes the various elements required to manage such a complex and diverse undertaking as a quality management program.

Chapter 1

INTRODUCTION TO AND PURPOSE OF PART II

210	Contents

This chapter introduces the concept of and context for quality management and describes this part's purpose and contents under the following major headings:

211. Purpose of this part
212. Contents of this part
213. Purpose of this chapter
214. Purpose and nature of quality management
215. Quality management in hospitals
216. Quality management system
217. The quest for quality
218. Origins of quality management
219. Forces driving toward health care quality management

211	**Purpose of this part**

Quality management (QM) is a new concept. It portends a revolution in health care's production function: what health care is provided and the way that services are delivered. Health care quality management represents the confluence of two hitherto quite distinct streams of evolution: the integrated manufacture of goods, most recently in factories distant from customers (often half a world away), and the custom provision of health care services, most recently in hospitals (which are still predominantly local, even though high-technology medical care, like manufacturing, is becoming global). The synthesis of these separate traditions forms this part's core.

Most hospital managers, doctors and other health care professionals are quite unfamiliar with quality management and the revolution it portends in health care. They can either help shape this revolution or allow it to shape their work. This part describes the concepts that underlie quality management, particularly those central to this manual's approach for its implementation in hospitals. This part intends to place the concept of quality management in the broad context of health care provision and to provide:

- a brief background to quality management and its constituent elements;
- a framework for the rest of the manual;
- a common reference to aid understanding and communication.

Quality management is a large, complex subject that lies at the heart of practice. This part provides a coherent view of health care quality management with particular reference to hospitals. It defines important terms to be consistent with this view and, consequently, definitions may vary from those with which readers are familiar. This part draws on industrial analogies because they are simple enough to understand and are good metaphors. Moreover, as this part explains, health care *is* a production function and industrial analogies are often as much material as they are metaphor. The following points deserve special mention.

First, this part covers a vast subject matter, far too vast to cover any of its multitudinous aspects in detail. It does not intend to be a textbook on quality management, nor a scholarly synthesis of information contained in the medical or other literature; nor to be exhaustive, nor to present all points of view. There are many ways to improve quality. This manual describes various useful concepts, methodologies and techniques, but necessarily stops far short of specifying a complete quality management system in a one-size-fits-all package or of providing a detailed how-to guide. A plethora of so-called quality improvement initiatives have been, and continue to be, proposed or pursued. Some are likely of dubious or limited value, despite pressures for their widespread adoption. This part describes several of these suspect initiatives and their conceptual flaws.

Second, one must distinguish macro (system-level) concerns, such as national health policy, from micro (production-level) considerations, such as the delivery of health care in hospitals. This manual describes system-level concerns only to provide a context for, and to distinguish them from, production-level considerations, which are the part's focus.

Third, quality management is a philosophy of, or approach to, management. Clearly, being a better manager of organisations, and even managing one's own time better, can only result in one being more productive. Further, one's attention on what one intends to achieve and trying to achieve it more perfectly can only result in improved performance. This manual does not intend to transmute organisations or managers. Rather, it intends to explain to hospital managers, and doctors and other professionals who work within them, why they should change their organisation and operations, describe what types of changes to make, and guide them in institutionalising these changes.

Fourth, quality management applies to everything that goes on within hospitals, including clinical and patient care (e.g. doctors' decisions, nursing, physiotherapy), clinical support services (e.g. imaging, laboratory), operational services (e.g. laundry, housekeeping), and administration (e.g. accounting, personnel). To date, quality management in hospitals—where it has been applied at all—has been limited generally to such operational services as the laundry, because they are simple situations and most resemble industrial operations. This manual focuses on clinical care—the heart of hospitals' production function—which hospitals have largely ignored or addressed inadequately. Nevertheless, the same quality management principles (described in this manual in relation to clinical care) apply to everything else that goes on in hospitals.

Fifth, health care quality management is complicated and so are, or appear to be, many of its underlying concepts, especially when encountered for the first time. This inherent complexity limits the amount of simplification that is possible without losing the concept being explained.

Sixth, quantification of both production and products is necessary to improve quality. Only in the last few years has it become possible to quantify the quality of health care in a practical way. This part describes the concepts that underlie and the methods that make practical the routine measurement and assessment of health care quality.

Seventh, quality management involves measurement—quantification of quality— which requires use of statistics. While knowledge of statistics is essential for effective quality management, this part deliberately minimises discussion of statistics to make concepts as accessible to as many readers as possible. Nevertheless, reference to statistical concepts is inevitable and, when mentioned, they are explained without going into detail.

Eighth, quality management requires a distinct body of knowledge and experience, beyond that required to practise medicine, for example. Effective quality management requires teams of managers, doctors, and health and social scientists working together. Some, and preferably all, team members must be trained specifically in QM principles and techniques. Quality management requires knowledge about measurement and decision making (e.g. biostatistics, epidemiology, systems theory and decision science) and management and organisational development (e.g. production systems, human factors, planned change). While this manual intends to provide an overview of quality management and may be useful as course material, it cannot substitute for formal instruction and guided experience.

212 Contents of this part

Part II consists of nine chapters, including this one.

- This chapter, *Introduction to and purpose of Part II*, states the part's purpose, defines and describes the origins of quality management and explains the forces driving inexorably toward its adoption in health care. The chapter intends to give the reader an appreciation for the part's subject matter and an overview of the most important aspects of quality management on which subsequent chapters elaborate.
- Chapter 2, *Total quality management*, describes the industrial origins of this management philosophy, on which this manual elaborates in the context of hospitals, and provides an introduction to the idea of the systematic improvement of products and production. The chapter intends to provide a brief background to the concept of the management of organisations, particularly the quality of their products and production function, and to highlight how, today, hospitals fail to match up to these requirements.
- Chapter 3, *The health system,* describes the concept of the health system (the totality of interventions that intend to maintain or to improve the population's health) and focuses on the largest of its components, the health care system (personal health services that respond to individuals who seek help, which account for the largest share of total health care expenditures). The chapter intends to provide a context for health care quality management and to show how it both is affected by and affects the health care system.
- Chapter 4, *Health as a production function*, expresses ideas that are fundamental to understanding health care quality management. The chapter intends to explain how, for quality management purposes, hospitals are health-producing facilities, and that a hospital's product—health status improvement—depends on the patients it treats, how it treats them and the environment in which treatment takes place.
- Chapter 5, *Quality and its measurement*, explains that quality is a multidimensional concept, that trade-offs may have to be made, and that customers (patients in the case of hospitals) must make them. The chapter intends to explain that health care quality can be measured, and to show how it should be measured and assessed for quality management purposes.

- Chapter 6, *Quality management, assurance and improvement*, describes how quality can be assured and improved. The chapter intends to explain quality assurance, utilisation review, risk management, and their interrelationships, and to describe the essence of a complete quality management system.
- Chapter 7, *Practice policies and criteria*, focuses on specifying health care's product for quality management purposes. The chapter intends to explain the pivotal role of practice policies and criteria in quality assurance and improvement, and to describe their essence and how to formulate them.
- Chapter 8, *Structured quality improvement*, describes how hospitals can operationalise two interlocking cycles: one to improve conformance to specifications and reduce variation in patient outcomes; the other, to improve specifications. The chapter intends to explain how hospitals can systematically identify and routinely resolve quality of care problems to improve the quality of their care.
- Chapter 9, *Management of quality management*, describes the process of implementing and improving quality management. The chapter intends to explain that quality management in hospitals can, and should, be subjected to the same scrutiny to which quality management subjects patient care.

213 | Purpose of this chapter

This chapter intends to give the reader an appreciation for the part's subject matter and an overview of the most important aspects of quality management on which subsequent chapters elaborate. The remainder of the chapter describes:

- the purpose and nature of quality management and its essential attributes, with reference to industry and to health care, noting the most significant specific differences between them;
- aspects of, and the essential elements of a system for, quality management in hospitals;
- the quest for quality, and origins of quality management;
- forces driving inexorably toward its adoption in health care generally and hospitals specifically.

214 | Purpose and nature of quality management

214.1 | Background

Total quality management (TQM) has become the latest term in the quest for quality and productivity. This management philosophy is customer centred, product focused, measurement oriented, improvement driven and all pervasive. It stresses the long-term view. Quality-focused organisations are totally dedicated to satisfying current and anticipated customers' present and future needs and wants, and to exceeding their value-for-money expectations. Their organising principle is product quality.

Quality-mature organisations strive ceaselessly for excellence and have institutionalised mechanisms to improve continuously the quality of their product and production processes (and its inseparable twin, productivity). Quality management encompasses all of the forms and functions necessary to achieve quality maturity. Its principal outcome is quality improvement. It requires leadership and strong management—not merely a tool-kit of TQM/CQI methods.

Hospitals have a long way to go to achieve quality maturity. Present-day hospitals are not organised for quality-focused production. They do not measure up because they do not measure. Consequently they can neither assure, nor document any improvement in, the quality of their care. Recent breakthroughs in quality measurement technology—

described in this part—permit, for the first time, quantification and systematic improvement of health care quality. Quality-mature hospitals continuously improve quality and patients' health status, at least cost and with greatest patient satisfaction. They measure quality and use results to review and if necessary revise practice and process policies and change production systems and processes to improve quality. Changes in culture, organisation, incentives and the hospital's operating environment are needed to facilitate progress toward this end.

Health care quality management promises to fulfil a cherished dream: knowing realistically what one can expect from medical intervention and being sure of getting it. Quality management can be as liberating for hospitals and doctors as it is reassuring for patients.

214.2 The meaning of quality

The meaning of quality and the means for its improvement vary by health system level. Production-level quality is concerned with production outcomes; it involves patient–provider interactions. At the system level, access to care is clearly an important quality consideration and may obviously influence a population's health. However, it is irrelevant at the production level.

Health care's purpose is to improve maximally patients' health status, using interventions consistent with their preferences, providers' circumstances, and society's resources and mores. Health status is an integrated measure of the health quality of life. It encompasses mortality, institutionalisation, morbidity, ability to carry out activities and, in principle, mental and emotional wellbeing. Health status measurement from onset of treatment permits the outcomes of radically different treatments—for example medical and surgical interventions—to be compared validly.

For quality management purposes, health care quality (provider performance) has four dimensions:

- technical quality—measured by patients' health status improvement;
- resource consumption—measured by the cost of care;
- patient satisfaction—measured by patients' perceptions of the subjective or interpersonal aspects of care;
- values—measured by the acceptability of any trade-offs that must be made among the three previous outcomes.

In health care (unlike manufacturing), process specifications define the product because, in practice, it is impractical to routinely measure patients' health status improvement and virtually impossible to attribute reliably any measured improvement to specific interventions. Practice policies—pre-established clinical decision rules for treating individual patients that take into account their preferences regarding ends and means—are the starting point for defining these processes and their expected resultant outcomes. They are the basis for practice, providing direct guidance or instructions to providers about how patients should be managed, including who should manage them and where they should be managed.

Practice policies represent the best way to manage individual patients and may encompass sociopolitical constraints. They make explicit assumptions between health care processes (specific medical interventions) and patients' health status improvement. If available, which usually they are not, fully elaborated practice policies can be translated easily into practice criteria to assess retrospectively the quality of care. If not available, practice criteria serve this latter purpose. Conformance to practice policies will only improve patients' health status if they are effective. Conformance to effective practice policies will improve quality, but only to the limits of the underlying technologies. Further improvement in health status requires better technologies.

One must distinguish between an intervention's effectiveness and providers' performance—the extent to which providers use an intervention appropriately and implement it properly. Effectiveness is a statistical concept. An effective intervention improves a population of patients' health status. Measuring an intervention's true effectiveness depends on determining the difference between intervention and a disease's natural history in such a way that it can be attributed confidently to the intervention, for example through a well-designed, well-controlled randomised clinical trial. An appropriate intervention can reasonably be expected to benefit a particular patient because he or she fits the profile of patients for whom it is known or assumed to be effective.

214.3   Essentials of quality management

Quality management is a production-level tool for improving production units' performance and products' quality. It is useful to manufacturers in the production of goods and to hospitals in caring for patients. Key concepts include:

- Quality and costs are intertwined; one cannot be managed without regard to the other.
- The quality of goods (produced by manufacturers) or services (health improvement produced by hospitals) results from production systems, not from the efforts of individuals working in isolation (e.g. production workers or doctors).
- Quality management is synonymous with, and required for, good management: achieving an organisation's purpose by improving its products and production system.
- Quality management is an integral part of production or service delivery, not something separate.
- Quality management can, and should, be subjected to the same scrutiny and continuous improvement to which it subjects an organisation's production function.
- Concepts, techniques and tools needed to implement quality management exist already (but, as with all aspects of production, can be improved continuously).

Considered broadly, quality management encompasses three distinct, but inextricably related, aspects of products and their production:

- production—manufacturing or health improving processes;
- product—what is to be produced and how it is to be produced; that is, the design of products and the processes to produce them;
- product and process technology—know-how to design products to please customers and processes to produce them efficiently.

214.4   Essentials of industrial quality management

214.41 PRODUCTION

In manufacturing, most immediately a product's quality depends on the quality of the processes used in its production and the inputs to these processes. The ultimate measure of quality is customers' satisfaction with the product, which depends, at least in part, on the product's performance, both technically (e.g. its reliability and durability) and functionally (in terms of meeting customers' needs). Key concepts include:

- Products must be specified in measurable terms (and techniques must exist that produce reliable measures of specifications, e.g. the length of a bolt).
- The results of such measurements must be used to control production processes (e.g. statistical process control); the goal is zero defects (i.e. all products meet

specifications with as little variance as possible). Production systems and processes are organised toward this end.

- Products' performance and customers' satisfaction must be measured to provide the information necessary to improve production processes and products' design.

214.42 DESIGN

Product design is the key to, and an order of magnitude more important to ultimate product quality than, production: junk produced perfectly is still junk. Key concepts include:

- Products must be designed to meet customers' needs at a price that they are willing to pay (to offer value for money, especially in comparison to competitors' products).
- Customers must have a voice in product design. Their voices must carry through to the shop floor where the product is made (e.g. through the continuous measurement of customers' experience and satisfaction with current, and reactions to planned, products).
- Manufacturability (the impact of product design on production processes and hence on the quality of the finished product) must be considered explicitly.
- A product's expected cost must be an explicit design consideration. What customers pay for the product (which is determined partly by a product's design and the efficiency of manufacturing processes) is an important dimension of product quality.

214.43 TECHNOLOGY

Product and process design depend on technology; specifically, the limits of knowledge about how to design and produce products that satisfy customers' desires at a price they are willing to pay. Technology—advances in knowledge that permit the design of new products (product technology) or that improve the production of new or existing products that more perfectly meet customers' needs (process technology)—is an order of magnitude more important to ultimate product quality than product design (within the limits of existing technology). Key concepts include:

- Advances in product technology permit the design of products that allow customers to satisfy needs that hitherto could not be satisfied, to more perfectly satisfy needs that are being satisfied imperfectly at present, or to satisfy needs at a lower cost (thereby freeing resources to satisfy other needs).
- Advances in process technology permit the improved production of new or, particularly, existing products, for example products that more perfectly meet specifications (and/or meet them with less variance) or that cost less than those produced with existing processes.
- In the years ahead, relevant technological innovation will increasingly be the key to competitiveness, and, consequently, success will go to organisations that can systematically and rapidly exploit technology toward winning clients and meeting their needs and wants.
- In the years ahead, process technology, which is often embodied in production systems, is likely to be a far more important determinant of competitiveness than product technology, which rapidly becomes available to everyone.

214.5 | Essentials of health care quality management

214.51 PRODUCTION

In health care, product quality—patients' health status improvement—depends on perfecting the fit between patients' characteristics and the processes that, if implemented properly, would result in the greatest improvement in health status (patient–process fit) that is achievable within patient's preferences, with respect to both ends and means and society's resources. Providers' knowledge, skills and attitudes, and access to equipment, as well as the interventions for which health financing schemes are willing to pay, limit quality. Key concepts include:

- Health status improvement (technical quality) is often patients' overriding concern, especially with serious health problems (but other concerns include cost—especially those costs that patients must pay directly—and patient satisfaction with the interpersonal aspects of care).
- All dimensions of quality should be maximised to the greatest extent possible, although trade-offs must often be made, and the acceptability of these trade-offs to patients is the final dimension of quality.
- Achieving a perfect patient–process fit and ensuring that specified processes are implemented properly, thereby ensuring zero production defects, is far more difficult than achieving zero defects in manufacturing.
- Variance reduction must strive toward improving poor provider performance (and, secondarily, eliminating poor performers), while encouraging good performers to do even better. In health care, process variance reduction is a means for, but not necessarily the primary goal of, quality management. In manufacturing, process and product variance reduction is both means and end.
- Health care processes and patient outcomes must be assessed simultaneously and continuously to determine the extent to which processes conform to care specifications and produce expected outcomes. Results must be used (feedback) to change processes toward improving the quality of care.
- It is relatively easy to measure outcomes, but quite difficult to attribute them confidently to preceding interventions. Attributing outcomes to processes (or other factors) is the key to quality improvement, but it is far more difficult to do confidently in health care than in manufacturing.
- Systems must be in place to determine why practices vary from policies and why observed outcomes vary from expected outcomes—which might be the result of non-conformance to policies—and to decide whether or not such quality of care problems should be resolved and with what priority. Mechanisms must exist to change care systems and processes to resolve quality of care problems, and to determine that problems have been resolved (and remain resolved) and that their resolution can be attributed to changes to the care system or its constituent processes.
- Immediate and long-term outcomes (the end results of care) must be measured and variations investigated to determine if they resulted from inadequate implementation of practice or procedural policies (see following), from inadequate conformance to policies, from inadequate policies, or from inadequate technology. Outcomes encompass health status improvement (and a variety of immediate outcomes, e.g. nosocomial infection), and the cost of, and patient satisfaction with, care.
- Quality management activities' results must be used to improve implementation of care processes and conformance to policies (through improving care systems and their components), to improve policies (through their revision in light of new information), and to improve technology (through drawing attention to the inadequacy of existing technology and setting priorities for research and development).

214.52 PRODUCT

Health care's product—health status improvement—is embodied in practice and procedural policies. To date, such policies have been conspicuous by their absence. For all practical purposes, hospitals can assure and improve the quality of their patient care only by adopting and adhering to practice and procedural policies. In general, hospitals lack the resources to develop practice policies; they must either collaborate to develop practice policies or adopt or adapt those developed by others (e.g. professional colleges and societies). Key concepts include:

- For production purposes, practice policies define health care's product. They specify what providers should do for patients and, by extension, who should do it (care processes), and what to expect as a result (outcomes). They make explicit assumptions between health care processes (specific medical interventions) and individual patients' health status improvement. This part focuses on practice policies and their use to define and, through structured quality improvement, to assure and improve the quality of care.
- Procedural (or process) policies operationalise elements within practice policies and thus specify them in greater, operational, detail. If a practice policy indicates that total hip replacement is the treatment of choice for a particular patient, for example, procedural policies would describe in relevant detail exactly how the operation is to be conducted, including, for example, operative preparation, type of prostheses, technique of insertion, postsurgical nursing care, discharge planning and rehabilitation.
- Quality improvement depends not only on the proper implementation of and conformance to practice and procedural policies, but also on improving them (e.g. through feedback generated by outcomes measurement and accommodating new product and process technology).
- For the immediate future, proper use of existing knowledge (process technology) manifest in adoption of and adherence to practice and procedural policies (e.g. for the treatment of colon cancer) can improve patient outcomes (the quality of care) to a far greater extent than any so-called breakthroughs that might be anticipated— the quixotic quest for incremental improvement in product technology. It also harbours the hope of containing health care costs.

214.53 TECHNOLOGY

Ultimately, quality improvement depends on better practice and procedural policies which, in turn, depend ultimately on better product and process technology. In health care, product technology is knowledge about disease processes and interventions to alter their course or cause. Process technology is knowledge about how to deliver interventions most cost-effectively. Key concepts include:

- To date, investments in research to improve health care technology have been inadequate to the task; virtually nothing has been spent on improving process technology. More money needs to be spent, especially on process technology.
- Only a fraction of funded health research has been immediately relevant to practice and only a fraction of that research has produced useable results.
- Traditionally, hospitals have funded little research, although they may have participated in projects funded by others (e.g. government). Hospitals, as health care providers, should fund research to improve health care technology, particularly process technology, and play a greater role in influencing what research is done (e.g. by government) to ensure that effort is directed to solving the most pressing problems—those that would confer the greatest ability to improve patients' health status (which would likely alter present research priorities).
- The information hospitals could generate from their quality management activities (outlined above) is essential to improve practices and to set research priorities.

215 | Quality management in hospitals

215.1 | Context

Hospitals have yet to come to grips with the quality revolution. In this decade quality management—rational decisions about health care's products and how best to produce them—will be one of the hospital's most significant challenges. Quality management is, or should be, an essential component of hospital management. Everything that hospitals do must be geared to improving patients' health status, reducing the cost of its attainment, and increasing patient satisfaction with the interpersonal aspects of care. Quality improvement depends on describing through data, understanding through analysis and improving through action.

Quality management is useful for improving the quality of hospitals' care. Quality management must include all of the hospital's activities, especially clinical care—the core of its production function. Improving the hospital laundry, while useful, will make very little difference if the quality of clinical care remains unaltered.

Health care system policy decision makers and hospital managers must provide the will, the means and the incentives to measure care processes and their outcomes and to use the resultant information to improve quality. There are no quick-fix solutions. Managers must stay the course and avoid sounding the retreat at the first sign of resistance. Managers must back demands with deeds. They must recognise excellence and reward success. Managers' failure to change can doom quality management efforts every bit as much as their lack of commitment to the structures and processes necessary to implement quality management.

215.2 | Aspects of quality management in hospitals

Quality assurance (QA), utilisation review (UR) and risk management (RM) are distinct but integral aspects of quality management (QM). However, QM encompasses far more than QA, UR and RM. Traditional quality assurance intends primarily to ensure that care conforms to specifications, and to provide information to validate and improve them. Utilisation review intends primarily to ensure that resources are used appropriately by ensuring that patients receive only needed interventions, in the least expensive setting, for the shortest effective duration; and that they do not receive unnecessary tests and procedures or days of care, and that all needed interventions are given (although the latter has traditionally been an aspect of QA rather than UR). Risk management intends primarily to reduce hospitals' exposure to financial loss consequent to providing care, including that which may result from employment of care providers. In practice, review of the utilisation of resources is part of the overall assurance of quality. Hence activities to assure quality of care will include utilisation review and by so doing will reduce the risk of financial loss.

215.3 | Quality assurance and improvement

Traditionally, in North America the term quality assurance (QA) has been associated with postproduction (retrospective) review of care, sometimes called medical audit. This activity has been confined largely to episodic, sporadic, or haphazard case-by-case review of medical records and, if deficiencies were found in care or its documentation, feedback to the doctor who was as likely to argue about the so-called deficiencies as to reflect on or change his or her practices to prevent their recurrence. Almost certainly there was no follow-up to see if problems recurred or not.

Three factors virtually precluded meaningful efforts to change practice and improve the quality of care:

- limiting QA to doctors' activities, with its implicit, erroneous assumption that doctors alone produce patients' health status improvement and that they are the cause of, or their (re)education would resolve, all problems;
- lack of pattern analysis to identify problems and investigate their root causes; and
- absence of systems to rectify any problems for which causes could be elucidated.

In Australia the term quality assurance has been applied inappropriately to any kind of review of any aspect of clinical or non-clinical activities. In this manual the term quality assurance denotes a cyclical process involving retrospective quality assessment— retrospective review of care outcomes and processes based on documentation in the patient's medical record—and subsequent steps to improve care processes to close any performance gaps. In health care organisations the terms quality improvement and, influenced by TQM, continuous quality improvement (CQI) have begun recently to supplant the term quality assurance.

Quality assurance (QA) and quality improvement (QI) are important but distinct aspects of production and product quality; continuous quality improvement (CQI) is merely performing QA/QI on a continuous basis. Arguments about the superiority of CQI over QA are vacuous. In reality, quality assurance is necessary to improve quality. Quality is improved both by better conformance to specifications and by better specifications (those that produce more health status improvement, or the same improvement at less cost or with greater patient satisfaction, and/or less variation in outcomes). This manual refers to the process of perfecting conformance to specifications as the conformance improvement (CI) cycle; that of reviewing and revising product specifications (practice policies that are the basis for QA activities) as the specifications improvement (SI) cycle. For all practical purposes, the conformance improvement cycle is synonymous with the quality assurance cycle. We refer to the combined continuous operationalisation of the CI/SI cycles as the quality improvement spiral.

215.4 | The bottom line

Managing quality costs money. But the lack of quality (quality-cost) can be, and almost invariably is, even more costly. Initially, quality management may increase costs because a hospital must pay for its quality management program and, in some cases, doctors may be undertreating patients now (in comparison to best practices). But in principle a quality-mature hospital can expect lower costs from: reduced liability insurance premiums, malpractice claims and monetary damages; reduced iatrogenesis, specifically preventable errors and clinical complications; reduced unnecessary tests and treatments; improved clinical efficiency resulting from quicker diagnosis, better treatment selection and so on; improved operational efficiency, with resultant better use of resources; and improved productivity through enhanced employee job satisfaction and morale.

Quality management's main benefit is improving the quality of care and reducing variability, giving patients more health status improvement with greater certainty. If quality-oriented care costs the same as or less than present care, that is an added benefit. Certainly, it provides better value for money.

216 | Quality management system

216.1 | Production of health

Health care is a production system that consists of a series of processes shaped by structures, each of which may be a production subsystem with its own process elements. The output of one process is an input to the next or a subsequent process. Health care processes intend to produce patient health status improvement. An effective medical intervention (process) transforms patients (input): patients' postprocess health status (outcome) is greater than it would have been at that point in time without the process. Three sets of variables—and their interactions—produce patient outcomes: health care production processes (producer), the patient's characteristics at the time of entering the process and the environment in which production takes place (coproducers). Attribution of patient outcomes to care processes is the key to quality improvement.

Hospitals are health care's principal production facilities, organisations designed to 'produce' health. They must put in place a complete quality management system—the structures and processes necessary to improve continuously the quality of their products and production processes. Quality management involves principally the design and evaluation of health products and production systems and of their constituent processes, such as coronary artery bypass grafts.

Outcomes must be measured, not assumed. The measurement of outcomes provides information on the end results of care in relation to care processes and patient characteristics. This information can improve the design and content of practice policies, confirm or cast doubt on interventions' effectiveness, point to the need for better interventions and help set research priorities. Research studies, especially randomised controlled trials, provide the best information for formulating practice policies and designing medical interventions and care processes. Such studies must include the cost of practices. The often encountered quest for incremental effectiveness at any price must yield to the search for more cost-effective interventions.

216.2 *Purpose and scope of a complete quality management system*

An effective quality management system assures and improves continuously the treatment of individual patients and the effectiveness of treatments. It encompasses mechanisms to:

- control or assure product quality at each of production's three phases: preproduction (e.g. admissions policies, credentialling, practice policies), intraproduction (e.g. decision support technologies) and postproduction (e.g. quality assessment and quality assurance);
- generate the information needed to validate and improve practice policies and their constituent product and process technologies (e.g. outcomes measurement and research and development);
- manage and improve the quality of quality management.

216.3 *Controlling quality*

216.31 OVERVIEW

Quality control takes places at two levels: the organisation and the workface. Organisations design production systems to produce products to specifications. What occurs at the workface determines products' quality. Ideally, organisational quality control mechanisms promote workface quality and workface experience shapes organisational quality control mechanisms.

For all practical purposes, in the immediate future quality management relevant to clinical care will be limited in most hospitals to adopting and adhering to practice and procedural policies and to ensuring conformance to these policies. To achieve these ends, hospitals must establish a system that includes the following quality control mechanisms—described in this manual—which are classified by their temporal relationship to production processes: preproduction, intraproduction, and postproduction.

216.32 PREPRODUCTION QUALITY ASSURANCE

Hospitals can assure the quality of patient care by controlling the inputs to care process. These inputs include:

- the types of services offered—controlled by hospital service policies;
- patients treated—controlled through admissions policies;
- doctors who treat them—controlled by credentialling;
- how they are treated—controlled by practice and procedural policies.

216.33 IN-PROCESS QUALITY ASSURANCE

In-process quality control—the ability to assure conformance to specifications (practice policies) during care processes—is generally beyond hospitals' present capability. Due to the complexity inherent in useful practice policies, they are best computerised and embodied in expert systems—a type of decision support technology (DST). Expert systems are already available to screen cases for quality of care issues—described in this part—and in the next thirty years DSTs are likely to play an increasing role in all phases of medical practice.

DSTs will provide the means to assist doctors and other health care providers to select the most appropriate diagnostic and therapeutic interventions for the patient's circumstances, and to implement and document them properly. Consequently, the quality of care should improve immensely. Robots will be used increasingly to implement care processes, thereby facilitating further improvements in the quality of care. The introduction of practice info-mation (information-controlled automation such as DSTs and robots) will permit greater attention to the interpersonal aspects of care, creating additional opportunities to improve further the quality of care and produce greater value for money.

216.34 POST-PROCESS QUALITY ASSESSMENT, ASSURANCE

Essentially, retrospective quality assurance mechanisms compare practice policies (what should be done and achieved) to performance (what was done and achieved), and indicate whether or not corrective or improvement action should be taken to change processes toward improving outcomes. By extension, these mechanisms must encompass ways of identifying the appropriate corrective or improvement actions to be taken, the means to implement them, and incorporate feedback mechanisms to monitor the results of such improvement actions to determine if additional corrective action should be taken and to attribute any improvement to changes. An ideal system would also contain elements to ensure the quality of the quality assurance mechanism.

Quality assessment—measuring and monitoring provider performance—is presently the key to quality improvement in hospitals. Through the quality assurance cycle hospitals can compare what is being done and achieved to what should have been done and achieved, and take steps to close any performance gaps. Quality assessment results can inform admissions policies, credentialling decisions and practice policies—the starting point for quality assessment and hence of the quality assurance cycle.

216.4 | *Measurement and feedback are keys to quality improvement*

Quality management means meaningful measurement. Health care has been devoid of meaningful feedback to improve its quality. Actions may be hit or miss, and without feedback no one will know that anything has really improved. Feedback of results to improve practice policies, care processes and quality control elements is the principal missing link to integrate systems and improve the quality of care.

Quality management's central goal is to improve product quality and to reduce production variance. Variation in patient outcomes or deviations from specified processes or expected outcomes may signify a quality problem. Hospitals' goal is to reduce the variation in the fit between what patients need and want, and what they receive. They must implement interventions, for example a surgical operation, as uniformly as practical. Uniformity of process facilitates assessment of variation in outcome by eliminating the obvious factor—variation in process. Variation in outcomes detracts from quality because it represents risk to patients. Quality managers must reduce variance in outcomes while simultaneously increasing average patient health status improvement. In some circumstances they may face trading-off increased average health status improvement and reduced variation in such improvement.

Quality managers can improve average health status improvement and reduce variation in individual outcomes for a given type of patient by:

- measuring distributions of patient outcomes—to know the shape of the curve;
- improving conformance to processes (product and production specifications), including removing underperforming providers who prove to be incapable of improving their performance despite the hospital's best efforts to help them to do so—to 'shift the curve to the right';
- improving product and production specifications—to 'lift the curve to the right'.

216.5 Quality improvement strategies

All strategies for improving the quality of care depend ultimately on analysing variation in production performance and resultant outcomes:

- Structured performance benchmarking is based on variation in performance, usually among, but also within, quality-immature hospitals.
- Structured quality improvement is based on variance (deviation) from what should have been done and achieved, or from expectations.
- Structured outcome measurement is based on such variation and variance in long-term outcomes.

Structured performance benchmarking refers to the strategy of measuring competitors' (colleagues') performance to identify the best performers, to discern what processes, patient flows and organisation seem to produce this performance, and to establish where one's performance stands in relation to the best. Consequently, one can align one's production system with that of the best performers toward improving one's performance. Today, structured performance benchmarking is beyond the means of all but large-scale hospital systems. However, the introduction of mechanisms to share valid comparable performance data among the hospitals will make benchmarking a practical reality for even the smallest hospital.

Structured quality improvement refers to a hospital-wide strategy to systematically identify quality problems, discover their root causes and routinely eliminate these causes. Quality-focused hospitals must design and deploy mechanisms for these purposes. It is the basic strategy for improving hospitals' quality of care and it is now practical.

Structured outcome measurement refers to the strategy of measuring the long-term outcomes (end results) of health care interventions. It examines the extent to which conformance to specifications actually improves patient health status and produces information to improve them. It is not a substitute for, but may help prioritise, needed research. Only the largest hospitals are likely to have the resources necessary to launch a structured outcome measurement program or conduct the clinical trials that its results suggest.

216.6 Structured quality improvement

Structured quality improvement (SQI) operationalises the quality improvement spiral. It pertains mostly to conformance improvement (getting done what needs to be done in the way it should be done each and every time), but also informs specifications improvement. Structured performance benchmarking and structured outcome measurement provide information mostly for specifications improvement (what to do and how to do it).

Structured quality improvement involves a hospital-wide system for:

- Structured problem identification—to identify systematically quality problems and their root causes. It involves:
  — defining and measuring or assessing quality;
  — identifying quality problems;
  — determining quality problems' root causes.
- Structured problem resolution—to resolve routinely quality problems and eliminate their root causes. It involves:
  — evaluating and selecting among alternative improvement actions to remedy quality problems and eliminate their root causes;
  — planning and implementing chosen improvement actions;
  — measuring quality to ascertain if it has improved, attributing any observed improvement (or its lack) to improvement actions, and to identifying any other problems that they may have created.

216.7 | Identifying quality problems

Hospitals can employ the following problem identification mechanisms (described in this part):

- systematic review of care or cases (patient records that document care processes and outcomes);
- systematic surveys of people's perceptions and suggestions;
- incident reports, including patient complaints and allegations of malpractice, and compliments;
- quality assurance studies;
- group problem-solving techniques, for example, quality circles.

At a minimum, hospitals must perform hospital-wide systematic surveillance of care or cases, using either, or preferably both, of the following methods (described in this part):

- structured quality assessment—reviewing care case by case—for example structured quality review or unaided structured medical record review to identify and characterise quality problems;
- structured quality monitoring—population based screening—that is, watching rates of events in populations of cases to trigger review of providers' care if rates exceed pre-established limits.

216.8 | Structured quality review

Structured quality review (SQR)—described in this manual—is a practical way to identify quality of care problems in a case. By aggregating results, hospitals can create a quality score to monitor quality improvement. Because it can be implemented easily, with minimal commitment of resources, SQR is likely to be the initial method for, and remain the mainstay of, problem identification in hospitals in Australia and elsewhere for the foreseeable future. Structured quality review involves the following three steps necessary to identify, confirm and illuminate quality of care problems and to reveal patterns of care:

- screening—use of automated outcome/process assessment screens (described in this part) to identify cases that harbour potential quality problems and that thus require further review;
- review—use of structured medical record review, a process for examining medical records to assess the quality of care (of cases failing screens) and to characterise quality problems;

- analysis—use of statistical (pattern) analysis of screening information and medical record review results to reveal patterns of care (the distribution of quality problems), to illuminate their causes and to guide subsequent investigations.

To fix problems and ensure they remain fixed, hospitals must establish the problem's root causes—those that if eliminated would prevent the problem's recurrence; not only their apparent causes, which are merely the problem's antecedent manifestations.

216.9 | Resolving quality problems

Hospitals must put in place a system for fixing quality problems and checking that they stay fixed. Hospitals that attempt to identify quality problems without institutionalising the means to resolve them are wasting their resources. Hospitals' structured problem resolution mechanisms should involve actively all relevant organisational levels in the process and devolve decisions to operational units to the greatest extent possible. Usually, existing organisational units can plan change and implement quality improvement actions. Exceptions include changes in organisation and the redesign of hospital-wide care systems or processes or those that transcend organisational units.

Resolving quality problems may require changes in one or more of the following three areas:

- care processes—how doctors and other health care providers treat or manage patients;
- patient flows—how patients are routed into and from clinical processes, how the hospital manages care delivery and the interrelationships among care processes;
- organisational management—how the hospital structures the production system or enterprise and how it manages people and processes.

217 | The quest for quality

217.1 | Essential quality

The quest for quality is eternal. The word 'quality' evokes a powerful and positive image that somehow encompasses the ideals of truth, beauty and abundance. The quest for quality is a crusade that is sometimes as compelling as the search for the holy grail; its attainment is elusive; its accomplishment ephemeral. Quality has become the watchword of the latter part of this century. Worldwide, industry has realised that it is quality or else. In the West many people attribute Japanese manufacturers' success to their relentless pursuit of quality. Their motto became 'if Japan can do it so can we!'

The idea that quality is the key to success has spawned a series of movements with various names such as TQM (total quality management), CQI (continuous quality improvement) and the Deming method. A host of management techniques—such as QCs (quality circles), SPC (statistical process control) and QFD (quality functional deployment)—support these philosophies of management. These movements have taken hold mostly in industry, although most companies have yet to implement effective quality management programs. Their quality management programs simply ground to a halt when they failed to produce expected results. Often they focused on the structure of quality management processes rather than on their outcome or effectiveness and failed to focus on what matters most to customers: the quality of goods and services. Undaunted, health care's motto became 'if industry can do it, so can we!'

217.2 | Health care in trouble

Health care is a troubled enterprise. In developed countries, health care has become one of, if not the, largest economic sectors, a consequence of what doctors order for patients and their ability to pay for care, either directly (out of their own pockets) or, most often, especially for high-technology interventions, indirectly (through socialised financing schemes). Many industrialised countries devote an ever-increasing fraction of their resources to health care. Rising health care expenditures threaten to crowd out those for education, housing and other beneficial social purposes and even to diminish the economic activities that have sustained them. Australia has capped public sector health care expenditures as a percentage of GDP (gross domestic product) at around 8%, putting various pressures on the system. Changes in technology and other factors could eventually lead to a cost explosion or force more explicit rationing of care. The United States spends over 14% of its GDP on health care and the proportion is growing inexorably.

Despite vast increases in health care expenditures and the supposed miracles of modern medicine, people are increasingly dissatisfied with the health care system. Quality to the rescue! In the United States, at least, a mass movement is underway to improve health care through TQM/CQI. Moreover, some people expect or at least hope that 'quality' can somehow contain seemingly uncontrollable increases in costs. Echoes of this movement are beginning to be heard in Australia. Hopes that 'quality' will solve the health care system's pressing problems are faint indeed. Many of its problems lie beyond the reach of quality management. Industrial TQM/CQI approaches offer little insight into improving clinical care. Hospitals are ill-prepared, and the environment in which they operate is ill-suited, to adopt quality management. Nevertheless, an effective quality management program can improve hospitals' production function and hence the value they provide for the money they expend.

217.3 Health care's ends and means

Health care's central purpose has remained constant for millennia. In ancient times it might have been expressed as curing the sick and preserving the healthy; today we might express it as improving health status. In the first century the Roman physician Asclepiades promised: '*curare tuto celeriter, et jucunde*—to cure safely, swiftly and pleasantly.[1] People also want that promise fulfilled today, although now they might also be forced to add the caveat 'at reasonable cost'.

The ancients, like Hippocrates, believed that 'nature cures. The doctor's business, therefore, must be to increase the healing force of nature, to guide that force, to avoid counter-acting it.'[1] This same sentiment survives today. Hippocrates relied on regulating diet, used a few drugs to enhance its effect and, if diet and drugs failed, resorted to surgery. But now we have more and more powerful means to affect diseases' course or cause for the better—and for the worse.

Hippocratic physicians were itinerant practitioners, travelling from place to place. There were few doctors and only the greatest cities of the day (fifth century BC) had settled physicians, salaried by the community.[1] Hospitals, places of refuge run by religious orders for sick and weary travellers and the poor and impaired, emerged as early as 200 BC. The oldest hospital in continuous use, Hotel Dieu in Paris, was founded in the 600s. Doctors did not practise in these early hospitals; when they did enter them, they treated only the poor there. Hospitals were decidedly unhealthy places; a prelude to death more than a promise of life. Only recently have hospitals become centres of healing, bastions of medical technology. As patients began to pay for their hospital care, the hospital's charity image faded. People wanted access to hospitals and medical technology regardless of their ability to pay.

Growth in health care expenditures provided the means to develop and deliver medical technology, which in turn stimulated demand for more health care services. The health sector not only accounts for an increasing fraction of nations' output but also increases government's role in the economy, because government accounts for or controls most health care expenditures. The increasing amounts spent on health care have created important secondary objectives: equity, employment, careers and social status. Increasingly, health care is a matter of public debate rather than private decision; political considerations dominate the debate.

217.4 | *Origins of quality assurance activities*

Interest in formal quality assurance activities has waxed and waned throughout history. In recent times, 1858, the English founder of modern nursing, Florence Nightingale, was concerned about the outcomes of hospital care and with statistical adjustment of mortality data to permit proper comparisons, although she lacked the technology to make the necessary measurements. In the United States early this century, 1917, a Boston surgeon, A.E. Codman, wanted to tally patient outcomes (the end results of care) to give credit for success and to fix responsibility for failure, although he too lacked the necessary technology. These activities may be characterised by a desire to measure performance and identify what works in order to improve care. Clinical research, which intends to identify effective interventions that medical practitioners should use in their practices, supplemented these efforts.

Few studies to measure the quality of care were done during the thirty years from the 1920s to the 1950s.[2] Interest in quality assessment and quality assurance heightened in the late 1960s and early 1970s. The establishment of the federal PSRO (Professional Standards Review Organisation) program in the United States in 1972 was a manifestation of this interest that continues to the present, even though the PSRO program was supplanted, in 1982, by the Peer Review Organisation (PRO) program. In Australia, interest in quality of care became manifest in the middle to late 1970s. By the late 1980s health care was mimicking industry's quest for quality, which had raised 'quality' from technical concern to political imperative. Now, in the 1990s, concern about health care quality has reached a crescendo everywhere.

218 | Origins of quality management

Virtually all quality management experience stems from manufacturing, necessitating constant reference to industry and industrial analogies. Health care, however, represents a more complex quality management challenge, even though the same basic principles apply. Industrial quality management techniques cannot be applied uncritically, and have limited applicability, to clinical care. Health care quality management requires use of more sophisticated techniques (outlined in this part) than those used in industry; industrial techniques can play a part, especially in improving operational efficiency. The greatest difference between manufacturing and health care is what constitutes and how to achieve quality.

Integrated industrial process control concepts were developed 5000 years ago by a physician, Imhotep.[3] Imhotep was minister of state to Zoser, the ancient Egyptian pharaoh who ruled in the opening of the third millennium BC. Ultimately, in death, Imhotep was to be deified as the Egyptian god of healing and his identity fused later with that of the Hellenic mythical deity Aesculapius, who came to represent the mythical underpinnings of Western medicine. In life, Imhotep may have been best known as the architect of the Step Pyramid at Sakkara, which stands today as the forerunner of the great pyramids of Egypt.[1] Through attention to end product quality and the processes that produced it, Imhotep was able to produce, at quarries far distant from the assembly point, huge blocks of stone that fit together so perfectly that it is impossible to pass a knife blade between them. Now, 5000 years later, we are poised to apply systematically concepts first elaborated by Imhotep to improve the activity that resulted in his deification: health care.

219 | Forces driving toward health care quality management

219.1 | Renewed interest in quality

In the late 1980s hospitals and other health care facilities began to notice the success of quality management in industry. Industry's motivation is clear: increased profits, created by avoiding the cost of reworking or fixing defective products and by increasing customer satisfaction. Hospitals' interest in quality is motivated by a desire to follow the fashion, by regulatory requirements and by a desire to market themselves as high quality providers. This interest in quality is also motivated by a desire to reduce malpractice and other risks, to counter external quality assurance initiatives and cost containment pressures and, at least in some cases, to improve practices.

To date, hospitals' renewed interest in quality has resulted in more talk than action, especially at the clinical level where it matters the most. The current quest for quality, inspired by industrial example, is only one of a number of historical forces driving health care toward quality management. Others, described in this section, include: payment strategies, utilisation management, risk management, quality assurance, medical technology assessment and, most recently and perhaps most importantly, the ability to quantify quality.

Necessarily, this section predominantly reflects experience in the United States, where most of it resides, and can only highlight some relevant aspects of each driving force. Nevertheless, it shows some of the trends evident to some extent throughout the world, and Australia can reasonably be expected to see some of these pressures in the years ahead. Moreover, these forces are likely to continue to shape health care quality management for the foreseeable future. Each driving force has its own rationale; sometimes one force intensifies, and at other times diminishes, the effects of others. The relative strength of each force varies dynamically and spatially and depends on various environmental factors.

219.2 | Health policy context

During this century, national health care policy initiatives have involved primarily financing reforms, designed to assure everyone's access to health care free of insuperable financial barriers. The general assumption was that hospitals and doctors would provide the best care of which they were capable if patients could only pay for all the care that was necessary. Concerns about runaway costs (which jeopardise everyone's access to adequate health care) and overservicing (which diminishes quality) soon followed and were attributed, in part, to the way providers were paid for their services. Consequently, health care financing schemes (payers) placed emphasis on such case-based payment strategies as DRGs (diagnosis related groups)—in which hospitals receive a fixed sum for a given type of care—and on utilisation management or managed care—in which payers assure themselves that requested medical care is necessary at the time of the request and that the procedure will be done in the least expensive setting in the minimum amount of time possible (to contain the cost of health care and to encourage efficiencies in its delivery). Such strategies have engendered concern about the resultant quality of care and have led to initiatives intended to strengthen quality assurance.

In addition to breaking down financial barriers to care, national policy initiatives have been directed generally toward increasing knowledge with a view to better preventing, diagnosing, treating and ameliorating diseases and their sequelae. This century, medical research became a distinct activity and, especially during the second half of the century, government increased its support for training and employing researchers. The resultant technology explosion propelled costs skyward, increasing pressure for further financing reforms to maintain people's access to health care. Recently, in the United States, vast (and in Australia more moderate) increases in health care expenditures have been associated with relatively modest increases in life expectancy. This situation has caused more and more people to question the value of much high-technology medicine (reinforcing a trend that began in the 1970s) and the efficiency of health care delivery.

The rise of medical science and concomitant technological advances produced increasingly powerful interventions. As interventions become more potent, the appropriateness of their use becomes more important, for all of the following reasons:

- A person who could benefit from the technology will only benefit if he or she receives it.
- The technology must be implemented properly if potential benefits are to be realised and potential harms avoided.
- A person who receives the wrong technology may be harmed more than helped, if only because he or she is precluded from receiving the right technology.

219.3 *Noble motives but no means to measure or to manage quality*

The medical and other health professions have traditionally espoused concern for quality. However, beyond the noble motive doctors have always had few incentives to improve the quality of their care and, until recently, very few efforts were made to measure their performance. In large measure, the lack of required technology was an important limiting factor. Moreover, until comparatively recently medical interventions were as likely to harm as they were to help.

Without a practical means of measuring quality and because people had few expectations for medical care, quality was simply assumed or left in the hands of the profession. Moreover, with open-ended payment schemes that characterised social policy until the latter part of this century, there was little reason to question the assumption that patients would receive high quality medical care. Although there have always been studies that questioned this assumption, it has been only recently that such studies have begun to drive the quest for quality. Among other things, in the United States such studies have found:

- There is a high, unexplained variation in surgical operations, for example hysterectomy.[4,5]
- A substantial proportion of hospital admissions are inappropriate, seemingly independent of the actual rate.[6–8]
- A significant fraction of elective operations, for example for carotid endarterectomy, are unnecessary.[9]
- Many patients under care are not receiving needed interventions.[10]

Some of these findings held out the hope that health care costs could be contained with better quality management. Others suggested that people were not receiving all of the care that would benefit them. Whatever the question, there is the sense that the in-vogue answer is 'quality management'. The danger, of course, is that people see quality management as a panacea rather than a helpful production tool to improve value for money.

219.4 *Payment strategies*

Originally, people paid for medical care mostly from their own pockets, although since ancient times government has provided some care to the poor. Since the late 1700s and particularly in this century there has been a trend toward some form of socialised prepayment for health care, referred to often as health insurance (which is an unfortunate misnomer). Since World War II government has come to dominate health care financing in all industrialised countries by making the rules, if not collecting and disbursing most of the money, which it does in many countries, including Australia, Canada and the United Kingdom.

The term 'payment strategies' refers to the way that third party payers (e.g. government, insurance companies) pay providers for their services. Traditional, fee-for-service medicine links providers' (hospitals' and doctors') services directly to payments from patients' pockets. Providers can adjust prices to patients' ability to pay. Patients can decide whether or not they can afford the care and, to some limited extent, if it is worth the price asked. However, as care becomes more expensive, major illness could result in financial catastrophe or no care or both. Over the years, medical care has been socialised to distribute risk. The most prominent schemes are those of government and private insurers.

Initially, in many countries these schemes kept the fee-for-service method of paying providers (although, for example, the British National Health Service provided its hospitals with annual budgets and entered into contracts with consultants—hospital-based medical practitioners—and paid general practitioners a fixed sum annually for each person who was registered with the practitioner). Providers either set their prices on the basis of customary-and-usual charges or cost-reimbursement or negotiated a fee schedule. These mechanisms provided no incentives to individual providers to deliver services more efficiently, let alone improve the quality of care. Because all medically appropriate services were covered, patients could theoretically receive all the care they needed at no, or little, out-of-pocket cost. On the other hand, with open-ended payment schemes, providers had positive incentives to overservice patients and to introduce unproven technology.

To control costs, third party payers have begun various initiatives, including the following: exclusion of specific interventions; limited coverage (e.g. to 100 days of hospitalisation per year); increased deductibles (the amount a patient must pay before the financing scheme pays) and copayments (that fraction of costs which patients must pay); utilisation management (e.g. requiring preauthorisation of surgical operations); prospective payments based on diagnosis related groups (DRGs); and alternative delivery systems, most notably HMOs (health maintenance organisations). Health maintenance organisations accept a single monthly payment (sometimes referred to as capitation) in return for providing all contracted services, including hospitalisation. The incentives here may include those to accept only healthy patients and to underserve those in the plan, to minimise expenditures. Importantly, in HMOs primary care practitioners act as gatekeepers, controlling access to specialists' services. The British NHS, which from its inception capitated payment to general practitioners, has begun an experiment in which general practitioners buy hospital services for their patients, influenced presumably by their quality and cost, in an effort to improve care.

Under case-based payment schemes, such as the DRG system that the US Health Care Financing Administration uses to pay for the hospital care of its Medicare beneficiaries, hospitals receive a fixed amount for delivering a particular type of care, for example cholecystectomy for gallbladder disease, irrespective of the hospital's actual costs. The DRG payment scheme differs from a fee schedule in that diagnoses are classified according to their propensity to consume resources. Some costs, for example capital, research and teaching, are excluded from DRG payments and are passed through separately. Such a scheme encourages efficiency because the hospital keeps the difference between income and expenditures. However, it favours hospitals with low costs for reasons other than efficiency, for example lower wage rates, and those hospitals with favourable case mixes, the types of patients treated within a given DRG that affect resource consumption.

Theoretically, DRG payment schemes also retard the introduction of cost-increasing (and encourage the introduction of cost-reducing) technology. New technology that both increases costs and provides health benefits to patients places policy decision makers, and hospitals, on the horns of a dilemma. Increasing DRG payments to accommodate new technology undermines policy decision makers' ability to contain costs; providing the new technology without an increase in payment undermines hospitals' financial stability. Further, DRG payment schemes introduce incentives to cut corners, to select profitable patients (referred to sometimes as creaming) and to reject others (referred to sometimes as dumping), and to discharge patients quickly (which is intended), and perhaps prematurely (which is not intended), and to readmit (prematurely discharged) patients (because hospitals are paid per admission). In the United States, specific anti-dumping laws, external review programs and concerns about malpractice liability moderate these incentives.

Payment strategies offer incentives that influence the effectiveness and efficiency of medical care. Their influence may be obvious or it may be subtle. Unintended effects may become more troublesome than the problems that changes in strategies were intended to alleviate. To date, payment strategies' influence on quality has been unintentional. In the near future, quality may become their principal target.

219.5 | Utilisation management

Utilisation management is of major concern to third party payers of care, such as government and insurance companies. Because of their importance in the marketplace, in the United States they have been able to insert controls on the utilisation of services. With respect to hospitals, such controls may include:

- preadmission certification—an agreement by the payer that an admission or surgical or other intervention is appropriate;
- continued stay review, in which payers agree that patients whose stay exceeds norms should be in the hospital;
- case management, in which the payer agrees in advance with the provider's treatment plans, used especially for high-cost care;
- review and denial or adjustment of payment claims, particularly for services not rendered, such as unbundling (breaking out individual interventions that comprise a coherent clinical treatment and billing them as separate services), and services provided inappropriately.

Claims review is as old as insurance. However, the other forms of utilisation management are new and are often referred to as managed care. Essentially, for certain interventions for all patients or all interventions for some types of patients, the payer must agree in advance with the necessity, timing, place and duration of care. Such schemes introduce burdens on providers for which they feel they are not compensated. Further, payers are injecting themselves into the patient–provider relationship, with all of its attendant costs and benefits; among these are liability for denied treatments and alienating patients and providers. Savings depend on avoided expenditures for unnecessary interventions exceeding the cost of program administration. As the volume of disputable care diminishes, savings can evaporate and leave a residual increase in financial and other costs.

219.6 | Risk management

Risk management is of concern primarily to providers. However, since they pass on to patients the cost of professional liability insurance and of defensive medicine that fear of malpractice suits engenders, everyone pays as health care costs are propelled skyward. The greater the number of successful malpractice claims and the larger the amounts awarded, the higher costs go.

For doctors, the major risk to avoid is financial disaster from successful malpractice suits. In addition, they are interested in winning suits to uphold the correctness of their practices. The classic response has been malpractice insurance in order to spread this risk and thereby avert financial ruin. Its existence, however, may encourage patients to sue (because insurers have deeper pockets and are more impersonal than doctors) and may discourage providers from paying close attention to quality (because their insurance pays claims and premiums become a cost of doing business). Nonetheless, both providers and professional liability insurers have a residual vested interest in reducing the risk of patients bringing malpractice suits, judges and juries finding in their favour and, if suits result in monetary awards, reducing resultant awards for damages, leading ultimately to reduced indemnity costs.

For doctors, the threat of a malpractice suit can translate into defensive medicine. Here the doctor, ever cautious of being criticised for not doing something that could have been done, does everything that he believes a jury would see as being reasonable. Doctors are rarely criticised for doing too much or leaving no stone unturned, although, of course, they are sued for using inappropriate interventions. The net results of defensive medicine have been increased costs and risks to patients from interventions that would not otherwise have been done.

In addition to malpractice avoidance, risk management in hospitals is concerned with minimising risks to staff (through occupational health and safety programs) and to society (through environmental engineering programs).

219.7 Quality assurance

219.71 OVERVIEW

Generally, quality assurance is concerned with ensuring that health care meets standards. To date, health care's product has been largely undefined (and certainly unquantified). Formal quality assurance efforts are a relatively new phenomenon. Earliest efforts focused on professional education and later ones on care settings, principally hospitals. Today these trends have converged with a resultant emphasis on provider performance—the outcome of care—which depends on care structures, including doctors' qualifications, and care processes, including how doctors treat patients.

219.72 REGISTRATION OR LICENSURE

Registration or licensure ensures that practitioners meet minimum educational and certain other requirements. License revocation offers a way of controlling who can continue to practise. Increasing specialisation among practitioners has paralleled the increasing complexity of medical practice. Formal postbasic education requirements have also expanded, as have specialty certification bodies. The increasing pace of change in medical practice has led, in some countries, to continuing medical education requirements to maintain a license to practise, and toward time-limited specialty certification to ensure that specialists remain current. Various schemes to relicense periodically or recertify medical practitioners have foundered on the means by which these ends can be accomplished meaningfully and practically. In hospitals, credentialling and privileging systems have further delineated who can practise, what they can practise, and how they can practise. Increasingly, recertification and recredentialling decisions are being based on performance rather than relying solely on formal qualifications.

219.73 ACCREDITATION

Hospitals (and other health care facilities) now undergo increasing scrutiny and regulation, principally through accreditation. Traditionally, surveyors undertake periodic inspection of hospitals to make sure they meet published standards, which encompass quality assurance mechanisms, and can thus be accredited. In the United States, the Joint Commission on the Accreditation of Health Care Organisations (JCAHO), a private body, undertakes hospital accreditation and in Australia the Australian Council on Healthcare

- Many TQM programs were form over substance. Chief executives paid lip-service to quality but never instituted meaningful programs to effect its improvement. Companies hid behind TQM activities to avoid the hard work of managing quality and failed to focus on what their customers wanted. They also failed to realise that fixing quality meant fixing the entire organisation. They confused ends and means, and mistakenly believed that if they carried out enough of the right improvement activities, performance improvements would inevitably materialise.

- True quality improvement takes ten or more years because of the need to change an organisation's culture. Many TQM efforts simply ground to a halt when they failed to fulfil their original promise. Bureaucratic TQM programs produced a prodigious amount of red tape and created as many problems as they solved. Failed TQM programs have spawned a new business: cleaning up the resultant mess.

- Corporate re-engineering has replaced TQM as the latest management fashion. Its basic premise is the need to continually redesign and rebuild organisations' production processes. Corporate re-engineers forget how things are done now, and decide how best to do them. They eschew quick fixes and incremental changes because they believe they often create as many problems as they solve. Relentless technological advances result in the constant need to re-engineer.

- To date, experience with TQM/CQI in hospitals is extremely limited and, in the United States at least, an anti-TQM backlash is beginning to develop. Few hospitals have attempted to apply TQM/CQI to clinical care. Hospital TQM programs suffer from the same types of defects as beset those in industry.

- Hospitals have a long way to go to achieve quality maturity. Being generous, the average Australian hospital scores about 80 out of a possible total of 1000 points according to TQM/CQI criteria. Present-day hospitals are not organised for quality-focused production. They do not measure up because they do not measure.

- A quality-mature hospital would be organised to improve quality and patients' health status at least cost and greatest patient satisfaction. Quality would be measured explicitly and results used continuously to review and if necessary to revise product specifications and change practices to improve quality. Changes in culture, organisation, incentives, and the hospital's operating environment are needed to facilitate progress towards these ends.

- Hospitals must both adopt a production perspective and customer focus to succeed in the quest for quality. Hospitals must focus on the value of their services to patients. Present incentives militate against a value-for-money focus.

- Hospitals do not measure, and consequently can neither assure nor document any improvement in the quality of their care. To begin to focus on quality, hospitals must measure their performance and compare it to others and to what is possible. To achieve quality maturity, they must measure patient outcomes and conduct research to identify better and more cost-effective practices.

- Government must guarantee, and society must support, the incentives needed to ensure that hospitals and doctors institute quality management.

223 | Industrial analogies: total quality management

223.1 | The quality revolution

Japan has led the quality revolution. How could a country known for its shoddy, cheap imitations of Western products surpass the best in the West? Joseph Juran, a leading quality guru for the past fifty years, explains. After World War II, 'I suggested that the Japanese try to find ways to institutionalise programs within their companies that would yield continuous quality improvement.'[1] Many of them took this advice to heart, producing a massive change in direction that added up to an unprecedented quality revolution. To launch their quality revolution, senior executives took personal charge of managing and trained managers in how to manage for quality. They trained their engineers to use statistical methods for quality control, provided their workforces with the means to participate in quality improvement and enlarged their business plans to include quality goals.[2] The results speak for themselves. For example, the Japanese auto industry progressed from an also-ran to world leader in product quality. In the 1950s Japanese cars were of such poor quality that they could not be sold successfully in competitive markets such as the United States. After more than twenty years of effort, in the mid 1970s they caught up and subsequently surpassed US auto-makers in customers' perceptions of the quality and value of their automobiles.

Western companies failed to follow Juran's advice 'because they saw no reason to do so. . . . To the West it was simply inconceivable, even laughable, that Japan of all countries could become the world's quality leader.'[2] Xerox offers a case study of how the quality revolution caught Western companies flat-footed and even threatened the survival of industrial giants that dominated their market. Instead of succumbing, Xerox fought back and regained market share that it had lost to the Japanese.

With markets for its traditional products in decline, in 1959 Haloid Corporation (which changed its name to Xerox in 1961) launched the world's first commercial xerographic copier. Sales boomed from US$40 million in 1960 to US$1.7 billion in 1970. In the 1970s Kodak and IBM started to erode Xerox's market share for high-volume copiers and Japanese companies that for low-volume copiers.[3] Xerox knew that its machines broke down regularly; its response was a service force to repair them. Customers wanted reliable machines, not repairs.[2] The Japanese saw and seized the opportunity. They grabbed such a large share of the market that Xerox's survival was in jeopardy. Xerox launched its own quality program in order to survive and to regain its competitiveness.

In 1983 noting that: 'We are no longer the company we once were, and are not yet the company that we must be,' David Kearnes, Xerox president, introduced Xerox Leadership Through Quality Strategy. Xerox compared its processes to the best in the world, reduced its suppliers, introduced systematic customer satisfaction measurement and took other steps to reorganise manufacturing in accordance with the strategy's quality principles.[3] Xerox's success was considerable.[4] In 1982, 92% of parts that suppliers shipped to Xerox were defect free. By 1988 the percentage had increased to 99.97% (300 defective parts per million), with a target of 125 defective parts per million.[5] In 1989 Xerox Business Products Systems division won the Baldrige national quality award (described later in this chapter).

Xerox has gone further toward satisfying customers' needs. In introducing its latest generation of copiers, Xerox simplified their operation and instructions for taking care of inevitable problems. 'Where it once took twenty-eight minutes on average to clear a paper jam, it now takes twenty-eight seconds with the new design.'[6] High-end Xerox copiers now include an expert system (an on-board computer) that forecasts breakdowns and automatically notifies the service department so that it can effect a repair before the expected failure. Product innovation at Xerox promises to take the photo out of copy. The company plans to replace lenses with scanners, creating digitised images that can be printed immediately, stored, edited and printed again later or in the same or other locations. The result will be a versatile all-in-one copier, fax and computer printer.[6]

Global competition is the principal force driving quality improvement. Competitiveness is often the rationale for companies' introduction of TQM/CQI. Critically, TQM/CQI stresses the long term and acknowledges that its employees are a company's greatest asset. Paradoxically, at the same time, in the United States at least, companies' quest for competitiveness results in right-sizing, often with its resultant elimination of jobs and organisational flexibility, and frequently with the loss of job security for those who remain. Whether or not the existence of more globally competitive companies leads to a more productive economy or a better quality of life is a much-debated question—one beyond this manual's scope.

223.2 | Origins and development of TQM/CQI

Total quality management (TQM) has become the latest term in the quest for quality and productivity. Like so many terms its origins are uncertain. Its roots lie in the early work on quality in the United States in the 1920s and 1930s. Walter Shewhart, a statistician at Bell Telephone Laboratories in New York, developed statistical control techniques for industrial processes and described what became known as the Shewhart (or more commonly the PDCA, plan-do-check-act) cycle. Shewhart's work was later extended by Edwards Deming in the 1940s, providing the foundation for SQC (statistical quality control) or SPC (statistical process control), as it is now known more broadly. Deming introduced these methods into Japan in the 1950s.

In 1951 Joseph Juran published the first edition of his *Quality control handbook.* Juran noted rightly that quality consists of wasted (defective) production and quality control (QC) efforts and that wasted production was gold waiting to be mined by better QC efforts. In 1957 Armand Feigenbaum introduced the concept of total quality control (TQC) to signify the need to broaden the purview of quality beyond production into product design. He saw the need for designers to be concerned with manufacturability. In 1961 he published his book *Total quality control: engineering and management.* In the 1970s and 1980s product quality assumed strategic importance, governing the development of new products; TQM had arrived. Now TQM/CQI is expanding into research and development (R&D) activities that produce the technological innovations and enhance the core competencies that permit companies to compete based on quality-focused design and production.

223.3 | Economic enterprise and the long-term view

Quality-focused economic enterprises or companies take a long-term view. Japanese managers assume that their enterprises will exist in perpetuity and therefore management must be concerned with long-term profit maximisation, which might require acceptance of lower short-term profits than would a short-term view. Thus, for example, in the short run market share maximisation may be of greater interest than immediate profits. In contrast, US managers for example, if not Western managers generally, have been criticised for being too focused on short-term results.

An enterprise's central or top managers must organise for long-term profit maximisation within their cultural context, which compared with other social contexts may help or hinder their efforts. Among other things, the cultural context determines who becomes managers in economic enterprises, how enterprises may influence the cultural context, and how profits are shared among or used by managers, employees, shareholders and other stakeholders. The profit potential of individual enterprises and entrepreneurs collectively depends in part on how enterprises divide profits among stakeholders and society in the form of taxes. Taxes can be viewed as a due to society because of the investments it makes in activities and infrastructure that support enterprises—such as education and transport systems—or for permitting the enterprise to exist. The amount of taxes and how government raises and spends them determines, among other things, how enterprises reward their employees.

Profit is the central measure of an enterprise's success. It integrates both the extent to which the enterprise has fulfilled customers' inherent or imagined needs and its management has fulfilled those needs efficiently within the enterprise's environment. Profit may be viewed as a reward for risk, the pay-off for investing oneself or one's resources in the enterprise or its technology. In a competitive world, enterprises that take little risk may be taking the biggest risk of all: seeing others win customers through product and process innovation. Under these competitive circumstances, low risk may be associated with failure rather than with success. High risk enterprises may fail or be wildly successful. Enterprises that take prudent risks have the greatest chance of long-term survival.

The task of managers is to improve performance through innovations that represent technological or other improvements to the enterprise's products and processes, those that add value in terms of meeting customers' needs or reducing costs or, preferably, both simultaneously. Profits permit managers to reward themselves, employees, shareholders and other stakeholders in the enterprise's success. They also permit them to invest in developing technological innovations and products to better fulfil customers' needs or new processes to do so more efficiently, and even to invest in new enterprises in order to remain competitive and ensure future profits. Enterprises with well paid, motivated employees, who prefer making useful products than worthless junk, have a distinct advantage in recruiting and retaining able employees. These enterprises can afford to invest their profits in their employees. Success begets success.

223.4 | Variation in quality

We know that quality varies. But by how much? Actually measuring quality can be illuminating. David Garvin, for example, studied the production operations of all but one of the manufacturers of room airconditioners in the United States and in Japan.[7] Each manufacturer used a simple assembly-line process and much the same equipment to make an essentially standardised product; thus quality comparisons are meaningful and not obfuscated by differences in technology or products.

> The shocking news, for which nothing prepared me, is that the failure rates of products from the highest quality producers were 500 to 1000 times less than those of products for the lowest. The 'between 500 and 1000' is not a typographical error but an inescapable fact.[7]

223.5 | Manufacturers' quest for quality and profits

From its humble beginnings, the concern and impetus for quality and its management has moved from the shop floor to the boardroom. David Garvin has divided this progression into the following four stages: inspection, statistical quality control (both of which are concerned with production), quality assurance (company-wide quality control and improvement) and strategic quality management.[8] Improvements in quality did not occur linearly. However, in general terms the frontiers of quality improvement have moved progressively from inspection to prevention—from identifying defective products to investigating their causes and preventing their occurrence. This section focuses on quality management's functional progression: from production to product to technology (that permits product and production innovation). (See Figure II-2-1 on page 81.) The text describes the evolution of quality in manufacturing and in product design and, increasingly, in product innovation.

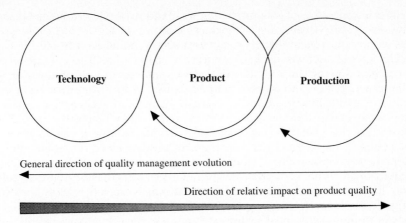

Figure II-2-1 *Quality management's evolution: through the interlocking cycles from production to product to technology*

223.6 *Product manufacture*

The central problem in manufacturing is producing a product to specifications with as little variation as practical—referred to often as manufacturing quality control. Over a period of about thirty to forty years, from the 1920s to the 1960s, manufacturing quality management progressed from inspecting products to weed out defects to instituting mechanisms to prevent their occurrence. Defect-prone processes were converted to those that were virtually defect-free. As part of this progression, manufacturers began working closely with their suppliers to ensure delivery of defect-free parts.

Customers who buy products that work are happier than those who have to return a defective one. A simple approach to assuring quality is to inspect products before they leave the factory, shipping only those that meet specifications. Inspecting every product could prove costly, not to mention the cost of reworking or scrapping rejected products. Product sampling is often used to reduce inspection costs. However, sampling products could mean that some defective products are shipped, in batches passing inspection for example. This means that in effect the customer performs the final quality inspection.

Customer service is the final extension of manufacturing. Customers' return of defective products is an additional expense to the company. Not only must the product be repaired or replaced, but customers are left with a poor image of the company, especially if it did not handle the return quickly and courteously. This sequence illustrates a quality maxim: the later in the production/use chain that a defect is discovered, the more costly it is to the company. Stated simply, it costs a great deal more to fix a defective product already in a customer's hands than it does to avoid use of the defective part that caused the problem. The inspection of incoming parts or ingredients to make sure they are fit to incorporate into or produce products is manufacturers' first line of quality defence. Obviously, if suppliers were to deliver parts guaranteed defect-free, manufacturers could eliminate this inspection cost. Thus quality conscious manufacturers either buy from quality conscious suppliers or, if need be, help them become so or ultimately seek alternative suppliers if they do not measure up.

According to another quality maxim, product quality cannot be inspected-in; it can only be assured by control of processes. Spending more money on inspectors to weed out defective products does not improve the manufacturing processes that produced them; some defective products will inevitably slip through the inspectorial net. This realisation led to a variety of preventive techniques to ensure that manufacturers produce only products meeting specifications. If this goal could be met completely, inspection would be unnecessary because every product made would meet specifications.

While progress has been made toward error-free production it is still impossible, of course, even though defects can be reduced to parts in millions. Inspection is still necessary to find defects, not only to avoid incorporate them into products or shipping them to customers but also to investigate their causes and prevent their recurrence and, importantly, to assure that products are actually produced according to specifications rather than assume that they meet them. However, quality-focused manufacturers can reduce the number of quality inspectors to one-seventh of what it was formerly.

Measurement is the key to quality. Manufacturing processes can be monitored using statistical process control (SPC). Manufacturers either measure all products or sample them, as appropriate. Whenever processes produce products outside of pre-set tolerances, production stops and the problem is ascertained and corrected. Clearly, detecting and eliminating defective parts is cheaper than finding them in finished products. This approach can result in substantial savings through less rework, less scrap and less waste. Given that up to 30% of a product's cost may be accounted for by waste in its production, quite a lot of money could be spent on SPC and slower production rates, if that was required for quality. The relationship between quality and productivity is obvious, but is often missed or confused.

Better measurement, that resulted in early detection of defective parts and prevention of defective finished products, also resulted in a better understanding of the reasons for defects. These reasons are often divided into special causes—intermittently-seen variation produced as a consequence of process implementation, for example from the blunting of cutting tools, which workers could be alert to and prevent (by replacing blunt tools)—and common causes—continuously-seen variation that is inherent in the process, which individual workers cannot prevent. Variation data often exhibit the Pareto effect: 80% of the defects result from 20% of problems. By following yet another quality maxim—focusing attention on the 20% of problems that caused 80% of defects—production quality can be improved economically.

Quality-focused manufacturing emphasises reduction in product variation. Manufacturers realised that it was important not only to produce parts or products to specifications but also to produce them with as little variation as possible in quality-critical parameters.[9] Stated simply, it is more important that at least 95% of widgets should be as close as practical to a single value than it is for all widgets to fall broadly within specified tolerance limits. This single value must fall within—and is preferably, but need not be, the central point of—specified tolerance limits.

SPC (statistical process control) quickly identifies processes tending or actually out of control, that is, producing products outside of their pre-set limits. However, batch production, the usual mode of manufacture and measurement, often means that some defective products are produced before they are discovered. Manufacturers must rework or scrap these defects. One solution is to inspect every part as soon as it is made—an expensive proposition unless made an integral part of the manufacturing process. Producing small batches and using them right away allows any remaining defects to be identified, and defective production processes to be corrected, quickly. Thus, kanban, or JIT (just in time) inventory methods can have as profound an impact on quality as on inventory costs.[10] With such methods, production line workers double as quality control personnel once they have mastered the basics of SPC and product quality measurement.

In manufacturing, set-up times can be extensive. To make frequent small batches requires reducing set-up times to a minimum to avoid increasing production costs. Thus to implement kanban successfully, attention focused on reducing set-up times. An added benefit of substantially shorter set-up times is still lower manufacturing costs. These techniques led to improved manufacturing quality with fewer defects and less waste.

Another challenge was to reduce the inherent cost of manufacturing the product. Through such techniques as value engineering, manufacturers began looking at every aspect of the manufacturing process to answer a single question: how can we produce the product for less without degrading its essential quality? One material might be substituted for another, a change made in the production process, workers trained appropriately and so on. Using this approach, manufacturers can change processes with a view to increasing reliability or performance characteristics, reducing variability and reducing costs.

Beginning in 1962 in Japan, companies formed quality control circles—small groups of production line workers—to discuss quality control activities and to suggest ways to improve operations.[11] These approaches exemplify continuous quality improvement, incremental progress towards meeting production specifications at least manufacturing costs. Thus quality is measured both in terms of product performance and cost.

223.7 *Product design*

The factory was now producing products to specifications reliably and at less cost. But was it the right product? As any successful entrepreneur knows, the customer is always right. In the 1970s quality-focused manufacturers began paying particular attention to systematically discern customers' functional requirements and incorporate them into product design systems. They progressed from making what they thought they could sell at a profit to producing products that customers wanted at the price that they were willing to pay.

What customers will buy is the right product, assuming one can sell it profitably at a price customers are willing to pay. Market-driven manufacturing is a well-established idea, to which the existence of market research attests. Manufacturers that produce what customers will buy are the most likely to be successful. Not surprisingly, customers are responsible for suggesting more product innovations than manufacturers. However, only manufacturers can actually produce innovations. Customers know what they want or need to accomplish. Tapping into this wellspring of innovation allows manufacturers to tailor existing products and to develop entirely new ones.

Involving customers in determining products' quality (i.e. their functional characteristics) proved to be yet another source of profit. Money was not wasted on producing goods people would not buy in economical quantities. Product performance more closely matched performance requirements. With advances in computer-controlled tools, shorter set-up times and similar innovations, manufacturers could produce a given product in endless varieties to meet customers' exact needs. Customers' needs and wants change dynamically, in part influenced by what manufacturers produce. The faster one can adapt to market needs, the more successful one can be, at least according to Asia-Pacific manufacturers. Emphasis shifted to the rapid adaptation of existing products and the introduction of new ones. The key problem was translating customers' wants into product designs and then into finished products. The right materials must be selected and procured, and the right process for the selected materials must be designed and set up. This difficult task was solved by QFD (quality functional deployment), developed originally in 1972 at Mitsubishi's shipyards in Kobe, Japan.

Essentially QFD is a set of planning and communication routines that focuses and co-ordinates an organisation's skills to design and produce desired products. The attributes and benefits of a good design process are similar to those of a good manufacturing process. For example, it is far cheaper to find out in advance that a customer likes this or that rather than when one rolls out the prototype. The prototype is the affirmation of a winning design in the same way that final product inspection is the confirmation that a product meets specifications.

Deciding all design aspects at the beginning—for example which customer needs to satisfy, performance characteristics and trade-offs including that with cost—is QFD's greatest advantage. Making these decisions together, at the beginning, permits design and hence product integrity. The result is a better, cheaper product. Moreover, manufacturers could reduce dramatically the time between conception and production.

Use of QFD not only permits more rapid introduction of better products but also cheaper product introduction and hence cheaper products. For example, after the introduction of QFD Toyota reduced its start-up and preproduction costs by 60%. Moreover, with QFD a Japanese automobile maker was able to freeze its design before production. A US company without QFD introduced many more design changes, most of them at a later point in the design–production cycle.[12]

Following these approaches to product design and manufacture permitted order-of-magnitude improvements in quality and reductions in cost. Another innovation further consolidated the advantage of companies adopting the quality management approach. It was to take a long-term view of profits. Products are introduced at a low price, even at a loss initially. This approach permits a company to build a large market share from the beginning. By manufacturing large quantities, through their continuous quality improvement mechanisms, quality-focused manufacturers can both realise improvements in products—which stimulates sales and retains or expands market share—and reduce manufacturing costs sufficiently to ultimately derive profits from subsequent sales. This never ending cycle of fast introductions, with high product quality and low product costs, gives established quality-focused companies an overwhelming advantage.

223.8 | Product and process innovation

With the institutionalisation of quality-focused product design and manufacture, competition shifted to breakthroughs in product and process innovation—discontinuities that mean huge advances in performance or reduced costs or both. Such innovation depends, of course, on the quality and productivity of research and development (R&D) and on the resources devoted to technology development and assessment.

To remain competitive, companies must continuously out-innovate their competitors.[13] Quality-focused manufacturers have progressed from using whatever technology researchers came up with to focusing on innovations needed to produce products of greatest value to customers and, particularly, on those to improve production processes and work practices. They have also charged their R&D departments with designing the technological and organisational forms (or architectures) and functions that facilitate quality management, including continuous innovation.[6]

Quality management principles apply as much to R&D as they do to product design and manufacture, a point that researchers and their sponsors have yet to grasp sufficiently. Because product technology (e.g. the idea of a widget) diffuses quickly, success in the twenty-first century will likely belong to those enterprises that develop and deploy innovative process technology to deliver quickly, reliably and at low cost defect-free widgets that meet customers' functional specifications.

224 | Quality management framework

224.1 | Quality management is an organisation-level tool

Quality management is a production-level (micro-), and not a system-level (macro-) management tool. Quality management applies to individual organisations, such as manufacturers and hospitals, and not the economy (economic enterprises collectively and their interrelationships) nor to the nation's health care system. Chapter 3 in this part elaborates on this point.

224.2 | Quality as organising principle

Quality management's purpose is to ensure that organisations are—and remain—competitive to ensure their survival and success in an increasingly competitive global marketplace. Quality management offers a philosophy of or perspective on management: organising for performance. Quality management is concerned primarily with an organisation's production function: what it produces and how it produces it. Stated simply, an organisation's production function is its raison d'être.

What an organisation produces, and how well, defines that organisation to the world and especially to its customers. For example, Mercedes-Benz is known for producing high quality, expensive motor cars. Qantas is known as the only major airline never to have suffered a fatal crash. Quality-focused organisations are totally dedicated to satisfying current and anticipated customers' present and future needs and wants, and to exceeding their value-for-money expectations. In quality-focused organisations, product quality is the organising principle, the one that shapes the organisation.

Quality-mature organisations strive ceaselessly for excellence and have institutionalised mechanisms to assure and improve continuously the quality of their products and production processes. They establish and evolve the management structures and processes, and employ the tools and techniques necessary to achieve quality maturity. Quality maturity is the end result of implementing quality management. However, quality management neither creates an organisation's purpose nor specifies its policies and practices. Quality management helps pose the right questions and provides the means to answer them correctly. However, it does not—and cannot—guarantee the right answers. For example, quality-oriented companies periodically ask such crucial questions as: What business should we be in? What are the right products for this business? How do we produce these products competitively? Effective leadership and strong management—not merely a tool-kit of TQM/CQI methods—are necessary to answer these questions.

Quality improvement is quality management's principal outcome. This improvement must be continuous because customers' expectations, and hence notions of value-for-money, change continuously. Quality-mature hospitals, for example, would be producing more and more health status improvement for patients, reducing the time needed to produce and the cost of producing any given level of health status improvement, increasing patient satisfaction with care, and perfecting the acceptability of any trade-offs that they might have to make to produce more and more health status improvement.

224.3 | Quality management's dimensions

Quality management has three dimensions, to which we refer as entirety, totality and continuity. Their common origin is production—the system of processes that an organisation uses to produce its defining goods or services. (See Figure II-2-2 on page 86.) Current concepts of quality management have expanded the notion of production from workers' activities on the shop floor to encompass the entire organisation—everything of concern to directors and top managers in the boardroom. Quality-focused organisation includes not only the systems and processes that produce goods and services but also those that determine and support their production.

Entirety refers to the technical dimension of production (technology–product–production). Original concern about quality was confined to producing products to specifications as economically as possible. Later it was recognised that product specifications determined quality more than production, although, of course, quality-focused organisations still produce products to (improved) specifications. Now quality management's frontier lies in improving the generation of technology that enables organisations to improve products' specifications and production processes.

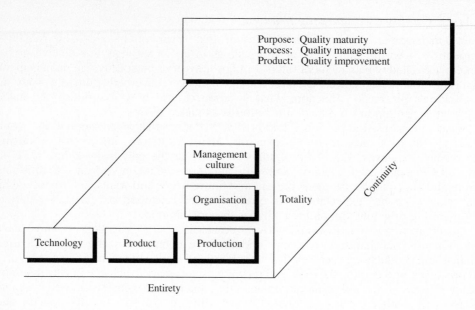

Figure II-2-2 *Dimensions of quality management*

Totality refers to the human resource dimension of quality (production–organisation–culture). Originally, management viewed quality as something of concern to production people (or, worse, only to quality control engineers). Then it realised that the organisation of which the production people were part determined products' quality. Finally, management realised that an organisation reflects the culture that it creates—the ethos that pervades an organisation determines the quality of its goods and services. Quality management is an organising principle; it is not an aspect of organisation.

Continuity refers to the dynamic dimension of quality. Satisfying customers' needs today is no guarantee that an organisation will satisfy them tomorrow. Customers' expectations change, influenced in part by how well the organisation—and more to the point its competitors—satisfy current and anticipate future needs, if not expectations. Continuous quality improvement requires not only changing an organisation's products and production processes but also the organisation itself to adjust dynamically to satisfy changing customers' needs and wants (referred to sometimes as reinventing the organisation). The idea of catching up to quality-mature organisations—those practising quality management—is illusory because they are constantly trying to perfect the fit between what they produce and what customers need and want.

224.4 Some characteristics of quality-focused organisations

The keys to successful quality management are knowledge, technology and information employed by empowered, motivated, competent, trained management and workers. Quality-focused organisations create systems and employ methods that produce quality maturity. These methods include: applying the necessary tools and techniques (e.g. statistical process control), managing people (the behavioural and organisational aspects of work) and creating and co-ordinating the various elements (including leadership and other aspects of strategic management) necessary to produce a coherent production system that is dedicated to satisfying external customer's needs.

Quality-focused organisations satisfy their external (true) customers—in contrast to focusing on satisfying the organisation's internal needs and wants. Nevertheless, they apply the same logic to their internal 'products' that they apply to manufacturing products for (external) customers. The 'customers' for these internal products are other people in the company. In a production line the person downstream represents a customer of the person upstream. Similarly, the employee can be viewed as a customer of the payroll department, for example. Improving the quality of payroll services with fewer mistakes and more courteous handling of complaints helps the company by improving worker morale and can save the company money.

Quality-focused organisations emphasise self-management, and relevant information and communication systems; they de-emphasise hierarchies. An organisation's managers and workers are the means for satisfying customers' needs. It must encourage them and must provide the necessary positive incentives to improve their own and the organisation's performance through personal and organisational development. Managers spend little time supervising and considerable time listening, reading, studying, learning and introducing new ideas in the constant pursuit of better and more efficient production. People work systematically in co-ordinated teams to identify customers' needs and to perfect the means for satisfying them, adding more and more value.

Morale in quality-mature organisations is high because people perform only demonstrably useful work (since anything else detracts from quality or increases cost). Moreover, they know why they are doing their work and are provided the means to do it well. However, while satisfied workers may be productive workers, employee satisfaction is neither an aspect of quality (which rests entirely on customers' perception) nor quality management's purpose. In fact, emphasising internal customers' needs is self-satisfying and can be counterproductive if they are at odds with those of the external—true—customers—the only needs that really matter in the long run.

The idea that quality management can somehow be grafted onto or incorporated into an existing organisation is bound to disappoint and may be a recipe for disaster. Quality management requires reorganising for total quality. Failure to grasp this fundamental reality will doom from the outset efforts to achieve quality maturity. Use of quality management tools and techniques—above all else meaningful measurement of quality— is necessary but insufficient to achieve quality maturity. Organisations must also pay attention to behavioural and organisational change and strategic management. Managers must reinvent or renew their organisations to adjust dynamically to new realities and must never let up, lest competitors' better performance doom them to extinction. This vision may appear utopian, but those organisations that can realise it more completely than others will survive and prosper. Survival and success stem from competitive advantage, not from the impossibility of achieving the ideal.

225 | Management, leadership and vision

225.1 | Management's essence

Definitions of management are as numerous as managers. Indeed, management has been defined as what managers do. The concept of management, as the term is understood today, is less than a century old. Peter Drucker, one of the world's best known and respected management gurus, believes: 'Management explains why, for the first time in human history, we can employ large numbers of knowledgeable, skilled people in productive work.'[14] Management depends on knowledge and, in turn, the systematic generation of knowledge depends on management. 'The emergence of management has converted knowledge from social ornament and luxury into the true capital of any economy.'[14] In the last forty years the concept of management has been broadened from business to all social organisations, including hospitals. 'Management worldwide has become the new social function.'[14]

Management can be viewed from at least two perspectives: liberal art and system science. The liberal art view stresses management's people dimensions; system science, its technical aspects, including information generation, analysis and evaluation, and its use in practice.

225.2 │ Management principles

Peter Drucker, for example, suggests that management is about a few, essential principles. They are:

- Management is about human beings. Its task is to make people capable of joint performance, to make their strengths effective and their weaknesses irrelevant. This is what organisation is all about . . .
- Because management deals with the integration of people in a common venture, it is deeply embedded in culture. What managers do in different countries is exactly the same. How they do it may be quite different . . .
- Every enterprise requires commitment to common goals and shared values . . . Management's first job is to think through, set and exemplify those objectives, values and goals . . .
- Management must also enable the enterprise and each of its members to grow and develop as needs and opportunities change. Every enterprise is a learning and teaching institution. Training and development must be built into it on all levels . . . training and development that never stops . . .
- Every enterprise . . . must be built on communication and on individual responsibility . . .
- Neither the quantity of output nor the 'bottom line' is by itself an adequate measure of the performance of management and enterprise . . . an organisation needs a diversity of measures to assess its health and performance. Performance has to be built into the enterprise and its management; it has to be measured—or at least judged—and it has to be continuously improved . . .
- (an enterprise's) results exist only on the outside. The result of a business is a satisfied customer. The result of a hospital is a healed patient. The result of a school is a student who has learned something and puts it to work ten years later. Inside an enterprise there are only costs.[14]

225.3 │ Management tasks

The technology of management is often equated with analytic techniques and tools, considered in isolation. The systems science view places them in the context of the organisation and its environment.

Management has three essential tasks: (1) to set objectives and policy; (2) to allocate resources for the achievement of objectives within policy constraints; and (3) to achieve objectives through other people or agencies . . . Good management depends upon solid information . . . For the most part, managers' information comes from what they have learned in training or from experience. Rarely does it derive from research.[15]

225.4 │ Management's role

The most important role that an organisation's central management, its board and, particularly, such top managers as the chief executive officer (CEO) and his or her immediate subordinates, play is setting the tone for the organisation, referred to often as management's philosophy. Tone can be set in two interrelated ways: hiring, and policies (including objectives) put into practice. Hiring the right staff is crucial; but so is setting the right policies and, more to the point, putting them into practice. Actions speak louder than words.

What is the right philosophy for today's successful organisation? Increasingly, the answer is seen as 'quality'—not product or production quality, where the term originated, but total quality. Ishikawa, a Japanese quality guru, believes:

Quality means quality of work, quality of service, quality of information, quality of process, quality of division, quality of people, including workers, engineers, managers and executives, quality of system, quality of company, quality of objectives, etc.[1]

225.5 | Leadership: the vision thing

Contemporary management (or leadership) theorists make much of the difference between management and leadership, much as earlier pundits distinguished administration from management. Leadership is about coping with change and empowerment; management is about coping with complexity and compliance.[16] Leaders do the right thing; managers do things right.[17] Leaders express vision; managers either have none or keep it to themselves. Leaders dedicated to excellence focus on the long term, think things through and avoid quick fixes.[18]

Leaders create and communicate the big picture to be painted; managers create the numbered canvas and supervise workers painting by numbers to produce the envisioned picture. Leaders take charge of the organisation's future. They produce change, often dramatic change, in the form of new products and production systems. They establish direction through vision; align people by communicating their vision; and motivate and inspire people to achieve the vision. Managers focus on current activities and produce results. They maintain order, the status quo with which they identify. They plan and budget, allocate resources, create structures necessary to carry out plans, organise and staff these structures, monitor progress and match it to plan, and resolve discrepancies and problems.[19] The distinction between management and leadership becomes more important as the speed of change increases. To succeed, organisations must be future-oriented and choose the right direction.

Leaders envision things to come; but unlike dreamers they also envision how to bring them about in a way that serves stakeholders' interests. At the critical boundary between leadership and management, they translate their vision into reality. Leadership complements, and does not replace, management.[16] Leadership and management are as inseparable as yin and yang; they must work harmoniously to produce results. Unbridled vision leads nowhere; management of ideas is needed to transform them into useful action. Creating and implementing plans to close the gap between the present and desired futures often involves changing the corporate culture (referred to sometimes as the social architecture) that confirms meaning on activity. This challenge is often a formidable undertaking—one that requires leadership.

Complacency, reluctance to change and blind adherence to a winning strategy are quality's nemesis. Managers may believe that 'if it ain't broke, don't fix it'; leaders know that when it ain't broke may be the only time when you can fix it.[20] Things are supposed to work—and to continue to work; because they work today does not mean that they will work tomorrow. If presently working things are likely to fail in the future because of anticipated changes in the organisation's environment, for example, it is better to replace them while they are working than to wait until they break, because then one might not be able to fix them. What is true of production processes and systems is also true of entire organisations.

Leaders challenge managers to change. Most organisations are managed, not led.[16] Good general (top) managers are leaders. They possess a vision of where the organisation is headed and how to steer it there, and can communicate this vision to gain its acceptance among lower echelon staff and can guide them toward its fulfilment. Creating a quality-mature organisation requires leadership. This manual provides a compelling vision of quality maturity and how to achieve it. Hospital managers' leadership role is to adapt this vision to their hospitals' circumstances, communicate the resultant vision to everyone in the hospital, and to motivate and empower them toward its realisation. Their management role is to create the structures and processes necessary to achieve this vision, monitor performance and reward success.

225.6 The vision statement

Quality-focused organisations and TQM/CQI practitioners often start with a vision statement—a way of expressing an organisation's purpose, its raison d'être and its desired future state. This statement expresses intentions, sets an agenda and specifies intended outcomes. It describes a long-term future and encapsulates values. The vision statement must describe attainable end-states and, by extension, plausible means to attain them. To prepare a good vision statement, the vision must be clear, easily understood, simple to communicate, desirable and energising.

226 TQM/CQI specifications: the Baldrige Award

226.1 Available TQM/CQI specifications

The principles of quality management or TQM/CQI are manifest in various criteria and standards, for example Q-90 criteria (American Society of Quality Control), ISO-9000 (International Standards Organisation), and several well known awards for which companies can compete. The oldest quality award is the Deming Prize, named for W. Edwards Deming, an American whose quality principles, especially of statistical quality control, were taken to heart by Japanese manufacturers. It was established in 1951. The prize is given by the Japanese Union of Scientists and Engineers (JUSE) and is the highest form of industrial recognition in Japan. The JUSE now offers a special category for foreign companies. In 1989 Florida Power & Light, an American utility, became the first special category Deming Prize winner. Enterprise Australia administers the Australian Quality Awards (and Australian Quality Prize which is open only to award winners).[21] In the United States companies compete for the Malcolm Baldrige National Quality Award, which increasingly exemplifies current quality management (TQM/CQI) specifications throughout the world.

226.2 Baldrige Award origins and purpose

The US Congress created the Malcolm Baldrige National Quality Award (Baldrige Award) in legislation signed into law in 1987. The award is named for a former Secretary of the US Department of Commerce, who served from 1981 until his death in 1987 in a rodeo accident. The award program, responsive to the legislation, led to the creation of a new public–private partnership. The National Institute of Standards and Technology (NIST), a unit of the US Department of Commerce, is responsible for the award. The American Society for Quality Control, under contract to NIST, assists in administering the awards program. The costs of administering the award are met by application fees and The Foundation for the Malcolm Baldrige National Quality Award that was founded in 1988 for this purpose and is supported by industry. A Board of Overseers, appointed by the US Secretary of Commerce, evaluates all aspects of the award program, including the adequacy of the award criteria and the process for making awards.

The Baldrige Award intends to promote:

- awareness of quality as an increasingly important element in competitiveness;
- understanding of the requirements for performance excellence;
- sharing of information on successful performance strategies and the benefits derived from implementation of these strategies (among other activities, awardees participate in a public 'quest for quality' conference held annually).[22]

Awards are made annually to recognise companies for business excellence and quality achievement. Awards may be given in each of the three elegibility categories: manufacturing companies, service companies, and small businesses (that have up to 500 full-time employees). Every year, up to two awards are made in each category. Fewer than two awards may be made in a category if applicants do not meet standards. Traditionally, the President of the United States presents awards in a special ceremony in Washington, DC. The Baldrige Award was first given in 1988. In the first seven years of its existence twenty-two awards have been made.

226.3 Baldrige Award process

Companies nominate themselves for a Baldrige Award. They provide a written description of their business and of their quality improvement processes and results, structured according to award criteria. Applicants must submit sufficient information on management of products and services to permit a rigorous evaluation, and to demonstrate that their approach could be replicated or adapted by other countries. Applications are limited to seventy pages (reduced from eight-five pages previously). The award's Board of Examiners evaluates applications, prepares feedback reports and makes recommendations for awards. The Board consists of 270 members, of whom nine are judges and about fifty are senior examiners. The NIST selects examiners through a competitive process, and all of them must complete a preparation course.[22]

Evaluation consists of the following four-stage process: (1) independent review and evaluation by at least five members of the Board of Examiners; (2) consensus review and evaluation for applications that score well in stage 1; (3) site visits to applicants that score well in stage 2; and (4) judges' review and recommendations.[22]

To apply for a 1995 Baldrige Award manufacturing and service companies must pay a US$4000 entry fee; small businesses, a US$1200 entry fee. For those companies making it to the site visit stage, there are site visit fees to cover site visitors' costs including their preparation of the site visit report. Small businesses pay half the fees charged of manufacturing and service companies.

The application consists primarily of a 'business overview'—to describe the applicant's business, what is most important to the business, and the key factors that influence how the business operates—and responses to the award criteria (see below). In the business overview, the applicant must describe its:

- business: products and services;
- principal customers and their special requirements, and special relationships with customers;
- major markets (local, regional, national and international);
- key customer requirements, noting any significant differences among customers or markets;
- market position (relative size, growth) in the industry and key competitive factors;
- number, type and characteristics of employees;
- equipment, facilities, technologies;
- number and types of suppliers of goods and services, including their relative importance and any special relationships;
- regulatory environment, including occupational health and safety;
- any other important factors.[22]

The business overview sets the context for the examination because the nature of the business and its customers is clearly important for determining quality and promoting business success. For example, if the applicant says that on-time delivery is a key customer requirement, then to convince examiners that it deserves an award the company, among other information, might show trends in its *measured* on-time delivery performance in comparison with the industry average, the industry best, and 'world-class' performance from another industry with similar activity.

226.4 | *Baldrige Award precepts and criteria*

Baldrige Award criteria 'are designed to help companies enhance their competitiveness through focus on dual, results-oriented goals: delivery of ever-improving value to customers resulting in marketplace success; and improvement of overall company performance and capabilities.'[22] The award criteria are built upon the following eleven core values and concepts:

- Customer-driven quality—quality is judged by customers . . .
- Leadership—a company's senior leaders need to set directions and create a customer orientation, clear and visible quality values, and high expectations . . .
- Continuous improvement and learning—achieving the highest levels of performance requires a well-executed approach to continuous quality improvement . . . both incremental and 'breakthrough' improvement. The approach to improvement needs to be 'embedded' in the way that the company functions . . .
- Employee participation and development—a company's success in improving performance depends increasingly on the skills and motivation of its workforce . . .
- Fast response—success in competitive markets increasingly demands ever-shorter cycles for new or improved products and service introduction . . .
- Design quality and prevention—business management should place strong emphasis on design quality—problem and waste prevention achieved through building quality into products and services and into production and delivery processes . . .
- Long-range view of the future—pursuit of market leadership requires a strong future orientation and willingness to make long-term commitments to all stakeholders—customers, employees, suppliers, stockholders, the public and the community . . .
- Management by fact—a modern business management system needs to be built upon a framework of measurement, information, data and analysis. Measurements must derive from the company's strategy and encompass all key processes and the outputs and results of those processes . . .
- Partnership development—companies should seek to build internal and external partnerships to better accomplish their overall goals . . .
- Corporate responsibility and citizenship—a company's management should stress corporate responsibility and citizenship . . .
- Results orientation—a company's performance system needs to focus on results . . . [22]

These core values and concepts are embodied in seven categories, used for scoring purposes. Figure II-2-3 (on page 93) shows the framework that interconnects and integrates them. Each category consists of a number of 'items' (there are twenty-four in all), and each has a number of 'areas to address' (there are fifty-four in all). Scoring is by item and the maximum overall score is 1000 points. The seven categories (and their respective number of points, items and areas to address) are as follows:

1.0 Leadership (90 points, 3 items, 7 areas)—examines senior executives' personal leadership and involvement in creating and sustaining a customer focus, clear values and expectations, and a leadership system that promotes performance excellence. Also examined is how the values and expectations are integrated into the company's management system, including how the company addresses its public responsibilities and corporate citizenship.

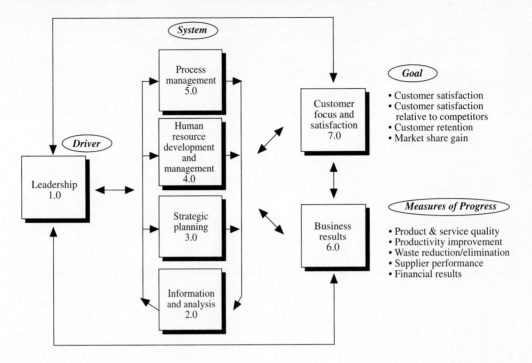

Figure II-2-3 *Baldrige Award criteria framework. Source:* Malcolm Baldrige National Quality Award: 1995 award criteria. Gaithersburg, Maryland: US Department of Commerce, National Institute of Standards and Technology, 1994

2.0 Information and analysis (75 points, 3 items, 6 areas)—examines the management and effectiveness of the use of data and information to support customer-driven performance excellence and marketplace success.

3.0 Strategic quality planning (55 points, 2 items, 3 areas)—examines how the company sets strategic directions and how it determines key plan requirements. Also examined is how the plan requirements are translated into an effective performance management system.

4.0 Human resources development and management (140 points, 4 items, 9 areas)— examines how the workforce is enabled to develop and utilise its full potential, aligned with the company's performance objectives. Also examined are the company's efforts to build and maintain an environment conducive to performance excellence, full participation, and personal and organisational growth.

5.0 Process management (140 points, 4 items, 10 areas)—examines the key aspects of process management, including customer-focused design, product and service delivery processes, support services and supply management involving all work units, including research and development. The category examines how key processes are designed, effectively managed and improved to achieve higher performance.

6.0 Business results (250 points, 3 items, 3 areas)—examines the company's performance and improvement in key business areas: product and service quality, productivity and operational effectiveness, supply quality, and financial performance indicators linked to these areas. Also examined are performance levels relative to competitors.

7.0 Customer focus and satisfaction (250 points, 5 items, 14 areas)—examines the company's systems for customer learning and for building and maintaining customer relationships. Also examined are levels and trends in key measures of business success—customer satisfaction and retention, current trends in and levels of customer satisfaction and retention, market share and satisfaction relative to competitors.[22]

Scoring takes place on the following three dimensions and there are specific scoring guidelines:

- Approach—refers to how the applicant addresses the item requirements—the *method(s)* used.
- Deployment—refers to the *extent* to which the applicant's approach is applied to all requirements of the item.
- Results—refers to *outcomes* in achieving the purposes given in the item.[22]

Award examination items are classified according to the kinds of information and/or data applicants are expected to furnish. The two types of items are: Approach/ Deployment; and Results.[22]

Table II-2-1 (on page 95) shows the scoring guidelines for the two types of items.

226.5 | Baldrige Award effort and reward

The Baldrige Award criteria are intended to permit a rigorous self-assessment, whether or not a company applies for an award. The effort needed to compete for the Baldrige Award varies substantially. For example Xerox (which won in 1989) created a twenty-person task force and spent US\$300 000 to gather the necessary data. In contrast a vice-president of Globe Metallurgical, the first small company to win a Baldrige Award (in 1988), completed the application in one long weekend because all of the needed data was already in his computer.[5]

The impact on quality of implementing quality management to the level needed to win a Baldrige Award can be substantial. For example Motorola (which won an award in 1988) practises six-sigma quality control—tolerating no more than 3.4 defects per million (the area under the normal statistical distribution beyond six standard deviations, denoted sigma). However, the award has its critics, whose number include several well known quality gurus.[23] The extent to which the award captures companies' potential for long-term success is controversial. Proponents see the award as a challenge to companies, a set of guiding principles and recognition of success.[24] Some critics suggest that the award focuses too much on results rather than on the value of methods and their linkage to success; any company could look good at a single point in time for reasons beyond the soundness of its methods and its intrinsic performance. Others suggest that the award bureaucratises quality management and stifles creativity, and that the criteria have little to do with final quality in products or services.

226.6 | Evolution of the Baldrige Award criteria

Since its inception, Baldrige Award criteria and processes have evolved in response to experience and criticism (although not sufficiently to mollify all critics). Within the award's framework (assuming that adherence to its criteria does promote quality improvement and business success, and that based on written applications and site visits examiners can separate wheat from chaff), the NIST has modestly attempted to practise what it preaches—to institute a process of continuous quality improvement. The award has progressed from an emphasis on product or service 'quality' (now the price of entry into world markets) to managing for success in competitive markets (indicating, implicitly at least, that quality is an essential attribute of management and managers' performance). There is also an increasing emphasis on methodology—how the business discerns and tracks relevant measures of quality and performance and uses these measurements to promote success.

The criteria continue to evolve in four major ways:

Table II-2-1 *Scoring guidelines for Baldrige Award examination items*

Score	Approach/Deployment	Results
0%	• no systematic approach evident; anecdotal information	• no results or poor results in areas reported
10% to 30%	• beginning of a systematic approach to the primary purposes of the item • early stages of a transition from reacting to problems to a general improvement orientation • major gaps exist in deployment that would inhibit progress in achieving the primary purposes of the item	• early stages of developing trends; some improvements *and/or* early good performance levels in a few areas • results not reported for many to most areas or importance to the applicant's key business requirements
40% to 60%	• a sound, systematic approach, responsive to the primary purposes of the item • a fact-based improvement process in place in key areas; more emphasis is placed on improvement than on reaction to problems • no major gaps in deployment, though some areas or work units may be in very early stages of deployment	• improvement trends *and/or* good performance levels reported for many to most areas of importance to the applicant's key business requirements • no pattern of adverse trends *and/or* poor performance levels in areas of importance to the applicant's key business requirements • some trends *and/or* current performance levels—evaluated against relevant comparisons *and/or* benchmarks—show areas of strength *and/or* good to very good relative performance levels
70% to 90%	• a sound, systematic approach, responsive to the overall purposes of the item • a fact-based improvement process is a key management tool; clear evidence of refinement and improved integration as a result of improvement cycles and analysis • approach is well-deployed, with no major gaps; deployment may vary in some areas or work units	• current performance is good to excellent in most areas of importance to the applicant's key business requirements • most improvement trends *and/or* performance levels are sustained • many to most trends *and/or* current performance levels—evaluated against relevant comparisons *and/or* benchmarks—show areas of leadership and very good relative performance levels
100%	• a sound, systematic approach, fully responsive to all the requirements of the item • a very strong, fact-based improvement process is a key management tool; strong refinement and integration—backed by excellent analysis • approach is fully deployed without any significant weaknesses or gaps in any areas or work units	• current performance is excellent in most areas of importance to the applicant's key business requirements • excellent improvement trends *and/or* sustained excellent performance levels in most areas • strong evidence of industry and benchmark leadership demonstrated in many areas

Source: Malcolm Baldrige National Quality Awards: 1995 Award Criteria. Gaithersburg, Maryland: US Department of Commerce, National Institute of Standards and Technology, 1994.

1. toward comprehensive coverage or overall performance, including customer-driven quality peformance;
2. toward better integration of overall performance, including employee performance, with business strategy;
3. toward further strengthening of the financial and business rationale for improvement priorities;
4. toward increasing emphasis on results . . .

The 1995 criteria are more future oriented, and more directed toward business strategy and competitiveness requirements. At the same time, the criteria requirements are more focused (24 items in 1995, compared to 28 in 1994) and aligned, permitting a 40% reduction in the number of areas to address (from 91 to 54).[22]

227 | Some TQM/CQI tools and techniques

227.1 | Perspective

There is a vast array of well known and widely-used tools and techniques that are useful in implementing quality management. Not surprisingly most of them have evolved in production, where manufacturers have placed most emphasis; fewer in product design; virtually none in technological innovation. They deserve, and are the subjects of, their own manuals. Consideration of their use is beyond this manual's scope. Nevertheless, certain techniques have become so closely associated with TQM/CQI that they are often equated erroneously with quality management. TQM/CQI techniques are merely tools; they do not provide or ensure quality. Technique can never substitute for judgment; however, judgment can be improved by technique. We have chosen to mention some of the techniques below, both to satisfy the reader's curiosity and, for those with some knowledge of TQM/CQI, to enhance their sense of the manual's completeness.

227.2 | Production

227.21 TYPES OF TOOLS

A vast number of tools and techniques exist to assure and improve the quality of manufactures. This section describes the following three types of tools that have become hallmarks of TQM/CQI programs: benchmarking, selective production methods and analytic charts.

227.22 BENCHMARKING

Benchmarking, a key aspect of TQM/CQI, was invented in the late 1970s and has evolved ever since. Essentially, benchmarking involves searching for, comparing oneself to, and learning from the best. Pryor defines benchmarking as:

> Measuring your performance against that of best-in-class companies, determining how the best in class achieve those performance levels and using the information as the basis for your own company's targets, strategies and implementation.[25]

One can benchmark any function or process, including quality management methods. For example Milliken (a textile manufacturer in Spartansburg, South Carolina, which won a Baldrige Award in 1989) benchmarked Xerox's approach to benchmarking.[26]

Camp defines four types of benchmarking:

- internal (e.g. comparing different manufacturing systems in the same company that produce a common product);
- competitive (e.g. comparing your manufacturing system to that of another company that produces the same type of product);
- functional (e.g. comparing your inventory system with others' systems, even though they manufacture different products); and

- generic (e.g. comparing such common business processes as invoicing with how other companies handle them).[27]

Benchmarking involves studying the factors that influence performance in order to identify those that are most and those that are least important:

> Benchmarking is a disciplined process that begins with a thorough search to identify best-practice organisations, continues with careful study of one's own practices and performance, progresses through systematic site visits and interviews, and concludes with an analysis of results, development of recommendations and implementation.[26]

Benchmarking requires substantial effort, not 'industrial tourism' (characterised, for example, by casual visits to companies that have won quality awards). AT&T (the United States' largest long-distance telephone carrier) estimates that a moderate-sized benchmarking project takes four to six months and costs US$40–60 000, including the cost of staff time.[26]

Benchmarking has several advantages. Firstly, one can know what level of performance is possible. Secondly, comparing one's production operations, structures and processes with those of the best performers, one can identify and analyse differences and hopefully identify those that make the difference. Clearly, benchmarking requires: measured performance, even if only categorically; knowing who is, and where one stands in relation to, the best; careful description of one's production structures and processes; willingness of the best performers to share their similar descriptions with others and/or allowing others to analyse their operations; ability to spot the differences that make the difference; and commitment to change what one can change to improve one's performance.

In medicine, knowledge of performance-influencing factors is usually limited and studies to identify them are often expensive. Moreover, there is no simple, measured way of identifying who is the best. Certainly, one can identify 'the best' by consensus opinion, but the result would only be opinion and not fact. Lacking any real measures, one cannot easily know where one stands in relation to the best or know if any changes one made would improve performance. One might be willing to analyse one's own operations, but whether or not 'the best' performers would be willing to subject themselves to rigorous analysis is open to question. Certainly, there are few people with enough training to benchmark meaningfully the production of health status improvement.

227.23 PRODUCTION METHODS

There are many techniques for manufacturing products to specifications and reducing product variance. Most techniques have only limited application to medicine, which involves state transformation, not manufacture (as Chapter 4 of this part explains). Among the best known manufacturing quality control techniques are: SPC (statistical process control); JIT (just in time) inventory or kanban; and poka-yoka (fool-proofing production to avoid operationalising Murphy's Law—what can go wrong will go wrong). The goal is error-free production through proper product specification, process design and in-process quality control. The latter is sometimes known as zero quality control because no additional, routine postproduction, quality control is needed. If error-free production is not possible, cost-effective mechanisms are needed to monitor production processes, shutting them down when they exceed pre-set limits, and to inspect finished products to identify and remedy production problems as early as possible. Inspection may also be necessary to check that any in-process quality control mechanisms are functioning correctly.

227.24 ANALYTIC CHARTS

Quality management methods emphasise use of graphics to communicate quality-oriented information. The following types of analytic charts have become integrally linked to TQM/CQI. They are referred to often as 'seven helpful charts'. (See Figure II-2-4 on page 99.) Doubtless these charts are helpful when applied appropriately. However, knowing how to use a hammer to hit a nail or a screwdriver to drive a screw is essential to build a house, but it is not sufficient to build one. So it is with these charts. We describe them here to provide readers with an appreciation of the quantitative thinking that underlies TQM/CQI. Some may be familiar to doctors, nurses and other health care workers. They are very simple analytic tools compared with those used by health systems researchers, epidemiologists and social scientists, for example. But they do embody an important point: proper use of simple techniques can produce useful information; wrong use of techniques can produce misleading information; use of no techniques will produce nothing. Graphics, visual presentation of information, are especially useful for quality assurance or improvement because trained people can comprehend their meaning easily and quickly.

- *Histograms:* simple graphic presentation of a frequency distribution, for example distribution of length of stay for patients undergoing cholecystectomy in 1990. In nature, distributions often exhibit a symmetrical bell-shaped 'normal' distribution.
- *Pareto chart:* a categorical frequency distribution, for example the number of injuries from different causes; showing that 80% of injuries result from 20% of causes.
- *Scatter diagram or plot:* a graphic presentation of the relationship between two variables, for example length of stay versus incidence of nosocomial infection.
- *Run or trend chart:* a graphic representation of a variable over time (time series), for example case fatality rate for each year in the past decade.
- *Control chart:* graphic representation of a variable over time (time series) showing the upper and lower limits, for example three standard deviations, to be used to monitor a process. An operator samples periodically a product quality variable, for example percentage of salt, or a variable that affects product quality, for example process temperature. As long as the measure falls between the control lines (determined by product specifications and sample sizes) the operator lets the process run. However, if it falls outside of the limits the operator shuts down production and looks for the cause. Production may be shut down if there is a clear trend toward a control limit before it is exceeded.
- *Flow chart:* a graphic technique used to describe a process. It usually shows operations and the events or decisions expressed in a binary (yes/no) form that initiate and connect them and result in a final event or product.
- *Cause-effect (fish-bone) diagram (Ishikawa-gram):* a graphic representation of the 'causes' that lead to or influence an 'effect', that is, the relationships among coproducers of an outcome such as nosocomial infection.

227.3 Design

TYPES OF TOOLS

The best known TQM/CQI design technique is QFD (quality functional development), to bring customers' voices to the shop floor. Another is the use of orthogonal arrays to discern the most important design factors affecting product performance. There are many others, but these two techniques serve to illustrate TQM/CQI principles.

227.31 QUALITY FUNCTIONAL DEPLOYMENT

Quality functional deployment (QFD) is an unusual name—a consequence of the direct translation of its Japanese origins—for a useful tool for facilitating product design quality control. Conceived in 1972, QFD offers a systematic way of listening to customers to

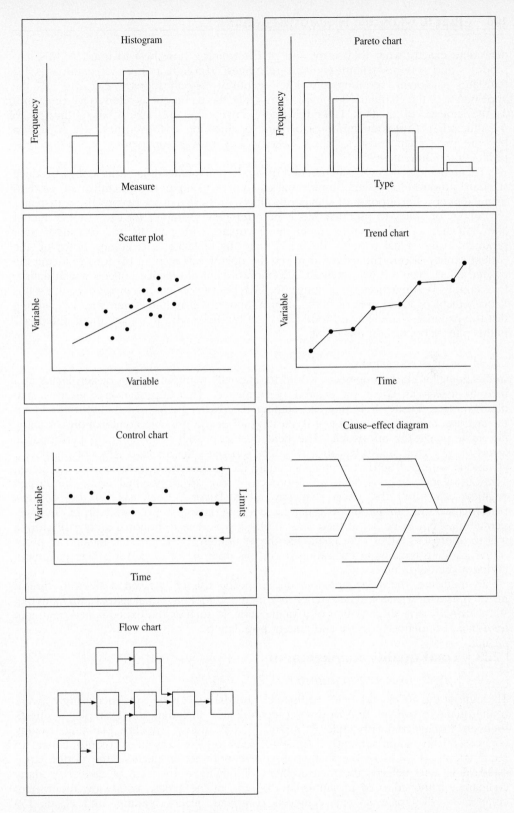

Figure II-2-4 *Total quality management/continuous quality improvements' 'seven helpful' analytic charts*

determine exactly what they want and of determining how best to translate this into products and services within available resources. Through a series of matrices, QFD translates customer requirements into technical specifications.[28] Because of the appearance of the charts used to implement QFD, the technique is referred to sometimes as the 'houses of quality'. Linked houses convey the customer's voice through to manufacturing. Customer attributes become engineering characteristics, which in turn become parts characteristics, which become key process operations, which become production requirements.[12]

Techniques such as QFD are needed by modern manufacturers because they produce standard products for distant, impersonal customers. Compared with craftsmen, modern manufacturers offer superior or cheaper products, or those that are beyond the craftsman's technology or ability to produce. Medicine offers few examples for use of QFD. Rather like craftsmen of old, doctors are in direct contact with patients and can tailor their products to individual patients' desires. Unlike the craftsmen's customer, however, the patient cannot discern the extent to which the doctor was responsible for producing the desired effect even if it was attained. Adoption of clinical practice policies which define, for example, best practices for treating specific types of patients can increase health status improvement or lower cost or both. Their adoption will require some way of ensuring that the patient's voice is heard loud and clear by those who formulate them. Chapter 7 in this part elaborates on this point.

227.32 ORTHOGONAL ARRAYS

In designing products, engineers would traditionally manipulate one design factor at a time to assess its effect on desired performance. This approach has at least two disadvantages. Firstly, it is time consuming. Secondly, performance may depend on interactions among factors. Obviously, testing all of the possible combinations of many factors is practically impossible. The next best approach is to compare performance levels of all factors under test in a way that separates the average effect of one factor at various settings. The design engineer could then select the best setting for that factor. The orthogonal array is such an approach. Using an orthogonal array the design engineer can distil the effect that any given factor setting has on the system's performance and can determine which factors have little effect on desired performance, permitting them to be set at their least costly levels. The orthogonal array is merely a tool to approach, rather than guarantee the attainment of, the design ideal. The proof of the pudding remains in the eating or, in this case, proof of performance remains in testing a prototype product.

In medicine, the same principle underlies the use of factorial designs in clinical research. However, medical researchers use them infrequently. Clinical trials, for example, still usually involve the isolation of a single variable such as the experimental treatment for a narrowly defined disease and patient population.

228 | Total quality management

228.1 | TQM: from fad to failure

Throughout the 1970s and 1980s companies and their CEOs became increasingly aware of the quality revolution and its driving technologies, including, for example: Deming's fourteen management principles;[29] Juran's quality trilogy (quality planning, quality control, quality improvement);[30] Crosby's four quality absolutes (conformance to requirements, do it right the first time—prevention not inspection, the performance standard is zero defects, the measurement of quality is the cost of quality).[31] Many companies launched TQM programs. By the end of the 1980s, worldwide about eight companies—all Japanese—had achieved complete quality maturity and about 150 companies had progressed far enough to be considered world-class in quality—the level needed to win the Deming Prize or Baldrige Award.[32] Most companies' TQM programs failed; quality improvement rates were depressingly low.[26]

In 1991 a survey of 300 electronics companies by the American Electronics Association found that 73% had quality programs underway; but of these 63% said that they had failed to improve quality by even as much as 10%. 'The performance improvement efforts of many companies have as much impact on operations and financial results as a ceremonial rain dance has on the weather.'[33] Winning a national quality award is no guarantee of success. The Wallace Company, an oil supply firm (Houston, Texas) that won a Baldrige Award (in 1990) went bankrupt when the oil industry recession overwhelmed its strong customer support. The bloom was off the rose. At most companies the flower had wilted. Why had most companies' TQM programs failed to thrive?

Many TQM programs were form over substance. They never progressed beyond slogans on managers' coffee mugs. Chief executives paid lip-service to quality but never instituted meaningful programs to effect its improvement. One survey of 100 top managers from Fortune 500 companies (the world's largest) found that almost 90% of them believed delivering value to customers was critical. But over 80% of these same companies did not tie compensation to customer satisfaction.[34] Companies:

- hid behind TQM—a set of initials without definition or formulation—to avoid the hard work of managing quality;[35]
- failed to focus on what their customers wanted. Their top managers were ignorant about quality. They tried to delegate their entire action plans to middle managers and failed to realise that fixing quality meant fixing the entire organisation—a leadership task that cannot be delegated;[2]
- confused ends and means, processes with outcomes, and assumed falsely that if they carried out enough of the right improvement activities, performance improvements would inevitably materialise.[33]

True quality improvement take ten or more years because of the need to change an organisation's culture. Many TQM efforts simply ground to a halt when they failed to fulfil their original promise. Bureaucratic TQM programs produced a prodigious amount of red tape and created as many problems as they solved. Failed TQM programs have spawned a new business: cleaning up the resultant mess. These post-TQM consultants suggest that successful change programs begin with results.[33] Forget about abstractions and generalities such as organisation-wide consciousness-raising, empowerment, teamwork and TQM's other trappings. Focus on palpable problems, such as production bottlenecks. Solving them brings immediate and measurable improvement. Institutionalise changes that work and create the context for continuous performance improvement.

In industry, TQM is a fading fad. Companies that embraced the quality revolution have made TQM their way of doing business; those that tried and failed, or that missed the boat, are left asking: What comes after TQM?

228.2 | Corporate re-engineering: TQM with an attitude

Classic TQM's prevailing ethos is everyone wins: glad tidings for all. Corporate re-engineering makes a virtue out of suffering: no pain, no gain. Aptly-named corporate re-engineering guru Michael Hammer advises: 'Don't automate, obliterate'.[36] The need to continually redesign and rebuild organisations' production (and that means all) processes is corporate re-engineering's basic premise. At best, organisations' production processes (that convert inputs into outputs to meet customers' needs) are built according to theories and practices relevant at the time of their construction. With technological advances, they rapidly become outmoded—and the rate of change is increasing.

Corporate re-engineering starts from scratch: How should production best be organised to take advantage of today's technology? Corporate re-engineers start by identifying and describing processes that are vital to business success. Then they simplify and streamline them and, best of all, identify the elements that can be eliminated entirely. The key perspective is outcomes: what customers want from processes. The key focus is success-determining processes that consume the most resources. The key technique is to substitute automation and info-mation (the automation of the generation of information and its use to control production processes) for labour to reduce costs and increase quality. The result is an organisation built for maximum business success; one that is often unrecognisable when compared to the original organisation.

In 1980 Ford (a leading US auto-maker) set about streamlining its accounts payable process, among others, in an attempt to reduce its costs. At first it expected its plans for a new computer system to reduce staffing by 20%, from 500 to 400 clerks. When Ford discovered that Mazda (a leading Japanese auto-maker) employed only five people to perform this same function, it began to think its accounts payable department was five times the size it could be. Ford opted for radical change, not modest improvement. It reduced its accounts payable staff by 75%, to 125 people.[36]

Taco Bell, a purveyor of Mexican-style fastfood (Irvine, California), is an oft-cited corporate re-engineering success story.[37] While competitors focused on trying to reduce the cost of ingredients—27% of dollar costs—Taco Bell focused on the other 73% of costs and was able to shave 7¢ from overheads. These cost savings permitted Taco Bell to increase employees' wages, cut prices and turn a profit (previously it had lost money). Rather than have employees prepare ingredients in costly retail space, Taco Bell opened regional commissaries and shipped prepared ingredients to its outlets. This production mode permits Taco Bell to peddle food from carts—opening new markets for its products on street corners and at other outlets such as at airports.

When new technology appears, organisations usually graft it into their existing operations, rather than building the organisation around it: the industrial equivalent of paving footpaths (rather than rethinking the best routes for automobiles). Existing ways of business may be computerised rather than designing new ways of doing business that take full advantage of computer technology. Existing electronic medical records, for example, are often no more than the equivalent of sheets of paper on a video display terminal; they need to be redesigned free of the sheets-of-paper constraint that computerisation permits. Corporate re-engineering starts with technological capabilities and builds the organisation on this foundation.

Successful corporate re-engineering depends first on acceptance of total transformation. Only organisations that are prepared for total transformation are good corporate re-engineering candidates. Corporate re-engineers forget how things are done now and decide how best to do them. They eschew quick fixes and incremental changes because they believe they often create as many problems as they solve. Relentless technological advances result in the constant need to re-engineer. Corporate re-engineering is a lot like painting the Sydney Harbour Bridge: as soon as you have finished, it is time to start again. While corporate re-engineering may displace lots of workers, corporate re-engineers' jobs are secure—at least until the next management fad comes along.

229 QM/CQI in hospitals: What would it take?

229.1 Experience to date

To date, experience with TQM/CQI in hospitals is extremely limited. In Australia there has been much talk but little action. Few hospitals have attempted to introduce TQM or CQI methods. In the United States, hospitals noticed the TQM/CQI movement at a time when industry's enthusiasm was beginning to wane. According to a study conducted by and published in the journal *Hospitals* (in June 1992), by the end of the 1980s about one in five hospitals had a TQM/CQI program. A majority of hospital CEOs, 58.5% (of 781 respondents), said they were implementing a TQM or CQI program; 84.6% of the rest said they planned to do so (96.7% of them in the next two years). Of existing programs, 68.8% were one year or less old. Only 1% of respondents said that they did not have a program because TQM/CQI was a fad.[38] CEOs reported that senior management was the most, and medical staff the least, enthusiastic about TQM in their hospital.[39]

Another, later, and much larger and more comprehensive suvey, reported in 1993/94,[40–42] found that 68.9% of responding hospitals indicated that they have undertaken a formal TQM/CQI effort to improve the quality of care; the rest had not. The survey was mailed to 5492 hospitals; 3033 responded (about 60%). Hospitals' CEOs and persons in charge of quality management efforts completed surveys. Of TQM/CQI hospitals, 87% have assigned their TQM/CQI efforts to a specific individual, but less than half of them (48%) were senior managers. About half of TQM/CQI hospitals (48%) had established a separate unit for TQM/CQI. At most hospitals (73.4%), TQM/CQI activities were less than two years old; at only 4.1% were they more than four years old.

Major barriers reported to TQM/CQI efforts fell into two classes:

- senior management (principally, lack of commitment and focus, insufficient resources, lack of training, and too many other changes going on);
- organisational barriers (principally, inability to use personnel in new ways or to work together, inadequate organisational structure and information systems, and lack of realistic goals).

Survey findings also included the following:

- Few doctors at TQM/CQI hospitals (16.2%) had received training in quality improvement and fewer still (10.1%) had participated in quality improvement teams. Non-TQM/CQI hospitals reported that 9.5% of their doctors had received such training and that 8.4% of their doctors had participated in QI teams.
- With respect to fifteen procedures, TQM/CQI hospitals reported using quality of care data in QA/QI project teams for 20.3% of those that they performed. For non-TQM/CQI hospitals the comparable figure was 11.8%.
- Half of TQM/CQI hospitals reported using practice policies of some type (such as clinical algorithms, protocols or pathways); 30% of non-TQM/CQI hospitals said they did so.
- About 35% of TQM/CQI hospitals reported using clinical and cost data in reviewing doctors' privileges and credentials; 21% of non-TQM/CQI hospitals said they do so.
- The biggest need at TQM/CQI hospitals was clinical data assistance. Non-TQM/CQI hospitals said that what they needed the most was TQM/CQI training assistance, but clinical data assistance was almost as important here too.

With respect to quality improvement, TQM/CQI hospitals reported greater impact on human resource development and financial outcomes than did non-TQM/CQI hospitals. There was no difference with respect to reported improvement in patient care outcomes. A higher percentage of TQM/CQI hospitals reported cost savings, although most TQM/CQI and most non-TQM/CQI hospitals reported that they had yet to realise any net savings.

Reports of benefits from TQM/CQI projects are different from substantiated attribution of improvements to TQM/CQI efforts, and from organisation-wide quality improvement efforts that result in organisation-wide performance improvement.[43] While TQM/CQI efforts have the potential to improve hospital-wide performance, realising such improvement requires the management will to effect the necessary organisational changes and a culture that supports quality improvement activities. Hospitals have a long way to go in this direction.

Just as the majority of hospitals were jumping on the TQM/CQI bandwagon, a backlash against TQM/CQI was beginning to emerge among some hospital CEOs.

According to Donald Berwick, one of the founders of the health care TQM/CQI movement in the United States, an emerging voice is saying that: 'quality management isn't fulfilling its initial promise, or that it's not going to be an important factor in health care as people might have thought.'[44] Berwick says the following factors are behind the anti-TQM voice:

> (people do not) really understand the degree of change involved in applying TQM methods . . . people will say that TQM doesn't work, when referring to efforts that really don't have much to do with it . . . No (information) currently exists that will allow us to learn from what we were doing . . . a lot of the activities now in quality management aren't yet really driven by purpose . . . We just keep shifting the deck chairs around.[44]

One of the most daunting aspects of introducing TQM into hospitals is obtaining the medical staff's co-operation. So far hospitals have concentrated on facility operations and other non-clinical aspects of care. Few hospitals have attempted to apply TQM/CQI to clinical care and some admit they are not sure how to do so. Other rationale advanced for starting with non-clinical aspects of care include a desire to test out and refine the concept first and the need to demonstrate improvement prior to involving medical staff. Some hospitals have also expressed the concern that once doctors get involved they will suggest many improvements, necessitating that well-worked out systems be in place to respond to them. One apparent result of the TQM/CQI movement seems to be greater integration of quality assurance, utilisation review and risk management activities under a single umbrella.

As industry has found, quality management is not a panacea and its implementation often requires a complete revamping of an organisation's business and the way it conducts it. Hospital managers are even more likely to fall prey to fads than their industrial cousins for the same reasons: constant change and competitive concerns. Their TQM programs suffer from the same types of defects—and hospital managers exert less control over their organisation's production function than industrial chief executives. The biggest problems are form over substance, failing to reorganise for quality, focusing on structures and process devoid of results, and lack of persistence and perseverance. Hospitals have become bogged down in TQM process. They are focusing too much of their effort on mastering CQI tools and not enough on cultural transformation. Their TQM efforts lack heart because they focus on the intellectual rather than the personal. Few hospitals actually focus their quality improvement efforts on the customer.[45] 'Hospitals spend too much time on theory and not enough on practice. Hospitals have to show . . . how CQI . . . makes a difference to patient care. Unfortunately, it can take a long time to see initial results.'[46]

In implementing quality management programs, hospitals must solve the same two paradoxes that face industrial companies: the desire for quick results that take a long time to achieve, and the wish for major effects from manageable beginnings. Firstly, to continue the initial level of enthusiasm for the promised results, they must show results, but it takes a long time to see initial results. Secondly, people want to implement large-scale programs, to do something really worthwhile, but initially at least such programs are often unmanageable; manageable programs produce small initial changes that do not seem worth the effort (although their cumulative number and effects may be substantial).

229.2 *Quality management in hospitals: a long way to go*

Quality-focused organisations fulfil customers' needs. They decide who are their customers, discern their needs, organise to fulfil them and determine the extent to which they are fulfilling them. They create the management structures and information systems to direct quality improvement efforts; possess the will, ability, and incentives to organise their activities to this end; and develop some way of gauging management success. Table II-2-2 (see page 106–7) compares the situations one might encounter at a typical TQM manufacturer and at the usual hospital with respect to critical quality, production and organisational characteristics. These situations do not compare on any fundamental characteristic; gaps are often of chasmic proportions.

Hospitals have a long way to go to achieve quality maturity. They spend virtually nothing on enabling technology, do not specify products and pay scant attention to improving production systems. They are not organised to maximise value for money and their culture is inimical to its achievement. Historically, health care's customers—patients—had no way of knowing if hospitals' or doctors' services benefited them beyond providers' (often erroneous) assertions that they did so. Consequently there could never be any real competition among providers based on quality's central attribute—patient health status improvement.

Quality management means meaningful measurement of improvement. This aspect of quality management alone will revolutionise medical care and, for the first time, will focus attention on patients' perception of value-for-money—the ultimate quality metric. Until recently, health care providers lacked the methods needed to improve quality. What methods existed were compartmentalised, for example under quality assurance, utilisation review, risk management, or were referred to as epidemiology, biostatistics, or decision science, or planned change.

Applying Baldrige Award criteria (described in a preceding section) to Australian hospitals reveals just how far they have to go to measure up. Being generous, the average hospital would score about eighty out of a possible total of 1000 points; thus a ten-fold improvement would be needed to even approach being a quality-mature organisation. Present-day hospitals are not organised for quality-focused production. They do not measure up because they do not measure.

We could be criticised for applying industrial TQM criteria to hospitals. After all, it is obvious that hospitals are very different from manufacturers, not only in what they do but also in how they do it—and that the relationship between what and how determines an organisation's character. Furthermore, hospitals are complex organisations—far too complex to discuss here in detail. Such a criticism would be valid, except that quality management principles apply more or less to all types of organisations, even if the practice of health care quality management is far more difficult than that of industrial quality management. In any case, this section intends only to demonstrate just how far hospitals have to go to achieve quality maturity, to set the scene for the rest of the manual, which provides a map for this long and arduous journey.

229.3 *Leadership for quality: customer focus*

229.31 HOSPITALS AS PRODUCTION FACILITIES

There is no leadership for quality in hospitals. Typically, hospitals do not see themselves as production or state-transforming facilities. Certainly, they are not organised to transform patients from one state to a predetermined alternate state at least cost and greatest patient satisfaction. Without adoption of this perspective, hospitals will make little real progress toward quality maturity.

Table II-2-2 *Comparison between quality-focused manufacturers and hospitals on various aspects of quality management*

Aspect	TQM manufacturer	Usual hospital
QUALITY PROCESS		
Essential product quality, value	Readily appreciated by customer and manufacturer; measurable, measured	Not always readily apparent to patient, or to doctor; not measured easily; often not at all measured
Warranties (of quality)	Usual, increasing	Unheard of; alien
Attribution of outcome (quality)	Usual straight forward; heuristic changes to process relatively easy	Difficult, expensive, experience may be misleading
Process	Manufacturing	State transformation
Process design	Substantial attention, knowledge, R&D; knowledge can be generated by manufacturer	Very little attention, knowledge, or R&D; essential knowledge generation beyond providers' resources
Production	Integrated; unified goals	Fragmented; various goals
Costs	Minimise	Little or no concern; sometimes (unintended) incentives to add cost
Information systems	Many, often integrated; substantial concern, investment	Few or none; medical record is inadequate base; little concern, virtually no investment
CUSTOMER/PRODUCT		
Coherence, congruence of purpose, interests among parties	High	Variable; sometimes conflicting
Customer	Is subject: chooses, uses product to satisfy needs or wants; advertising shapes choices	Is object: product is changed patient; doctor shapes choices
Payment–preference linkage	Customer pays; direct value-for-money concern	Patient pays rarely; maximise outcome regardless of cost
Product differentiation	Goal is high differentiation in performance, cost, other factors	Goal is low or no differentiation in performance; cost irrelevant; other factors marginal
Customer segmentation	High; match customers' needs to profitable products	Usually none: treat everyone
Product design	Substantial investment; customer pull	Little or none, particularly at provider level; technology push
Development strategy	Identification, development of competencies that underlie innovative products	Usually none; amorphous products

continues

Table II-2-2 *continued*

Aspect	TQM manufacturer	Usual hospital
Enterprise/environment		
Culture	Production	Professionalism
Central measure of management performance	Long-term profits	Various or none
Management preparation	Reasonably good	Usually poor
Competition	Real, may be intense; include substitution	Virtually none; little substitution possible or desired
Incentives	Winning products, efficiency of production; market share; profits	Reputation, prestige, income or budget

Hospitals are not customer-focused. At best they focus on units of service rather than on patient outcomes: health status improvement, the cost of its attainment and patient satisfaction with care. Hospital managers are more like workshop custodians than leaders of production facilities. In fairness, compared to industrial companies, hospitals face some difficult problems with respect to discerning who are their customers and responding to their needs. Nevertheless, they must adopt both a production perspective and customer focus in order to succeed in the quest for quality.

229.32 CUSTOMERS

An automobile manufacturer, for example, can target its customers and produce a car intended to satisfy their wants at a price they are willing to pay. However, this situation does not exist for all organisations, including hospitals. Who is a prison's customer? Certainly not the prisoner, a person convicted of a crime against society. One could decide that a prison's customer is society or the state. Prisoners are not autonomous. They cannot choose whether or not to go to prison, or even to which prison to go. And, of course, they do not pay for their stay. If prisoners are not a prison's subjects or customers, they are certainly its objects on which the prison is intended to act. What voice should prisoners be accorded in determining a prison's quality? Patients fall somewhere between automobile customers and wards of the state and, depending on one's views, closer to one than the other. Hospitals cannot always choose their patients and patients cannot always choose among hospitals. Moreover, patients face considerable difficulties choosing among hospitals based on their quality of care.

229.33 HOSPITAL MANAGERS: CUSTODIANS OF DOCTORS' WORKSHOPS

Hospitals, especially in the United States and to a lesser extent in Australia, have often been conceived as doctors' workshops. In Australia, private hospitals operate much like doctors' workshops, while in public hospitals doctors may be viewed as contracted providers of service; although if something goes wrong in either a public or private hospital both hospital and doctor may be held jointly responsible. This same situation pertains in other countries and in some circumstances doctors are hospital employees or part of a government agency that operates the hospital, such as in the case of military hospitals.

Essentially, in private practice, patients are doctors' customers. Doctors order whatever services patients need from the hospital on their behalf. In marketplace medicine, this agency leads hospitals to view doctors as their customers and to compete for doctors' business. One could imagine 'automobile doctors' who took customers' orders, negotiated with suppliers and delivered cars that would meet individual customers' specifications, modified by the automobile doctor based on what he or she thought was possible and other factors such as how much the customer could afford.

In the sale of automobiles, there is no doubt who is the customer. The automobile purchaser is the manufacturer's customer; dealers act as distributors. The manufacturer is the parts suppliers' customer. In the United States, at least, some hospitals, even those purporting to be following TQM/CQI principles, see patients *and* doctors as customers. This view is inconsistent and leads to inherent contradictions.

Suppose a hospital has several up-to-date operating theatres. It decides to build more, not because its present theatres cannot handle the workload but because they are full at the time doctors prefer to operate. Faced with a similar capacity problem, an electric utility for example, might decide to offer off-peak rates to better utilise expensive generating equipment. Both customer and utility benefit. The customer could make adjustments, running appliances at off-peak times for example, and save money. The utility company would make higher profits than if it built more capacity to meet unfettered peak demand. Hospitals do not offer off-peak operating theatre rates.

In Australia, even if private hospitals, which charge patients for operating theatres, were to offer off-peak rates, what incentive does the surgeon have to change the time he or she wishes to use theatres? Neither patient nor surgeon would even bother to consider a change in the use of theatre time. In the case of public hospitals, the cost of theatre time would not be a matter for consideration by anyone. In the end, of course, we all pay. The hospital's additional capital expenditures for extra operating theatres contribute to the cost of health care without any plausible commensurate improvement in patients' health status. The hospital, faced with patients' desire for lower costs and doctors' desire to operate only at certain times, must decide who is its customer. Fundamentally, it must decide if its central purpose is to improve patients' health status as cost-effectively as possible or to be a doctors' workshop, for example.

229.34 FOCUS ON VALUE

Hospitals do not focus on the value of their services to patients. In fairness, present payment arrangements and incentives either discourage or militate against a value-for-money focus. Consideration of value is central to quality management.

When DRGs were introduced in the United States everyone was concerned that the incentives involved to cut lengths of stay would reduce quality. In the event, lengths of stay were reduced and 'quality' does not appear to have deteriorated, although costs of care have been shifted to others, so that perhaps no net savings have really been effected. From a quality management perspective, the concern about reduction in quality (health outcomes for patients) from the introduction of DRGs was miscast. The proper question is: how can we reduce length of stay without reducing patient outcomes?

Manufacturers realise increasingly that the time it takes to develop new products or manufacture existing ones is the key to success. Moreover, they also realise increasingly that they are making something that meets customers' needs rather than physical specifications, and thus service is an integral part of the product. Hospitals following this line of thinking, for example, may realise what people understand: time is money. But they do not always realise that time is more valuable than money. The extra profits to be made by Australian private hospitals in reducing throughput times may be manyfold the cost of the reduction. Posthospital care is part of the total product. If a hospital could reduce length of stay significantly, the cost savings may enable it to pay for home care (including cash payments to the patient's relative to offset expenses) and still reduce total per episode costs. The problem, of course, is that present mechanisms may not even permit hospitals to follow this course, let alone provide them with the incentives to try to do so.

229.4 Information and analysis

229.41 HOSPITALS DO NOT MEASURE, AND THUS CANNOT MANAGE QUALITY

Hospitals do not measure the quality of their care. Consequently, they can neither assure the quality of their care nor document any improvement that may result from changes to practices; some of these practices may worsen quality, but they will never know. Hospitals neither compare their performance nor strive to do better than others in any meaningful sense. They also do not strive to be the best that they could be by, for example, benchmarking their performance and practices. Hospitals do not specify their products, nor strive to improve product specifications, nor make any meaningful efforts to improve practices through research. To begin to focus on quality, hospitals must measure their performance, and compare it to others and to what is possible. To achieve quality maturity, they must measure patient outcomes and conduct research to identify better and more cost-effective practices.

229.42 MEASURING QUALITY

Presently, health care's product is amorphous or is often defined in such trite or banal terms as 'not merely the absence of disease but a positive feeling of wellbeing'. Quality management means meaningful measurement and hence measurable quality. Hospitals must define their product in measurable terms that are acceptable to patients. Health status improvement is the appropriate central measure of provider performance, or quality.

Since hospitals have never defined quality in operational terms, it is not surprising that they have never measured quality operationally. In ordinary practice, actual measurement of health status improvement (the preferred health care product measure) is extremely difficult if not impossible. Instead, hospitals must measure conformance to individuated process and outcome criteria and population-adjusted standards. Only recently has even this degree of measurement become possible. The inability to measure quality parameters directly is not unusual. The problem in health care is the weakness of the link between what can be measured, such as care processes and outcomes, and the desired product (health status improvement). This link can be strengthened only by generating knowledge and information useful for practice. We are presently spending virtually nothing to provide this information, despite expending trillions of dollars worldwide on health care.

229.43 FEEDBACK: LEARNING TO IMPROVE QUALITY

Feedback is essential to improving quality. Despite this obvious need, and valiant efforts by the few, medicine today is still best characterised as an open system of efforts to produce good. Clinical information systems are virtually non-existent and the few that exist do not produce information designed to improve practice. Quality management is information based. Early pioneers lacked the technology to measure and the organisational structure to improve quality. Today the technology has emerged. The organisation must now be created to use it effectively.

229.44 IMPROVING PERFORMANCE

Measurement alone cannot improve quality. Once hospitals have identified production deficiencies they must investigate their root causes and, once elucidated, take action to eliminate them. Sometimes root causes are obvious and hardly bear investigating.

However, in medicine this is often not the case. Not only is the systematic identification of problems difficult, but so too can be identifying their causes. Hospitals must employ clinical epidemiologists and other research-trained specialists in quality management. Today there are few trained health care quality management specialists of any type. A substantial investment in training them, either in formal academic settings or on the job, is essential if health care quality is to be improved. Perhaps the greatest barrier to quality improvement is the existing organisation of health care, specifically the lack of mechanisms to implement improvement strategies. Unless hospitals, for example, organise themselves for improvement it cannot happen.

229.45 IMPROVING TECHNOLOGY, PRODUCTS, PRODUCTION

Systematic attention to the development of technological innovations, new products and production processes is an essential aspect of quality management. Present health care research and development efforts are both too meagre and too divorced from practice to be effective. The essential goal is to produce knowledge to improve practice, to create greater health status improvement per dollar spent on care. Cost-effectiveness can be improved by reducing cost as well as improving effectiveness by more than its marginal cost. Both strategies require knowledge which must be generated and used in practice to improve quality.

Hospitals rarely engage in research and development to design improved health care technologies (e.g. diagnostic and therapeutic interventions), or products (e.g. practice policies), or production systems (e.g. health care delivery processes). Where such research does exist in hospitals, it is generally funded and directed by others (e.g. government agencies), and usually involves product development technology, exemplified by clinical trials to assess drugs' effectiveness, the results of which are published in the medical literature. Research on processes is rarely done anywhere. We give car manufacturers incentives and sanctions to produce more efficient, less polluting cars even while funding research on new forms of transportation. We cannot afford to let manufacturers conduct business as usual while hoping for a new form of transportation that would make cars obsolete. Quality management demands the same logic be applied to health care.

By organising for quality and investing in well-conceived clinical and administrative information systems, hospitals can improve the extent to which they utilise existing knowledge and generate information to improve process design (health care practices). Similarly, they can expand product design knowledge (how to diagnose and treat patients). Research on product technology (cures for diseases), which seems to have preoccupied us for centuries, is important but not paramount. We should spend at least as much, if not even more, on trying to improve process technology (care delivery) to ensure the cost-effective use of the trillions of dollars spent on health care, as we do on chasing cures for disease—quests which in some cases at least may ultimately turn out to be as futile as the search for the holy grail.

Due to the cost and complexities of generating new knowledge, individual hospitals acting alone can make only limited contributions to improve products, for example in the form of better practice policies. Meaningful progress in this area requires concerted action among clinicians in hospitals and other production facilities rather than reliance on lone scientists working in ivory towers funded by remote government agencies.

229.5 | Strategic quality planning and human resource development and management

The simple truth is that hospitals have no strategic quality planning. Few have any meaningful human resource planning and management, and what little there is in hospitals is not integrated with their overall operational and performance goals—because they have none. Hospitals may engage in isolated TQM/CQI training or employee involvement activities, but their lack of quality-focused management structures means that such activities more often than not represent wasted effort. We have yet to find any hospital that bases staff members' pay on quality-focused performance, let alone patient's health status improvement. Clearly there is a great deal of room for improvement.

229.6 | Process management and business results

The idea of actually designing health care products and processes is foreign to hospitals. There is virtually no explicit design of products (manifest in practice policies, for example) or of processes to implement them (manifest in planned workflows, for example). Lacking relevant information hospitals cannot maintain and improve key production processes, let alone support services to enhance them. Hospitals do not have a prevention mentality. Hospitals must seek out and remedy quality problems before they surface, rather than pretending that because they are not painfully obvious they do not exist.

Actively seeking improvement opportunities would further enhance hospitals' performance and provide greater value for money to their customers (patients). Ideally hospitals should generate real-time information to monitor results of, and to improve, their production processes. Presently, hospitals are about as far from approaching this ideal as they can be. Since hospitals do not know the quality of their products they cannot know whether or not they are improving! Doing virtually anything along these lines would represent a significant step forward.

229.7 | Customer focus and satisfaction

As mentioned previously, hospitals are not customer-focused. They make virtually no efforts to determine customers' expectations nor patients' satisfaction with care in any meaningful fashion. Most hospitals do a poor job of even handling patient complaints and maloutcomes when they occur. Lacking basic information, charting trends or making comparisons among hospitals is out of the question. There is room for enormous improvement.

229.8 | Resources for quality management

Attentive readers would have realised by now that to improve quality requires considerable investment in quality measurement, assurance and improvement mechanisms, information systems, and knowledge generation. Where is this money to come from, especially when the health care system, in Australia at least, seems to be under considerable financial stress? Stated simply, it takes money to save money. Quality can be improved only if resources are devoted to this end. Either additional, spend-to-save funds are provided initially, or less must be spent on existing activities. Eventually, improved productivity would finance quality improvement. Along the way, some interventions might be reduced while others would be increased.

This process has to be managed. Suppose an expensive intervention consuming billions of dollars was found to be indicated in only one-tenth of cases in which it was used presently. Implementing strict payment criteria immediately would result in catastrophic loss of income for providers who specialise in doing the procedure, if they were unprepared to perform other services. Proper policies might include paid retraining or time-limited payment for *not* performing the procedure while providers adjusted their practices or lifestyles. Managing the practice environment through proper incentives is vital to quality management's success.

| 229.9 | *Incentives for quality management*

People learn to do things a certain way, become comfortable with these ways and find it hard to change. The medical profession has an unrivalled history of noble concern about patients and their outcomes. The spirit to improve is strong even if at times the will is weak. Medicine, however, often confuses means with ends. The intention to do good is confused with actually doing good and questioning outcomes is interpreted falsely as impugning motives. Lack of objective measurement of how much good is being done only reinforces these tendencies. Quality management depends not only on the will to do better but also on ways to measure progress and the means to change. Ultimately, it must also depend on comparing results with costs. Most people can do better with unlimited resources. It takes a resourceful person to achieve the same results with less, and an innovator to do better with less. Without such comparisons it is quite easy to spend more but do no better, or even to achieve less while deluding oneself that by spending more one must be doing better.

Where are the incentives and sanctions to apply quality management to health care? Without them quality management efforts are doomed to fail. They simply cannot succeed through the devotion and altruism of good men and women. Presently, hospitals and doctors have no incentives beyond altruism to improve quality. In fact, they have many incentives *not* to adopt quality management practices. Quality improvement requires measuring performance, changing practice and becoming more efficient. Who would voluntarily subject themselves to scrutiny, change and accountability? Quality improvement is only possible by sustained, systematic and systemic action.

Weeding out bad doctors, for example, will meet a hospital's fiduciary responsibility and help improve quality, but only marginally. Much greater improvement requires changing what everyone does and/or the way that they do it. It requires management, information systems and, above all, incentives. Payments based on results such as conformance to process and outcome criteria would encourage quality improvement. Allowing providers to keep the savings from efficiencies would also stimulate quality improvement, provided that quality (conformance to process and outcome criteria and standards) were monitored.

By measuring and publishing quality scores, patients would be able to pick and choose rationally among providers. Given such valid information, health care would become a market-based enterprise and consumers could once again be given choices. They could decide what treatments to seek. Providers in turn could differentiate their products and customers would make quality decisions. Given the current health care environment, this may seem somewhat too fanciful to some readers. But which has greater social utility: spending $250 000 on treating a terminal cancer patient or allowing that patient to accept less heroic treatment (perhaps with little or no loss of health status) and creating an annuity for his or her family with the balance? Certainly, a choice for conservative therapy would enrich the family, not health care providers. Such choices require information.

The primary concern of policy makers should be creating mechanisms to provide patients with the information to make choices, to whom they rightly belong, and empowering patients to effect their choices. Hospitals and other health production facilities would respond appropriately and quality would be assured and improved. That is quality management's essential message. Government must guarantee, and society must support, the incentives to ensure that providers hear it and respond appropriately.

References

1 Juran JM. What Japan taught us about quality. Washington Post 1993; Aug 5: H1.
2 Juran JM. Made in USA: a renaissance in quality. Harvard Business Review 1993; Jul/Aug: 42–50.

3 Tenner AR, DeToro IJ. Total quality management. Cambridge, Massachusetts: Addison-Wesley Publishing Company, Inc., 1992.

4 Detouzoz ML, Lester RK, Solow RM. Made in America. Cambridge, Massachusetts: MIT Press, 1989.

5 Main J. How to win the Baldrige Award. Fortune 1990; Apr 23: 101–16.

6 Brown JS. Research that reinvents the corporation. Harvard Business Review 1991; Jan/Feb: 102–11.

7 Garvin DA. Quality on the line. Harvard Business Review 1983; Sep/Oct: 65–75.

8 Garvin DA. Managing quality. New York: Free Press, 1988.

9 Taguchi G, Clausing D. Robust quality. Harvard Business Review 1990; Jan/Feb: 65–75.

10 Schoenberger RJ. Japanese manufacturing techniques. New York: The Free Press, 1982.

11 Ishikawa K, Lu DJ (trans). What is total quality control—the Japanese way. Englewood Cliffs, NJ: Prentice-Hall, 1985, p. 45.

12 Hauser JR, Clausing D. The house of quality. Harvard Business Review 1988; May/Jun: 63–73.

13 Moore, JF. Predators and prey: A new ecology of competition. Harvard Business Review 1993; May/Jun: 75–84.

14 Drucker PF. The new realities. New York: Harper & Row, Publishers, 1990.

15 Goldschmidt PG. Health Services Research and Development: The Veterans Administration Program. Health Services Research 1986; 20: 789–824.

16 Kotter JP. What leaders really do. Harvard Business Review 1990; May/Jun: 103–11.

17 Bennis W, Nanus B. Leaders: The strategy for taking charge. New York: Perennial Library (Harper & Row), 1986.

18 Hickman CR, Silva MA. Creating excellence: Managing corporate culture, strategy, and change in the new age. New York: Plume (Penguin Books), 1986.

19 Kotter J. A force for change: How leadership differs from management. New York: Free Press, 1990.

20 Zaleznik A. Managers and leaders: are they different? Harvard Business Review 1992; Mar/Apr: 126–35.

21 Australian quality awards 1995. St Leonards, NSW: Australian Quality Awards Foundation [69 Christie Street, St Leonards, NSW 2065—61–2–901 9967].

22 Malcolm Baldrige National Quality Award: 1993 award criteria. Gaithersburg, Maryland: US Department of Commerce, National Institute of Standards and Technology, 1993.

23 Does the Baldrige award really work? Harvard Business Review 1992; Jan/Feb: 126–47.

24 Garvin DA. How the Baldrige award really works. Harvard Business Review 1991; Nov/Dec: 88–93.

25 Pryor LS. Benchmarking: A self-improvement strategy. J. Business Strategy 1989; Nov/Dec: 28–32.

26 Garvin DA. Building a learning organization. Harvard Business Review 1993; Jul/Aug: 78–91.

27 Camp RC. Benchmarking. Milwaukee, Wisconsin. Quality Press, 1989.

28 Guinta LR, Praizler NC. The QFD book. New York: American Management Association, 1993.

29 Walton M. The Deming management method. New York: Dodd, Mead & Co, 1986.

30 Juran JM. Juran on leadership for quality. New York. Free Press, 1989.

31 Crosby PB. Quality is free. New York: Mentor Books (new American Library), 1979.

32 Williams R, Bertsch B. Stages in the management of quality improvement programmes. Rotterdam: Erasmus University Department of Business Organization, 1989; quoted in Tenner AR, DeToro IJ. Total quality management. Cambridge, Massachusetts: Addison-Wesley Publishing Company, Inc., 1992.

33 Schaffer RH, Thomson HA. Successful change programs begin with results. Harvard Business Review 1992; Jan/Feb: 80–89.

34 Total quality management. Washington Post 1993; Jun 6: H1.

35 Crosby PB. Completeness: quality for the 21st century. New York: Dutton, 1992.

36 Hammer M. Reengineering work: don't automate, obliterate. Harvard Business Review 1990; Jul/Aug: 104–12.

37 Hammer M, Champy J. Reengineering the corporation. New York: Harper Business (Harper Collins Publishers), 1993.

38 TQM/CQI. Hospitals 1992; Jun 5: 24–36.

39 CEOs say hospitals must learn from each other for TQM success. Hospitals 1992; Jun 20: 42–50.

40 The quality march: National survey profiles quality improvement activities. Hospitals and Health Networks 1993; December 5: 52–5.

41 The quality march: Part two of a national survey of quality improvement activities. Hospitals and Health Networks 1993; December 20: 40–6.

42 The quality march: Part three of a national survey of quality improvement activities. Hospitals and Health Networks 1994; January 5: 45–8.

43 Shortell SM, Levin DZ, O'Brian JL, Hughes EFX. Assessing the evidence on continuous quality improvement. Is the glass half empty or half full? Hospital and Health Services Administration 1995: 40(1); 4–24.

44 Berwick DM. TQM backlash prompts questions. Hospitals 1992; Jun 5: 30.

45 Albrecht K. Hospitals need kinder, gentler TQM. Modern Healthcare 1993: 23(1): 29.

46 Clinical quandaries: getting MDs to buy into CQI means making adjustments. Hospitals 1993: Jan 5; 29.

Chapter 3

THE HEALTH SYSTEM

---

231 | Purpose of this chapter

The practice of medicine may be as old as humankind. Certainly, doctors existed in ancient civilisations, such as those of Mesopotamia and Egypt. Hippocrates of Cos lived 2500 years ago and was an itinerant physician who went from town to town to ply his trade. Hospitals too have a long history, and have changed dramatically from a respite for the sick and weary to bastions of medical technology. As spectacular as these changes have been, they have been eclipsed by another: government's guarantee that all citizens should have access to health care and the concomitant rise of the health system.

Growth in health care expenditures provided the means to develop and deliver medical technology, which in turn stimulated demand for more health care services that resulted in spiralling expenditures. In industrialised countries, costs spiralling out of control now threaten to destabilise their health systems and force far-reaching changes. Health care expenditures now threaten to crowd out those for education, housing and other beneficial social purposes, and even to diminish the economic activities that have sustained them. Vast increases in health care expenditures have been accompanied by relatively modest gains in health, measured inadequately by life expectancy at birth. Paradoxically, increasing health care expenditures may soon become one of the greatest threats to people's quality of life and even to their health. Quality management may be the last best hope of improving value for money, controlling costs without losing benefits, and permitting rational trade-offs when necessary.

This chapter provides the broad context necessary to comprehend quality management's role in the production of health and in hospitals. It describes:

- the purpose, nature and components of the health system, including the distinction between public health programs and personal health services;
- quality at the system and production levels, and the difference between health policy and quality management;
- determinants and measurement of, and health care's impact on, health;
- health research and development, including medical technology assessment;
- the concept of health care interventions' effectiveness;
- the economic appraisal of health care, including the elements of cost-effectiveness analysis.

Most doctors are unfamiliar with the macrolevel perspective that this chapter presents, but are nonetheless subject to its forces and will likely be more so in the future. The nature of the health system, its role in society, and such extensions as national health policy, are extremely complicated matters that involve the philosophy of government and the individual, and other ideological or value-laden subjects. Necessarily, this chapter covers them selectively and somewhat superficially. It intends to provide readers with a big picture perspective and quality management's place in it. Later chapters in this part amplify on many of the concepts mentioned here.

232 | Key concepts

This chapter elaborates on the following key concepts essential to understanding the health system, quality management's role in it, and the quantification of health—the measurement of effectiveness—and the calculation of cost-effectiveness.

- The health system is a conceptual system, one in the mind of the beholder. It consists of all elements (and their interrelationships) that intend to maintain and improve people's health. Different groups, including government, each with its own sociopolitical traditions, controls or influences system elements. A conceptual system is not the result of rational design efforts to achieve its perceiver's purpose. It cannot be managed in the organisational sense. It has no identifiable clients (or customers); merely everyone collectively, regardless of philosophy, purpose and desires.
- The health system may be viewed as consisting of the following five principal components: public health programs; personal health services; research and development; resource development; and system policy management.
- Public health programs target populations and intend to protect people from health threats. Personal health services (often referred to collectively as the health care system) intend to maintain and improve the health of those individuals who seek health care. They account, by far, for the largest share of total health care expenditures.
- The health care system is also a conceptual system; hospitals are among its elements. Government influences the environment in which hospitals operate. Policy decision makers influence events through health policy—an instrument to promote the achievement of health goals in the same way that economic policy intends to achieve economic goals. Health policy may include incentives or sanctions that encourage or limit certain behaviour on the part of individuals, health care providers, corporations and other social institutions, to achieve socially desirable ends.

- Historically, wealth has been a source of health. Now, health care has become a source of wealth. Health care is one of the largest economic sectors. The resources devoted to health care continue to grow, both absolutely and relative to other sectors. Health care financing schemes have expanded to ensure citizens' access to health care.
- Growth in health care expenditures provided the means to develop and deliver medical technology, which in turn stimulated demand for more health care services. The health sector not only accounts for an increasing fraction of nations' output but also heightens government's role in the economy, because government accounts for or controls most health care expenditures.
- The meaning of quality and the means for its improvement vary by health system level. Production-level quality is concerned with production outcomes; it involves patient–provider interactions. At the system level, access to care is clearly an important quality consideration and may obviously influence a population's health. However, it is irrelevant at the production level.
- Quality management is a production-level tool, useful for improving production units' performance and products' quality. It applies only to organisations, which are managed systems that exert command and control, including the ability to hire and fire managers and workers.
- Policy management refers to the mandates, prohibitions, incentives and sanctions that health system actors, particularly government, intend to alter the functions of various elements in the system, their interrelationships, or the environment to achieve policy objectives. System-level policy may influence production-level management and vice versa.
- Maximising production units' (e.g. hospitals') outcomes will not necessarily improve the population's health maximally: only people with access to hospitals can benefit. Interventions may not be very effective; the last units of achievable health status improvement may be gained at considerable cost. The population's health status might be improved to a far greater extent by increasing access to care for people who have no or only limited access, or by diverting some resources elsewhere, thereby yielding more population health status improvement per dollar expended.
- System-level (global) effects are the result of production-level (local) interactions: results of provider–patient interactions that express individual choices, constrained by system policies that promote or prevent actions. Effecting positive change in complex dynamic systems is difficult. Concentrating resource allocation decisions in few hands politicises them and increases the difficulty of breaking the mould. Smooth dynamic adjustment of complex systems depends on distributed decision-making.
- Accountable health schemes (referred to as 'plans' in the United States) both collect payments for and deliver health care, overcoming the fundamental flaw of separating health care financing from its delivery. They represent a significant shift in the health care paradigm from payment for services to responsibility for patient outcomes.
- A person's health status is the result of four sets of interrelated factors and their interactions: biology (genes or genetic programming); behaviour; the prenatal and postnatal environments, encompassing the physical (e.g. climate, pollution), biological (e.g. viruses, bacteria), economic (e.g. food, shelter, clothing), and social (e.g. population aggregation, workplace factors, social support systems) environment; and the health system.

- Life expectancy at birth is an established way of measuring the population's health, but tells us nothing of the health quality of life. Health status is a measure of a person's health throughout life (or for a defined period) and includes the number of years lived and the health quality of life, taking into consideration morbidity, institutionalisation and functional ability. Health status provides the common metric necessary to evaluate all of the health effects of alternative, disparate interventions.
- Most gains in life expectancy seem to have come from improved socioeconomic circumstances that improved nutrition, public health measures that separated man from microbe, and preventive interventions such as vaccination that reduced threats to health or increased resistance to them. Public health measures are often credited with improving life expectancy because, until recently, effective specific medical interventions are thought to have been lacking.
- The role of specific medical interventions in improving health is controversial, with opinions arrayed against inadequate facts; yet, each day worldwide we spend trillions of dollars on medical interventions on the presumption that they are effective. The widespread failure to evaluate health care's impact on populations' health and to assess interventions' effectiveness—and the general lack of concern about this failure—may be one of the twentieth century's most important social phenomena.
- One must distinguish between health care's impact on the population's health and specific medical interventions' effectiveness. Medical interventions may greatly improve some individuals' health, but their impact on the population's health may be small.
- People have long presumed that medical care is effective; questioning its effectiveness is a relatively new phenomenon. Two principal perspectives cast doubt on the effectiveness of modern medical interventions: vast increases in health care expenditures have produced modest gains in life expectancy; and well-designed studies show that most interventions tested are ineffective, whereas inadequately-designed studies show them to be effective.
- Good intentions do not necessarily produce good results. For far too long we have simply assumed that: health care services resulted in health status improvement; the ability to palliate translates into the ability to cure; and advances in medical science result in more effective interventions. What is plausible is not necessarily valid.
- Rational quality management depends not only on the practice of scientific medicine but also on scientific methods for assessing (measuring) the quality of care and improving practice.
- Little is spent on science; little is known scientifically. Too little useful research is being done, too few research results are useable, and information that is relevant and valid is too hard to find. We know little about the diffusion of innovation or the best way to transfer technology, to disseminate information to practitioners.
- Medical technology assessments are needed to determine interventions' cost-effectiveness, to inform choices among alternatives and to improve practice. Such knowledge is essential for setting practice policies and thus for meaningful quality management programs. Most interventions are introduced in practice without scientific assessment of their effectiveness; costs are rarely measured.

- Interventions have both general (placebo) and specific effects. An intervention's specific effects define its effectiveness.
- An effective intervention produces a desired effect or outcome: patients' health status improvement, the difference between intervention and a disease's natural history. True effectiveness refers to this difference determined in such a way that it can be attributed confidently to the intervention. Assumed or observed effectiveness refers to what one has observed in practice; attributing any observed 'improvement' to the intervention usually overestimates true effectiveness, and the intervention might not be effective at all. Studies that compare one treatment to another demonstrate interventions' marginal, but not their true, effectiveness.
- Effectiveness is a statistical concept; it describes the results of interventions applied to populations of patients, a statistical distribution. For patients, the mean expresses an intervention's expected health benefits; the variance, its inherent risks. Understanding the statistical nature of interventions' effectiveness is critical for quality management.
- One must distinguish between an intervention's effectiveness and providers' performance—the extent to which providers use an intervention appropriately and implement it properly. An effective intervention improves a population of patients' health status. An appropriate intervention can reasonably be expected to benefit a particular patient because he or she fits the profile of patients for whom it is effective.
- The economic appraisal of health care intends to answer one or more of three questions: Do benefits exceed costs?—cost-benefit analysis. Which intervention is most cost-effective?—cost-effectiveness analysis. Is the intervention's effect worth its cost?—cost-worth analysis.
- Cost-benefit analysis weighs all of an intervention's costs against all of its benefits, measured in monetary terms, usually, from society's perspective. Even if benefits do exceed costs, distributional effects—who benefits and who pays—are also important considerations. Cost-effectiveness analysis involves choices among alternative interventions; not deciding whether or not any intervention is worthwhile. Cost-worth analysis involves comparing the value of an intervention's effectiveness to the cost of its production.
- A cost-effectiveness analysis produces data about alternative interventions' discounted streams of effects and the direct costs of producing them. Cost-effectiveness analysis differs from cost-benefit analysis in three important ways: only specified program effects, for example health status improvement, are of interest and they are not valued in money terms; only the direct costs (valued in money terms) of the intervention or program are considered; and 'net' benefit is not calculated.
- Decision makers may want to achieve: a fixed level of effectiveness at lowest cost; the maximum level of effectiveness for a fixed cost; or a given unit (rather than level) of effect at least cost (the cost-effectiveness ratio). A cost-effective intervention produces a specified unit of effect at a lower cost than practical alternatives.
- Medical science has emphasised the quest for more effective interventions. The net result is ever-increasing health care expenditures. In an era of increasing scarcity, cheaper treatments that are as effective as those that exist now may be more valuable socially than marginally more effective treatments whose cost is so high that few people or health financing schemes can afford them.

- Quality and costs are intertwined. Quality managers must facilitate production of patient health status improvement at least cost and, when necessary, make trade-offs between quality and cost.
- The coming era of quality management promises to fulfil a cherished dream: knowing realistically what one can expect from medical intervention and being sure of getting it. Quality management can be as liberating for doctors as it is reassuring for patients.

233 | Industrial analogies

The economy is a conceptual system that produces, distributes and consumes goods and services. Converting the value of these goods and services into money terms provides a measure of economic activity and of nations' wealth. The economy encompasses, for example, factories and other types of production units, facilities for financing the production and consumption of goods and services, government and other regulatory mechanisms, and their interactions. Basically, the economy consists of a myriad of transactions intended to satisfy human needs and wants. From these local interactions emerge global properties that are manifest in the economy's performance. In turn, these global properties may affect local interactions, creating the dynamics that are characteristic of complex systems. These dynamics shape the economy's evolution and its long-term success or failure. The economy is so large, interactions among its elements so numerous, and its dynamics so complex that it is difficult to describe fully, let alone understand completely, even though it is a product of human activity.

The economy is a conceptual—not a managed—system, even though its principal constituent production elements (business organisations) are managed systems. Government policy decision makers cannot manage the economy in the same sense that directors of industrial enterprises manage the manufacture of goods. Through industrial, fiscal and monetary policies, and exhortations to spend or to save or to export, government policy decision makers may try to influence the economy, but these actions can only affect the economic environment. They are not linked directly to the operation of business organisations. Many economists would say that government policies are as likely to hurt as they are to help the economy.

In the West, Japan's success is often ascribed to government co-ordination of 'Japan, Inc'. In Japan, such 'co-ordination' is often viewed as unwarranted, unwelcome and unhelpful meddling. The idea that the government can actually run the economy has been discredited, at least for now, with the breakdown of the economies of the Commonwealth of Independent States (the former USSR) and its former Eastern European satellites, and the worldwide movement toward the privatisation of the production of goods and services, including health care.

In most industrialised countries, the health system has, or is about to, become the economy's largest sector, accounting for 7–14% of nations' output of goods and services. The health sector's growth has increased its salience. Health care employs a lot of people, from highly educated doctors to less skilled orderlies and labourers, and this type of employment is expected to grow at a time that traditional sectors, for example agriculture and manufacturing, are shrinking. In the United States, General Motors spends more on health care than on the steel that goes into the cars that it produces. The cost of health care now exceeds all of the profits of US businesses. Nations' economies and their international competitiveness depend increasingly on heath care and its cost. Health care holds the key to populations' wealth as well as to their health.

234 | The health system is a conceptual system

234.1 | Perspective

Beginning in about the middle of the nineteenth century, there was a renewed and heightened belief that medical intervention could affect people's health for the better. This belief grew and society's major concern was how to assure everyone's access to health care and to bring them the benefits of medical research. Financed or encouraged by government, health care exploded. In the 1960s increasing scepticism confronted the so-called miracles of modern medicine: To what extent did modern health care improve health? However, during the 1970s health care expenditures continued to grow at an increasing rate, generating concern about the cost of health care: Were expenditures sustainable? In the 1980s, even though expenditures continued to grow rapidly, the focus of concern shifted to the quality of care: Were people getting what they should have been getting from medical care?

Since the early 1990s concern has centred on, and well into the twenty-first century will in all likelihood continue to centre on, three key issues: What is value-for-money? Who decides? And how? The next section describes the nature of the health system and health care's rise to economic pre-eminence in developed countries. Necessarily, the section provides a broad-brush perspective relevant to this manual's purpose rather than the photographic analysis that these complex subjects deserve.

234.2 | Nature of the health system

The health system (referred to sometimes as the health sector) is a conceptual system that consists of the totality of entities (and their interrelationships) that intend to maintain or improve people's health. Activities of other social sectors, for example agriculture, construction or transportation, may affect people's health, positively or negatively, but people do not perceive the maintenance or improvement of health to be their primary purpose. A conceptual system is one that people can form in their minds but does not exist in a tangible form. A conceptual system is not the result of rational design efforts to achieve its perceiver's purpose. It simply exists as it has evolved. Different groups, each with their own sociopolitical traditions, control or influence each of the system's disparate elements. Unlike an organisation, for example a government office, a company, or a hospital, a conceptual system cannot be managed. Management implies the ability to command and control—to hire and fire—inherent in organisations but lacking in conceptual systems. In managed (as opposed to conceptual) systems, decision makers control system boundaries, the operations of their various constituent elements, and elements' interrelationships, even though the environment—including system-level policy decisions—influences these systems. In conceptual systems, government policy decision makers are merely one of the myriad of elements that comprise the perceived whole; they do not manage it in the organisational sense. In the case of government-run health services, government manages these systems as well as being an element in the conceptual health system.

Policy decision makers may view the production and consumption of health care services from various perspectives, for example as a right, as an investment, or as a source of employment. Nevertheless, their major concern must be the extent to which health care expenditures translate into health status gains. System-level policy decision makers may talk about or set goals or targets, for example for reducing mortality, and view resultant levels in the population as outcomes. They may establish policies intended to affect system performance, including, for example, resource allocations toward achieving goals (in the same way that economic fiscal, monetary and industrial policies are intended to achieve economic goals). They may also provide incentives or sanctions that encourage or limit certain behaviours on the part of individuals, health care providers, corporations and other social institutions, thereby altering the way that they act. To these decision makers, the health system may be a black box. They may be able to measure inputs (e.g. resource expenditures) and outputs (e.g. life expectancy), but they have few, if any, plausible ways of knowing, let alone influencing, what goes on inside the box. Policy decision makers may alter the environment in which system elements operate, but they lack the degree of control necessary to change their operations directly.

234.3 Health system components

The health system may be viewed as consisting of the following five principal components:

- *Public health programs*—health protection for populations or communities, including, for example, health education, product safety, consumer protection, sanitation, occupational health and safety, recycling and environmental programs;
- *Personal health services*—the delivery of health care to individuals at primary and higher levels by doctors, nurses and other health workers—and, through decision support technology, by individuals themselves—and the organisation, financing and management of such care;
- *Research and development*—the generation of new knowledge, development of technology, assessment of existing and new health policies, practices and programs, transfer of technology and dissemination of information, and development of methods and mechanisms for these purposes;
- *Resource development*—the provision of system inputs encompassing, for example, production of health workers, construction of health facilities, and the manufacture and distribution of health care products;
- *Policy management*—setting objectives and formulating policies for the system, its components and their interrelationships; obtaining resources for the health system and allocating them among its components; monitoring health conditions and outcomes; evaluating system performance and economic, ethical and social impacts; assessing prospects.

234.4 Public health programs

Public health programs target populations, either the general or specific communities. They intend to protect people from potential or actual threats to health by, for example, changing people's behaviour or their environment. Sanitation, health education and mass vaccination activities have long been staple public health programs. Over the years, public health programs have expanded to encompass the work, social and physical environments. For example, government inspectors may visit employers to ensure that they provide workers with safe work sites, and government may prohibit employees accepting additional monetary compensation for occupational risks if employers can reduce them by changing processes—even if such changes incur greater costs—because society has determined that such exchanges are not ethical.

Violence in society is now increasingly seen as a public health problem; certainly it takes an increasing toll of young lives. However, the means to implement effective preventive measures, even were they to exist, are presently beyond health workers' sphere of influence, let alone control. Undaunted, doctors with a concern for social responsibility campaign against violence, nuclear war and for environmental protection, as their forebears in the last century did for hygiene and public health. The medicalisation of social problems is not without its attendant dangers, of course; however, discussion of this issue is beyond this manual's scope.

Traditionally, public health programs have been, and mostly still are (although need not be inherently), government-run. However, private community agencies, for example, may attempt to educate the public of the dangers of smoking tobacco, to prevent non-smokers from starting and to persuade smokers to quit. These types of activities by voluntary associations and other non-government agencies are also public health programs. Some traditional public health activities, notably mass vaccination and screening programs, work directly on individuals and thus intersect with personal health services. The difference is that public health workers carry out their activities on a mass scale and go out into the community, while doctors wait in their surgeries or offices for individuals to seek their advice or assistance.

Increasingly, public health programs and personal health services work in a two-step process. For example, the national cancer society may encourage women to get a mammogram. Health financing schemes may pay for this diagnostic test. Activated women request this test from their doctors. The cancer society's goal may be seen as motivating as many women at risk for breast cancer as possible to undergo periodic mammography; the health financing scheme's, as reinforcing motivation and facilitating testing; the provider's, as helping the activated woman assess the test's risks and benefits, if needed and desired, performing the test properly, and acting promptly on its results. Health education efforts cost money and may induce additional demand for health services thereby increasing health expenditures further. They can also reduce demand for health services by, for example, educating patients when (and when not) to visit the doctor.

Government may deliver health care to individuals. In Australia, for example, government runs hospitals, although private visiting medical practitioners may provide patient care in public hospitals. Such care represents government-provided personal health services (because government controls directly the terms and conditions of their delivery), not a public health program. This manual is concerned only with personal health services; the other components of the health system are beyond its scope.

234.5 | Personal health services

Personal health services (referred to sometimes as health care) target individuals. They intend to maintain and improve the health of those individuals who seek health care. They deliver preventive, diagnostic, therapeutic and rehabilitative interventions to these individuals, who are also usually the interventions' object (although in some cases, for example certain psychiatric interventions, patients' family members may be the intervention's object).

With the advent of sophisticated decision support technology (DST), individuals may increasingly become providers of their own health care. While individuals have long followed the nostrums of the day and have relied on their own intuitions to attempt to prevent, and even to cure, disease, decision support technology promises fundamental empowerment. Enterprises' provision of and individuals' access to personal health DSTs will increasingly challenge traditional ideas of personal health services' provision. Here, however, we focus only on traditional, provider-mediated personal health services to provide a context for later discussions of quality management's role in their improvement.

Providers—individual health professionals or institutions such as hospitals who employ or contract with them—deliver personal health services. Health care professionals, medical doctors and others who are trained explicitly for and derive their living from health care practices, intend to relieve pain and suffering and, if possible, to extend life; secondarily, they intend to prevent mortality and morbidity by counselling patients in health (about keeping well) and in sickness (about aiding recovery and preventing further deterioration if complete recovery is not possible). Their activities may be divided into:

• caring, exemplified by the old-style family general practitioner or the hospice;

- advice and counsel, including education that permits better self care, for example the information primary care workers offer mothers about well-baby care;
- specific medical interventions—what patients allow doctors and other providers to do to them, the most sophisticated and expensive of which take place in hospitals.

Medical care refers to those personal health services that medical doctors deliver traditionally. Medicine is the art and science of promoting, maintaining and restoring individual health, of diagnosing and treating disease, and of predicting the course of disease with and without intervention. A sick person visits the doctor who diagnoses the patient's health problem and, for example, may prescribe a drug for the patient to take, in the expectation that it will restore the patient to health within a few days.

The health care system refers to the aggregate delivery of personal health services, including their financing and organisation. Like the health system of which it is part, the heath care delivery system is almost always a conceptual system, as it is in Australia. Its elements include production units that deliver health care services, such as doctors' offices, hospitals and nursing homes; health care financing schemes; professional and trade associations; and government policy decision makers. Existing health care organisations and their interrelationships may represent rigid barriers to innovation.

In most industrialised countries, health care is largely financed publicly and is mostly delivered privately. Government or other social institutions, such as employers or provident associations, socialise health care expenditures and, in the case of government, there may be only a single payer. These health care financing schemes pay individual doctors and institutions for the care that they provide to their patients. In Australia, as in Britain, general practitioners and specialists are nominally private practitioners but are heavily dependent on government for their income and terms of service. They work in their own offices, surgeries or clinics. Government may run hospitals in which private practitioners deliver care, the usual situation in Australia, or employ health professionals to provide health services, for example to the poor. In the United States, almost all health care practitioners, hospitals and nursing homes are private, but government pays for about 40% of health care expenditures, and it exerts considerable influence on the medical market.

Sociocultural traditions or political considerations may limit severely the extent to which government can produce effective, efficient and acceptable health care service, even when it runs hospitals and employs health care providers. Government operation or control of health services does not assure outcomes; often it militates against them. In industrialised countries, government does not run most economic enterprises, yet the environment in which they operate (which government does influence) has allowed them to produce unprecedented wealth to citizens' benefit.

Personal health services account, by far, for the largest proportion of health care expenditure, and hospitals account for a large share of these expenditures. Thus, for almost all practical purposes, health sector expenditures are synonymous with spending on personal health services. In 1989/90, the latest year for which figures are available, personal health services accounted for 91.8% of Australia's total health care expenditures (A$28.7 billion), and hospitals accounted for 42.0% of these expenditures (38.6% of total health expenditures).[1] In 1990 the United States spent US$666.2 billion on health care, of which 96.6% was for personal health services and 37.1% (38.4% of total health expenditures) went to hospitals.[2] Due to differences in national accounting, these figures may not be strictly comparable.

234.6 | Growth in and vastness of the health care system

The practice of medicine is virtually as old as humankind, but the concept of the health care system is a modern invention. The health care enterprise has grown enormously, fuelled by the rise of the nation state, the industrial revolution, government financing of medical care and the concomitant explosion in medical technology, and the enduring human desire to remain healthy and, when sickness strikes, to be restored to health. Consequently, industrialised countries have created a vast health care system that has already, or is about to, become their single largest economic sector. Government involvement has now become so great that in virtually all countries, including the United States, its hand controls the health care system's growth and direction. The health sector's increasing size and economic importance is of concern not only because it accounts for so much of nations' economic output but also because it is controlled by government, thereby continuously increasing government's role in the economy.

In ancient Greece, medical practitioners like Hippocrates were itinerant tradespeople who provided medical services to small communities. Cities that wanted a doctor to settle there offered him an annual salary, for which the money was raised through a special tax. To a large extent, the community doctor served the needy. The doctor was guaranteed an income even when there was not much work.[3] By the second century AD, ancient Rome also had a public medical service. In imperial Rome many doctors were in private practice, and some were attached to a few families who paid them an annual sum for all attendances throughout the year. Roman infirmaries for slaves, which also appear to have been used by free Romans, were the foundation of hospitals for the sick and indigent. This century, hospitals have been transformed into bastions of medical technology.

With the rise of the modern nation state between the sixteenth and eighteenth centuries, the idea arose of a national health policy and all that it implies. Government's concern with the people's health stems from the idea that society's and the state's welfare were one and the same. In continental Europe, with its tradition of absolute monarchy, these ideas led to government-created medical policy implemented through regulation in the interest of protecting the people's health and fostering the ruler's wealth. This movement culminated in the German physician Johann Peter Frank's system of a complete medical policy, of which the first of six volumes was published in 1779.

Improvements in agriculture freed people from having to work on the land. They moved to cities to work in the factories created by the industrial revolution. Factories produced an unprecedented flow of goods that materially improved people's lives. Continuous improvements in agricultural and industrial productivity permitted people to produce more for the same or less effort. Incomes rose and people could buy the plethora of goods and services that they produced. Rising wealth permits countries to devote more resources to health care. Historically, countries have tended to spend a disproportionate fraction of their rising national wealth on health care.

234.7 Government's role in expanding the health care system

Governments' greatest role in health care has been to generate the flow of funds that has fuelled the system's growth, motivated by the desire to ensure citizens' access to, and the presumed benefits of, the latest advances in medical care. Universal, mandatory government-guaranteed, health care financing is both a cause and consequence of the enterprise's vast size and increasing cost. The explosion in medical technology—brought about by general advances in science and specific increases in public financing of research and development, and relatively unfettered payment for (or incorporation into government-run health services of) resultant technologies—both increased the cost of care and promoted further expansion in health care financing schemes. Government's expanding role in financing medical care began over 200 years ago and continues to the present.

In 1789 in the United States, the federal government instituted compulsory insurance for sick and disabled seamen, which led eventually to establishment of the US Public Health Service. In 1793 the British parliament passed an Act that facilitated the establishment of friendly societies among wage-earners, and by 1801 they numbered more than 7000 (in England and Wales). Beginning in 1883, Bismarck introduced a system of comprehensive social insurance in Germany that included medical care. In Britain, by the beginning of the twentieth century: 'Doctors had won full freedom to prescribe and manage treatments, both among their private patients and their dispensary and hospital inmates, regardless of the social costs of the resources they used.'[4] The culmination of this trend in Britain was the introduction, in 1948, of the National Health Service.

In the United States, amendments to the *Social Security Act* in 1965 created Medicare and Medicaid—the government's principal programs for directly financing medical care. In February 1993, for at least the seventh time this century, the United States once again began debating how to ensure all of its citizens were given universal, government-guaranteed access to health care, with, so far, the same ambiguous results. In November 1994, while the public ostensibly favoured universal access, voters repudiated the Clinton Administration's approach as too bureaucratic and as giving government too large a role in health care. In Australia, in 1952 the Commonwealth government introduced the first national health insurance scheme. Initially, it was a tripartite system paid for by the Commonwealth government, voluntary health insurance, and the individual through membership of a health insurance fund. In 1984 the Commonwealth government introduced tax-funded universal health care. While access to care and all services for all citizens was the original aim, government is now trying to find ways in which it can limit its financial commitment to health care.

Some of the architects of the British National Health Service thought that while it might prove expensive initially, ultimately—by improving individuals' health—it would reduce the cost of health care.[5] They were wrong—for at least two reasons. Firstly, the longer people live, the more health care services they can consume. Secondly, there is an infinite amount that one can spend on virtually anything, especially health care which seems to require, or is at least capable of absorbing, limitless infusions of wealth.

234.8 Growth in health care expenditures

Throughout the world, and especially in industrialised countries, health care expenditures have increased markedly in recent decades, consuming (or accounting for) an ever-increasing fraction of nations' gross domestic products—the sum of their outputs of all goods and services. Resources devoted to health care are vast and, in industrialised countries, are still growing more rapidly than the economy as a whole. In the United States for example, in 1993 health care accounted for over 14% of the nation's output, by far the world's largest percentage. However, in many industrialised countries the percentage is approaching or has exceeded 10%. In Australia, in 1992/93 it was 8%. This lower percentage reflects a conscious government decision to limit health care expenditures. Further, while the United States has the world's highest per capita health care expenditures, in the last twenty-five years those of other industrialised countries, for example Canada, France, Japan and the United Kingdom, have increased at a greater rate.[6,7]

Historically, nations' wealth has been a source of their populations' health. Now, health care has become a source of individuals' wealth. Material improvements, manifest in rising average per capita incomes for example, have long been associated with better health—more to do with better nutrition, living conditions and public health programs than specific medical interventions. Nevertheless, the associations between rising wealth, increasing health care expenditures and improving health, undoubtedly reinforced pre-existing beliefs in the effectiveness of medical care, which further fuelled its expansion as fast as rising wealth would permit. The introduction or expansion of health care financing schemes meant that providers were paid to take care of patients whom they had previously treated free of charge as charity cases. Patients were guaranteed financial access to health care; providers were guaranteed incomes. Although providers' incomes increased, their productivity did not increase commensurately. Price inflation followed, as surely as night follows day.

Unlike other industries, where increased demand and/or prices brings forth increased supply and price stabilisation, increasing the supply of doctors leads to additional health care expenditures. The more doctors, the greater the increase in expenditures, because doctors generate their own demand. Further, while doctors' fees account for about 20% of health care expenditures, they control about 80% of such expenditures, at least in the United States. The magnitude of health care expenditures is not an inherent consequence of disease but of doctors' and patients' responses to disease. Cardiac myopathy might be treated conservatively or by a heart transplant. Patient outcomes might not be much different but there may be a vast difference in the resultant cost of care.

The principal factors underlying increases in health care expenditures are: population changes; price inflation; and product changes such as the intensity with which services are provided. In the United States for example, in recent years about 10% of health care expenditure increases have been due to its ageing population; about 70% to price inflation; and about 20% to product changes.[8] As the population ages, health care expenditures tend to rise because disease and disability increases with age. In industrialised countries, the continued ageing of the population promises to propel health care expenditures to new heights. General price inflation increases nominal health care expenditures, of course, but the special factors fuelling medical cost inflation are of most concern. In the United States for example, the medical care consumer price index has consistently increased at double the rate of consumer prices generally.

In the past fifty years, the content of medical care services has changed markedly. The ceaseless flow of new technologies has driven costs skyward. New technologies expand medical practices and tend to be more costly than existing ones and rarely replace them completely. The increasing rate of ever-more-costly medical innovations threatens to rocket medical care expenditures out of sight. The combined effect of these engines of medical care expenditure growth promise to transform industrialised economies. In the United States, for example, in 2040 health care expenditures may account for 35% of its gross domestic product, compared to 11.6% in 1990 and about 4% in 1940.[9,10]

There is nothing inherently wrong with spending an ever-greater fraction of national resources on health care. However, the size and rate of increase of these expenditures may make them unsustainable, intensifying competition for resources, both within the health care sector and between it and other sectors. At some point health care expenditures may crowd out those for such desired and desirable ends as housing, education and industrial investment, may threaten the very economic activity on which they depend, and may result in a diminution in the general quality of life and, paradoxically, in population health status as well.

235 | Quality by the level

235.1 | *System-level quality differs from production-level quality*

The meaning of quality and the means for its improvement vary by health system level, although health care quality's principal considerations remain constant. They are: health status, cost, satisfaction and trade-offs among these attributes. (See Table II-3-1 on page 127.)

Table II-3-1 *Quality by the level*

Characteristic Level:	Health system, social subsystem	Health care system, health subsystem	Production unit, health care subsystem
System type	Conceptual	Usually conceptual; concrete, if government run or mandated	Concrete
Purpose	Promote population's welfare	Ensure people's health security—availability of, access to health care; finance, organise, deliver personnel health services	Produce health status improvement
Central goal	Maintain, improve populations' health	Maintain, improve people's health, peace of mind	Improve patients' health status
Targets	Usual, e.g. —to reduce infant mortality by 10% by the year 2000	Sometimes, e.g. —to provide basic health care to everyone; —to provide primary care within 1 km of residences	Rare —usually expressed implicitly as maximal health status improvement
Interventions	Various policy initiatives	Various strategies for financing, organising, delivering personal health care services; health-producing facilities	Specific medical interventions
Effects	Indirect, through mandates, suasion, education, incentives, etc. to engender subsystem change	Usually direct, depends on various factors, constraints	Direct, but extent of health status improvement usually unknown
Effectiveness	Usually low	Variable, depends on system's organisation, mandates, etc.	Variable, with great variation by problem, provider, etc.
System elements' integration	Low	Low to high, depending on system's organisation, mandates	Moderate to high, depending on system's culture, organisation
Quality measures	• Population health status • Mortality, morbidity rates • Health care expenditures, lost income, reduced productivity • Felt fairness, political contentment	• People's, enrollee's access to, availability of health care • Enrollee's health status • Cost, health plan premiums • Satisfaction with plan, providers, acceptability of trade-offs	• Patient health status improvement • Cost of care • Patient satisfaction • Acceptability of trade-offs
Quality means	Policy management	System management	Quality management
Key features	• Complexity • Ideological differences • Conflicting policy objectives • Lack of political will • Resource allocation conflicts • Lack of knowledge	• Dynamic adjustment difficulties • Sociopolitical traditions • Historical lack of systems • Lack of local political will • Economic vested interests • Lack of experience, know-how	• Requires paradigm shift • Culture, resistance to change • Lack of political will • Lack of incentives • Lack of knowledge, technology

People rarely distinguish clearly between these two distinct perspectives: system-level and production-level quality. This distinction is poorly understood by many policy decision-makers, managers and doctors and, consequently, is an endless source of confusion. People rarely appreciate the fundamental differences that are crucial to managing the health care system and to improving the quality of care. People might imagine, for example, that if every hospital were to improve the quality of its care, the health care system's quality would improve. Indeed it might, but not necessarily. It depends on how hospitals improve the quality of their care and how one judges the health care system's quality. Maximising outputs of a system's elements does not necessarily maximise the system's output. This idea may be difficult to grasp and appear counter-intuitive. This section examines this fundamentally important concept.

This section describes the essential characteristics of quality at the system and production levels and their interrelationships. It juxtaposes the health care system and its individual production elements, including hospitals. Necessarily this section is superficial. It intends only to provide a context for and better understanding of quality management in hospitals. Production-level quality is this manual's focus and the rest of this part discusses it in detail.

235.2 | *Production-level quality*

Production-level quality is concerned with production outcomes, production units' performance in terms of the quality of their products. Health care production performance refers to the extent to which providers, for example hospitals, improve patients' health status, at what cost and with what patient satisfaction (and the acceptability of any trade-offs).

Health production takes place in, and hence health care outcomes result from, production units. Presently, health production units are organisations based on specialised facilities, such as hospitals and doctors' offices or surgeries, even if patients' homes are the actual site of care. These production units are managed systems because their managers can, and to some substantial extent do, define the system's boundaries and control what goes on within them, although they may use few modern management techniques to improve their production quality, for example.

Traditionally, health care providers have assisted only those who demanded their services. Individuals in need of care seek out providers, who treat them, and then they slip away to become once again part of the environment in which providers operate. At the production level, outcomes pertain to patients—individuals whom providers have treated. Production level outcomes depend on patient–provider interactions. Medical practitioners treat most patients in their offices or surgeries. With the advent of larger production units, such as hospitals, their organisation—the system of care—affects outcomes directly or by influencing patient–provider interactions.

In vertically integrated health care systems (described later, and referred to sometimes in the United States as accountable health care plans), in which all providers function as part of a managed health care system, the organisation is designed to influence the nature and outcomes of provider–patient interactions toward improving health care quality. These systems of care give providers the information, tools and environment necessary to improve patient outcomes—conditions that they could not obtain outside of such a system with its integrated information systems, network of interrelationships and other factors that are intrinsic to such managed systems. Nevertheless, the production-level outcomes of such vertically integrated systems consist ultimately of patient–provider interactions, albeit they are influenced by the managed system of care in which they are embedded.

235.3 | Quality management is a production-level tool

Quality management is a production-level tool, useful for improving production units' performance and products' quality. Health care quality management's success is gauged by the extent to which it assures and improves production outcomes. Quality management applies only to organisations. Organisations are concrete systems whose managers are accountable, or should be, for the quality of their products. These managers also should have the authority to change the system to improve its performance, that is, the quality of the organisation's products. An organisation's boundaries, which may be influenced by system-level policy, define its quality management efforts, as the following example shows.

Hospitals can only improve admitted patients' health status to the maximum extent they can within their walls. Patients may be admitted to hospital because of failed outpatient management. Improving the quality of these patients' care would require changing the practices of community practitioners. Even assuming the hospital could identify such quality of care problems, given the health care system's present structure, there is no way for the hospital to resolve them and no mechanism to transmit this information to any other entity to take action. On the other hand, if the hospital were part of a vertically integrated health care system, with unified management, its quality management program would pass the information to someone who could take action to confirm the quality of care problem, investigate its root causes, eliminate them and thus resolve the problem.

235.4 | System-level quality

The health care system (which delivers and finances personal health care services), like the larger health system of which it is part (which consists of all elements that intend to improve people's health), is a conceptual system. There are no managers who can be held accountable for the quality of its products, in the organisational sense, and no customers—merely the population collectively.

At the health care system level, quality cannot be managed in the sense it can be managed within individual production elements, such as hospitals or vertically integrated health care delivery systems. The term quality management does not apply to conceptual systems because they are not managed in the organisational sense. We use the term policy management to refer to individuals', groups' and, especially, government's attempts to influence the nature, operations, interrelationships among, and the environment of conceptual systems' elements.

At the system level, quality considerations are quite different from those at the production level. For example, access to health care is clearly an important quality consideration at the system level and may obviously influence a population's health. However, it is irrelevant at the production level, which involves patient–provider interactions. At the production level, patients have already gained access to care, and health status improvement accrues only to patients, individuals who receive care.

One can measure production-level quality simply in terms of patients' health status improvement (the amount of health improvement that production units produce) and, for quality management purposes, compare what was produced with what could have been produced. But how is one to judge the quality of the health care system? How much could it be improved? How could any achievable improvement best be realised? These are complex questions, answers to which are either lacking or difficult to articulate, and on which it is almost impossible to reach any meaningful or lasting consensus.

One might judge the quality of a nation's health care system based on the population's health status. However, the health care system may play a relatively minor role in, or may not be a particularly efficient means for, maintaining and improving people's health. Can a system that provides excellent care for 85% of the population but little or no care to the rest be considered high quality? To what extent should differences in distribution of health care resources or people's access to health care be a factor in deciding system-level quality? If some of the 85% of the people who have access to health care gave up some marginal benefits to the 15% who do not, thereby increasing aggregate health status without increasing costs, would the system's quality be increased? Can a system in which rising costs threaten to crowd out investments in other vital social areas and to reduce access to care for many be considered high quality?

One might measure the extent of system-level quality improvement as the difference between current population health status and that which is achievable within that nation's sociopolitical traditions. Cynics might argue that what is being achieved is all that is achievable, not necessarily technically but certainly within sociopolitical traditions. Of course sociopolitical traditions, as well as technology, evolve thereby affecting what is achievable. Short of revolution, sociopolitical traditions change slowly. Technology changes relatively quickly, but true breakthroughs occur infrequently and their effects take time to propagate. Ultimately, policy decision makers, which in a democracy means the public, must decide whether or not what is being achieved is all that can be achieved within sociopolitical traditions. Such decisions may involve one group giving up something to benefit another, the very essence of politics.

235.5 | Policy management is a system-level tool

Policy management refers to the mandates, prohibitions, incentives and sanctions that health care system actors, particularly government, intend to alter health care system elements' functioning, their interrelationships, or environment to achieve explicit or implicit policy objectives. Policy management is fundamentally different from quality management. There may be diverse policy objectives, which may reflect different interest groups' goals or ideologies, or inherent contradictions in a particular group's position. Thus resultant policies may be incoherent; one conflicting or interfering with the accomplishment of others. Such conflicts, which reflect political realities, are inherent in policy management but would be disastrous in quality management.

Policy management seeks primarily to influence health care providers' environment, to shape their organisations and influence their performance. The environment legitimises some organisational forms and practices, and may prohibit certain others, and includes incentives and sanctions that affect providers' behaviour. These influences include, for example, laws regulating medical practice, establishing and running health care facilities, and financing health care services. Health care financing mechanisms provide powerful incentives that shape what is offered, by whom to whom. Conspicuously lacking, however, are command and control features inherent in organisations that can hire and fire their employees to shape the organisation and give incentives to employees toward achieving the organisation's goals. Policy may have little direct influence on performance or may produce perverse incentives, for example, that for political reasons are hard to change. Such weak linkages and difficult-to-change perverse effects that are inherent in policy management would be disastrous in quality management.

An important aspect of health policy is the extent to which production units should be responsible for patient outcomes and even the population's health (or at least that of those people who choose it as their health care provider). Presently, hospitals or doctors may do the best they can for people who seek their services. However, they are not held accountable in any meaningful sense for their patients' outcomes, let alone their health. They are like garages which repair cars but are not accountable for the condition of people's cars, let alone their driving. Ultimately, individuals are responsible for their own health. Government can only empower individuals by, for example, encouraging them to make informed choices, providing them with the information to make choices, and facilitating resultant decisions through, for example, ensuring the availability of and access to health care. When believed politically to be necessary and possible, government can provide incentives and sanctions to convince people or providers to act in what government (and its constituencies) believes to be socially desirable ways. Holding providers accountable for patient outcomes, thereby promoting effective quality management, for example, is one such way.

235.6 *Production-level and system-level interactions*

System-level policy may affect production-level management and vice versa. For example, government promotion of quality management in hospitals could be expected to encourage its adoption. The public's reaction to problems in hospitals could encourage the government to adopt such a policy. Production-level quality management and improvement can have positive and negative system-level consequences. Quality management may provide better value for money or reduce access to care for some people. Similarly, system-level policy management can have beneficial and adverse production-level consequences. Coping with these effects begins by recognising the possibility of their occurrence.

If providers' quality were measured validly and known widely, how would access to the best doctors and hospitals be controlled? Would the highly prized be highly priced? If a hospital did not measure up, would it be forced to close even if it was the only one in town? Would patients choose to go to a distant, but better quality, hospital? Should the health financing scheme pay for their transportation costs? If a hospital decided it could not deliver certain services to standards and stopped offering them, where would patients who needed those services go? If health care financing schemes decided a certain oft-performed surgical operation was not effective or not worth its cost and stopped paying for it, what would happen to providers' incomes? Would they go quietly out of business or search vigorously for alternative sources of income, for example by increasing the frequency with which they performed other procedures? What effects would patients' and providers' decisions have on system-level quality?

Hospitals' efforts to improve quality for their patients, by treating only those cases they can treat to standards, for example, may reduce the population's access to some types of care. The health status of those treated is better than it would otherwise have been, and their treatment may also cost less as the result of the hospital's quality management efforts. What happens to those people that the hospital no longer treats is a system-level concern. While the hospital has no direct responsibility for access to its care, which is a system-level issue, it may be affected by whatever decisions system policy decision makers take to deal with what they perceive to be any problems in access to hospitals' care.

Maximising production units' (e.g. hospitals') outcomes will not necessarily improve the population's health maximally. Firstly, only people with access to hospitals can benefit. Secondly, the interventions may not be very effective, that is, even if used when indicated and implemented properly, patients' health status may not be improved very much. Finally, the last units of achievable health status improvement may be gained at considerable cost. The population's health status might be improved to a far greater extent by increasing access to care for people who have no or only limited access, or by diverting some resources elsewhere, for example to health promotion and disease prevention programs, or to jobs creation, education or housing, if these programs would yield more population health status improvement per dollar expended.

Some benefits for some individuals may be traded-off for greater benefits to others, especially if public money is involved. Inevitably, this might mean that a rich octogenarian could buy at great cost a few units of health status improvement that a poor person could not afford. The government, through taxes, could buy these benefits for the poor octogenarian but, if tax revenues are limited (which they are inevitably even if the limits are not fixed), only at the cost of forgoing some other expenditure, for example feeding the hungry, housing the destitute or educating poor children.

Health care funding depends on competing uses for resources and the maximum aggregate amount that people are willing to pay directly or through health care financing schemes or taxes to maintain and improve their own and other people's health. People may neither agree to forgo some potential or actual benefits nor to pay increased premiums or taxes to provide services to those without access to them. At death's door, would someone with means be willing to forgo a chance to extend life? Should that person even have the option to decide, if the cost of the treatment would be borne by taxpayers, a social insurance scheme or an employer? Who should decide? Ultimately, these decisions, like taxing the rich to support the poor, are political and depend on one's views of consequences, of both means and ends. These are profound questions, examination of which is beyond this manual's scope. Nevertheless, answers to such questions shape notions of health system quality and influence the extent to which it can be achieved. They also may affect providers' incentives to adopt quality management.

National health care expenditures are the aggregate results of individual decisions, principally by doctors and their patients. Government policies, health care financing schemes and financial incentives affect providers' willingness to deliver and individuals' abilities to consume health care. Sometimes frustration with the state of affairs and the seeming inability to influence them leads to direct government control. But problems may stem from fundamental factors not subject to such control and the situation may deteriorate. Faced with escalating costs, government may attempt to stem rising health care expenditures by, for example, price controls, rationing and other bureaucratic mechanisms that may turn out to promote inequity, inefficiency and stagnation, leaving society worse off than it would have been if other policies had been adopted toward this same end. On the other hand, pouring money into the health care system in an attempt to provide access to those who do not have it may stimulate medical care cost inflation, increase costs and, ultimately, reduce access to and satisfaction with the system.

System-level (global) effects are the net results of production-level or local interactions: results of provider–patient interactions that express individual choices, constrained by system policies that promote or prevent actions. (See Figure II-3-1 on page 133.) Given any perceived measure of system performance, policy decision makers may want to change system policies in an attempt to influence local provider–patient interactions. However, evolved interconnections among system elements may make it hard to implement planned policies (e.g. because they are unacceptable to powerful interest groups) or produce perverse effects (e.g. because people may try to subvert them or their intent). Effecting positive change in complex dynamic systems is difficult even if the public, for example, were to agree on what changes are desirable and how they should be brought about. Smooth dynamic adjustment of complex systems depends on distributed decision making. Concentrating resource allocation decisions in few hands politicises them and increases the difficulty of breaking the mould. Over time, pressures on and inherent contradictions within the system may cause cracks to appear that may be difficult to patch. Cracks may become chasms that break the system, creating political turmoil. The dynamics of health care systems are complex and their consideration is beyond this manual's scope.

235.7 | Accountable health schemes or plans

In most industrialised countries, government finances most health care, although its provision is nominally in private hands even if government sets medical practitioners'

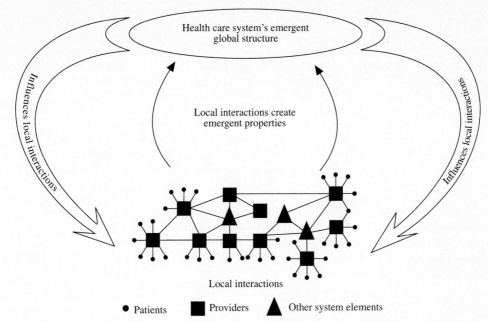

Figure II-3-1 *System-level effects result from, and affect dynamically, production-level interactions. Model after Chris Langston in Lewin R.* The science of complexity: Life at the edge of chaos. *New York: Macmillan Publishing Company, 1992.*

terms and conditions of service. In some countries, including Australia, government runs hospitals, although private visiting medical practitioners treat patients. The evolution of health care has resulted in the separation of health care financing from the provision of health care services. Government's goal of ensuring citizens' financial access to health care has perverted the means to an end. There is no accountability for health care outcomes; the provision of health care services is only one of the means of maintaining and improving health.

Recognition of this fundamental flaw, and emerging technologies to measure and manage health care quality, have given rise to the concept of the accountable health scheme (or plan as it has become known in the United States, and is referred to here). Essentially, accountable health plans are responsible for both collecting people's money and delivering their health care. These plans operate vertically integrated health care systems that provide, directly or under contract, primary (general practitioner), secondary (specialist), and tertiary (subspecialist) care, and may also provide long-term and other types of care, in peoples' homes, doctors' offices (surgeries), clinics, hospitals and other settings. The primary purpose of plans is to maintain and improve enrollees' health status by providing the services that they want and need in the most cost-effective and acceptable way practical. They are accountable to their enrollees for both costs and the quality of care. The rest of this section describes the authors' vision of an accountable health care plan, which has yet to be realised anywhere.

Accountability can be achieved in one or more of the following ways: only plans meeting government standards can continue to operate or to receive government payments; enrollees elect the plan's directors and officers, who manage the plan; and people are free to choose among alternative plans. To allow people to choose among plans, in addition to describing the usual benefits covered and services offered, they must annually report their financial conditions and care outcomes, and the extent to which they improved them, for example, enrollees' standardised health status, the cost of the plan and patient satisfaction. Table II-3-2 below provides an example of such a 'report card'. They may also publish verbatim enrollees' complaints (while not revealing their identity) and what the plan did to answer each complaint and, if appropriate, reduce the chances of a recurrence of the care that led the enrollee to complain. To ensure truth in advertising, external auditors conduct patient satisfaction surveys, and certify financial statements and all claims of outcomes' improvement. Auditors are liable for their opinions and face civil and criminal penalties if they are negligent in carrying out their duties.

The key shift in the health care paradigm is from payment for services to responsibility for outcomes. The shift comes in three strengths: accountability for improving production outcomes (whatever the base level); accountability for achieving production outcomes; and accountability for enrollees' health status. The first strength provides incentive for health care plans to improve patient outcomes; the second, to achieve minimum patient outcomes; the third, to consider what mix of interventions acceptable to enrollees would achieve best value for money, that is, most health status improvement per dollar expended. This paradigm shift puts the consumer back in the driver's seat. Government's role is reduced to empowering consumers to make inherently difficult choices and to monitoring the entire health care system to ensure it is working as its 'designers' intended.

Table II-3-2 *Example format of an accountable health plan report card*

Beneficial accountable health plan subscribers' report card for 1999

Your plan is pleased to report that subscribers' health status is at an all-time high. Because of our aggressive quality management program, we have been able to reduce the cost of the federally-mandated minimum benefits package for the second straight year. Our market share continues to grow, showing consumers' confidence in our ability to deliver the kind of health care they want. Here's how we're doing on some key performance measures. Remember to watch our award-winning television series *Tips for Healthier Living* each Sunday night at 8.00 pm on Channel 2. Beneficial's staff wish you a healthy 21st century!

Measure	1998	1999
Enrollee health status years	68.3	69.5
Cases treated according to practice guidelines	94.3%	95.2%
Expected health outcomes realised	83.2%	84.5%
Effective annual cost of federally-mandated minimum benefits package for a family of four	$15 250	$15 125
Salaries and cash value of perquisites of the plan's ten top highest paid individuals* ($ million)	$2.75	$2.75
Staff turnover	10.2%	9.8%
Market share	25.6%	27.8%
Complaint's per 1000 enrollees (includes malpractice and other suits)	2.8	2.4
Re-enrollees	85.9%	88.7%

* The ten individuals included in this group for 1999 were . . .

These data were collected according to industry standards and were certified by Health Care Plan Auditors, Inc. Subscribers can receive free-of-charge a copy of our complete annual report by calling **800-123-4567**.

In this idea's fullest incarnation, consumers—not government or employers—control funds. Government's responsibility is to ensure all citizens access to health care; not what services should be provided, nor who should provide them, nor how they should be provided, nor how much they are worth. Government no longer finances the majority of care, does not provide health care services, does not micromanage care delivery, does not check on providers' quality of care, and does not conduct research that is better conducted by these health care plans. For example, plans' internal quality management systems would monitor and strive to improve care outcomes, through, for example, changing delivery systems, educating providers, and conducting or co-operating with others to conduct needed research. Private external auditors certify these systems' compliance with professional standards and all claims of outcomes' improvement. Private professional bodies develop standards for auditors. Consumers choose among various plans based on certified performance. Government provides the incentives and sanctions to make the system work. Discussion of how a health care system based on accountable health plans might look, and how to facilitate the transition from the present to this future—even assuming that such a transition is feasible now—are both subjects beyond this manual's scope.

To improve the quality of care and to bring value in line with expenditures, thereby ending the perception of a crisis in health care cost and quality, consumers must be in charge at all levels; not subjected to a health care system over which they have little or no control and which they perceive to be a political football of special interests and unresponsive to their concerns. Advances in information technology, for example, permit the substitution of nineteenth century solutions to health care financing and quality assurance problems with those relevant to twenty-first century circumstances and expectations. For example, in the twenty-first century consumers will be front line health professionals. Some time in the twenty-first century they will have access to the same expert systems as health professionals to diagnose their health problems and to select among treatment options based on measured outcomes. These systems will outperform today's unaided health professionals.

236 | Health care's impact on health

236.1 | Perspective

In the United States in the forty-year period between 1950 and 1990 average per capita health expenditures increased over 450% in real terms (adjusted for general price inflation); life expectancy at birth increased 10.6%. Increased life expectancy at birth seems to have been accompanied by increased disease and disability among those alive; health status, which includes the number of years lived and the health quality of life, may have improved little. In the 1980s, a time when life expectancy grew slowly, US health care expenditures soared, sharpening questions about health care's impact on populations' health. This section describes the determinants of health, explains measures of health, and explores the extent to which health care improves health.

236.2 | The determinants of health

A person's health status is the result of four sets of interrelated factors and their interactions.[11] They are:

- biology (genes or genetic programming);
- behaviour;
- prenatal and postnatal environments, encompassing the physical (e.g. climate, pollution), biological (e.g. viruses, bacteria), economic (e.g. food, shelter, clothing), and social (e.g. population aggregation, workplace factors, social support systems) environments;

- health system, including public health programs and personal health services (the health care system).

The extent to which any one set of factors affects an individual's health is controversial, as exemplified by the long-standing debate between nature (genetic make-up) and nurture (environment). Beliefs about the determinants of health, how much one can—and should—influence them and the acceptability, to decision makers and those subject to their decisions, of effective interventions are important determinants of health policy.

236.3 Health status and its measurement
236.31 THE NEED TO MEASURE HEALTH
Quality management means meaningful measurement; one can only manage what one can measure. Since the health care system's central purpose is the maintenance and improvement of health, its management requires quantification of the amount of health improvement that the system produces. Health is intangible and subjective. Its quantification is difficult but nonetheless essential, for example, to:

- describe meaningfully a population's health;
- assess meaningfully interventions' effectiveness;
- quantify meaningfully patient health outcomes for quality assessment and quality management purposes;
- choose meaningfully among alternative interventions.

This section describes the importance to quality management of the basic ideas underlying, and how health can be quantified by, health status measurement. Detailed discussion of how to measure health status, and its implications for patients' preferences and their choices among alternative interventions, are subjects beyond this manual's scope.

236.32 ESSENTIAL CONCEPTS
The population's health is a summation of individuals' health. Historically, mortality rates (and life expectancy, a statistical measure based on them) have been the only measures of a population's health (or rather of its lack). As the length of life lived increases, measuring the burden of illness becomes more important. Ultimately, the population's health must be measured in terms of people's health status, an integrated measure of the length and health quality of life.

Life expectancy is a calculated value that assumes people born in a given year will experience the same age–sex specific mortality rates as those experienced by people alive during that same year. It has the virtue that it is relatively easy to tell if someone is alive or dead, and to count the dead and relate the number of deaths to the size of the population. However, it was only at the close of the seventeenth century that advances in social organisation and mathematical science coincided to the point that people could construct reliable life tables. While present-day life tables are extremely reliable, especially in industrialised countries, they tell us nothing of the health quality of life and are thus poor measures of health during life. Health status is more difficult to measure, and even in the most advanced industrialised countries such data are still not available routinely. Health status is the preferred measure as it encompasses mortality and morbidity.

Health status is a measure (quantification) of health that includes the number of years lived and the health quality of life, taking into account morbidity, institutionalisation and functional ability. It can be measured for an individual or for a population (health status experienced, comparable to years lived) or estimated from population data (health status expectancy, comparable to life expectancy). Such measurements or estimates may pertain to a lifetime or to a defined period, for example ten years after a surgical operation.

Health status measurement depends on ascertaining the length of time spent in various health states (e.g. institutionalised, unable to do activities). This idea is referred to sometimes as quality adjusted life years (QALYs) or disability adjusted life years (DALYs). A person's health status may vary not only as a function of the amount of time spent in a given health state but also the value he or she (or someone else) places on that state. Finally, the value of each state can be discounted depending on when in the future it occurs. The resultant product is expressed as 'health status years' (HSY).

236.33 AVAILABILITY OF HEALTH STATUS DATA FOR QUALITY MANAGEMENT

Interventions' effectiveness and patients' outcomes should be measured in health status terms. As appealing as health status data are, virtually no information exists about such outcomes. In fact, there is a dearth of any type of information on outcomes.[12] In practice, when measured at all, outcomes are usually expressed in terms of five-year survival or mortality rates, or even less satisfactory measures. Mortality is an inadequate measure of outcome because most interventions are likely to alter the quality, and not necessarily the quantity, of life. Five-year survival rates, for example, tell nothing about the shape of the survival curve nor about the quality of life lived. Both types of information may influence patients' choices among alternative interventions.

236.34 HEALTH STATUS IN QUALITY MANAGEMENT

Health status provides the common metric necessary to evaluate all of the health effects of alternative, disparate interventions, for example a good-for-life surgical operation versus lifelong medical therapy. Measuring health status from onset of treatment permits the effect on health of different treatments to be taken into account. Health status measurement enables proper comparison of interventions' effectiveness. Such information results preferably from well-designed, well-controlled, randomised clinical trials so that observed improvement can be attributed confidently to the intervention, or, if empirical data are lacking, must be assumed based on experience. Patients can use this information to assist most meaningfully their choices among alternative interventions. Further, patients can use their own preferences to weight health states and to discount them.

Ideally, for quality management purposes, providers' performance should be measured by the extent to which they improve patients' health status compared to the extent to which they could have improved it constrained by patients' preferences and society's resources. Practically, it is difficult and expensive to measure long-term outcomes and to attribute observed outcomes to interventions. Hospitals are usually limited to measuring care processes, for example adherence to required diagnostic interventions, and acting on their results; process outcomes, for example duration of surgical operation; and immediate patient outcomes, for example discharged alive. The underlying rationale for practice policies (and for practice criteria) is their known or, more likely, assumed relationship to patient health status improvement. Quality managers, therefore, must understand the basis of health status measurement. Moreover, to the extent practical, they must validate assumptions linking interventions (practice policies) to health status improvement through structured outcomes measurement and health systems research, particularly medical technology assessment.

236.35 NATURE OF HEALTH STATUS

Health status is an integrated measure of the health quality of life. It encompasses mortality, institutionalisation, morbidity, ability to carry out activities and, in principle, mental and emotional wellbeing. Measurement of health status is the result of integrating three dimensions: (1) states of health; (2) prognosis of health state; and (3) the value of health states at each moment.[13] Thus a patient's health status can be determined by measuring his or her health at various moments, weighting the states' value relative to other states and moments, and summing the products. Operationally, measuring health status depends on:

- defining a series of mutually exclusive health states into which a person (patient) may be categorised at any given moment, for example able to do activities, can do limited activities, institutionalised, dead;
- deciding over what period to measure health status, and into how many moments to divide the chosen period;
- ascertaining (estimating) the person's (patient's) health state at each moment;
- deciding the value of that state at that moment;
- doing the necessary sums.

Any number of health states can be defined. Ideally, measurement procedures would be the same for persons (patients) of all types and at all ages. Practically, different methods are needed for babies and the aged, for example. Thus the challenge is operationalising measures for a given state—for example, able to do activities—at different ages, and ensuring their reliability and comparability. Presently, there is no universally agreed way to categorise or measure health states. However, tested, acceptable and accepted instruments are beginning to emerge.

The period over which health status is to be measured or extrapolated (the time horizon) is important for several reasons. Firstly, the longer the period, the more points there are to measure or estimate. Secondly, the longer after intervention one makes such measurements, the harder it is to attribute observed outcomes to preceding interventions. Thirdly, the time horizon may affect an intervention's apparent effectiveness. For example, some patients may die from surgical intervention, but those who survive do much better over five years than those treated medically and, after ten years, the aggregate health status of patients treated surgically may exceed that of the same number treated medically. The number of intervals into which the health status period is divided for measurement purposes affects precision. Daily measurement of health state (365 measurements per year) obviously gives a better picture of the patient's course than determining it once in a year. However, 36 500 000 measurements (and weights) is more burdensome than 100 000 (e.g. in a study of 10 000 patients for ten years).

The weights applied to each health state to make them commensurable (to quantify patients' health quality of life), depends on patients' discount rates and their values. Each state of health can be weighted relative to the other. The best state, that is, being healthy, measured, for example, by being able to do all activities without restriction, is given full weight (1.0); lesser states, for example being institutionalised, less weight (e.g. 0.5); being dead counts zero. States that people may deem to be worse than death, for example persistent vegetative state, can be given negative weights.

Health states (outcomes) can also be discounted (weighted depending on when they occur after intervention begins). Being able to do activities tomorrow might be more important than being able to do them in ten years' time. Generally, people discount distant outcomes, often quite steeply. Obviously, people may vary in the weights they attach to different health states. Further, health state weights and discount rates may not be independent. Once one has ascertained a person's health state at each future moment and the weight that the person (or someone else) accords each state at each moment, one can sum the resultant values to produce a quantified measure of health that encompasses mortality, morbidity and functioning.

236.36 ON SUBJECTIVITY

Health status measurement is inherently subjective. There are two kinds of subjectivity: one relates to determining a patient's health state; the other to the value of any given state at any given moment. To some extent one can assign patients to health states on objective grounds. However, to some irreducible extent one must rely on the patient's subjective assessments to determine his or her functioning (e.g. able to do usual activities), and especially his or her effect (e.g. feelings of wellbeing). Ideally, a health status instrument should be able to reliably assign individuals with similar functioning (and affect) to a given state. Practically, however, different instruments may be needed to assign different types of people—for example, babies, young adults, mature adults— to one of several health states in a given set, which makes health state assignment less reliable than mortality data, for example. Nevertheless, instruments are emerging that can assign people to health states for the purpose of measuring health status.

The second kind of subjectivity deals with people's values. Different people may value a given health state differently. Moreover, even if they value identically the same health state at one moment, they may differ on its value at another. This kind of subjectivity is inherent in health status measurement and is one of its strengths. In choosing between alternative treatments, for example, patients can determine individually the value to them of alternatives' streams of health benefits (expected future health state, moment to moment). For example, given the choice of living ten years with limited mobility or five active years the patient may forgo the five extra years for the ability to play with his young children. Since the patient is almost certain to die before they are grown, it is more important to the patient to think that his children will remember him actively than as a helpless cripple. Another patient in different circumstances may choose the treatment that offers greater longevity.

236.37 ON RATIONALITY

Doctors and their patients' perspectives and values may differ; therefore doctors sometimes see patients' choices as irrational. Certainly, patients may be irrational. However, unless the patient has deranged mentation, necessitating a guardian for example, doctors must inform patients about alternative interventions and their expected health outcomes and allow the patient to choose. Health care providers must resist the temptation to impose their values on patients and to shape information to produce an outcome that they desire.

Doctors who believe in a new therapy, for example, may tell a patient that it is his or her last hope. Indeed, it may be, but the intervention may also be very risky (and shorten rather than lengthen patients' lives), and the patient may not want to take the risk. The doctor must fairly represent the risk and help the patient make an informed decision.

The rationality (and hence legitimacy) of choices is often debated and is frequently in the mind of the beholder. For example, with surgery the patient's health status in the next ten year looks better than with conservative medical therapy. However, the chances of leaving the hospital alive are greater with conservative therapy. The patient must trade-off greater long-term benefit for greater immediate risk. Sometimes a patient may rule out surgery, for example, because he or she fears going under the knife rather than because it would produce a worse outcome. While the doctor may view the patient's fear of surgery as irrational, it may be no more irrational than some of the patient's other (and some of the doctor's own) fears. Ultimately, patients (and not doctors) must live (or die) by their decisions.

236.4 *The population's health*

Life expectancy at birth seems to have increased steadily since the 1700s,[14] and has almost doubled in the last 130 to 150 years. In the United States, life expectancy increased annually by an average of almost half a year between 1900 and 1925 (three times the rate of the previous fifty years), and almost 0.4 years annually between 1925 and 1950. Such high rates of gain were not seen again until the 1970s, when life expectancy gains averaged 0.3 years annually (over twice the average annual increase observed in the period 1950–70). In the 1980s life expectancy has increased on average less than 0.2 years annually,[1,11,15,16] at a time when health care expenditures have been increasing at unprecedented rates.

In the United States, institutionalisation rates and prevalence of disease and disability rates (among the non-institutionalised population) have both increased—for all age groups.[11,17–20] Recent evidence, however, suggests that the prevalence of chronic disability among elderly Americans may now be declining.[21] Studies in other industrialised countries have found similar results among their populations.[22] However, in Australia and Canada disability rates are rising. Between 1951 and 1978, Canadian's life expectancy increased by six years, but almost five of these years were in a state of disability.[23] The extent to which health status has increased is far from clear. Future trends are also in doubt. As life expectancy continues to grow, some people see a flood of increasingly disabled aged while others see an expansion in the number of functional old people. Both views may be correct: both the number of disabled and the proportion of functional aged may increase. If the proportion of functional aged declines, the number of disabled aged will be that much greater.

'While ... (people's) health ... has improved ... during the past 150 years, it is not too clear how this has been brought about.'[24] Traditionally, public health measures have been credited with improving life expectancy, at least to recent times, because effective medical interventions are thought to have been lacking.[25] Public health measures began in the seventeenth century, for aesthetic reasons, with the clean-up of malodorous messes, and continued into the eighteenth century. The nineteenth century saw such major public undertakings as the provision of potable water, the removal of waste and the inspection of factories. However, recent evidence suggests that life expectancy in European populations began improving about a century before the great Victorian sanitary reforms, possibly related to nutrition, '(making) one wonder whether (they had much impact) upon a situation which was already improving for other reasons.'[14]

McKeown, for example, argues that the available evidence suggests strongly that most gains in life expectancy seem to have come from improved socioeconomic circumstances that improved nutrition, public health measures that separated man from microbe, and preventive interventions such as vaccination that reduced threats to health or increased resistance to them. He notes the decline in industrialised countries of respiratory tuberculosis death rates from the mid nineteenth century (when it was a leading cause of death) until its virtual elimination as a cause of death a century later.[26] By the advent of specific chemotherapy (in the late 1940s), the tuberculosis death rate was a mere fraction of that observed earlier. Unfortunately, in the United States, at least, drug-resistant tuberculosis is making a come back, especially among HIV-positive individuals and people with AIDS. In Australia, likewise, in recent years the incidence of tuberculosis has been on the increase. Worldwide, tuberculosis is still a major cause of death and disability.

Our understanding of the dynamics of death and disease is limited. Natural phenomena, basic biology and its interaction with the environment, may affect life expectancy more than we realise. For example, sunspot activity at the time of one's mother's conception may affect one's length of life by about four years.[27] A mother's nutritional status and its effect on her developing foetus seems to affect her offspring's health throughout his or her later life.[28] Genetics determines species' life spans (the maximum period that individuals who are spared from accidents and self-inflicted mortality and morbidity live). The human life span seems to be limited to about 115 years, with relatively few people living past 100 years, and most not surviving as long as eighty-five years. Natural ageing processes lead inexorably to death. Chance, individuals' behaviour, and their social circumstances, including health care, determine how long individuals live within their biologically determined limit.

The following changes have contributed to improving people's health: the agricultural revolution—which stabilised and increased food supplies; the industrial revolution—which increased productivity and wealth and improved nutrition, social circumstances and public health measures; and, most recently, personal health services. The information revolution, on which quality management depends, provides the means to increase the relevance, validity and accessibility of information available to policy decision makers, providers and patients. This change will further contribute to improving individuals' and the population's health status.

236.5 | Health care expenditures and life expectancy at birth

In 1990 the world spent about US$1700 billion on health care—about 8% of global income. Worldwide, there is tremendous variation in per capita health expenditures and substantial variation in life expectancy at birth. 'At any level of income and education, higher health spending should yield better health, all else being equal. But there is no evidence of such a relation.'[29] In general, 'at any time, the higher a country's average income per capita, the more likely its people are to live long, healthy lives.'[30] According to recent World Bank data, in 1900 in the richest and healthiest countries, life expectancy was about 59.5 years; by 1990 it had reached about 78.8 years. Yet, in 1990, in some countries with the same average annual per capita income as the richest countries in 1900, about US$4500, life expectancy stood at about 75.5 years. Average annual per capita income in the richest country was about five times as much—about US$22 500.[30] In developing countries, at least, 'many of the most cost-effective health interventions are preventive in character or fall into the category of primary care.'[31]

In industrialised countries, in the last twenty years, health care expenditures have increased by about 10% per annum and life expectancy at birth by about 0.3% per annum—despite substantial differences in their average per capita health expenditures and their health care systems. (See Figure II-3-2 on page 142). During the period 1970–90 per capita health expenditures in Australia grew at an average rate of 9.8%, compared to 12.1% for Japan, 10.8% for the United States, 10.5% for France, 10.3% for Canada, 10.0% for Germany, 9.7% for the United Kingdom and 7.9% for New Zealand. However, actual expenditures per capita vary tremendously. They correlate highly with these nations' average per capita GDP,[32] and reflect differences in their health care systems and the morbidity burdens of their populations. In 1990, for example, Australia spent US$1127 per capita on health care—less than half the amount of the United States, US$2566; New Zealand spent only US$850 per capita (based on purchasing power parity conversions).[33]

During this same period, life expectancy at birth increased by 6.9% in Australia, compared to 6.5% for the United States, and 6.1% for New Zealand. In 1990 life expectancy for Australian men was 71.9 years and for women 80.0 years,[34] compared to 75.4 years for US males and 78.8 for US females (which has the world's highest per capita expenditures),[2] and 72.4 years for New Zealand males and 78.3 years for New Zealand females (of those analysed, the industrialised country with the lowest per capita health expenditures).[35]

> In industrial countries, life expectancy depends much more on income distribution than on income per capita, and it has been rising faster in countries with improving income distribution. Japan now has the highest life expectancy in the world (76.1 years for men and 82.2 years for women, in 1992) and a highly egalitarian income distribution.[30] In 1990 Japan spent US$1113 per capita on health care, about the same as Australia and less than half that of the United States.

Life expectancy at birth (years), multi-year averages prior to 1975

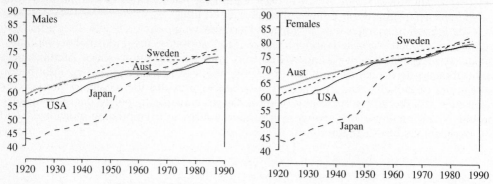

Health expenditure per person for four OECD countries, purchasing power parity conversion, 1969–70 to 1989–90
Because of differences and changes in national data collection mechanisms these data may not be strictly comparable

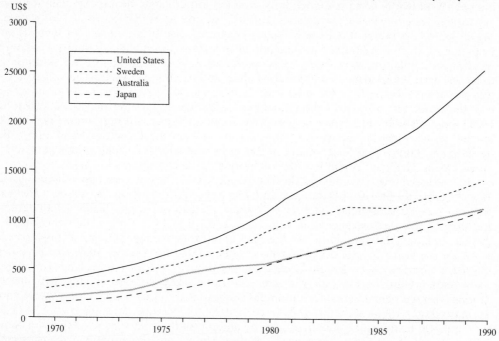

Figure II-3-2 *Trends in life expectancy at birth and health care costs in selected industrialised countries* (courtesy of the Australian Bureau of Statistics)

Industrialised countries are experiencing unprecedented increases in health care expenditures, while life expectancy at birth stagnates or grows only slowly. Medical care may provide great benefits to some but at great expense to all. The health of the many remains largely unaffected by the improved health status of the few.

236.6 | Medicine's effect on health

One must distinguish between health care's impact on the population's health and specific medical interventions' effectiveness (the extent to which they improve patients' health status). For example, individuals' robustness at birth influences their life expectancy. To the extent that medicine permits the birth of individuals who would not have been born in earlier times but cannot assure them the same life expectancy as others, it reduces the population's health. There is no implication that such interventions are not worthwhile, merely that what one chooses to measure and how well one can measure it influences one's perception of reality. Medical interventions may greatly improve some individuals' health, but their impact on the population's health may be small. Social and other forces beyond the health system's control may determine the population's health to a far greater extent than health care. The presumption that observed improvements in the population's health are attributable to health care, or to specific medical interventions, may lead to erroneous decisions on the part of policy decision makers, providers and patients.

To some people, modern medicine's accomplishments are self-evident; to others, especially in recent decades, they are much more elusive. People have long presumed that medical care is effective in improving health. Erasmus, for example, wrote: 'Medicine ought to be praised because it had, among bringing many other benefits, allowed more men to attain great age with less infirmity.'[36] Erasmus held this belief at a time (1518) when we would consider medicine synonymous with quackery and in a place (the Netherlands) where life expectancy may have actually been decreasing. These same sentiments were expressed strongly in Victorian times and echo to this day in the popular phrase 'medical miracles'. Questioning medical care's effectiveness is a relatively new phenomenon.[4] Beginning in the 1960s, some people began to question anew medical interventions' effectiveness, 'partly because of the great increase in the cost of medical care, and also because some major causes of disability and death have as yet been little affected.'[37]

The extent to which specific medical interventions have contributed to improved health is controversial, and compounded by what is measured—mortality or morbidity, or disease or discomfort. Opinions are arrayed against inadequate facts. One might be tempted to conclude: 'As we haven't the statistics we shouldn't make the judgements.'[38] However, each day worldwide we spend billions of dollars on medical interventions on the presumption that they are effective. The widespread failure to evaluate health care's impact on populations' health and to assess the effectiveness of specific medical interventions—and the general lack of concern about this failure—may be one of the twentieth century's most important social phenomena.

McDermott points out that present health indicators—concentrating as they do on mortality rather than health status—underestimate the value of modern medicine.[29,40] Beeson argues that medicine is the cause of recent health improvements,[37] a view shared by most US health system leaders.[41] However, two principal perspectives cast doubt on the effectiveness of many modern medical interventions:

- Vast increases in health care expenditures have produced modest gains in life expectancy (and perhaps even less health status improvement).
- Well-designed medical research studies show that most interventions that are tested are ineffective, whereas inadequately-designed studies show them to be effective.[42] Detailed discussion of the evidence on the effectiveness of medical care (or its lack) is beyond this manual's scope.

Advances in medical knowledge and practices began to take off in the middle of the nineteenth century. The age of modern medicine, with its attendant explosion of medical technology and rising health care costs, dates only from the 1950s. Because of modern medical intervention, few women now die in childbirth. Advances in surgery, such as anaesthesia, aseptic techniques, natural and artificial blood product transfusions, antibiotics, and new materials and methods have made surgical intervention relatively safe and painless. Surgeons can set broken bones, repair wounds, save the lives of trauma victims, even if they cannot restore them to health, and remove stones and blockages, providing symptomatic relief, even if leaving the underlying disease unaffected. Insulin gives a new lease of life to diabetics; haemodialysis saves thousands from certain death. In many large and small ways medical interventions save lives and improve health. But in recent decades, why have health care expenditures increased so much and health so little?

Patients, their behaviours and circumstances, may have changed adversely, sapping interventions' potency. Patients may not comply with (otherwise effective) treatments. Treatments may not be very effective (and increasingly costly). As one health problem is solved those revealed may be harder (and more costly) to treat. A biological wall may exist that is impervious to incremental medical technologies; breaching it may require distant technological breakthroughs, if it can be done at all. Many medical interventions, such as the treatment of infertility and breast implants for cosmetic reasons, may have little effect on such traditional measures of health as life expectancy, although they may improve individuals' sense of self-worth, which, in principle, health status measurement might encompass.

Until recently, communicable diseases were the principal cause of death and the greatest threat to health. Better nutrition and hygiene, public health measures and antibiotics stemmed the tide. For example, in the early 1950s smallpox killed five million people annually.[29] In 1976 the World Health Organization (WHO) reported the last known naturally occurring case of smallpox: the first, and so far only, disease to be eradicated. Celebrations were short-lived. In 1981 medical scientists recognised HIV infection and its sequelae, AIDS. While in principle AIDS is preventable, it threatens to devastate human populations. WHO expects AIDS will kill millions of people annually after the year 2000. Other old, new, and as yet unknown pathogens lurk, poised to threaten people's health. Chronic, degenerative diseases (heart attack, cancer, stroke, etc), from which persons spared from infectious diseases and accidents now suffer increasingly, remain stubbornly defiant to medical advances. Some result mostly from behaviours or lifestyles, for example smoking-related deaths.

New plagues such as violence (homicide, suicide, accidents, family member abuse, rape) and drug abuse (tobacco and alcohol as well as illicit substances and the misuse of medications) take their toll on health. Iatrogenesis (health care induced mortality and morbidity) may threaten patients' health, the result of ever more ubiquitous, complex and powerful treatments. Medical care would have to improve immensely to recoup, and may be incapable of offsetting or overcoming, the population health status loss from such causes. What help medicine does offer comes at increasingly higher prices. The increasing cost of medical intervention reduces funds available to prevent disease, promote health and improve other aspects of people's quality of life.

Good intentions do not necessarily produce good results. The provision of health care services does not necessarily result in health status improvement. For far too long doctors, patients and the public have simply assumed that advances in medical science result in more effective interventions; that the ability to palliate translates into the ability to cure. What is plausible is not necessarily valid. When tested, some interventions based on supposedly sound logic have harmed rather than helped patients. Meaningful measurement of patients' long-term outcomes—end results of health care—is necessary to know which interventions are effective, that effective interventions are being used properly in medical practice, and that quality management efforts produce cost-effective improvements in the quality of care.

236.7 *Medical care's effectiveness and quality management*

Since the first doctor treated the first patient, patients have been concerned about treatments' effectiveness. However, determining interventions' effectiveness and ensuring that doctors provide only effective care is easier said than done. Effective systems to assure and improve patient outcomes have yet to be implemented anywhere. They require a way to measure interventions' effectiveness and to assure patients' outcomes, and the will to implement quality management.

In 1913, following a series of revolutions in manufacturing, E.A. Codman, a Boston surgeon, made the case for studying and improving the end-points (outcomes) of medical care. But he pointed out that: 'It is against the individual interests of the medical and surgical staffs of hospitals to follow up, compare, analyse, and standardise all their results.'[43] Although Codman's work in the United States led to an investigation into the quality of surgical care (in 1918) and ultimately (in 1952) the Joint Commission on the Accreditation of Hospitals (now Healthcare Organisations), very little was done to assess and improve the outcomes of medical care. And so it remained for almost sixty years, for the same reasons that Codman cited: lack of concern, lack of incentives and lack of resources. Today, heightened concern about health care outcomes once again follows another revolution in manufacturing (the quest for quality). How does the last decade of this century differ from its first decade?

For the first time we have the means to measure interventions' effectiveness, assess the quality of care and take the steps necessary to improve it. They result from the organisation and bureaucratisation of care manifest in regulatory requirements, records keeping and management information systems. They also include computers to collect and analyse data economically, sound concepts and analytic models necessary to measure care processes and outcomes and to interpret resultant data meaningfully, and strategies to manage change in health care delivery organisations, whose creation makes quality management a practical possibility. Now that there is a way is there a will? Advances in education, social democracy and autonomy may provide the political will to collect, analyse, and use quality of care and effectiveness data to reshape health care. The coming era of health care quality management promises to fulfil a cherished dream: knowing realistically what one can expect from medical intervention and being sure of getting it.

237 | Health research and development

237.1 | Information for decision making

Decisions must be made in practice whether or not solid information exists. Uncertainties abound. Doctors may be uncertain about which diagnostic interventions to use or the order in which to use them or how to interpret the resultant information. Nevertheless, they must diagnose the patient's health problem in order to treat it. Interventions must be matched to patients. Doctors may be uncertain about the patient's treatment goals or which treatment would best accomplish them. If complications occur, doctors may be uncertain as to why they occurred or how best to manage them.

Traditionally, doctors have learned how to treat patients through education—which has become longer and more rigorous; continuing medical education—which has become more formal; and practice experience—which has become more systematic. Information conveyed through education may not be valid or appropriate; that derived from practice may be subject to misinterpretation. Moreover, it is one thing to learn something at one point in time and quite another to apply it correctly in practice at another. At the moment one may forget, or misremember, or misjudge the circumstance. Practice is increasingly difficult because of patients' heightened expectations, the explosion of medical information, the bewildering array of interventions and the complexity of the health system. Paradoxically, concerns about the quality of care have increased as resource consumption has grown. Rising costs and increasing complexity have driven these concerns.

Quality management reduces these uncertainties by specifying practice policies, which are standing rules on how to treat patients. To be most useful, practice policies must be based firmly on sound scientific knowledge. Existing technology limits health status improvement. Ultimately, better practice policies require advances in medical technology. Medical care can only improve health status if it employs effective interventions. Health systems research intends to develop and assess new medical technology. Medical technology assessment is essential to determine if a new intervention, or an existing intervention used in a new way, is effective.

Rational quality management depends not only on the practice of scientific medicine but also on scientific methods for assessing (measuring) the quality of care and improving practice. This section describes this type of research and summarises the present state of affairs. Necessarily, it paints a broad picture sufficient to provide a context for quality management and does not cover in depth this complex, and sometimes philosophical, subject.

237.2 Some basic concepts

237.21 SCIENCE VERSUS TECHNOLOGY

Science is the generation of (scientific) knowledge through systematic observation and experimentation to establish and systematise facts, principles and methods for their generation. Science's purpose is to describe, explain and predict phenomena, and, ultimately, to make such knowledge available for humanity's purposes. Technology is the application of knowledge and science to achieve a practical end. In the case of health (or medical) technology that end is the maintenance and improvement of health. In practice, science and technology are inseparable: advances in science require better instruments to measure phenomena; better instruments depend on advances in technology.

237.22 RESEARCH VERSUS DEVELOPMENT

Research is systematic, scientific inquiry. As a necessary first step, an investigator prepares a protocol that describes the research question to be answered, the methods to be used to answer it and a plan for implementing the methods. The investigator reviews his or her protocol prior to implementing it. Peers may also review it as a means of assuring that the proposed methods are practical, that they will answer the question posed, and that the question is worth answering. Usually a separate body reviews the ethical aspects and implications of the research, especially if there is any potential to harm human subjects, which is almost always the case. Studies that are not sound scientifically cannot be ethical. Yet another body may be responsible for the welfare of any animals used in the study, and it will also review the research protocol. When the investigator intends that someone else fund the research a protocol becomes a proposal.

The principal quest of research is new knowledge, and by extension better technology (know-how)—the application of knowledge to achieve practical ends. Since science is knowledge substantiated by scientific methods, research also encompasses the verification (or refutation) of existing information (the basis of practice). Synthesis of information is a critical element of science, an important type of research, and a prerequisite for development.

The aim of development is to improve existing interventions or design entirely new ones by stating explicitly the ends to be achieved and evaluating scientifically the evidence for claims that existing or planned interventions will achieve them. By extension, development encompasses the empirical assessment of the extent to which a modified or new intervention actually achieves its objectives. Scientific assessment begins with a research protocol, demonstrating the inseparability of research and development when applied to health care.

237.23 TYPES OF HEALTH RESEARCH AND DEVELOPMENT

Health research and development encompasses generation of new knowledge; development and assessment of proposed, new, or existing technology health policies, programs and practices; transfer of technology and dissemination of information; and development of methods and mechanisms for these purposes. For quality management purposes, it comprises two broad fields that, while distinct, conceptually overlap in practice. They are:

- biomedical research, the scientific foundations of medicine: research into the basic patho-physiological, biological, cellular or molecular (including biochemical and biophysical) mechanisms of function and derangement, and natural or artificial ways of preventing dysfunction, altering its course or responding to its manifestations;
- health systems research and development, the scientific and technological underpinnings of medical practice, quality management, health care organisation and health policy.

237.24 HEALTH SYSTEMS RESEARCH AND DEVELOPMENT

Health systems research and development has many different branches (supported by such disciplines as biostatistics, epidemiology, psychology, sociology) but, in relation to quality management, the principal branches are:

- At the system level:
  —policy analysis or management research (referred to sometimes as health services research), concerned with the goals, economics and organisation of health care delivery.
- At the production level:
  —medical technology assessment, encompassing clinical research, concerned with the content of health care or medical services, practice policies, interventions or practices;
  —health services research, concerned with the delivery of health care or medical services, practice policies, interventions, practices or processes including the design and evaluation of quality management mechanisms.

Health systems research and development informs choices among alternative interventions. Examples of these choices must be faced by patients (in deciding, for instance, whether or not to seek or use services); by providers (in diagnosing health problems and in selecting and administering treatments); by researchers (in selecting among projects and methods); and by anyone else whose decisions are intended to maintain or improve health through or by means of direct or indirect health system interventions. Correspondingly, health systems research projects may range from those seeking to determine the cost-effectiveness of treatments for a health problem to those aimed at developing an improved method of measuring health status.

In formulating a health systems research project, one must be able to propose the information to be generated and to articulate its value in improving health or health care delivery, its users and ways in which it can be used. Only research relevant to the health system for which the usefulness of the intended or generated information can be articulated is health systems research. A corollary of this idea is that any research meeting this criterion is health systems research. Use of information substantiated by research requires that the research results be valid to be useable; be relevant to be useful; and be accessible (to those who could use it to inform their choices among alternatives) to be used. Only when used in practice are health systems research results of any value.

237.3 Medical technology and its assessment

237.31 ABOUT MEDICAL TECHNOLOGY

In the last twenty to thirty years medical technology has increased markedly; its further rapid expansion is anticipated. Applications of technology raise concerns because of their economic, ethical, legal and social implications that increase interest in its assessment. Assessments can be concerned with: benefits and costs; implications, for example whether or not the technology should be used, even if cost-effective; and policies needed for appropriate use and to ameliorate deleterious impacts. We need medical technology assessments to inform choices among alternatives as the health services we could provide begin to outstrip our ability to provide them all. This information is critical to improving practice. Today, however, too little useful research is being done, too few research results are useable, and information that is relevant and valid is too hard to find. We know little about the diffusion of innovation or the best way to transfer technology, to disseminate information to practitioners.

237.32 MEDICAL TECHNOLOGY ASSESSMENT

The US Office of Technology Assessment, a research arm of the US Congress, defined medical technology as:

> Techniques, drugs, equipment, and procedures used by health-care professionals in delivering medical care to individuals, and the systems within which such care is delivered.[44]

The US Institute of Medicine (IOM) defines medical technology assessment as:

> Any process of examining and reporting properties of a medical technology used in health care, such as safety, efficacy, feasibility, and indications for use, cost, and cost-effectiveness, as well as social, economic, and ethical consequences, whether intended or unintended.[45]

237.33 THE COMPREHENSIVE VIEW

Classically, medical technology assessments have been viewed as comprehensive policy analyses, focused on a class of or particular existing or anticipated technology, such as the comprehensive study of the ethical, legal, social implications of advances in biomedical and behavioural research and technology, mandated by the US Congress.[46] The IOM captures this view as follows:

> Technology assessment ideally would be comprehensive and include evaluation not only of the immediate results of the technology but also of the long-term consequences. A comprehensive assessment of a medical technology—after assessment of its immediate effects—may also include an appraisal of problems of personnel training and licensure, new capital expenditures for equipment and buildings, and possible consequences for the health insurance industry and the social security system. Technology assessment provides a form of policy analysis that includes as potential components the narrower approaches to technology evaluation. Most assessments stop with a partial effort. Not all technologies warrant the full assessment, nor is it feasible to provide comprehensive assessments for all technologies.[45]

237.34 A PRAGMATIC VIEW

Knowledge about what practitioners can achieve in practice, and how they can achieve it, is quality management's foundation. This knowledge derives from medical technology assessments and health services research. Pragmatically, medical technology assessments must inform choices among alternative interventions for a health problem or disease, or the use of a particular technology for one or more health problems. For assessment purposes, a technology's key properties are effectiveness and costs. Axiomatically, results of conforming to practice policies can equal but cannot exceed those of the best practices (which practice policies embody).

237.4 Aspects of medical technology assessment

237.41 UNDERTAKING MEDICAL TECHNOLOGY ASSESSMENTS

The assessment of medical technology is a complex endeavour, one requiring considerable expertise and experience. Techniques for assessing diagnostic interventions differ from those for assessing therapeutic interventions, for example. Presently, few people are trained to conduct adequate assessments. This section is intended only to inform readers of some key aspects of medical—primarily therapeutic—technology assessment; not as a guide for conducting assessments. It describes the importance of defining the intervention to be assessed, the focus of the assessment, the stage of a technology's life cycle at which the assessment is conducted, the assessment's content, and methods for conducting assessments.

237.42 DEFINITION

Careful definition of an intervention is a prerequisite for its assessment.[47] An intervention comprises two parts: technology and its delivery mechanism. The technology is the active ingredient that produces the desired effect. The delivery mechanism may be inseparable from the technology, or, if separable, it may, and often does, interact with the technology, affecting outcomes. An intervention's definition must encompass both the technology, for example practice and practitioner, and its milieu, for example the time, place and conditions of its use.

237.43 FOCUS

An assessment's focus may be a health problem or disease, or a particular technology. One can envision a matrix consisting of two dimensions: health problem and technology. The intersections would permit identification of either those technologies that are effective for a particular health problem or those health problems helped by a particular technology. The cells would contain definitions of the interventions and descriptions of their use in practice.

237.44 STAGE

Technologies have been envisioned as having life cycles.[44] For example, a technology's life cycle may be viewed as consisting of the following seven stages:

- idea—nascent technology, born of knowledge and ingenuity;
- first use—emerging technology, not yet used in practice;
- diffusion and adoption—beginning use in practice;
- use and acceptance—widespread and growing use in practice;
- maturity—general use in practice;
- obsolescence and decline—beginning to be replaced by alternative technology;
- disuse and death—replaced by alternative technology.

Technology assessment is customarily thought of as a formal process that usually occurs before a drug, device or procedure is first used, the result of an experiment or clinical trial. Testing the safety and efficiency of drugs or devices to win regulatory approval to market them is perhaps the best example of this concept of technology assessment. However, most technologies are not assessed formally prior to use in practice. Nevertheless, people do assess technologies at the various stages of their development, with the assessment's purpose and criteria varying by stage as well as by assessor.

The progression of a technology from one point to another in its life cycle involves at least an implicit assessment. Early on the inventor must decide whether or not he or she can profitably develop the concept into workable technology. The prototype technology may be assessed to determine whether or not it should be introduced into practice. A regulatory body may have to decide if a drug can be marketed. An insurance company or government may have to decide if it should pay for a surgical operation. A hospital may have to decide if it should buy a new imaging system. A doctor may have to decide if he or she should prefer the technology for treating patients.

Initial stage assessments are often parochial, encompassing predominantly the developer's view. At later stages regulatory bodies may control a technology's use. Ultimately, the number of decision makers broadens when individual practitioners or consumers choose among alternative interventions for health problems. At these stages, decision makers must rely mostly on information provided to them by developers, regulatory bodies, or researchers who have become interested in the technology, or, very often, colleagues' opinions.

The incorporation of a new technology into practice may alter why and how it is used, affecting patient outcomes as well as staff roles, satisfaction and wellbeing, for example. Over time, new technologies may supplant old ones. The comparative assessments of old and of new technology may hasten the idea that the old technology is obsolete and should not be used, or used only in specially defined circumstances.

237.45 CONTENTS

Medical technology assessments must be concerned not only with technical performance, but also with clinical results. New imaging technologies, for example, may provide better images. However, use of such technologies in practice can only be justified if such better images are translated into improved outcomes for patients. To decide among alternative interventions, at a minimum technology assessments must be concerned with an intervention's effectiveness for a specific population with a given health problem that the intervention was designed or intended to affect. They should also evaluate its cost-effectiveness, and may analyse the intervention's net social benefits and impacts. Administrators must also be concerned with the distribution of medical technologies, for example siting, personnel, budgets; policy decision makers with access, and financing.

237.46 METHODS

Information for a technology assessment may be derived from any one of the following sources or a combination of all of them:

- empirical, observational research that produces research findings;
- information synthesis that evaluates and summarises research findings;
- group judgment that produces expert opinions, either interpreting research findings for practice or quality assurance purposes or filling gaps in knowledge.

The best (or by some people's definition, the only) knowledge of interventions' effectiveness comes from scientific (well-designed, well-controlled) trials. In such trials, investigators define and describe precisely the intervention and its use, assign randomly those patients who meet criteria for inclusion in the study to treatment and control groups, and, preferably, neither patient nor provider knows to which group randomisation has assigned him or her (double-blind trial). Further, an impartial third party analyses results (triple blind trial) to eliminate the inherent bias of the person who invented or is a proponent of the intervention, especially if he or she also conducts the trial.

Although randomised controlled trials, which isolate the intervention being tested from other factors that could affect outcomes, offer the best means to gauge effectiveness, they are not always feasible or practical. Other technology assessment designs offer less certain information. Information syntheses are essential for specifying what should be known, what is known with what certainty of validity, and consequently what gaps in knowledge exist.[48] Group judgment methods must be used to fill knowledge gaps until more solid information is available from research. The methods appropriate for a particular technology assessment depend on the technology and its stage of development; the assessment's purpose, focus and contents; and the desired certainty and timeliness of results. Consideration of these issues is beyond this manual's scope.

237.5 Limits of effectiveness as a decision criterion

Decisions about which interventions to permit or to use may depend on considerations other than their effectiveness, or even their cost-effectiveness. These other considerations may include: distribution of costs, benefits and power; affects on values; expectation of personal responsibility; humaneness of treatment; and individual rights versus social good. For example: Should people be free to select the sex of their offspring? If a technology can only be offered to a select few, is it better to offer it to no one? These are very important questions that depend mostly on considerations other than effectiveness. Health technologies can alter our conceptions of ourselves, our values and the way we behave, and raise ethical dilemmas. Finally, we have to be concerned with the kinds of policies and incentives that are needed for appropriate use of a technology or to ameliorate its deleterious impacts if it is used. Some impacts may be indirect, delayed or even unintended. We must balance these impacts with those that are intended, including their magnitude, probability of occurrence, and when in the future they are expected to occur. This picture, already complex, is further complicated when one realises that an outcome one person views positively another may view negatively.

237.6 The state of affairs

237.61 LITTLE IS SPENT ON SCIENCE; LITTLE IS KNOWN SCIENTIFICALLY

Given the health care system's size and its importance far too little is spent on research and development to improve health and the interventions that would make such improvement possible. Most health research expenditures are directed toward understanding human biology and pathophysiological processes. No matter how laudable the quest for such knowledge may be, nor how useful it may prove to be ultimately, it is simply not helpful for coping with the serious problems facing current medical practice. To date, very little money has been spent on health systems research to improve medical practice. The cost-effectiveness of most medical interventions is unknown.[31]

Most interventions are introduced in practice without scientific assessment of their effectiveness, let alone their cost-effectiveness; costs are rarely measured. Virtually no one pays any attention to finding better, cheaper ways to deliver effective interventions or to improving medical practice. Moreover, according to one evaluation, despite researchers' best intentions, most studies that are published are invalid or scientifically inadequate in terms of their design, data, statistical inferences or documentation.[42] Consequently, we know scientifically little or nothing about the effectiveness of most medical interventions or about improving medical practice.

237.62 THE STATE OF MEDICAL TECHNOLOGY ASSESSMENT

The ideological basis of modern medicine is scientific practice: from scientific knowledge we can understand disease processes and fashion technology to prevent disease, cure illness and enhance functioning. Through scientific inquiry we can judge whether or not a plausible treatment fashioned from theory is effective. However, most medical practice has no scientific basis. The United States spends more money than any other country on health R&D and publishes more articles in journals. In the United States, however, expenditures for all types of health research and development have fallen as a fraction of health expenditures, from a peak of 4.9% in 1965, to 2.9% in 1984; being about 3.5% in 1992.[45,46,49] Further, even our biomedical research expenditures have not been directed to the problems that truly ail us.[50] 'Paradoxically, our knowledge is often most incomplete with respect to disorders that affect mankind with the greatest frequency.'[51]

Even though we have invested heavily in biomedical research to try to understand basic biochemical and pathophysiological mechanisms, we have spent virtually nothing on finding out if medical tests and treatments are effective in improving health. In its latest report on technology assessment, the Institute of Medicine (IOM) estimates that US expenditures for medical technology assessment amounted to US$1.3 billion in 1984, 'a generous estimate . . . (representing) a nearly vanishing 0.3% of the money that is spent for health care'.[45] Moreover:

> By far the biggest item was US$1.1 billion for clinical trials (US$750 million of which was spent by the drug industry). Health services research expenditures hardly amounted to US$200 million. Spending for the rest of medical technology assessment (to synthesise and interpret primary evaluation data for determining how to best apply in practice new and currently available technologies) will not reach US$50 million for 1985.[45]
>
> These amounts are less than one-tenth of what we should be spending, according to an expert panel.[46]

The US Institute of Medicine summed up the present situation regarding medical technology assessment as follows:

> The nation requires a systematic approach for technology assessment. We need to have a strategy and an organisation for setting priorities. Given the priorities, we need mechanisms for actually making the assessments and implementing the findings. And finally, we need a method for paying for many of the needed assessments. As with any large-scale technological enterprise, we need to maintain a strong body of professional personnel to carry out the assessments, and they must be encouraged to conduct work of high quality and develop new techniques as required. Although some parts of this overall process are in place and are contributing well to the health of Americans, the system as a whole has major gaps and deficiencies.[52]

The diffusion, adoption and abandonment of interventions has been little studied.[44]

237.63 T<small>HE STATE OF PUBLISHED RESEARCH</small>

Medical practitioners gain their primary store of medical knowledge from medical school and early training. They modify their practices through experience and continued learning. Most medical practitioners' continuing medical education comes from reading medical journals. In fact, medical knowledge is first reported in print in medical journals and is later compiled in reviews and textbooks that serve as the basis for medical education and practice reference.

The number of medical journals has exploded in recent years; more papers are being published than ever before. Abstract services and computerised databases for citations, such as Medlars of the US National Library of Medicine, have been developed in response to this proliferation of literature. Nevertheless, it remains inaccessible to the practitioner, most of it is irrelevant to practice, and the data it contains are unsubstantiated scientifically.[53] According to one meta-evaluation, only a fraction of studies assessing medical interventions and procedures produce scientifically substantiated findings. Moreover, the stronger the author's claim of effectiveness, the weaker the study scientifically:

> Eight assessment articles correlated the frequency of positive findings with the adequacy of the methods used to obtain these results; this rate was 80% in 449 inadequately-designed studies and 25% in 305 adequately designed studies.[42]

237.7 | Health systems research and quality management

Knowledge of medical interventions' cost-effectiveness is essential for setting practice policies and thus for meaningful quality management programs. In the long run, only with substantial, sustained expenditures on relevant, valid health systems research and the use of results in practice can we expect to improve the quality and productivity of health care.

The entire cycle of research to improve medical practice should ideally be use-driven. Practitioners need to make decisions: what decisions would most benefit from better information? Quality management systems (described later in this part) can help answer this key question. After setting priorities for what research is needed, improved mechanisms must be put in place to ensure that researchers generate useable data. Further, mechanisms must be devised to permit routine knowledge synthesis and its active dissemination to those who can use relevant, valid information to improve practice. First and foremost doctors and other health care professionals are practitioners, not researchers or knowledge synthesisers. They should be able to seek and obtain reliable information, for example to choose among treatments, without having to worry about the quality of the information. Decision support technology is the preferred way to make relevant, valid information available to practitioners when they need it, a point discussed later in this part.

238 | Effectiveness

238.1 | Importance of effectiveness in quality management

This section describes the concept of effectiveness and hence an effective intervention. In the broadest sense, health care quality management's goal is to design and document effective interventions, to ensure and document their proper application in clinical practice, to measure and document health care outcomes, and to use the resultant information on process and outcome variation to improve conformance to cost-effective health care processes and interventions' effectiveness in producing health outcomes.

The term effectiveness applies to diagnostic as well as to therapeutic interventions (referred to here generally as interventions). The term therapeutic includes preventive, curative, palliative and rehabilitative interventions (referred to here generally as treatments). The terms interventions and treatments apply singly and in the aggregate. Most people associate the terms effective and effectiveness with therapeutic interventions, which is the topic on which we focus here.

Knowledge about interventions' effectiveness is crucial for health care quality management. Providers need effective interventions to maintain and improve patients' health status. Providers, quality managers and patients must be able to distinguish effective from ineffective and harmful interventions. Practice polices, the key to successful quality management, must be based on sound information about interventions' effectiveness. Despite the obvious need to know, very little money has been spent finding out about interventions' effectiveness. Quality managers must overcome this lack of knowledge by using structured expert judgment until more solid, scientific information becomes available.

Effectiveness is a much used, but also much misunderstood, term. This section defines effectiveness for quality management purposes. It describes the essence of the effectiveness of diagnostic and, particularly, therapeutic interventions, and addresses a number of contentious issues. They include: the placebo effect, the nature and importance of risk, and the fallacy of efficacy.

238.2 *Effectiveness of diagnostic interventions*

An effective diagnostic intervention correctly classifies a person or patient, for example, as having a particular disease or not. Diagnostic interventions (diagnostic tests) provide information to classify patients for purposes of treatment selection and prognosis. Realising achievable patient outcomes depends on correct diagnosis: an effective treatment for a particular disease is unlikely to benefit, and may harm, a patient with a different disease, if only because use of an ineffective intervention for the patient's health problem precludes use of an effective one. Inadequate diagnostic performance—missed or misdiagnoses, as well as delays in diagnosis—is one of the greatest quality management problems, as it precludes timely use of effective treatments. Given its critical importance, correct diagnostic classification often receives too little quality management attention. Often very little scientific information is available about individual diagnostic tests' performance, not to mention diagnostic strategies—that is, sequences of diagnostic tests that determine diagnosis' cost-effectiveness.

For different types of patients the same treatment may be indicated (because it is the most effective for their health problem), but they may differ in their prognosis. To the extent practical, patients should know what likely awaits them without and with alternative treatments, so that they can make informed choices. Further, for quality management purposes patients should be classified into groups that are homogeneous, for example with respect to outcomes and preferences. In this way practice policies can be developed which match expectations of long-term patient outcare with observed patient outcare.

Studies of diagnostic intervention may relate to an entire diagnostic strategy, including the rules used to draw inferences from the resultant information, although they relate usually to a single diagnostic test, for example an electrocardiogram. To assess diagnostic interventions' performance one must compare it to that of a 'gold standard', which may be a single diagnostic test or information determined from data gathered from several sources, including, for example, autopsy data, which increases the certainty that patients did (or did not have) the particular disease. Determining who truly has (and does not have) a disease (or other characteristic) may be difficult, so that some uncertainty may remain about tests' accuracy.

Three related measures indicate how well diagnostic interventions classify patients as having, or not having, a disease or other characteristic. They are: false positives and false negatives rates; sensitivity and specificity; and positive and negative predictive value. Technical Appendix A of this chapter defines these terms. Doctors may use diagnostic classifications to estimate patients' prognosis, their health status with and without treatment, for example. While one may assess the predictive accuracy of such classifications, different considerations apply than those for assessing diagnostic accuracy. They are beyond this manual's scope.

238.3 *Effectiveness of therapeutic interventions*

Therapeutic interventions come between diseases' causes and their courses. An intervention is designed to achieve a desired objective (e.g. health status improvement), and generally consists of several elements and their interrelationships. Ideally, all elements are necessary and sufficient to achieve the desired objective, and their interrelationships are as efficient as possible. In practice, some of an intervention's elements may not be needed to achieve (or may hinder achieving) the desired effect, others that would enhance effectiveness are missing, or elements' interrelationships may not be as efficient as possible (reducing effectiveness or increasing cost, or both). A subsequent chapter on the production of health elaborates on these points. The remainder of this section describes the concept of effectiveness and the difficulties of measuring it.

| 238.4 | *The nature of effectiveness*

238.41 EFFECTIVENESS DEFINED

An effective intervention produces a desired effect or outcome. This desired effect is manifest in an intervention's objective. Objectives state or suggest measures of effectiveness. Since health care's objective is to maintain or improve health, an effective health care intervention maintains or improves patients' health status. Effectiveness is the extent to which intervention is superior to no intervention in maintaining or improving patients' health status. Operationally, it is the difference in health status improvement between intervention and a disease's course if untreated (its natural history). (See Figure II-3-3 below.) Thus, an intervention's effectiveness may be defined in terms of health status improvement gained over doing nothing. (See Figure II-3-4 on page 156.) An ineffective intervention does nothing: it neither improves nor worsens patients' health status. A harmful intervention reduces patients' health status from what it would have been without intervention.

238.42 EFFECTIVENESS IS A STATISTICAL CONCEPT

Effectiveness is a statistical concept: it describes the results of interventions applied to populations of patients. Effective interventions transform the health status of some patients to some average extent with some variance. In other words, an effective intervention results in greater aggregate health status for a specified patient population suffering from a given health problem than no intervention, even if the intervention results in no health status improvement, or even its deterioration, for some patients. Any intervention will produce a statistical distribution of health status improvement, with a mean and variance. For patients, the mean expresses an intervention's expected health benefits; the variance, its inherent risks. Understanding the statistical nature of interventions' effectiveness is critical for quality management.

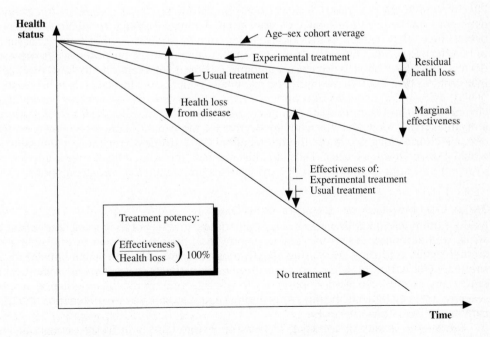

Figure II-3-3 *Calculation of treatment effectiveness and selected other measures*

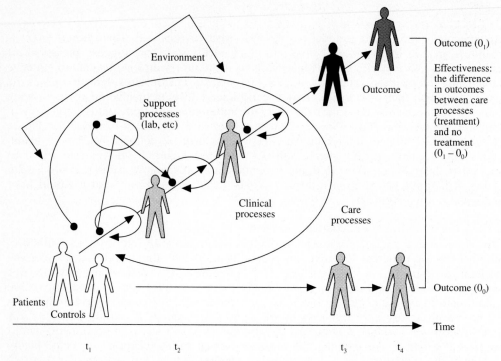

Figure II-3-4 *(True) Effectiveness is the difference in patient outcomes between treatment (O_1) and no treatment (O_0)*

238.43 EFFECTIVENESS IS A CHARACTERISTIC OF INTERVENTIONS

Effectiveness applies to, and is derived from, population-based measurement. One cannot determine an intervention's effectiveness from a single patient. In treating patients, doctors may select treatments that, based on research or experience, they know or assume to be effective for that type of patient. For quality management purposes, assessment of doctors' treatment choices involves comparing chosen interventions to best practices, interventions that would have improved maximally patients' health status. For this reason, quality assessment refers to appropriate treatments (those that fit patients' needs and circumstances) and inappropriate treatments (those that do not). Clearly, if a doctor selects an inappropriate treatment it is likely ineffective for the patient's condition. However, the doctor's choice does not affect the intervention's effectiveness (for those patients who would benefit from its use). Thus, in this manual, the term effectiveness applies to interventions; appropriateness, to doctors' choices among alternative interventions.

238.44 EFFECTIVENESS SUBSUMES SAFETY AND EFFICACY

Analysts often refer to interventions, especially drugs, in terms of their safety and efficacy. While well accepted, the terms are less precise than they may appear at first sight and are potentially confusing. Measuring effectiveness in terms of health status improvement subsumes the notion of safety (absence of unwanted effects that adversely affect health status). For quality management purposes, a safe intervention exhibits a small chance of severely reducing patients' health status during or, if a long-term or maintenance therapy, early in the intervention's course.

Safety—the quality or condition of being free from danger or injury—is a judgment about the acceptability of risk. All medical interventions can cause injury, and so none can be absolutely safe, although they can be relatively safe; some interventions carry considerable risk. Risk is a population-based estimate of the chances for harm. Harm can be measured in terms of reduced health status. If effectiveness is measured in terms of health status improvement—as it should be—any harm that the intervention may cause is counted automatically and thus safety need not, and cannot, be considered separately, as the same measure captures both gains (in health status) and losses (injury or harm to patients' health), to yield net health status improvement (or deterioration).

238.45 EFFECTIVENESS IS A RELATIVE MEASURE OF TREATMENT POTENCY

An effective intervention improves patients' health status compared to doing nothing. Effectiveness is a relative measure of an intervention's treatment potency. Operationally, treatment potency is an intervention's ability to restore patients' health status to that enjoyed by the average person of the same age and sex (quantified, for example, as the percentage of health status loss recouped). (See Figure 11-3-3 on page 155). These data are generally not available presently.

238.46 EFFECTIVENESS IS MORE THAN OBSERVED IMPROVEMENT

Measuring outcome variables tells one nothing about what produced resultant readings. The observation that particular patients' health improved does not mean that the preceding intervention produced the improvement. To attribute outcomes to intervention one needs a point of comparison. Ideally, this comparison would be of outcomes for patients meeting defined criteria assigned randomly to treatment and control groups. In the absence of such data, attribution must be assumed or inferred. The strength of the inference depends on the strength of the measurement system (e.g. randomised controlled trial, opportunity sample of cases, quality assessment, personal opinion), and the extent to which plausible mechanisms are known scientifically or can be inferred plausibly to connect interventions to outcomes. All too often assumptions are wrong and inferences weak; treatments believed to be 'effective' are not.

True effectiveness refers to the difference in health status (outcomes) between patients who received and those who did not receive the intervention, determined in such a way that any difference can be attributed confidently to the intervention. Assumed or observed effectiveness refers to what one has observed in practice, for example the difference between a patient's preintervention and postintervention condition. Simply attributing any observed 'improvement' to the intervention usually overestimates true effectiveness, and the intervention might not be effective at all.

Effectiveness refers to interventions' specific capability to alter diseases' courses or causes. Any medical intervention may improve a patient's health status if only by making him or her feel better for a time, but may not alter the course or cause of his or her disease. Treatments' general (non-specific) beneficial effects are often attributed to doctors' healing properties or referred to as interventions' placebo effect. While any intervention may improve health status compared to doing nothing at all, an effective intervention has specific (rather than only general or placebo) effects that alter the course or cause of patients' health problem or disease. Of course, it may be difficult to distinguish a placebo from a specific effect unless one measures an intervention's effectiveness in a well-designed, well-controlled randomised clinical trial, and measures outcomes for a sufficiently long period after the initiation of intervention.

Patients' postintervention health status may be worse than their preintervention health status, even if an intervention is effective, that is, alters the course of their disease for the better. Patients' health status may have been even worse without the intervention. Just because patients' observed health status is worse after the intervention does not mean that the intervention was ineffective. Pre-and post-intervention comparisons cannot measure an intervention's true effectiveness. The only valid comparison is between health status improvement with intervention (experimental) and that without (control). True effectiveness is the difference in outcomes between experimental and control patient populations, for example the difference measured between patients who do and those who do not receive the intervention that can be attributed confidently to intervention— for example in the manner of a well-designed, well-controlled randomised clinical trial.

238.47 MARGINAL EFFECTIVENESS

For making comparisons, almost invariably one has outcome data only on patients who experienced alternative interventions; there are no untreated controls. Often it is not possible or permissible to leave patients without treatment. Studies that compare one treatment to another, for example an experimental one to a usual or accepted treatment, demonstrate the marginal or additional effectiveness of one treatment over another. From this type of study it is not possible to determine scientifically the extent to which the most 'effective' intervention produced observed outcomes. In this circumstance, one must either assume that the most 'effective' intervention produced observed outcomes, while recognising the possibility that it is not truly effective, or one must adjust observed outcomes to account for what would have occurred without intervention, if valid information exists to permit such adjustments to be made (which it almost invariably does not). If knowledge of natural history (natural outcomes) is lacking, one can easily overestimate therapeutic effectiveness, as was the case with the use of penicillin to treat syphilis.[54]

238.5 | *Effectiveness is a specific, more than the placebo, effect*

238.51 THE PLACEBO EFFECT

Many conditions for which patients consult doctors are self-limiting; some resolve themselves; for others the doctor is the treatment. Doctors' healing powers and the hope they engender in patients have been known for centuries. The patient wants a cure and needs hope; the doctor obligingly supplies both. Hopeful patients' outcomes may actually be better than others without hope who receive the same treatment. Yet, an intervention's supposed effectiveness may be no more than the placebo effect.[55]

The placebo effect is manifest when an intervention improves a patient's health status without having a known specific effect on the health problem or its manifestations. The patient feels better, for a time at least, but the intervention affects neither the course nor the cause of the patient's disease. A disease's course may be altered by affecting either the resultant deranged physiology or its manifestations, for example symptoms. An intervention may affect a disease's manifestations without affecting its course, or its course without affecting its cause. Interventions that affect a disease's underlying cause may prevent its (re)occurrence. Placebos cannot affect directly a disease's underlying processes and their effect is thus transitory; long-term outcomes are unaffected, except that treatment-engendered hope may affect the patients' physiology and indirectly affect disease processes and thus outcomes. Simply being in treatment may affect the patient's condition for the better, irrespective of the intervention used.

A patient with low back pain with no obvious (or, following investigation, revealed hidden) cause may be helped simply by being in treatment; any intervention the doctor prescribes may have no discernible specific effect on the disease. If the doctor prescribes aspirin for pain, this drug has a specific effect against one of the disease's symptoms (unless it is entirely psychological in origin). It is extremely unlikely that aspirin affects the disease's course or its cause, whatever it may be. Similarly, it is unlikely that surgery, radiation, chemotherapy or any other treatment for cancer affects the disease's cause although it may affect its course, and, conceivably, could eradicate the cancer (i.e. it would be undetectable, at least for a time, and the patient may die ultimately of some other disease).

Correct use of antibiotics will resolve infections caused by bacteria, for example pneumonia, which might have killed the patient, or, if self-limiting, may have taken longer to resolve without their use or have resulted in permanent impairment. These effects will be realised whether or not the patient believes in the treatment's effectiveness. Placebo effects may enhance these specific effects. Antibiotics have no specific effects on the course of an uncomplicated common cold, a virus. Their use, however, may have placebo effects and the patient may feel better. People who have undergone sham operations, for example simply opening their chest and closing it again, have reported beneficial effects comparable to those reported by patients who underwent the definitive cardiac procedure (which might have had only a placebo effect).

238.52 SEPARATING FACT FROM FAITH
The placebo effect manifests itself best when both doctor and patient believe in an intervention's effectiveness. The power of illusion and for delusion are obvious. If patients question an intervention's effectiveness its placebo effect is lost. If doctors know an intervention has no specific effect, his or her ability to heal, through the placebo effect, may be diminished. Patients' hopes spring eternal. Almost everyone can convince themselves that an intervention might do some good, especially if the patient wants and has the means to pay for it. Zealots for a particular treatment may achieve apparently good results precisely because they believe, and can convince their patients to believe, in its effectiveness; avoiding scientific studies of the intervention's effectiveness bolsters their beliefs, of course.

Only well-designed, well-conducted scientific studies can validly measure interventions' effectiveness and differentiate specific (technological) effects from general (placebo) effects. Simply because a placebo has no specific effects does not mean it has no effect on patient outcomes. In randomised clinical trials, control patients may be given a placebo (in this context a harmless, supposedly medically inert preparation, e.g. sugar pill) to disguise the fact that they are not receiving the experimental intervention. Conceivably, their outcome may be better than that which would have been observed in true no-treatment controls. Thus, the placebo may be 'effective' in this sense. However, the study may show that the experimental intervention is no more effective, that is, lacks specific and demonstrates only a non-specific (placebo) effect. Since any treatment may have a placebo effect, an intervention's specific effect can be discerned only in comparison with that observed among controls. Without adequate controls, an intervention without a specific effect may appear effective—when in fact it is not—because of its placebo effect. Subsequent use of the intervention in the mistaken belief that it is effective precludes the search for or use of an effective intervention, may harm patients directly, and wastes money that could be better spent elsewhere.

238.53 PLACEBO PLUS
People are becoming more educated and sophisticated, and hence more sceptical, and they are demanding a role in medical decision-making and informed consent which precludes deception. Paradoxically, their scepticism may limit the doctor's healing abilities. He or she must substitute interventions with specific effects for placebos and, where none exists, help the patient live with the knowledge that nothing can be done. People have come to expect use of sophisticated diagnostic instruments and potent therapeutic interventions. Today a patient may only be satisfied that there is nothing wrong with him or her after an expensive battery of medically unnecessary tests; the doctor's reassurance is not enough. The magic has shifted from the medicine man to the medical machine, exposing patients to potential harms and increasing health care costs.

Tomorrow's research may find much of our present medical technology, or the way that we use it, to be no more than placebo-plus. Use of an intervention with specific effects in patients for whom it is not effective may harm them. Further, money saved from reducing such inappropriate use of interventions (substituting instead the lowest cost acceptable treatment) can pay for effective interventions for other patients, and for research to find effective interventions for health problems where none exists now. Any resultant loss in the placebo effect can likely be made up quickly through application of more scientific medicine.

Many, if not all, doctors come to realise that their interventions may be less effective than they and their patients would like to believe. The resultant uncertainty about what to do creates anxiety about what should be done. This anxiety, coupled with the belief that if something goes wrong someone must be at fault and, consequently, should pay handsomely, fuels defensive medicine, engenders distrust and drives costs ever higher. Quality management can be as liberating for doctors as it is reassuring for patients.

238.6 *Evidence of effectiveness requires solid science*

Quality managers need access to the results of scientifically-sound, replicated research studies to be certain of interventions' effectiveness. Such studies are a rarity. Knowledge about interventions' effectiveness derives usually from far less sound studies, and often is little more than an assumption. Differences in outcomes between intervention and no intervention (the necessary comparison) can reasonably be attributed to the intervention to determine its true effectiveness if these measurements resulted from a well-designed, well-conducted randomised controlled trial involving true controls who receive no (or only a placebo) treatment. If outcomes' data resulted from poorly designed or poorly conducted trials, other less rigorous types of research, management information system, or other sources, attributing any observed 'effectiveness' to the intervention may be unwarranted.

Quality managers must guide clinicians in their rigorous review of the evidence for interventions' effectiveness in order to formulate practice policies. Practitioners should base their practices on sound practice policies, which, in turn, should be based on scientific studies. Where sound practice policies exist, medical practitioners would be well advised to follow them. Practitioners who devise new interventions or use existing interventions in a new way must assess them scientifically, lest they conclude they work when in fact they do not.

Quality managers face innumerable political, economic and technical difficulties in measuring interventions' effectiveness. Hope springs eternal and often with an irresistible force. Doctors believe in their interventions' ability to improve patients' health status. But their beliefs may be misplaced and engender false hopes. For example, innovators may be zealous proponents of their innovations and point to startling success in treating some, if not all, of their patients. Patients facing certain death may grasp desperately at any hope of a cure, even if it will probably shorten their lives. The combination of zealous proponents and desperate sufferers may produce unstoppable pressure to adopt untested innovations, often with tragic consequences to patients and the waste of health care funds.

There is neither the time nor the money to do all of the clinical trials that should be done. Further, randomisation of patient to treatment and control groups is not always possible or practical. Priorities must be set in order, to answer the most important questions. Finally, a number of technical obstacles face investigators who do set out to determine interventions' effectiveness. They relate to the design and implementation of clinical trials and other health systems research studies. Technical Appendix B of this chapter describes some of these technical difficulties for interested readers in the context of cost-effectiveness analysis. Their complete review is beyond this manual's scope.

238.7   *Effectiveness and risk*

Effectiveness is a statistical concept and depends on measuring an intervention's effects on a population of patients. As a group, patients are more helped than harmed by an effective intervention. However, variability (not certainty) characterises the patient outcomes of interventions. An effective intervention may (or may not) improve the health status of (be effective for) every patient of a given type. If there are no known characteristics to divide patients into those more likely to be helped than harmed, there is an inherent risk in the intervention. Obviously, one would not expect an intervention to be effective for patients who are not of the type that the intervention benefits.

Medical practitioners would like to recommend, and patients would like to select, the most effective intervention for their condition, that is, the one that produces the greatest health status improvement. However, in recommending or selecting interventions, at best one has only the results of effectiveness studies involving patients whose characteristics are identical to the patient who is placed in the position of having to choose among alternative treatments. Sometimes studies involve patients with similar, rather than identical, characteristics so that one must extrapolate study findings to particular patients. At other times there are no studies, so that interventions' effectiveness is based on experience or assumption.

If researchers have assessed an intervention's effectiveness, doctors can use these results to tell patients about the expected results of treatment. For example, the doctor may tell the patient that he or she has a 50–50 chance of surviving the operation, based on the results of an assessment of its effectiveness for similar patients. The patient, however, wants to know if he or she is going to survive the operation or not. To improve prognostic information, one must identify those patient characteristics that affect outcomes. These characteristics may be unknown initially, but emerge through research. Based on results of initial assessments, researchers can identify such outcome-influencing characteristics and repeat assessments to see if outcomes exhibit less variation for a given type of patient for which the intervention is effective.

Ideally, patients would be classified ultimately into groups that are homogeneous with respect to outcome. Such groups would exhibit low variability in outcomes; any observed variation would result from improper treatment implementation (variation in process and/or performance), or from the random variation that seems to be characteristic of all natural phenomena. In practice, patient preferences are an important source of outcome variation, complicating further the already difficult task of grouping patients into those who are homogeneous with respect to outcome.

In expressing an intervention's effectiveness, researchers revert usually to population means, considering variance only for purposes of statistical significance testing. However, variance is an important part of informing patients' choices among interventions. For example, without treatment patients with a hypothetical condition uniformly die within eleven to thirteen months. With treatment most patients live much longer, but the treatment kills some of them. Overall, the treatment would result in more health status than no treatment, if patients invariably chose the treatment. But suppose they refused to accept the risk of dying from the treatment. In this case it could hardly be considered effective in any practical sense. Suppose some patients chose the treatment and some did not. As a whole, it would be effective for the subset of patients who opted for the treatment as a group, unless they also happened to be the ones most likely to die from the treatment, in which case it might not.

This scenario highlights several points. First, patients should be classified according to outcome-influencing characteristics, to produce patient classes homogeneous with respect to outcomes (and patient preferences), and information of most value to patients. Second, variance in patient outcomes (effectiveness) must be considered explicitly. Third, patients should be informed about the distribution of outcomes of alternative treatments, not merely the mean (of some unspecified distribution). Fourth, patients' treatment choices should be monitored to examine the effect on their decisions of informing them of expected outcomes (determined in clinical trials, for example). Fifth, patient outcomes should to be measured in practice, to gauge providers' performance and to gain insight into interventions' effectiveness, for example to set research priorities.

Despite the dictum *primum non nocere* (first do no harm), during many treatments the patient may be in a lower health state than an untreated individual, simply because he or she is in the hospital and may undergo uncomfortable tests, a surgical operation, or other procedures. This expected immediate loss may be more than made up by the health benefits that treatment confers. However, for some patients the outcome of the treatment may be worse than that of the disease. Careful evaluation of interventions' effectiveness, in terms of their distribution of patient health status improvement, is essential to inform medical decision-making. Quality management intends to improve treatments' effectiveness and, especially in the hospital's context, improve providers' performance. Nevertheless, all treatment carries with it an element of irreducible risk.

238.8 Efficacy

238.81 THE TERM EFFECTIVENESS IS PREFERABLE TO EFFICACY

The terms efficacy and effectiveness are often used interchangeably and, when not, are an endless source of confusion. This section explores the basis for this confusion and explains why we prefer the terms effective and effectiveness, and why there is no need to, and why it is preferable not to use, the terms efficacious and efficacy. Over the years, analysts have created a distinction between efficacy and effectiveness. They base the distinction on the idea that what is achievable in a research laboratory may not be achievable in ordinary practice. With respect to medical interventions, however, this distinction is dogmatic rather than logical and, as we explain below, for quality management purposes may be misleading.

The term efficacy connotes the potential to produce an effect or result; effectiveness, the production of an effect or result. Pragmatically, only results matter. What is theoretically possible but not realisable has no practical significance (although it might be important to research reasons for such discrepancy). Stated simply, medical technology assessors use the term efficacy to describe a technology's (intervention's) benefit for a given medical problem under ideal conditions of use; effectiveness, its benefit under average conditions of use.[45] This distinction is between ideal and average conditions of use. Analysts have extended this idea to define efficacy as an intervention's achievable benefit and effectiveness as the extent to which this achievable benefit is actually achieved in community practice.[56] These ideas confuse measurement of an intervention's effectiveness with providers' performance—the extent to which providers use an intervention appropriately and implement it properly.

238.82 THE EFFICACY FALLACY EXPOSED

Effectiveness is a measured (or all too often an assumed) attribute or property of an intervention. There is a tendency to regard such measured effectiveness (e.g. a clinical trial of a surgical operation conducted by university surgeons at an academic medical centre) as an intervention's efficacy, and its maximal health benefit. This argument suggests that an intervention's efficacy is its potential to improve patients' health status, and, further, that what can be achieved in practice (e.g. by general practitioners using this surgical operation) represents the intervention's so-called effectiveness. In this view, implicitly at least, effectiveness is always less than or equal to efficacy; therefore the difference between efficacy and effectiveness represents improvement potential. This idea is, however, a fallacy, for all of the following reasons:

- Measured (true) effectiveness (results of controlled clinical trials) cannot be compared to observed outcomes (results in uncontrolled circumstances). Many factors—not only medical intervention—coproduce outcomes. Clinical trials are designed to eliminate their effects toward measuring an intervention's true effectiveness.
- Differences in outcomes that result from performance deficiencies (e.g. not implementing an intervention as its designers intended, the basis of its measured effectiveness) are not a reflection of an intervention's effectiveness, but rather of providers' performance.
- Even if GPs' patient outcomes were the results of a well-controlled, well-conducted clinical trial in which the intervention was otherwise used as its designers intended, the comparison is between two different interventions: the university surgeons in one practice setting and the GPs in another, so that one is comparing apples with oranges.
- The implied (and sometimes stated) difference in patient outcomes does not necessarily represent improvement potential, because of an unbridgeable gap: the difference between interventions.

These ideas may be hard to grasp, in part because the persistence of the existing dogmatic distinction between efficacy and effectiveness confuses an intervention's effectiveness (how well it does what it is supposed to do in defined circumstances) with providers' performance (how well they use an intervention), and fails to recognise the fact that practitioner characteristics define an intervention: one cannot divorce practice from practitioner.

238.83 THE NATURE OF AN INTERVENTION

An intervention is designed to achieve a desired objective (e.g. health status improvement) and, generally, consists of several elements and their interrelationships. In describing interventions one must identify all of the variables that influence their effectiveness. For example, surgeons' skill, training and experience may be an important determinant of a surgical operation's effectiveness. Operator characteristics, therefore, may differentiate one intervention from another. For quality management purposes, one must define an intervention on all such outcome-influencing variables; not rely on a label for a black box with unknown contents.

A proper description of an intervention's design includes, for example: what exactly is to be done and how; who is to do it, when and where; and on whom it is to be done (i.e. what types of patients the intervention is intended to benefit). Clearly, interventions' designers must—but often do not—specify these design elements in operational detail. Thus statements about interventions' effectiveness implicitly (or sometimes explicitly) encompass statements about the intervention (what it is, who performs it, under what circumstances), as well as on whom it is used (types of patients).

238.84 IDEAL USE—DESIGN CONFORMANCE

Confusion reigns over the notion of ideal (versus average) conditions of use. Ideals can be approached but never attained. Medical technology assessors must determine that practitioners use the technology or intervention as its designers intended. We refer to such use as design-conformance implementation. There is zero process variation (between what should have been, and what was actually done). Design-conformance encompasses, for example: characteristics of patients to be benefited (the health problem for which the intervention is effective); details of the intervention (e.g. the exact nature of the surgical operation that is the intervention's core medical technology, plus postsurgical care); its implementation (e.g. surgeon's training and experience); and the therapeutic milieu (e.g. type of hospital in which the operation is to take place).

An intervention's defining characteristics include all outcome-influencing parameters, such as practitioners qualifications and setting. In changing them—for example from an operation conducted by university surgeons in academic medical centres to one conducted by general practitioners in their setting—one is dealing with a different intervention. The idea that the academic setting represents ideal, and that general practice represents average, conditions of use is fallacious. One is simply dealing with two different interventions, each with its characteristic effectiveness. In either setting, deviations from design conformance would represent inappropriate or improper use of the intervention. They would have nothing to do with ideal versus average conditions of use. Thus the idea of ideal (in contrast to average) conditions of use is not helpful for understanding interventions' effectiveness; nor for quality management purposes.

238.85 MEASUREMENT PROBLEMS

An intervention's (true) effectiveness (the extent to which it improves patients' health status) is measured by the difference in health outcomes for populations of treated and untreated individuals of a given type, including the characteristics of their health problem. Measuring an intervention's true effectiveness is difficult and requires a well-designed, well-controlled clinical trial. Researchers specify in operational detail the intervention the effectiveness of which is to be tested, the patient population on whom it is to be tested, in terms of characteristics of inclusion and exclusion, and all of the other matters one would ordinarily expect to find in a research protocol. Further, qualified, competent providers would implement the intervention, and they may have been trained specifically in its implementation prior to the trial.

Patients meeting criteria for inclusion in the trial would be randomised in relation to the intervention to be assessed and in relation to its control (placebo) groups. Patients' health state would be determined periodically, and for a sufficiently long, predetermined follow-up period. After the trial, investigators would also check that patient inclusion/exclusion criteria and randomisation procedures were followed faithfully and did not result by chance in significant differences between patients assigned to experimental and to control groups. It will also be necessary to check that the intervention was implemented as designed and, if not, ascertain why not, and that experimental and control group intervention experiences did not differ materially (e.g. that controls did not supplement their treatments with over-the-counter medication to a greater extent than experimentals). Any resultant difference between the experimental group who received the intervention and the control group who did not would be the intervention's true effectiveness.

All one knows is what one measures scientifically. Without sound scientific studies it is not possible to know interventions' true effectiveness. Interventions are rarely tested with the required degree of rigour, if research studies are done at all. The result is that an intervention's true effectiveness may not be known scientifically, and has to be estimated from less certain information or simply assumed, both of which likely overestimate it. Given that one has determined an intervention's true effectiveness in an academic setting, how is one to determine results achieved in general practice, for example?

Simply observing outcomes would be misleading because they would be the result of uncontrolled circumstances, and many factors coproduce them. Comparing observed outcomes to true effectiveness is, of course, meaningless. One could conduct a well-designed, well-controlled clinical trial of general practitioners' use of the intervention. The results would show the intervention's effectiveness for the same type of patients. Comparison of academic surgeons' results with those of GPs would still likely be meaningless for quality management purposes because one is comparing the results of two different interventions, although patients would be able to use them to choose among interventions (academic surgeons versus general practitioners). There is no implication that any performance gap between the academic surgeons and GPs can be closed. One cannot say the university surgeons' performance represents an intervention's efficacy and the community surgeons' performance represents its effectiveness. To do so is meaningless and misleading, as the following scenario demonstrates.

238.86 THE FALLACY OF DIVORCING PRACTICE FROM PRACTITIONER

Effectiveness is a property of an intervention. One cannot divorce practice from practitioner. Take running, for example, as a technology to transmit a message from point to point. The goal is to run as fast as possible to cover the distance, say a mile, in the shortest time possible. Professional milers can run the distance in less than four minutes. Weekend athletes might take five or six minutes. Importantly, the variance in the professional milers' performance would likely be quite small; that for the weekend athletes, quite large. Given that one had to get a message from point A to point B in under four minutes, the professional milers are the clear choice. Moreover, the time of any professional miler picked randomly for the task would be close to the average, reducing the risk that the message would take longer than four minutes to deliver. Professional milers are both more effective and more certain in running messages over one mile than weekend athletes. However, a marathon runner would be a better choice if point A was a great distance from point B. Running's effectiveness is an attribute, and does not exist independent, of the runner.

How fast one can run depends on the runner, his or her training, state of readiness, and fit with the task, including the ground to be covered and environmental conditions. Medical technology assessors would suggest that professional milers represent running's efficacy (what is possible) and that weekend athletes its effectiveness (what is usual). Certainly, milers can run the distance faster than weekend athletes. But the performance gap has nothing to do with running and everything to do with the runners. One might be able to transform weekend athletes into professional milers but not often, and if one could they would likely be different people: professional milers.

For purposes of assessing interventions there is a general tendency to divorce the practice from the practitioner—to say, for example, that a hysterectomy is a hysterectomy, without reference to the type of practitioner who performs it. For quality management purposes, a hysterectomy performed by a gynaecologist in a university medical centre who performs the operation several times a week is a different intervention than a hysterectomy performed by a general practitioner in a cottage hospital who performs the operation occasionally. Gynaecologists' hysterectomies may be more effective, that is, improve patients' health status more than GPs' hysterectomies because gynaecologists' operations result in fewer complications, for example. This perspective avoids the fallacy of thinking that one can bridge an unbridgeable performance gap.

There may be no way that GPs can achieve specialists' performance without having gynaecologists' knowledge and experience. If GPs could achieve specialists' performance level, then they should perform all hysterectomies, presumably at less cost. Similarly, if nurses, assisted by decision support technologies and robots, for example, could achieve the same performance level, they should do the operations, presumably at still lower cost. This example does not suggest that specialists always perform better than general practitioners. The contrary is true. General practitioners perform primary care better than specialists. Practitioners' skill and working environment are integral aspects of health care interventions: one cannot divorce the practice from the practitioner; all hysterectomies are not the same intervention; and GPs delivering primary care are more effective than specialists operating outside of their domains.

238.87 DIFFERENTIATING INTERVENTIONS' EFFECTIVENESS FROM THEIR USE

The following scenario illustrates what may happen when a new treatment diffuses into widespread use in practice, and why it is not helpful to differentiate between an intervention's efficacy and its so-called effectiveness. A group of university surgeons invent oomphoplasty (a hypothetical treatment) for oomphosis (a hypothetical disease). In a well-designed, well-conducted clinical trial they find that this innovation improves oomphosis sufferers' health status from 2.7 hsy (with supportive therapy, which is tantamount to no specific intervention) to 5.4 hsy (health status years, an outcome measure described earlier in this chapter). They publish their results and the operation is adopted quickly by surgeons everywhere. The College of Surgeons (a hypothetical professional body) launches a review of the operation's use by community surgeons because of several sensational reports of patients' deaths and a concern about the number of oomphoplasties being done, at considerable cost.

The College reports that many community surgeons are:

- attempting the operation without proper training and exhibit great variation in surgical skills and experience (which would likely compromise, and increase the variability of, observed outcomes);
- not following the university surgeons' protocol—nondesign-conformance implementation—resulting in considerable process variation among surgeons; and individual surgeons vary what they do from patient to patient (which might improve or, more likely, would compromise and increase the variability of, observed outcomes);
- operating in a variety of settings (which would likely compromise, and increase the variability of, observed outcomes);
- operating on patients who do not have oomphosis because of misdiagnosis (which might improve observed outcomes because the natural course for patients without oomphosis is better than those who have the disease) or in whom the operation is contraindicated (which would likely impair the outcomes, and both situations would increase their variability);
- using oomphoplasty for other diseases, that is, broadening its indications to include patients for whom the interventions were not intended, with unknown effectiveness for these patients (which might increase or compromise observed outcomes for the community surgeons' patients in comparison to those measured for the university surgeons whose patients truly have the disease, and would increase their variability).

Variations in processes can—and often do—lead to large variations in patient outcomes. The College's report speaks to many quality management problems, including the appropriateness of the use of oomphoplasty. It says nothing about oomphoplasty's effectiveness: the extent to which it improves patients' health status (when used in design conformance—as intended by whom and on whom intended). If we found that nurses were using ordinary clinical thermometers to measure the temperature of hypothermia patients or recording body temperatures after ten seconds (when the manufacturer recommended one minute), we would not be surprised to learn that nurses' readings were in error. We would say that the nurses' performance was deficient—not the thermometers'.

238.88 LESSONS FOR QUALITY MANAGEMENT

Observed effectiveness (results in uncontrolled circumstances) is not true effectiveness (results of a controlled trial). With observed outcomes, one has the difficulty of attributing outcomes to interventions. Observed outcomes result from any and all of the following factors that affect patient outcomes, beyond unreliable measures and random variation:

patient preferences and other characteristics that affect outcomes (e.g. surgeons may operate on patients who do not have the disease for which the intervention is intended, because of misdiagnosis, for example); surgeons may not implement the interventions as its designers intended; they may implement elements improperly, for example because of lack of training or experience, or because their hospitals are less well-organised, less well-equipped, or less well-staffed than those which participated in studies to determine the intervention's effectiveness. Thus, when observed in ordinary practice (without the controls of a randomised clinical trial), one would not be surprised to find that patient outcomes are highly variable and that an intervention's effectiveness appears to be greater (and not, as efficacy dogmatists might lead one to believe, less) than its true effectiveness.

For quality management purposes, effectiveness defines what to expect from an intervention, defined according to all parameters that affect patient health outcomes. Clinicians of similar training and experience in similar practice settings may achieve better or worse results than those observed in a well-designed, well-controlled clinical trial. These differences in patient outcomes have nothing to do with an intervention's true effectiveness and everything to do with practitioners' performance.

Ordinary doctors working in ordinary circumstances may achieve less good results than the best doctors working in the best circumstances, even when they try to follow an intervention's protocol to the best of their ability. There may be no way to reduce the performance gap between the best and the rest. Faced with worse than expected, or large variations in, patient outcomes, quality managers must first ascertain their root cause: Do they stem from poor provider performance or from poor practice policies (or the interventions that they embody)?

When practitioners' performance (beyond design conformance implementation) influences patient outcomes, and differences between classes of practitioners and/or their settings (e.g. university surgeons versus general practitioners) represents an unbridgeable gap, for quality management purposes one is dealing with different interventions. In this case, quality managers must focus on ensuring that patients receive the right intervention, for example through credentialling or referral (from a GP to a university specialist); not on the impossible task of attempting to bridge an unbridgeable gap (e.g. turning GPs into academic specialists).

For quality management purposes, the relevant comparison would be the best that can be achieved by similarly qualified practitioners operating in similar circumstances; not with the best performers operating in the best circumstances. What could GPs achieve for their patients if they implemented an intervention as designed (its effectiveness)? What are they achieving now for patients on whom they use it (with whatever degree of design conformance), some of whom have the health problem that the intervention is intended to improve and some of whom do not? Any observed performance gap is, at least in principle, potentially bridgeable, although the costs of building the bridge may not be worthwhile if spending the money in other ways would yield greater health benefits for the population. However, one should not overlook the possibility that use of a different intervention, in GPs' or others' hands, would improve these patients' health status to a greater extent than improving GPs' performance with the intervention. Of course, one such alternative intervention would be university surgeons performing the operation in a university setting.

In quality management terms, improvement potential is the difference in health status improvement between what is achievable and what is being achieved for patients (referred to sometimes as ABNA, achievable benefit not achieved[56])—but not necessarily using the same interventions. Improvement potential is not linked inherently to a particular intervention. For example, university surgeons treating a health problem with intervention A at academic medical centres provide better outcomes than with intervention B. However, intervention A is complicated, requires special skill and extensive experience, and is expensive. Intervention B, on the other hand, is much simpler. In community practice, one may find that outcomes are better with intervention B. If one had to choose which intervention to promote, one would make a mistake in promoting intervention A (apparently the more effective based on results of a trial at an academic centre) because of the invalid assumption that these outcomes can be replicated by community practitioners.

From the patient's perspective, use of an inappropriate intervention (including an unqualified practitioner's use of an otherwise appropriate intervention) or improper implementation of an appropriate intervention, is ineffective. However, quality managers must focus on the process (intervention) used for the patient's health problem; not on trying to measure the effectiveness of some incoherent set of interventions used in uncontrolled practice. Variation in observed outcomes is a means to improve processes toward maximising patients' health status improvement and reducing variation in its attainment.

238.9 | *Effectiveness and appropriateness, and quality management*

An effective intervention is one that improves a population of patients' health status. An appropriate intervention is one that can reasonably be expected to benefit a particular patient because he or she fits the profile of patients for whom it is effective. Medical technology assessment is concerned with interventions' effectiveness for specified types of patients; quality assessment, their appropriateness for a particular patient. The difference between effectiveness and appropriateness is often another source of confusion, as the following situations illustrate.

A certain anti-neoplastic agent may be an effective intervention for patients with a certain type of malignant tumour, but only if the agent affects the tumour; such sensitivity might be indicated by a hormone assay. The patient's health financing scheme may cover the cost of this effective intervention but may not check that its use for a particular patient is appropriate, that is, the patient's cancer was assayed and found to be sensitive to the anti-neoplastic agent. (Inappropriate) use of the anti-neoplastic agent in a patient whose tumour is insensitive to it is a quality assurance problem, a failure to conform to or follow practice policies. For example, the provider may have misdiagnosed the patient (perhaps because he or she failed to do the assay), unknowingly selected the wrong treatment, or believed the patient had nothing to lose from a 'trial' with the agent. The patient always has something to lose: his money and his life, points we elaborate on later in this part.

Government and other third party payers may pay for certain interventions or services so that they become a 'benefit' of the policy, if not to the patient. The presumption is that receipt of the service will improve patients' health status. Recently, in the United States, payers have begun to evaluate the effectiveness of new, high-cost, high-risk procedures, using whatever evidence exists from medical technology assessments and other sources, as a means of containing rapidly rising health care costs. If a new medical technology is found to be effective, one might expect payers to cover its cost if it also meets their cost-worth standard (although this latter consideration, discussed later in this part, rarely, if ever, enters into coverage decisions). To date, payers have generally not specified the indications for use of a technology or intervention, relying instead on the idea of 'medical necessity', an implicit notion that a particular patient would likely benefit from it. Hence the dilemma created by the dichotomy between an effective intervention and its appropriate use in practice.

Based on whatever evidence they choose to review, payers may decide to pay for an intervention, but usually do not review individual decisions to use the intervention in practice (except in the United States, especially for high cost procedures, as the section on utilisation review in Chapter 6 in this part describes). Doctors may use the paid-for technology inappropriately, that is, where it is known not to be effective (but, obviously, not by the doctor in question unless he is perpetrating fraud) or where its effectiveness is unknown for a particular patient. To contain costs from inappropriate use, payers must review every case in which the technology is used, not merely assure themselves that the technology is effective for some defined class of patients before agreeing to pay for it. Alternatively, payers can certify providers to perform a procedure and monitor their performance (known sometimes in the United States as a centre of excellence program), with the explicit or implicit threat of withdrawing certification if they use the technology inappropriately. Withdrawal of certification could mean that the payer would no longer pay providers who were previously eligible to receive payment for performing the intervention, and patients who wanted it, and would genuinely benefit from it, would have to go elsewhere to receive it.

239 | Cost-effectiveness

239.1 | About the economic appraisal of health care

Quality and costs are so intertwined that one cannot be managed without regard to the other. Quality managers must facilitate production of products at least cost and, when necessary, make trade-offs between quality and cost. To do so successfully, they must understand the principles inherent in the economic appraisal of health care. This section intends to give health care providers an appreciation of such principles applied to quality management. The two principal methods of economic appraisal of health care are cost-benefit and cost-effectiveness analysis. While these techniques are now well established, one is often confused with the other and they are not well understood by doctors. This section describes the history of cost-benefit and cost-effectiveness analysis, the techniques highlighting their differences, and the use of cost-effectiveness analysis in clinical decision making. These subjects are vast, complex and value laden. Necessarily, this section touches only on some key points. Detailed discussion is beyond this manual's scope.

Economics is essentially about choices, the alternative use of resources. Considered broadly, the economic appraisal of health care involves the allocation of resources to and among competing health services or interventions. Rapid growth in health care expenditures has stimulated increased interest in the economic appraisal of health care and the use of cost-effectiveness analysis in decision-making, and this interest can be expected to increase further as resource demands and health care costs continue to grow.

Most health care providers, including hospital managers and, in particular, doctors, are unfamiliar with the principles of the economic appraisal of health care. In fact, they often are repulsed by the idea that 'economics' can have any part in what they do. The reality is that explicit economic considerations will play a much more important part in health policy decisions, will be an increasingly important aspect of clinical decisions, and, eventually, may be incorporated into medical practice policies and constrain patients' and doctors' choices.

Some economists see health care as an investment in human capital: healthy people are more productive. Others see health care as a consumption good, competing with ice-cream and automobiles. Clearly, health care has both attributes, to varying degrees, depending on one's perspective and purpose. Rulers have long been interested in their subjects' health as a means of increasing their wealth; principally the wealth of princes but also that of the people. National policy decision makers may consider investments in jobs, education and housing to be better bets for increasing wellbeing and even health. Social investments in children's health is clearly of economic benefit; expenditures for octogenarians are harder to justify in simple economic terms.

Individuals have a vested interest in their own wellbeing and, given the money, or, more to the point in industrialised countries, access to other people's money, have revealed their seemingly insatiable appetite for health care. Consequently, health care has, or will soon, become the single largest sector of industrialised countries' economies. Because financing has become largely socialised, either through government or private 'insurance' schemes, people's health care expenditures are often paid by others. Consequently, health care is increasingly politicised. As aggregate health care expenditures continue to rise, talk of the need to ration health care grows ever more insistent. Treatment decisions are increasingly a matter of public debate rather than private deliberation.

239.2 Types of questions to be answered

Essentially, the economic appraisal of health care intends to answer one or more of three questions:

- Do benefits exceed costs?—cost-benefit analysis (CBA).
- Which intervention is most cost-effective?—cost-effectiveness analysis (CEA).
- Is the intervention's effect worth its cost?—cost-worth analysis (CWA).

Cost-benefit analyses are most appropriate to decisions of 'how much, if any?'. Cost-effectiveness analyses are most appropriate to decisions of 'which one?'. Cost-effectiveness analyses which value central effects in monetary terms, to which we refer as cost-worth analyses, are most appropriate to decisions of 'which is worthwhile?'.

Cost-benefit analysis is usually applied prospectively (to investment decisions) and is often viewed as a program planning technique. While cost-effectiveness analysis can be used in much the same way, it is often applied retrospectively to evaluate programs. Cost-worth analysis can be used as a funding or clinical decision criterion.

239.3 Some basic concepts

239.31 SCARCITY

Choices, decisions among alternative use of resources, are necessary because resources available to a particular group, in a particular place, at a particular time are limited and insufficient to satisfy completely all of the group's wants. Economists refer to this reality as scarcity (of resources). Economics is about individuals' or groups' (community's or society's) use of resources. Economic appraisal of health care usually involves a community-oriented or public perspective about the appropriate uses of resources for planning purposes (which health services to provide, for example). Clinical decisions involve an individual-oriented or private perspective about the actual use of resources necessary for patient care.[57] Many of today's contentious issues arise because patients can no longer afford the cost of care, and their decisions involve allocating the community's resources.

239.32 CHOICES

Medical practitioners view their role, quite rightly, as serving their patients' best interests. Usually, practitioners view their patients one at a time rather than as a defined group for whom they are responsible (either medically or economically). Thus a surgeon may want to perform a third liver transplant on his or her patient after the first two have failed, as it offers the only hope of keeping the child alive. Society may object to providing the money for any, let alone third, liver transplants; not because they have no value, but because, from society's perspective, the resources could be used better elsewhere, for example for prenatal care, to better effect—that is, it would yield greater population health status improvement.

A practitioner may only have enough of an expensive medication to treat half of his or her patients who could benefit from it. He or she could dispense the medication to the first half of the group that walked through the door. Society, however, may insist on establishing criteria to decide who should and should not receive the medication. The option of giving all patients who could benefit half a dose is silly, because none of them would receive enough to realise the medication's benefit. Nevertheless, notions of social justice may demand that everyone receives something, even if a different allocation would produce greater aggregate tangible benefits to the community. These examples illustrate several key points. Firstly, economic efficiency (choices that result in maximum aggregate benefit from use of resources) is only one decision criterion. Secondly, aggregate benefits to the community are merely the sum of benefits accruing to individuals in that community. Thirdly, distributive effects—who benefits and who pays—are very important considerations.

239.33 BENEFITS AND COSTS

Economists have special notions of benefits and costs. To economists, a benefit is any positive effect for the individual or community that results from the consumption of resources. A program's benefits, for example, would include a treated individual's improved health status, his or her enhanced contribution to the nation's production, and all of the other benefits that flow from health status improvement. Often benefits can be cost averted as a result of the program. For example, prompt treatment may avoid the need for disability payments, a benefit to society (a cost averted). Obviously, what constitutes a benefit (or a cost) depends on one's perspective. Classic cost-benefit analyses assume a social perspective and try to identify and value in monetary terms all of the benefits and all of the costs to everyone in society. Regardless of the technical difficulties of totalling up all of a program's costs and benefits and valuing them in money terms, one could question whether anyone or any one group can speak for society. This issue of representative sociopolitical decision-making is beyond this manual's scope.

To economists a cost is the benefit that would result from the best alternative use of a resource unit (hence the term opportunity cost). To most people, cost means how much (cash) they have to pay for something (often referred to as its financial cost). The two are not necessarily the same. For example, a hospital may charge patients only a fraction of the true cost of an expensive new diagnostic test, subsidising it with revenues from routine laboratory tests. Economists would want to use the 'true' cost of providing the new diagnostic test (and routine laboratory tests as well) in appraising its (their) economic value. In competitive markets, where informed consumers can choose freely among many suppliers, one would not worry unduly about this distinction. In the long run, prices would reflect supply and demand for particular tests. If suppliers, for whatever reason decided to 'underprice' products, that would be their business (although government may be concerned because such a strategy, if adopted widely, could be ruinous if suppliers went bankrupt en masse, or because predatory pricing by a few firms could lead to monopoly). In any case, determining the 'true' cost of anything depends on many assumptions, for example about valuing resources and apportioning 'costs' to various activities. In health care, which does not operate generally within the context of market-based economics, the distinction between cost and cash can be very important.

239.4 Cost-benefit analysis

239.41 HISTORICAL PERSPECTIVE

Resources are limited. Competition for resources results in their allocation by markets, government, or some other mechanism. Cost-benefit analysis and cost-effectiveness are two related techniques intended to aid decision makers allocate scarce resources. The concept of evaluating strategies on the basis of their costs and benefits is likely as old as humankind itself. Applications to health care were made as early as 1667 by Petty, 'Of

Lessening Ye Plagues of London',[58] an example of his 'Political Arithmetic'.[59] In 1850 Shattuck used cost-benefit analysis to justify his proposals for sanitary reforms in Boston.[60]

In 1924 Pigou formulated the contemporary concept of cost-benefit analysis, a formal and systematic approach to choosing among investments in public projects, programs and policies.[61] However, the modern practice of cost-benefit analysis is about thirty-five years old, with very few references in the literature antedating 1958.[62] Present-day cost-benefit analysis is an outgrowth of public finance and welfare (or normative) economics, that branch of the discipline concerned explicitly with value judgments or norms.[63]

Early applications of the technique involved public works, particularly water resource projects, an outgrowth of the United States *Flood Control Act* of 1936 (PL 74-738) that led to standardisation of project appraisal procedures.[63] Cost-benefit and cost-effectiveness analysis were propelled into prominence as a result of the Programming Planning and Budgeting System (PPBS) adopted by the Executive Branch of the US federal government in the early 1960s. In 1965, the US president's Bureau of the Budget (later renamed the Office of Management and Budget) established a special unit to adopt and apply cost-benefit and cost-effectiveness studies to a broad range of government programs.[64] Analysis of health services in these terms is still at an early state of development. The difficulties inherent in cost-benefit analysis, particularly that of finding a satisfactory basis for the problem of making benefits commensurable,[65] has led to a concentration on cost-effectiveness analysis.[66]

239.42 ESSENCE OF COST-BENEFIT ANALYSIS

A worthwhile program is one in which total benefits exceed total costs.[67] However, distributional effects—who benefits and who pays—are also important considerations, even if total benefits do exceed total costs.[63,68,69] Moreover, resource and political constraints may preclude funding all worthwhile programs.

> Cost-benefit analysis is a practical way of assessing the desirability of projects, where it is important to take a long view . . . and a wide view . . . , i.e. it implies the enumeration and evaluation of all the relevant costs and benefits.[70]

In performing a cost-benefit analysis, one must essentially:

- be able to choose among alternative policies, programs, or projects for which the analysis is to be conducted (referred to here generally as programs), initiate only programs in which benefits exceed cost, and/or cease providing those in which costs exceed benefits;
- decide what constitutes the program of interest and separate it in some sensible way from other programs;
- identify all consequences, including so-called spillover (second and subsequent-order) effects, that is, a program's direct and indirect costs and all of its benefits; measure them as completely as possible; and value them commensurately in economic (i.e. money) terms;
- discount all monetised future costs and benefits to their present value;
- compare alternative programs (for investment purposes) to set priorities, or to determine which is best (or, for a single program, determine if benefits exceed costs and compare it to an implicit or explicit standard to decide if it should be funded) on the basis of some decision criterion, for example net benefit (net present value), cost-benefit ratio, or internal rate of return (the one economists prefer usually).

According to health economist Herbert Klarman, the following minimum criteria apply to a complete cost-benefit analysis:

- empirical data must form the basis of the analysis;

- both the benefits and costs of specified programs must be measured and valued simultaneously, with their respective present values juxtaposed and compared;
- benefits and costs must reflect a known link between program and outcome, that is, between inputs and outputs.[62]

239.43 APPLICATIONS OF COST-BENEFIT ANALYSIS IN HEALTH CARE

Cost-benefit analysis explicates, quantifies and analyses implicit judgments permitting decisions to be based on economic efficiency grounds, rather than made solely on political grounds. Although economists, and some doctors, have endorsed the use of cost-benefit (and cost-effectiveness) analysis in health care for many years, few such analyses have been performed, and those that have been performed are often flawed.

Application of cost-benefit analysis in health poses formidable obstacles in identifying, quantifying, valuing and discounting costs and benefits.[71] Rarely is sound empirical data about costs and benefits available and, where such measurements do exist, evidence that the program produced the 'benefits' (outcomes) is often lacking or weak. Since cost-benefit analysis is predominantly a planning tool, one could argue that it is impossible to know empirically the planned-for program's benefits and costs. Consequently, analyses must rely on experts' opinions supported by whatever empirical data exist, for example about outcomes of similar past programs. Deciding over what period to measure costs and benefits is also tricky. The further one extends the time horizon, the more speculative are measures of costs and benefits, and most importantly, their attribution to the program, especially for spillover effects. Valuing benefits in monetary terms can obviously be difficult and contentious; agreement about 'costs' might also be elusive. Selecting the appropriate discount rate is also not as simple as it may appear at first sight. Finally, how resultant data should be arrayed for decision purposes can also be an issue. For these reasons, attention has focused increasingly on cost-effectiveness analysis.

239.5 | *Cost-effectiveness versus cost-benefit analysis*

Cost-effectiveness analysis differs from cost-benefit analysis in three important ways:

- Only the direct costs of the program (intervention) are considered; they are valued in economic (i.e. money) terms.
- Only specified program outcomes, central effects, for example health status improvement, are of interest, with spillover, and second and subsequent order, effects either assumed to be equal for all programs evaluated or deemed unimportant for purposes of analysis.
- Program effects (i.e. outcomes) are not valued in economic terms; 'net' benefit is not calculated.

Cost-effectiveness analysis can be regarded as a special case of cost-benefit analysis, although studies that are technically cost-benefit analyses are often labelled cost-effectiveness analyses and vice versa. The advantages of cost-effectiveness analysis lie in the technique's directness (consideration only of a program's central effects and its direct costs), and avoidance of valuing effects in monetary terms. However, because cost-effectiveness analysis does not value costs and effects in commensurable (i.e. the money) terms, one can calculate neither a program's net benefit or value (which requires subtracting present value, discounted, costs from benefits) nor its internal rate of return (which requires finding the discount rate that equates its benefits' value to the program's present value cost).

Cost-effectiveness analysis requires that one measure the effects of the programs one wishes to compare in the same (i.e. commensurable) terms. Measuring them in health status terms (or valuing effects in money terms, as in cost-benefit analysis) makes them commensurable. Further, the need to discount programs' effects—to compensate for differences in the timing of their effects' streams—also requires that one measure them in the same, commensurable (e.g. health status) terms.

239.6 | *Essence of cost-effective analysis*

Cost-effectiveness analysis is concerned with the cost of achieving an objective by alternative means.[72] Classically, this approach has assumed that decision makers want to achieve a fixed level of effectiveness at lowest cost. However, decision makers may be interested in achieving the maximum level of effectiveness for a fixed cost. In reality, alternative means of achieving the same objective may vary both in terms of the extent to which they achieve the objective and the cost of what they do achieve. Also, decision makers may be interested in achieving a given unit (rather than level) of effect at least cost.

Given that the purpose of cost-effectiveness analysis is to select the program that produces a given effect at the lowest cost, the essence of cost-effective analysis is to calculate effectiveness and cost streams in such a way that programs can be compared meaningfully. To evaluate or compare programs on the basis of their cost-effectiveness one must:

- define the programs (interventions) in meaningful terms;
- identify a measure of effectiveness applicable to all programs to be compared, for example health status improvement;
- measure the effectiveness of each program such that different effects' streams can be compared meaningfully;
- determine or assume the fraction of measured effectiveness that can be attributed confidently to the programs (which may vary by program if each treats different proportions of patients with characteristics that affect outcomes);
- determine the cost of producing the measured effectiveness;
- discount costs and, if at all possible, effects to present values;
- calculate cost-effectiveness ratios (by dividing costs by effectiveness).

239.7 | *Mechanics of cost-effectiveness analysis*

An intervention or program can be viewed as incurring a stream of costs—the money needed to buy the intervention or provide the program—and producing a stream of effects, for example health status improvement. The stream of costs may be short, for example if the intervention is a surgical operation, or long, for example if the intervention is a rehabilitation program, or continuous, if the intervention is a maintenance program. Programs may also provide different streams of effects. How can one realistically compare programs' different streams of costs and effects? For example, how does the cost-effectiveness of a single intervention good for life compare with that of a lifelong maintenance program? A detailed model to answer such questions is described elsewhere.[73,74]

In common with cost-benefit analysis, cost-effectiveness analysis depends on the availability of data about programs' costs and effects, exhibits the difficulty of attributing effects to programs, and retains the need to decide over what period to measure costs and effects. Costs and effects must be measured simultaneously, in the same patients, for a predetermined period. This period, the time horizon, should be sufficiently long for all, or almost all, costs and effects to be realised. The time horizon may be two, five, ten or more years, depending on the program's nature and its expected outcomes. Technical Appendix B of this chapter summarises these and other difficulties of conducting and using the results of cost-effective analyses. Their complete consideration is beyond this manual's scope.

239.8 | Cost-worth analysis

What is a cost-effective treatment? Generally, a cost-effective intervention would be one that produces a specified unit of effect at a lower cost than practical alternatives. Popularly, the term 'cost-effective' conveys the idea of good value for money. However, because a particular intervention is the most cost-effective one does not necessarily mean its benefits exceed its costs or that it is worthwhile. For example, a particular treatment may improve patients' health status at an average cost of $20 000 per benefit unit, which is less than any alternative treatment for their condition. However, society (and/or the patient) may not view the gain as worth the cost. Whenever the cost of producing a unit of effect is compared to an implicit or explicit monetary standard, one is judging an intervention's cost-worth (and not its cost-effectiveness). When an intervention's cost per unit of effect is less than such a standard (which might be the cost of its production), we refer to it as a cost-worthy intervention.

Clinicians so inclined are fond of totting up an intervention's cost and equating it with some measure of effectiveness, 'clinical benefit', a fuzzy measure of health status improvement. They conclude that the intervention is or is not cost-effective. Instead of a cost-effectiveness analysis, they have performed an ersatz cost-benefit analysis. Cost-effectiveness analysis involves choices among alternative interventions; not deciding whether or not any intervention is worthwhile. Cost-benefit analysis weighs all of an intervention's costs against all of its benefits, measured in monetary terms usually, from society's perspective. The clinicians' analysis is a reduced form of cost-benefit analysis in which they weigh their perception of the treatment's direct cost (which they usually do not know) against their impression of some, albeit central, measure of benefit, for example health status improvement.

Whenever an intervention's effectiveness is compared directly to the cost of its production, we refer to this comparison as cost-worth analysis (CWA). Essentially, in this type of analysis, often referred to erroneously as cost-effectiveness analysis, effectiveness, for example units of health status improvement, are implicitly or, preferably, explicitly valued in monetary terms. For an intervention to be considered worthwhile, the cost of producing an effectiveness unit must not exceed an explicit or implicit standard. Thus if the cost of the effective treatment for the patient (that producing the greatest health status improvement) means that the ratio of effectiveness units to costs exceeded the standard it would not be considered worthwhile. If this criterion prevailed, the patient's choices would be limited to treatments whose effectiveness/cost ratios did not exceed the worth standard. If all of the available interventions exceeded this ratio, the patient may have to settle for the cheapest treatment, which might be supportive or palliative care.

239.9 | Overemphasis on effects, underemphasis on costs

Medical science has emphasised the quest for more effective interventions. Certainly, technological breakthroughs can produce interventions whose effectiveness is far superior to existing ones; sometimes they are only marginally more effective. Some so-called advances turn out to be no more effective than existing interventions; others may be harmful. They almost always, although not invariably, are more expensive, if for no other reason than producers must recover the cost of research and development that led to the innovation. Moreover, the production and delivery of the innovation may also be, and usually is, more expensive. The net result is ever-increasing health care expenditures. To counter this trend, researchers and technology developers must be given incentives to develop cheaper, but no less effective, interventions, rather than pursue only more effective ones. In an era of increasing scarcity, cheaper treatments that are as effective as those that exist now may be more valuable socially than marginally more effective treatments whose cost is so high that few people or health financing schemes can afford them.

Interventions' costs and effects must both be measured carefully. Doctors must be given this information and both doctors and patients should be given incentives to use the most cost-effective alternative. Stated simply, society may have an obligation to provide everyone with basic health care, but may not have a moral obligation, and certainly cannot afford, to provide everyone with every intervention that might offer some hope, no matter how uncertain, of improving health status, no matter by how small an amount, regardless of cost, no matter how high.

Various incentives could be self-reinforcing. For example, if technology developers know that health care financing schemes will pay only for those interventions that meet a certain cost-worth standard, they would have little incentive to pursue interventions that they expect to be costly and have only marginally greater effectiveness. As now, they would bear the risk of the reality of their assessments, and reap the rewards if innovative treatments save money and exhibit the same or greater effectiveness. In some instances, for example those in which only very expensive treatments are available, a new treatment that is very inexpensive but slightly less effective would also be a great social boon. Providers can expect to see increased use of cost-worth analysis to evaluate medical interventions, and the incorporation of results into practice policies.

References

1 Australian Institute of Health & Welfare. Health expenditure bulletin, April 1993; 8: Table 14.
2 Statistical abstract of the United States, 1992. Washington, DC: US Government Printing Office, 1993.
3 Rosen G. A history of public health. New York: MD Publications, Inc, 1958.
4 Smith FB. The people's health 1830–1910. London: Croom Helm, 1979.
5 Lindsey A. Socialized medicine in England and Wales: The National Health Service 1948–61. Chapel Hill, NC: The University of North Carolina Press, 1962, p.100.
6 Health Insurance Association of America. Source Book of Health Insurance Data, 1991. Washington, DC. HIAA, 1991.
7 Australian Institute of Health & Welfare. Health expenditure bulletin, Dec 1994; 10.
8 Health Care Financing Review 1991; 11(4):187.
9 Rich S. Sharp rise in health costs projected. Washington Post 1992; Jan 20:A23.
10 Moynihan DP. Don't blame democracy: the socialization of slow-growth jobs. Washington Post 1993: Jun 6; C_7.
11 Goldschmidt PG. Health conditions of the year 2000. In: Bezold C (ed). Pharmaceuticals in the year 2000: The changing context for drug R&D. Washington DC: Institute for Alternative Futures, 1983.
12 Najman JM, Levine S. Evaluating the impact of medical care and technologies on the QOL: A review and critique. Soc Sci Med 1981;15:107–15.
13 Goldschmidt PG. A model for measuring the health status of a population; application to the United States. Baltimore: Policy Research Incorporated, 1978.
14 Vandenbroucke JP. Survival and expectation of life from the 1400s to the present: A study of the Knighthood Order of the Golden Fleece. Am J Epidemiol 1985; 122:1007–16.
15 US Bureau of the Census. Historical statistical abstract of the United States: Colonial times to 1970. Washington, DC: US Government Printing Office, 1975.
16 US Department of Health and Human Services. National Centre for Health Statistics. Unpublished data. Hyattsville, MD, 1986.
17 Feinleib M, Wilson RW. Trends in health in the United States. Environmental Health Perspectives 1985; 62: 267–76.
18 Colvez A, Blanchet M. Disability trends in the United States population 1966–76: Analysis of reported causes. Am J Public Health 1981; 71:464–71.
19 Verbrugge LM. Longer life but worsening health? Trends in health and mortality in middle-aged and older persons. Milbank Mem Fund Q 1984; 62:475–519.
20 Newacheck PW, Dudetti PP, Halfon N. Trends in activity limiting chronic conditions among children. Am J Public Health 1986; 76:174–84.
21 Manton KG, Corder LS, Stallard E. Estimates of change in chronic disability and institutional incidence from the 1982, 1984 and 1989 National Long Term Care Survey. Journal of Gerontology 1993; 48(4): S153–66.
22 Shall age weary them? Economist 1993; Dec 4; 87–8.

23 Wilkins R, Adams O. Healthfulness of life. Montreal: The Institute for Research on Public Policy, 1983.
24 Dubos R. Mirage of health: Utopias, progress, and biological change. New York: Harper & Row (Perennial Library Edition), 1971.
25 McKeown T. The role of medicine: Dream, mirage, or nemesis? 2nd edition. Oxford, England: Basil Blackwell, 1979.
26 McKeown T, Low CR. An introduction to social medicine. Oxford, England: Blackwell Scientific Publications, 1966.
27 Juckett DA, Rosenberg B. Correlation of human longevity oscillations with sunspot cycles. Radiation research 1993; 133:312–20.
28 Barker DJ, Bull AR, Osmond C, Simmonds SJ. Fetal and placental size and risk of hypertension in adult life. BMJ 1990; 301 (6746): 259–62.
29 Jamison DT. Investing in health. Finance & Development 1993; 30(3):2–5.
30 Tan JP, Hill K. The foundation for better health. Finance & Development 1993; 30(3):14–16.
31 Bobadilla JL, Saxenian H. Designing an essential national health package. Finance & Development 1993; 30(3): 10–13.
32 Australian Institute of Health & Welfare. Health expenditure bulletin 1992; 7: 1.
36 Erasmus D. De lof geneeskunde (In praise of medicine). Eraut L (tr). Antwerp, Belgium: Standaard-boekhandel, 1950.
37 Beeson PB. Changes in medical therapy during the past half century. Medicine 1980; 59:79–99.
38 Morris JN. Are health services important to the people's health? BMJ 1980; 187–8.
39 McDermott W. Evaluating the physician and his technology. Daedalus 1977; 106:135–57.
40 McDermott W. Absence of indicators of the influence of its physicians on a society's health: impact of physician care on society. N Eng J Med 1981; 70:833–43.
41 Goldschmidt PG, et al. Health Prospects 1983/2003: A survey of US health system leaders. Baltimore: Policy Research Institute, 1985.
42 Williamson JW, Goldschmidt PG, Colton T. The quality of medical literature: An analysis of validation assessments. In: Bailor JC, Mosteller F (eds). Medical uses of statistics. Boston: NEJM Books, 1986.
43 Codman EA. A study in hospital efficiency. Boston: Published privately, circa 1917.
44 Office of Technology Assessment. Strategies for medical technology assessment. Washington, DC: US Government Printing Office, 1982.
45 Institute of Medicine. Assessing medical technologies. Washington, DC: National Academy Press, 1985.
46 Goldschmidt PG, Bordman S, Jillson IA. A comprehensive study of the ethical, legal, and social implications of advances in biomedical and behavioural research and technology. Baltimore: Policy Research Incorporated, 1977.
47 Goldschmidt PG. Assessment of the effectiveness of medical technology. In: Beaver L (ed). Technology Assessment: 9th annual FDA Science Symposium Series. Washington, DC: US Department of Health and Human Services, Food and Drug Administration, 1984.
48 Goldschmidt PG. Information Synthesis: A practical guide. Health Services Research 1986:21; 215–37.
49 Levit KR, Sensenig AL, Cowan CA, et al. National health expenditures, 1993. Health Care Financing Review 1994; 16(1): 247–94.
50 Strickland SP. Research and the health of Americans. Lexington, Massachusetts: DC Heath & Co, 1978.
51 Feigin RD. Otitis media: Closing the information gap. N Eng J Med 1982; 306:1417–18.
52 Institute of Medicine. Planning study report: A consortium for assessing medical technology. Washington, DC: National Academy Press, 1983.
53 Williamson JW, Goldschmidt PG, Jillson IA. Medical Practice Information Demonstration Project: Final Report. Baltimore: Policy Research Incorporated, 1979.
54 Gjestland T. The Oslo Study of untreated syphilis: An epidemiological investigation of the natural course of syphilitic infections upon a re-study of the Boeck-Bruusgaard material. Acta Dermatology and Venereology 1955: 35 Supplement; 34 et seq.
55 Skrabanek P, McCormick J. Follies and fallacies in medicine. Glasgow, Scotland: Tarragon Press, 1989.
56 Williamson JW. Medical quality management systems in perspective. In: Couch, JB. Health care quality management for the 21st century. Tampa, Florida: American College of Physician Executives, 1991.
57 Drummond MF. Principles of economic appraisal in health care. Oxford, England: Oxford University Press, 1980.
58 Fein R. On measuring economic benefits of health programmes. In: McLachlan G, McKeowan T (eds): Medical history and medical care. New York: Oxford University Press, 1971.
59 Pett W. Political Arithmetick. In: Hull CH. The economic writings of Sir William Petty. Cambridge, England: Cambridge University Press, 1899.
60 Shattuck L. Report on the Sanitary Commission of Massachusetts. Cambridge, Massachusetts: Harvard University Press, 1948 (facsimile edition of the 1850 report).
61 Pigou AC. The economics of welfare. London, Macmillan, 1924.
62 Klarman HE. Application of cost-benefit analysis to the health services and the special case of technological innovation. Int J Health Services 1974; 4:325–52.

63 Sassone PG, Schaffer WA. Cost-benefit analysis: A handbook. New York: Academic Press, 1978.

64 Maass A. Benefit-cost analysis: its relevance to public investment decisions. Quarterly J of Economics 1966; 8:208–26.

65 Gorman W. Some uses of quantitative analysis to improve the allocation of public funds. Washington, DC: US Department of Health and Human Services, 1968.

66 Glass NJ. Cost-benefit analysis of health services. Health Trends 1973; 5:51–6.

67 Barnes BA. Cost-benefit analysis of surgery. Am J Surg 1977; 133:438–46.

68 Weisbrod BA. Income redistribution effects and cost-benefit analysis. In: Chase SB (ed). Problems in public expenditure analysis. Washington, DC: Brookings Institution, 1968.

69 Layard R (ed). Cost benefit analysis. New York: Penguin Books, 1977.

70 Prest AR, Turvey R. Cost benefit analysis: A survey. Econ J 1965; 75:685–735.

71 Barnes BA. An overview of the treatment of end-stage renal disease. In: Bunker JP, Barnes BA, Mosteller F (eds). Costs, risks, and benefits of surgery. New York: Oxford University Press, 1977.

72 Glass NJ, Goldberg D. Cost-benefit analysis and the evaluation of psychiatric services. Psych Med 1977; 7: 701–07.

73 Goldschmidt PG. Cost-effectiveness model for evaluating health care programs; application to a drug abuse treatment. Inquiry 1976;13:29–47.

74 Goldschmidt PG. A model for measuring the cost-effectiveness of treatment programs. Baltimore: Dissertation for the degree of Doctor of Public Health, The Johns Hopkins University, School of Hygiene and Public Health, 1979.

Appendix A

MEASURES OF DIAGNOSTIC INTERVENTIONS' EFFECTIVENESS

This appendix defines various terms that measure diagnostic interventions' effectiveness.

A false positive results when a diagnostic test suggests that a patient has a disease when in fact he or she does not. *A false negative* results when a diagnostic tests suggests a patient does not have a disease when in fact he or she does.

Sensitivity is a measure of how well a test detects people who have a given characteristic, that is, the extent to which people who truly manifest a characteristic are so classified. It is measured by dividing the number of people the test says have the characteristic who truly have it, by the total number who truly have the characteristic.

Specificity is a measure of how well a test detects people who do not have a given characteristic (and hence does not label them as having a disease that they do not have), that is, the extent to which people who truly do not manifest a characteristic are so classified. It is measured by dividing the number of people the test suggests do not have the characteristic who truly do not have it, by the total number who truly do not have the characteristic.

Sensitivity (and specificity) can vary from 0% to 100%. A rate of 100% means a test identifies all people who truly have (sensitivity) or those who do not have (specificity) a disease (or other characteristic of interest). A rate of 0% means that a test perfectly misclassifies people (and if interpretation is simply reversed is equivalent to 100%). Randomly assigning people to 'having disease' and 'not having disease' produces sensitivity and specificity rates of 50%. Thus, practically, to be considered effective diagnostic tests must have sensitivity and specificity rates that exceed 50% and preferably approach 100%.

Diagnostic accuracy indicates the proportion of people that a test classifies correctly as having and not having a particular disease or other characteristic of interest. It is measured by dividing the sum of the people that the test suggests have the characteristic who truly have it and those the test suggests do not have the characteristic who truly do not have it, by the total number of people tested.

A *test's positive predictive value* is the probability that the people it suggests have a disease or other characteristic truly have it. It is measured by dividing the number of people the test suggests have the characteristic who truly have it, by the total number of people the test suggests have the characteristic (whether or not they truly have it).

A *test's negative predictive value* is the probability that people it suggests do not have a given characteristic truly do not have it. It is measured by dividing the number of people the test suggests do not have the characteristic who truly do not have it, by the total number of people the test suggests do not have the characteristic (whether or not they truly do not have it).

Positive (and negative) predictive values can vary from 0 to 1, certain to have (or not to have) the characteristic.

Sensitivity and specificity—and hence positive and negative predictive values—as measures of diagnostic tests' accuracy have a number of limitations. They include the following, for example:

- The population is simply divided into people who have and those who do not have a disease, implying a diagnostic certainty that might not reflect reality but nevertheless influences treatment selection and patient outcomes.
- The distribution of characteristics within a population, which may vary dynamically, affects the proportion stated to have and not have the disease, because, for example, a test may be better at detecting late-stage than early-stage disease; the more homogeneous the relevant population with respect to characteristics that affect diagnostic outcomes the better.
- Classification criteria and procedures adopted to implement them affect the proportion of people stated to have and not have a disease; the more structured the criteria and procedures the better.
- Interpretations—and hence classification as having or not having a disease—are subject to problems of intra- and inter-rater reliability; the more reliable the measurement system the better.
- The integrity of data inherently limits the accuracy of interpretations; the more reliable and valid the underlying data the better.
- The 'gold standard' (the reference used to determine a disease's presence or absence) is itself almost always an imperfect test; its reliability is less than 100%, and it cannot be more valid than it is reliable.

Another way to assess diagnostic tests is to compare the areas under their respective receiver-operating-characteristic (ROC) curves. A ROC curve results from plotting a test's sensitivity against one minus its specificity. Traditionally, to construct a ROC curve, test results are classified into the following five categories: definitely has, probably has, may have the disease, and probably and definitely does not have the disease. By using different arbitrary thresholds to determine a disease's presence or absence, one can plot four sensitivity/specificity points. A strict threshold (definitely has the disease) reduces sensitivity but increases specificity; a lax threshold (may have the disease) increases sensitivity but reduces specificity.

Appendix B

MEASURING INTERVENTIONS' COST-EFFECTIVENESS

23B.0 | Contents

This appendix provides more detail concerning the technical difficulties in measuring interventions' effectiveness and the mechanics of cost-effectiveness analysis. It intends to satisfy those readers who desire additional information on these complex subjects. Non-expert readers who desire to conduct effectiveness research or cost-effectiveness analyses would be well advised to consult professionals in these areas to avoid the many pitfalls that trap novices. This appendix covers the following ten difficulties:

23B.1. measures of effectiveness
23B.2. attribution of effects: patient selection bias
23B.3. measuring costs
23B.4. time horizon
23B.5. discounting
23B.6. decision indicators
23B.7. uncertainty of estimates
23B.8. observed versus true effectiveness
23B.9. marginal cost-effectiveness
23B.10. effectiveness versus efficiency—inputs and outputs

23B.1 | Measures of effectiveness

Interventions' objectives define or suggest measures of effectiveness. One must use reliable measures of effects otherwise they become the equivalent of using rubber bands to measure length, for example. Only with reliable measures can one distinguish effective from ineffective (or harmful) interventions with an acceptable degree of certainty of validity. Measurements cannot be any more valid than they are reliable. Outcomes (effects) are often difficult and expensive to measure. For medical interventions, health status improvement is usually the most (and often the only) relevant measure of effectiveness. An effective intervention improves patients' health status beyond what would have occurred without the intervention. Presently, few studies attempt to measure effectiveness in terms of health status improvement. Mortality rates are usually inadequate proxies for health status improvement, except if the natural history usually leads rapidly to death. Further, measuring differences in survival rates at a single point fails to account for the all-important shape of the survival curves.

For purposes of cost-effectiveness analysis, an intervention's central effects must be captured in a single measure. If decision makers want to compare interventions on multiple measures of effectiveness, they must weight the measures in accordance to their importance or develop other explicit rules for aggregating them, to create a single measure with which to compare interventions. Valuing effects in monetary terms in the manner of cost-benefit analysis is another way to make effects commensurable to permit explicit comparisons. Without explicit decision rules to aggregate multiple effectiveness measures, or valuing them in money terms, decision makers must weight the different measures intuitively, introducing an element of subjectivity into decisions.

23B.2 | Attribution of effects: patient selection bias

Not only are effects often difficult and expensive to measure, but they are also often even more difficult to attribute confidently to interventions. Even when measuring outcomes is relatively simple, for example mortality rates, attributing death (or its absence) to interventions may not be. The extent to which measured outcomes (observed effects) can be attributed confidently to interventions depends on the source of data. Information about interventions' effectiveness obtained from experiments in nature, rather than designed experiments such as randomised controlled trials, may exhibit patient selection bias.

When comparing interventions, such bias may lead to erroneous inferences about their relative effectiveness because they were used to treat different proportions of patients with characteristics that affect outcomes. In well-designed, well-conducted randomised controlled trials investigators enter only patients meeting predetermined (prerandomisation) diagnostic criteria into the trial. Patient selection bias is eliminated to the extent practical, and resultant outcome measurements are theoretically free of such bias (although are still susceptible to random variation, of course).

Information from well-designed, well-conducted, randomised controlled trials is best, but often difficult or expensive to obtain. Other study designs or sources of data, for example management information systems, provide less certain information. Even randomised controlled trials may not provide information on true effectiveness, which requires simultaneous measurement of outcome (effects) without treatment (often referred to as natural history), because they compare alternative treatments; there are no untreated controls. In this circumstance, one must either assume that the interventions produced the observed outcomes, while recognising the possibility that none of them is effective, or adjust observed outcomes to account for what would have occurred without intervention, if valid information exists to permit such adjustments to be made.

The requirement that effects be attributed confidently to interventions is a severe constraint on cost-effectiveness analysis because such information is almost always lacking. Conversely, cost-effectiveness analyses in which effects cannot be confidently attributed to interventions are of dubious utility. Obviously, assumed effectiveness may, and likely does, differ from true effectiveness. Generally, assumed effectiveness overestimates true effectiveness because whatever level of outcome would have resulted without the intervention is not subtracted from the observed level. However, if patients' postintervention status is observed to be the same or worse than their preintervention status, analysts may conclude erroneously that the intervention is not effective when in fact it is, because without the intervention patients would have been even worse off. A subsequent section in this appendix discusses the implications for cost-effectiveness analyses of assuming that interventions are effective.

Information on effects obtained from experiments in nature rather than designed experiments such as randomised controlled trials may be biased because the various interventions to be compared treat different proportions of patients with characteristics that affect outcomes. In these circumstances the cost-effectiveness analysis must either be conducted for the various classes of patients whose characteristics affect the outcome of interest, or adjustments made for the different proportions treated by each of the interventions. Assumptions that patients do not exhibit characteristics that affect outcomes or that interventions do not vary in the proportions of patients with such characteristics that they treat, are usually invalid. Further, the cost of treating patients may also depend on such characteristics. Thus costs may have to be calculated separately for each class of patients whose characteristics affect outcomes.

23B.3 Measuring costs

An intervention's cost is the money one would have to spend to obtain effects. One might imagine it is simple to measure the direct cost of care, for example the cost of a coronary artery bypass graft (CABG); however, often it is not. For example, prices that hospitals charge may not reflect costs. For example, a hospital may charge only $1000 for an experimental treatment whereas the true cost is $2000. Since it is doubtful that the hospital could (or even would) continue to subsidise the treatment were government to cover its cost, the $2000 cost figure would be used in any cost-effectiveness analysis. In a similar vein, donated services must be valued since they may have to be purchased if the intervention were implemented on a large scale. If decision makers were concerned only about how much they would have to pay, they might not be concerned with providers' costs. However, if charges were only a fraction of costs, they might be concerned with costs because purchasing from the cheapest hospitals might bankrupt them, and alternative suppliers might have failed for lack of business.

In cost-effectiveness analysis, one is not concerned about price changes brought about by funding the interventions being compared. If government were to fund new interventions that depended heavily on biochemists, for example, the demand for biochemists might be expected to increase; so would their salaries (at least until their supply caught up). Thus, the intervention's cost might be greater than calculated using present prices (e.g. for biochemists' salaries). Cost-benefit and cost-effectiveness analysis are microeconomic tools, and generally disregard changes in factor prices and other macroeconomic considerations.

23B.4 Time horizon

An intervention's cost-effectiveness depends on both a stream of effects and a stream of costs. Interventions may differ in their effect and/or cost streams. The time horizon, which defines the period over which effects and costs are calculated, affects interventions' apparent cost-effectiveness. This section considers the need to calculate effects and costs streams and the period over which such streams should be calculated.

Outcomes must be measured periodically from the initiation of treatment, and not just at the end of a pre-defined period, for example five years. At the end of five years, for example, the same, small percentage of experimental and control patients may be alive. However, the shape of the mortality curve and the quality of lives lived may distinguish the two groups. It is the difference in areas under the mortality curve that matters; not the difference in the percentage of patients alive at some point. This simple fact seems to elude most researchers and policy decision makers.

The time that an intervention begins is the correct point from which to measure effectiveness. Interventions may initially affect patients adversely compared to untreated individuals. Patients' experience in treatment must be included in the measurement. One cannot begin to measure 'effectiveness' after intervention processes have been completed, because patients' in-treatment experience would be lost and it usually varies among alternative interventions, and almost certainly varies from no intervention.

The period over which one calculates interventions' effects and costs may affect their apparent cost-effectiveness. For example, shortly after discharge treated patients' outcomes may appear better, only to be the same as the control group's a year later, perhaps because of the placebo effect or the delayed consequences of the treatment. Compare an expensive treatment intended to be good for life, for example a nine-month residential (therapeutic) community treatment for heroin abuse to a lifelong therapy, for example methadone maintenance. One intervention's cost-effectiveness may appear superior to the other's cost-effectiveness depending on the elapsed post-treatment period when the comparison is made, for example one, two, five, ten, twenty years.

There is no simple rule for selecting the appropriate time horizon for the analysis. It depends, for example, on the condition from which patients suffer, the types of interventions being compared, and their expected outcomes, for example, cure versus a small, sustained improvement in symptoms. Obviously, it need not extend beyond the point when streams of central effects and the cost of generating them have ceased flowing. Interventions' cost-effectiveness should be compared when all, or almost all, of their effects (and costs) have become manifest. But this point should not extend beyond that at which effects can be attributed confidently to interventions. The longer the follow-up period the more chance that other factors coproduce observed outcomes, and the treatment and control groups' experience may vary in this regard, introducing both noise and bias into measurements. A rule of thumb would suggest that the period should be sufficiently long to satisfy decision makers that at least 80% of effects that can be attributed confidently to interventions have been taken into account. The remaining 20% of effects might be omitted because they occur far in the future (and would be diminished substantially by discounting), their attribution to interventions would be less certain, and substantial sums of money would be needed to collect the additional data.

23B.5 | Discounting

Discounting to present value provides the means to compare cost and effect streams. Interventions may have cost and effect streams that differ in their temporal distributions. For example, one intervention may produce most of its central effects in the first three years of its five-years' life; another, in the last two (fourth and fifth) years. Because of the possibility of such differences in temporal distribution, one must discount cost and effect streams to present values in order, to permit proper comparisons. This idea is well accepted in evaluating investment decisions, but is not well understood in health care decision-making.

The idea behind discounting is common enough: a bird in the hand is worth two in the bush. Early benefits are preferable to later benefits. But by how much? For costs the situation is most straightforward. The discount rate can be the prevailing interest rate. The idea here is that if you put money into an interest-bearing account today you will receive more (principal plus interest) tomorrow. Thus the discount rate is reverse interest and results in the sum you would have to invest today at that interest rate to yield a dollar in the specified future year. Market interest rates define the cost of money, and hence reflect its perceived value. Thus they are affected by expectations about inflation— what the money you lend today (and the interest on it) will buy when you get it back tomorrow, and the riskiness of the investment (the chances that you will get the money back with interest). The 'true' value of money would be free of these expectations. Economists have various esoteric ways of estimating the true value of money, which is most important for cost-benefit analysis. For cost-effectiveness analysis, market interest rates are usually good enough.

There is no equivalent basis for discounting effects. We can recognise that an intervention that promises a quick cure may be preferable to one that slowly improves a patient's condition. Market interest rates can also be used to discount effects. This approach is simple but is not inherently correct. Distant effects may be far less certain than proximal ones. The discount rate can be set to reflect this uncertainty, and even increase with each future year rather than remain the same. Uncertainty aside, why should tomorrow's health status gains be appraised as less valuable than today's? There are at least two reasons. First is the general idea that proximal benefits are better than distant ones. Second, implicitly, the money used to generate them could be put in the bank and earn interest, that is, be used alternatively to generate other benefits.

23B.6 Decision indicators

A cost-effectiveness analysis produces data about alternative interventions' discounted streams of central effects and the direct costs of producing them. Through discounting, both effects and costs for a specified period can be reduced to present values. How are the resultant data to be arrayed for decision purposes? Essentially, one can look at the discounted costs, the discounted effects and the ratio between the two. Take the following example:

Intervention:	A	B	C
Cost	$100 000	$50 000	$20 000
Effectiveness	120 EMU	80 EMU	20 EMU
E/C ratio	$833/EMU	$625/EMU	$1,000/EMU

EMU = Effectiveness Measure Unit, a generic outcome measure.

Given no money restrictions, of the alternatives, 'A' has the greatest effectiveness, but 'B' produces an effectiveness measurement unit (EMU) at least cost; 'C' costs the least. If one can only afford 'C', because that is all one has to spend, one gets the corresponding effectiveness. If money is no object and one wants maximum attainable effectiveness, 'A' is the choice. Clearly, 'B' offers the best value-for-money if one is willing to forgo or cannot afford the extra effectiveness attainable with 'A'. This type of choice is familiar to consumers. A Rolls Royce motor car may be the 'best'; it is certainly the most expensive. A little known import may be the cheapest car, but may lack features that reduce its 'effectiveness', certainly if up-scale image is one of them. A solid middle-of-the-road automobile may represent the best value for money but it lacks the prestige of a luxury car and the economy of a cheap import, for example.

23B.7 Uncertainty of estimates

If one measured the costs and effects of a given intervention one would usually find some variation, especially in effects. The alternative interventions can, and usually do, vary in these regards. The resultant uncertainty can be analysed by calculating the range of cost-effectiveness ratios that each intervention exhibits. Unfortunately, one may find such an overlap in ranges that one cannot distinguish easily between interventions.

The data shown in the preceding section exhibit no variance, that is, the treatment is assumed to produce the same effect in, and cost the same for, each patient in the group. In fact, they may be means of distributions (i.e. average values). Using averages assumes homogeneity. This circumstance is unusual. Variability is the rule in nature; use of a population average denies this reality. Taking into account variances in effects and costs complicates the picture, especially if effects and costs are not independent. In this circumstance, the variance in costs associated with patients exhibiting effects at the ends of the effects distribution would have to be calculated before determining effectiveness-cost ratios (the high cost estimate for low effect patients divided by the low effect estimate, and the low cost estimate for the high effect patients divided by the high effect estimate, to yield the appropriate range of effectiveness/cost ratios). Technically, assuming that effects and derivative cost distributions were normal, for purposes of calculating the range of cost-effectiveness estimates, high and low effects (and derivative cost) estimates could be set at two standard deviations.

If effects and derivative cost distributions exhibit high variance, the resultant ranges of cost-effectiveness ratios for alternative interventions could well overlap to such an extent that one would be hard-pressed to tell which one was the most cost-effective (i.e. provided an effectiveness unit at least cost). On this basis, it might be hard to distinguish one treatment from another. Subdividing groups, for example based on tumour type, stage of disease, or other patient characteristic that affects outcomes, might make them more homogeneous with respect to outcome and thereby narrow the range of effectiveness/cost ratios. From a decision maker's perspective, 'cost' might be unvaried if, for example, a hospital charged the same amount for each CABG regardless of what it cost to provide care to a particular patient.

23B.8 Observed versus true effectiveness

Effectiveness is inherently a medical intervention's central effect, the observed outcome of interest to a decision maker less that which would have occurred without the intervention (the natural outcome). Thus, for example, if the observed outcomes for two treatments, 'X' and 'Y', for a given disease were 100 EMU (a generic benefit measure) and 80 EMU respectively, and the natural outcome were 50 EMU, the first intervention's true effectiveness would be (100–50) 50 EMU; the second's, (80–50) 30 EMU. If the two treatments cost the same—$1000—the first treatment would be seen to be more cost-effective than the second whether the observed outcome or the true effectiveness (observed minus natural outcomes) were used to calculate the cost/effectiveness ratios.

If a decision were to be made between funding treatment for the disease treated by 'X' or that for patients with another disease treated by 'Z' with a true cost-effectiveness ratio of $15/EMU, the differences in ratios would be significant. Using observed effectiveness, the cost-effectiveness ratio for treatment 'X' is $10/EMU; that using true effectiveness, $20/EMU ($1000/100–50 EMU)—twice as much, and 50% more than the cost-effectiveness ratio of treatment 'Z'. Thus using observed cost-effectiveness, decision makers may erroneously favour treatment 'X' over treatment 'Z'. Most of the time we have no idea what fraction of observed outcomes (even in those rare instances when measured) is attributable to the intervention. Randomised controlled trials in which effects and costs are measured simultaneously are needed to provide valid cost-effectiveness estimates.

23B.9 Marginal cost-effectiveness

The density of effects and costs may not be uniform. The last unit of effect may cost more to obtain than the first one. The cost of obtaining the last unit of effect is often referred to as an intervention's marginal cost-effectiveness and exists only if the intervention consists of separable elements. For example, a course of thirty daily treatments at $100 per treatment ($3000 total) may yield 300 EMU ($10/EMU). Reducing the course to twenty-five treatments, ($2500 total cost) may yield 280 EMU ($8.93/EMU). The last twenty EMU cost $500 ($25/EMU). Using this approach, we might find that the last treatment provided yields only one additional EMU; its marginal cost-effectiveness would be, therefore, $100/EMU. For simplicity, assume adding (a thirty-first) treatment would yield no additional effect.

Should we limit therapy to thirty, or twenty-nine, or some fewer number of treatments? The answer depends on who decides the issue. If the patient decides, the result would depend on whether or not he or she had access to other people's money. A patient who had to pay the $100 for the last EMU may decide to forgo it. If the government paid, the patient would have no incentive to decline the thirtieth treatment. We might not begrudge the patient a $100 EMU. But the government, assuming it footed the bill, could well have spent the money elsewhere to generate ten EMU for the same $100, albeit for someone else. Only if individuals, or government, had sufficient funds and were willing to spend without limit until no more EMU could be generated could such choices be avoided. This circumstance is unlikely ever to exist. How, to whom and in what amounts government dispenses its largess—and how it collects the requisite money to pay for it—is a matter of politics. Presently, we have virtually no information about interventions' marginal cost-effectiveness to inform such decisions.

23B.10 | *Effectiveness versus efficiency—inputs and outputs*

Cost-effectiveness analysis is often equated with economic efficiency because it directly relates inputs to outputs. However, the relationship between effectiveness and efficiency is not as simple as it might appear to be at first sight. Often effectiveness, the achievement of objectives under given constraints, must be traded for efficiency, the best use of resources to achieve objectives without these constraints. For example, a certain route may be the shortest (and quickest) one to pick up goods from six shops. However, if one were to follow this route one would arrive at some shops after they had closed. Thus, to pick up all goods from all of the shops one would have to travel from one to the other following a different route than the most efficient one that one could follow if closing times were not a constraint on achieving one's objective. Thus being effective (achieving objectives) means being inefficient (not using the most economical route), and vice versa.

If a decision maker wanted to achieve a given level of effect, he or she would have to spend whatever it costs to achieve this effect, even if the resultant cost-effectiveness ratio was less than an alternative intervention that could not achieve the desired effect. Obviously, if two or more interventions would achieve the desired effect, the decision maker could choose the one with the lowest cost. The lowest cost intervention might still not be the one with the best cost-effectiveness ratio. In this latter instance, the decision maker might not select the most cost-effective intervention because he or she does not value the additional effect commensurate with the additional cost.

HEALTH AS A PRODUCTION FUNCTION

---

241 **Purpose of this chapter**

A person's health depends on his or her environment, genetic make-up, behaviour and the health care he or she receives (and the interactions among these factors). Health care interventions are intended to alter a person's health status for the better, either by changing the environment (e.g. by separating man from microbe), the person's genetic make-up (e.g. by gene therapy), his or her physiology (e.g. by immunisation or drug therapy), his or her behaviour (e.g. by educating him or her to avoid drinking and driving) or his or her affect (e.g. by assisting him or her to cope better with terminal cancer). This chapter focuses on the production of health by means of personal health care services: the intent to improve individual patients' health status through specific medical interventions.

This chapter introduces the ideas that health care is a production function and that hospitals are health-producing facilities. A hospital's purpose is to improve patients' health status, to manufacture health. The idea that factories produce manufactures is well accepted, even if people do not know how they manufacture particular items. The idea that health can be 'manufactured' or that health facilities such as hospitals are health-producing 'factories' is a perspective on health care that is rarely articulated and foreign, if not repugnant, to most doctors. While quality management requires that hospitals be viewed as health-producing facilities, clearly they are not industrial factories. The production of health in hospitals differs markedly from the production of manufactures in factories. Producing health status improvement is far more difficult than manufacturing products. While industrial quality management principles may apply to hospitals, industrial quality management methods are only marginally useful for improving the production of health.

Industry has shown dramatically that quality management can improve quality. Today's television sets are far superior to yesterday's and, relatively speaking, cost far less. This quality revolution is spreading to services, including hospitals. Quality management views organisations as production entities geared to producing products that please customers. Health care quality management intends primarily to improve the production of health. For quality management purposes, hospitals are health-producing facilities. The quality manager's goal, as an integral member of the production team, is to assure and improve the quality of a hospital's many products. His or her role is to lead and co-ordinate all of a hospital's activities intended to achieve this goal.

Many people's view of factories stems from classic images that originated in the early part of this century: places where people mindlessly tighten nuts on ceaselessly moving assembly lines to mass produce products. Tomorrow's factories will employ fewer people than today's and increasingly they will be college graduates. They will work in teams, manage computer-controlled machines and industrial robots, and use statistics and other quality management methods. In these respects, factories will become indistinguishable from hospitals, and neither one will much resemble Henry Ford's turn-of-the-century assembly lines that revolutionised the production of automobiles, made possible mass production, and led to the consumer society in which we live today. In today's advanced factories, the future has arrived already. Hospitals must prepare for the quality revolution.

This chapter expresses the most central idea in this manual, an understanding of which is essential for effective quality management and hence for improving patients' health status:

- Outcomes (most importantly, patient health status improvement) depend on: inputs to processes (patient characteristics); processes, which are shaped inherently by structures (the health care production system, interventions and their implementation); the environment in which processes take place; and the interactions among inputs, processes and the environment.

The chapter describes:

- the nature of processes and outcomes, and models that explain outcomes in terms of processes;
- the production of health;
- the hospital as a health production system;
- production system design and evaluation;
- health care quality management's central goal: to change processes to improve, and to reduce variation in, patient health outcomes.

Readers may find this material new, somewhat theoretical and difficult to understand. They may be tempted to skip ahead. However, the material provides a framework in which to set subsequent chapters' contents. To facilitate comprehension, the chapter looks first at production systems and processes intended to produce desired outcomes. Then it looks at outcomes in terms of what may have produced them. Next, it explores issues in designing and evaluating, and then redesigning, health production systems, processes and practices. Finally, it introduces the important topic of variation in patient outcomes, health status improvement, and how hospitals can use this information to improve quality of their care.

242 | Key concepts

This chapter elaborates on the following key concepts essential to understanding the production of health.

- Health care's purpose is to improve maximally patients' health status, including physical, emotional and social aspects of health, using interventions consistent with their preferences, providers' circumstances and society's resources and mores.
- Hospitals are health care's principal production facilities, organisations designed to 'produce' health.
- Health care is a production system that consists of a series of processes, shaped by structures, each of which may be a production subsystem with its own process elements. The output of one process is an input to the next or a subsequent process.
- These processes give rise to economic, health, social and other outcomes with a given probability, magnitude and timing that accrue to patients, providers, other stakeholders and society. Outcomes may be intended or unintended; positive or negative.
- Patient health status improvement is health care processes' principal intended outcome. An effective medical intervention (process) transforms patients (input): patients' postprocess health status (outcome) is greater than it would have been at that point in time without the process.
- Three sets of variables and their interactions produce patient outcomes (health status improvement): health care production processes (producer); the patient's characteristics at the time of entering the process; and the environment in which production takes place (coproducers).
- An interactive effect exists when the state of one outcome-producing variable affects the effect on outcome of another. Interactions among variables may be paramount and are often little understood. Their number rises disproportionately to the number of variables.
- Measuring outcome variables tells one nothing about what produced resultant readings. It is one thing to measure postintervention patient health status (outcome) and quite another to attribute it to preceding medical interventions (process). A patient's recovery or death may have everything, nothing, or something to do with care processes.
- Attribution of patient outcomes to care processes is the key to quality improvement in two distinct circumstances: attribution of effect (to determine an intervention's effectiveness for particular patient populations, to formulate practice policies, for example) and attribution of maloutcome (to determine if an observed maloutcome in an individual patient was attributable to malprocess, to assess care's appropriateness).
- Attribution of outcomes to processes must either be assumed or inferred. The strength of the inference depends on the strength of the evidence and the extent to which mechanisms are known or can be inferred plausibly to connect processes to outcomes. Attribution may be based on experience or on research results. Quality managers must often rely on analyses or studies that produce uncertain results. Plausible mechanisms are not necessarily valid chains of cause and effect.

- Quality management involves the design and evaluation of health production systems and their efficient operations; the design and operation of health production facilities, such as hospitals, and their interrelationships, such as patient and information flows among them; and the design and evaluation of processes within facilities, such as coronary artery bypass grafts, which are the technologies that constitute their core production processes.

- Design presupposes evaluation. Designing new and redesigning established processes (practice policies and production systems to implement them) involves selecting from among available interventions and contexts those that are known or assumed to maximise patients' health status improvement (outcomes).

- Evaluating existing and experimental health production systems involves attributing observed health status improvement (outcomes) to preceding interventions and their inputs (patients) and environment. Only through scientific evaluation can one produce the certain knowledge necessary to (re)design health production systems to improve achievable health status improvement and to raise the level that is achievable.

- Industrial quality gurus often define quality simply as meeting specifications; zero defects as a quality absolute. Zero variation in products requires either zero variation in processes and inputs (the usual situation in manufacturing) or fitting processes to inputs if they are not and cannot be made uniform (essential in health care).

- Health care provides a far greater quality management challenge than industrial production. Manufacturers know how (otherwise they would not be able) to produce products. Doctors must manage patients whether or not they can determine what ails them and whether or not there are effective interventions for defined ailments. Patients vary. Instead of starting with uniform inputs to uniform production processes doctors must first classify patients into diagnostic categories for treatment selection purposes.

- Providers' goal is to reduce the variation in the fit between what patients need and want, and what they receive. It is not to treat all patients alike regardless of what is wrong with them. Nevertheless, for a given diagnostic category of patients, they must implement a specific intervention, for example, surgical operation, as uniformly as practical. Uniformity of process facilitates assessment of variation in outcome by eliminating the obvious factor—variation in process.

- If a manufacture fails, the task of finding out why is straightforward and root causes are likely relatively easy to eliminate. If a patient's postintervention health status is not all that was expected, the task of finding out why is complex and, even if problems' root causes are known, that of their elimination may be difficult even if it is possible at all.

- Health care quality management emphasises increasing the average health status improvement providers achieve for given types of patients, referred to often as 'shifting (and lifting) the curve [of the distribution of patient health status improvement that providers produce] to the right'. Shifting the curve to the right requires a more perfect adherence to practice policies and their proper implementation. Lifting the curve to the right requires better practice policies that provide greater health status improvement.

- Variation in patient outcomes detracts from quality because it represents risk to patients. It alerts quality managers to the possibility of improving quality.

They must reduce variance in patient outcomes while simultaneously increasing average patient health status improvement. In some circumstances they may face trading-off increased average health status improvement and reduced variation in such improvement.

- Variation in patient outcomes may result from the following interrelated factors:
  —patient factors—failure to classify patients into diagnostic categories homogeneous with respect to outcome given their complementary therapeutic interventions;
  —production factors—failure to follow practice policies when circumstances dictate that they should be followed, and their improper implementation;
  —product factors—ineffective practice policies, including their constituent interventions;
  —persistent factors—random events and their interactions with patient, production and product factors.

- Because one cannot usually measure health status improvement in quality management practice, production variance is often concerned with conformance to practices—practice policies and processes designed to implement them.

- Quality managers can improve average health status improvement and reduce variation in individual outcomes for a given type of patient by:
  —measuring the extent of conformance to product and production specifications (processes)—to know the shape of the curve;
  —improving conformance to processes—to shift the curve to the right;
  —improving product and production specifications—to lift the curve to the right.

243 | Industrial analogies

243.1 | Production

For most people, 'production' invokes an image of a factory producing manufactures, products designed to fulfil certain wants or needs. The automobile factory producing cars is an often-used example of manufacturing, here and elsewhere. Humans have been making artefacts for as long as they have existed; first in their homes, be they caves or cottages, and later in factories, places devoted exclusively to manufacturing goods. In today's most advanced factories, humans tend robots that actually make products, including more industrial robots.

Since the mid eighteenth century there have been five revolutions in manufacturing, all of which were exploited first in the United States, and resulted in improved product quality: the manufacture of interchangeable parts; the advent of scientific management; mass production; statistical quality control; and industrial robots, numerically controlled machine tools and CAD/CAM (computer assisted design and computer assisted manufacturing). Other countries, most notably Japan, have perfected these ideas and have added some of their own, including TQM (total quality management), JIT (just-in-time inventory) and QFD (quality functional deployment). Health care is at the beginning of its quality revolution. The use of artificial intelligence, including robotics, is only now beginning to emerge.

243.2 | Types of processes

For convenience, production processes can be divided into various types, based largely on tradition rather than concept, for example agriculture, extraction, manufacturing and services. At first glance, one may consider agriculture as nature's manufacture, with canny humans clever enough to reap the bountiful harvest. In reality, agriculture is one of man's greatest inventions, an area of continuing technological innovation whose output is intended clearly to satisfy human needs and wants. While agriculture once employed nearly everyone, in advanced industrialised countries it now employs a small fraction of the workforce. Extraction is exemplified by mining, in which valuable (useful) components are separated from the whole.

Manufacturing, which is characterised by production of goods, may be divided into various types, for example transmutation, fabrication, transformation. In transmutation, inputs are changed into outputs which bear no resemblance to them, exemplified by baking a cake, starting with flour, shortening, sugar and other ingredients to produce a tasty treat. In fabrication, parts are assembled into wholes, which can be disassembled into their constituent parts, for example automobile manufacture. In transformation, inputs are changed into outputs which are recognisably the same or similar to, but whose properties differ from, inputs, indicating a change of state, for example, creating gems from rough diamonds. Services, like health care, are essentially state transforming processes. A hotel transforms the weary traveller into a rested person. Automobile repair transforms a car that does not run into one that will.

For purposes of illustrating critical differences between classical manufacturing processes and health care we examine, in simple terms, two processes: manufacturing nuts and bolts and transforming a rough diamond into a gem. The key to quality assurance is variance reduction but its meaning differs by type of production, as these two illustrations show.

243.3 Manufacturing nuts and bolts

Manufacturing often involves making parts and assembling them into wholes. Quality of products depends both on quality of parts' manufacture and of assembly. Nuts and bolts are used widely in manufactures. Their characteristics, for example, strength, must be appropriate to their function in the finished product. Clearly, the nut must fit the bolt just right: not too tight, not too loose. The manufacturer intends to produce nuts and bolts to certain specifications. Inevitably, nuts and bolts exhibit variance in dimensions, for example. A too small nut fitted to a too big bolt and vice versa is sure to produce a poor fit. While a too big nut and too loose bolt might produce an acceptable fit, it is obviously chancy to rely on their meeting on the assembly line.

The best quality management strategy is to produce all nuts and bolts within specified limits and ideally with zero variation in their dimensions and any other characteristics that affect product quality. In this example, the quality control goal is zero variation, preferably achieved by in-process quality control that prevents production of defective nuts and bolts or, if not, by other means—for example selecting only nuts and bolts meeting specifications to be used in assembly (which is a costly strategy). One can control both the quality of the material fashioned and the shaping processes, which must be matched to the material being shaped. Well-controlled processes result in nuts and bolts that meet specifications with little variance. This approach—of direct variance reduction— cannot be used in many state transforming processes, such as health care, because of inherent variation in inputs.

243.4 Transforming a rough diamond into a gem

For purposes of illustration we can envision that the process for producing gem stones consists of three subprocesses, all of which take place in the diamond cutter's workshop: diamond selection, stone cutting and gem polishing. One step's output is another's input. Clearly, the result of one process may affect what can be achieved by the rest. If the cutter wants to produce a large gem he or she must start with a large rough diamond.

Similarly, if the cutter wants to produce a gem of exceptional brilliance and clarity, he or she could hardly start with a flawed stone.

To fashion the gem, after selecting the stone the diamond cutter decides what cuts to make, makes iterative cuts and controls the process through feedback. Finally he or she polishes the cut stone to bring out its brilliance. If the workroom is very hot, the cutter may sweat profusely. His or her hand might slip, affecting the cut and hence the quality of the product. The quality of the resultant gem could be measured in many ways, some more technical than others. To assess a gem's quality, one could poll people about its beauty, or measure its brilliance, clarity and weight, or determine if it deviated from what the cutter intended to produce. However measured, the gem's quality is a product of the cutter's skill, the rough diamond he or she started with, and the environment in which he or she worked.

243.5 | Zero defects, variation

Quality gurus often define quality simply as meeting specifications and advocate a zero defects policy as a quality absolute. Moreover, the tighter the specifications, the higher the quality. Thus, variation, deviation from an average within (tight) specified limits, is detrimental to quality. This formulation works best in manufacturing nuts and bolts, for example.

With diamond cutting, we find that variation is inherent in the raw material. We could sort incoming stones into classes or grades to make them as uniform as possible, but variation would still exist. We could accept this, and create uniformity in the process so that the resultant product uniformly met specifications for a finished gem. Indeed, this might be a perfectly acceptable approach for routine production. But suppose we found an exceptionally large stone. We could simply subject it to the standard process and produce one or more 'quality' gems. But this approach might not realise the greatest return. Instead, we could adjust the process to suit the size of stone and produce a magnificent, even unique, gem.

When inputs vary, in order to achieve high quality products one can either sort or shape them to create homogeneous inputs to processes, or accept heterogeneous inputs and vary processes to suit. The former produces uniform products that are high quality; the latter, high quality products that are unique. The key differences are the notion of quality and the extent to which the potential inherent in inputs is transformed (and hence realised) in outputs. Thus a 12 carat rough diamond might be transformed into ten excellent 1 carat gems or, alternately, into a single magnificent 10 carat gem. Certainly the latter is far more valuable than the former—which could have been produced from ten smaller, undistinguished rough diamonds—and realises its potential as a magnificent gem. Quality, as perceived by the customer's delight, is the magnificence of the gem not merely its sparkle.

In summary, production's goal is to maximise product quality. In most manufacturing situations, quality is maximised when there is zero variation in products, and is assured through standardisation (zero variation) in processes. Process standardisation requires input standardisation to produce zero product variation. If there is inherent variation in inputs which cannot be reduced by a production process without affecting adversely product quality or value, maximising product quality requires fitting the process to the input and hence results in process variation. Thus highest quality health care requires reduction in variance of the fit between patient and care process; not reduction in process variation regardless of patient heterogeneity.

243.6 | Process control

Statistical quality control is a technique for monitoring processes or products and, through feedback, for reducing or controlling variation in processes and hence minimising variation in finished products. It applies directly to manufacturing nuts and bolts, for example. However, its application to a diamond cutter who specialises in producing unique gems would be detrimental. The stones exhibit inherently large variation; the cutter must adjust his or her cuts to the stone; the resultant gem is unique. In transforming rough diamonds into gem stones, populations of rough diamonds (inputs), cuts (processes), and finished gems (outcomes) would all exhibit large, but (for rough diamonds) inevitable or (for cuts) appropriate variation.

To assess the quality of the diamond cutter's work, one must compare what he or she intended to produce with what he or she actually produced. There should be zero variation between the ideal and intended cuts, and between the cutter's intended and actual cuts. Thus the policy of zero defects, that is, no variation in finished products appropriate to nuts and bolts, must be transformed to one of zero variation between ideal and actual cuts. This transformation creates significant specification and measurement problems. Can customers' preferences for gems be measured and expressed in product specifications to guide their production? For any given rough diamond, what is the ideal finished product? What cuts and other processes will produce it? Can actual cuts be measured and compared to ideal cuts? If ideal–actual variation exists, how can production processes be changed to reduce this variation? In reality we would not be overly concerned. People can decide if the diamond cutter's gems are value for money. The diamond cutter's livelihood depends on how much his or her products delight customers in comparison to competitors' products. Measurement and knowledge difficulties have not allowed this discipline to work in medicine until now.

One can accept readily that patients vary in the extent to which their health status can be improved with existing knowledge and technology (which ultimately limits providers' performance). For any broad class of patients one could apply standard processes and produce acceptable outcomes, measured in terms of aggregate health status improvement. Alternatively, one could type each patient in the class and apply processes that were most appropriate to that type. The result would be greater health status improvement, both in the aggregate and for each individual patient. To achieve this happy result requires more knowledge than simply treating broadly defined patients and more sophisticated monitoring of doctors' performance. Rather than simply measuring whether or not doctors invariably follow process specifications and achieve expected outcomes one must measure the fit between what they should have done and achieved for the type of patient, defined narrowly, and what they did and achieved. In these regards, medicine is more analogous to creating gems from rough diamonds than manufacturing nuts and bolts; to automobile repair than to automobile manufacture.

244 | Production systems: processes and outcomes

244.1 | Perspective

Hospitals can be regarded as health-producing factories or production systems. Their production elements consist of imaging and other diagnostic services, operating suites, clinical, nursing and other therapeutic services, and various support services that inform or supply these units, nourish patients, and maintain buildings and grounds. Hospitals have evolved over time and are not necessarily designed to function optimally as production systems. For example, when Dr Smith wants to try out the latest imaging device, the hospital manager may install it in a spare corner of the basement without much regard for optimising patient flows or product throughput. In the future, hospital architects and managers will need to view hospitals as production systems, and design and operate them like the complex health-producing factories that they have become. This chapter focuses on the concepts of health production, an understanding of which is central to improving the quality of health care, especially its underlying technology. The design and operation of hospitals is beyond this manual's scope.

The practice of medicine is far different from the manufacture of goods. Stated simply, manufacturers specify products and design new or adapt existing factories or production systems to produce them. They know how to produce these products. If they did not, they would not be able to produce them with the desired quality. Doctors face great uncertainty. They must treat everyone who seeks their help. They may not be able to determine exactly what ails a patient or an ailment's cause. Even if they believe they know an ailment's root cause, at least with some level of specificity, they may not know which is the best therapy for the patient. Patients have different preferences for outcomes and interventions. Some may want to add years to life; others, life to years. Some patients may want the certainty of surgery; others may prefer medical intervention or holistic treatments. Surrounded by a sea of uncertainty, improving the quality of care depends on adoption of appropriate models of reality and more and better data to operationalise them. Importantly, improving health care quality requires different models and more complex methods than are used in industry.

244.2 | *About purposeful systems*

A purposeful system achieves desired ends. Choices arise in their design.[1] Designers may make these choices, or they may be made by chance (as in natural selection). Purposeful systems have elements that function as a whole to achieve the system's purpose: the whole is greater than the sum of its parts. None of the system's elements can achieve the system's purpose. The system's elements and their interrelationships are sufficient to achieve its purpose. Fundamentally, maximising each elements' output may not maximise the system's output. Usually, in artificial purposeful systems (those designed by humans), such as production systems, the system's elements and their interrelationships are believed to be necessary (as well as sufficient) to achieve its purpose.

In natural purposeful systems (whose purpose is implied by humans) and some artificial systems, elements or interrelationships may not be necessary to achieve the system's proximal purpose. These redundant elements and interrelationships may be superfluous (are not and never were necessary to achieve the system's purpose), vestigial (having lost their useful function), reserve or buffer elements (function only when primary elements or interrelationships fail), or duplicative (share other elements' functions and thereby add to the system's capacity or production potential).

Production systems' design and operation is simplified when all elements and their interrelationships are both necessary and sufficient to achieve their purpose. However, if elements fail they may have to be replaced or repaired. If interrelationships are interrupted, they must be re-established. Further, if the environment changes, the system may have to be redesigned if it is to continue to achieve its purpose. In systems that evolve by natural selection, redundant elements and interrelationships may permit the system to achieve its purpose even if some elements fail, some interrelationships are interrupted, or the environment changes necessitating use of different elements or interrelationships or the same ones in different intensities. Natural purposeful systems are replete with redundancy that makes them very robust. For example, humans can lose parts of their brain and still function. Destroy virtually any part of an ordinary computer and it will no longer function.

244.3 | *About production systems*

Production systems intend to produce goods or services. A production system consists of one or more elements, referred to usually as production processes, and their interrelationships, designed and arranged to function as a whole. A production system's defining purpose or product is something that none of its elements can produce, and every element is needed to produce it. The elements collectively constitute a complete system, that is, every part is necessary and in their arrangement sufficient to produce the desired product or effect. Some system elements function to manage production, including quality control that assures that products meet specifications. Production systems can include elements that determine what products to make in what quantities and when and where to make them. A key question is what elements to include within the system's boundary. For quality management purposes, a system's boundary must include all of the elements that materially influence products' quality.

An automobile manufacturer may make every part that goes into the finished product. Conceivably, the manufacturer could produce the raw material, energy, and all other components that go into the manufacture of the car's parts (a system known as vertical integration). However, this may not be the most efficient arrangement. The manufacturer might be able to buy raw materials or parts from suppliers at a much lower cost than it could make them itself. Further, buying rather than making provides the manufacturer with greater flexibility to use different or better parts from other suppliers as its needs or circumstances, or as technologies, change.

In buying parts the manufacturer loses some measure of control over their production. If the supplier provides substandard parts, in the long term the manufacturer might change suppliers, but in the short term must cope with the resultant quality problem. For this reason, quality-focused manufacturers emphasise working with suppliers to improve their products to ensure that they meet manufacturers' needs and specifications. Similar reasons lead to the emergence of *keiretsu*—groups of related companies that work together to produced a core group of products. Strategies for optimising long-term production efficiencies involve many considerations and are complicated. Over the years, a considerable body of knowledge has emerged to manage such matters.

244.4 | *About processes*

Processes produce products. A process may be defined simply as a particular method of doing something, generally involving a number of steps or operations, for example an industrial process. Process implies purpose: a desired product (its outcome) is expected to result from the process. It also implies structure: the physical, including informational (e.g. feedback), elements that define and determine the process. A process can be divided into a number of subprocesses, which in turn can be subdivided into the most basic elements that constitute fundamental processes.

Delineating a process implies an environment in which the process takes place. The boundary between a process and its environment may be inherent or maintained by the process: clear or fuzzy; static or dynamic. Further, it implies that inputs flow from the environment into the process and that the process consumes or alters them. A process' outputs may be released into the environment, be inputs into subsequent processes, or used to sustain the process, its supporting structures, or the process-environment boundary. Over time, processes may alter the environment, thereby affecting their viability or outputs. Processes, and hence outcomes, exist in space-time; they are dynamic.

For quality management purposes, one must distinguish process outcomes from patient outcomes. Process outcomes characterise the process, for example the length of a patient's surgical operation. In production systems, process outcomes may trigger subsequent processes; for example poor (characterisation) obstetrical management (process) may necessitate hysterectomy (subsequent process). Patient outcomes refer to processes' effects on patients, for example need for hysterectomy (effect on patient of poor obstetrical management), loss of uterus (end result of obstetrical management, including the effect of the needed hysterectomy), and amount of health status improvement or its deterioration.

244.5 | About outcomes

Outcomes are the results of production processes, which precede them in space-time, acting on inputs in a given environment. They are what occurs, but are neither necessarily processes' inevitable nor their perpetual result. Outcomes are always in doubt because many factors coproduce them. Not only is what may occur in doubt but the probability, magnitude and timing of any given outcome may be in doubt. Outcomes involve probabilities, not certainties.

Health care outcomes may accrue to patients, providers, other interest groups or stakeholders and society. Outcomes may be intended or unintended, positive or negative, and of various types, for example economic, health, social. Since health care's central purpose is to improve patients' health status, one's attention focuses naturally on this intended, positive outcome. Indeed, it is this manual's primary focus. However, despite its centrality, it is only one of a myriad of production system outcomes. A positive outcome for one person or group may not be so positive for others.

Health care financing schemes may dwell on the sky-rocketing cost of care. Providers may be concerned about their incomes. Social action groups may worry that the poor and disadvantaged cannot access the care they need. Patients may be troubled by the quality of care. Professional liability insurers may focus on risk, reflected in malpractice awards. Politicians may be faced with the results of technological advances, including salvaged, but not whole, babies, and a rapid increase in the very old and dependent, but also vigour prolonged into older years affecting retirement, social security and the very fabric of society.

In health care, the term outcome is tricky. For quality management purposes, it refers to postintervention measurements—the observed 'outcomes' of intervention—whether or not one can attribute these results to preceding interventions. There is no implication that observed outcomes are attributable to interventions. Restricting the use of the term outcome to health status changes attributable to interventions (which some people like to do) means we would have to invent a word to describe postintervention values of desired outcome variables (for which we use the term observed outcome or observed effectiveness), because scientifically supportable evidence of attribution is almost invariably lacking. We use the term true effectiveness to refer to health status improvement (patient health outcome) that is attributable to interventions. See Chapter 3 in this part for an explanation of interventions' effectiveness.

In production systems, outcomes are measured by statistical distributions, such as the percentage of products that are defect-free or the average amount of, and variation in, health status improvement observed in a given patient population. Quality management's purpose is to maximise the probability of achieving intended outcomes by, among other things, knowing how, and controlling the processes necessary, to produce them. In controlled processes in a defined environment intended outcomes can tend toward, but can never achieve, certainty.

In designing health production systems or processes designers must consider expected outcomes in such terms as their importance, probability of occurrence, magnitude, and when in the future they will occur, and whether or not they are intended (or unintended) and positive (or negative) in reference to their perception of the system's client and its decision makers. The client (whom the system intends to benefit) may or may not be the same person or entity as the decision maker (who may foot the bill, for example). For expected negative outcomes, designers must consider either changing processes to avoid them or developing policies or other mechanisms to ameliorate them. Such design considerations are beyond this manual's scope, however, and are not considered further.

245 | Models of reality: causality, production and interactions

245.1 | Perspective

Our perceptions of reality shape our choices and actions. They mould and are moulded by our models of reality. Purpose shapes our models for inquiring about and understanding events and their interrelationships. This section explains the idea of producer-product in the context of the more familiar cause-and-effect, and the concept of interactive effects and their importance to understanding attribution and/or production of outcomes or effects. People often find it difficult to comprehend interactive effects. However, in the ultimate analysis all outcomes can be viewed as being the result of interactive effects. Production systems involve many interactions among process elements and their environment. Uncertainty of outcomes dominates such complex systems. These emerging views of reality (explained below) explain why, particularly in health care, it is often difficult to determine producers' and coproducers' relative effects and to attribute outcomes to interventions.

245.2 | Cause and effect

We are all familiar with the idea of cause and effect. A cause is anything producing an effect; an effect, anything brought about by a cause! Defined precisely, the idea says that something (cause) precedes and is both necessary and sufficient to result in something else (the effect). For example, if 'X' causes 'Y', then the occurrence of 'X' (at one point in time) will result in 'Y' (at a subsequent point in time); and if 'Y' exists it must have been preceded by 'X'. However, as we have noted, processes exist in an environment and the environment can influence outcomes. If 'X''s environment can influence whether or not it causes 'Y', 'X' remains necessary but is no longer (inherently) sufficient to cause 'Y'. In this circumstance, the general notion of cause-and-effect must be superseded by the special case of producer-product.[2]

245.3 | Producer-product

An acorn produces an oak but only in a number of environments (and not in others). The acorn is the producer of the oak (its product); the environment coproduces the oak. All producers have at least one coproducer (the environment). But coproducers are not limited to the environment. Taken together, producer 'X' and its coproducers are sufficient to cause 'Y'. However, if 'Y' can be caused by various producers (and their coproducers), 'Y''s existence does not mean that 'X' inherently preceded it. The acorn is the unique producer of the oak. Death and disease may have various producers and each producer may have its own coproducers, some of which may be shared with other producers.

We may not know with any degree of certainty which factor is the producer and which factors are coproducers. Moreover, it is entirely conceivable that a given product could be the result of different production systems and that some factors may be common to them. Thus it is convenient to talk generically of 'coproducers' to encompass the producer (the necessary) and its coproducers (the sufficient). In health care, medical intervention is the intended producer of health status improvement. This idea presupposes the intervention's effectiveness. Ineffective interventions cannot be producers. In this case, observed outcomes must result from other production systems (producers and their coproducers) which may—or may not—include the intervention as a coproducer.

245.4 | Interactive effects

An interactive effect exists when the state of one outcome-producing variable affects the effect on outcome of another. Phenylketonuria (PKU), for example, is an inborn error of amino acid metabolism (genetic defect) that results in mental retardation. Treatment depends on knowing that disease results from the interaction between the affected person and his or her environment. Affected infants maintained on a phenylalanine-controlled diet are not mentally retarded.

Interactions between organisms' genes and their environment are good illustrations of interactive effects and of the difficulty of spotting the producer. A farmer owning several strains of certain fowl and feeding them only yellow corn would notice the presence of 'yellow shank' in some of them. He would conclude the trait is genetically determined. Another farmer owning genetically susceptible strains of the fowl and feeding some of them on yellow corn and some of them on white corn would notice the trait in the fowl fed yellow corn. He would conclude that the trait is environmentally determined.[3] In reality, the expression of the trait is an interaction between the fowl's genetic make-up and its environment. The trait will be expressed if, and only if, the fowl has a certain genetic make-up and is fed yellow corn. Fowl of the same genetic make-up not fed yellow corn and those of a different genetic make-up—whether or not fed yellow corn—will not exhibit the trait. In this example, there are two relevant states for each of two coproducers (susceptible/non-susceptible genetic make-up, and yellow/non-yellow corn), and two relevant outcomes (yellow shank/normal). In other examples, there could be more coproducers and multiple states for each one, and numerous outcomes that might not be distinct. As the number of coproducers and the possible number of their states increases so does the complexity of their interactions, disproportionately.

Interactions may be direct or indirect. A direct interactive effect exists when the state of one coproducer interacts directly with that of another coproducer to produce different outcomes. For example, a virulent organism encountering a susceptible, but healthy, host may cause disease but not death. An indirect interactive effect exists when something (indirect coproducer) affects a coproducer's state, and hence affects its effect an outcome. For example, a virulent organism encountering a susceptible, HIV-infected host may cause death: the HIV infection has compromised (altered) the host's immune system (state).

Knowledge about interactive effects is important to understanding outcomes and designing processes to produce them. Only certain combinations of factors (producers and their coproducers) in a particular space-time arrangement will produce the desired outcome; other combinations or arrangements may have lesser, no, or undesirable effects. In one environment the relationship between inputs, processes and outcomes may be different from that in another. For example, a surgeon operating in one hospital may achieve better outcomes than in another for a given type of patient and the same operation. In part, the difference may result from differences in other coproducers, for example, the skills and organisation of the nursing staff. But in part they may result from differences in expression of the surgeon's skills within the different environments.

If one knew all possible states of coproducers and the outcomes of all possible combinations of all coproducer states arrayed in space-time, one would know interaction-specific outcomes. Given this information, one could predict more accurately patient outcomes. However, given the large number of variables involved, this amount of information would be unimaginably large. Moreover, its generation and use depends on correct measurement and classification which will always be imperfect. Further, measuring something may alter its state, affecting the outcomes of the system of which it is an element. Additionally, prior to or during an intervention, for example, one would still have to predict or control the state of process variables. For example, the patient's outcome may depend materially on the surgeon's state at the time of operation, for example hung over, tired, alert. Ideally, in this instance, to assure outcomes surgeons would have to pass a 'readiness' test to preclude those from operating whose state militates against an acceptable outcome. Surgeons' states to be precluded might well vary by types of patient. For example, more states might be excluded for 'fragile' than 'robust' patients. This idea is merely an extension of that embodied in preventing junior doctors from operating unaided on complicated cases or referring patients to specialists whose greater skills and experience are expected to produce better outcomes.

245.5 | *Paradigm shift*

A paradigm shift occurs when people see the same facts in a new way, altering their view of reality, which often has profound implications. For example, a paradigm shift occurred when people realised that the earth revolved around the sun and was not the centre of the universe. People saw the same physical world in an entirely new light, with dramatic consequences. Nature can be viewed as a smooth progression or a series of discontinuities, and one may masquerade as the other depending on the phenomenon's scale and one's instrument's resolving power. For example, in 1962 Thomas Kuhn disputed the age-old view that scientific progress involves the accumulation of knowledge, with one discovery building on previous ones.[4] He distinguished normal science from scientific revolutions. Normal science consists of puzzle solving within a given scientific paradigm rather than innovation. True innovation involves a paradigm shift, a new way of thinking about nature that represents a scientific revolution. Within a given paradigm only so much progress can be made. Further progress requires a new paradigm.

Health care is in the midst of an important paradigm shift: from its current focus on plying processes to one of optimising outcomes. Stated simply, patients desire health status improvement (outcomes), not health services (processes). This idea is this manual's central premise. It represents a paradigm shift in health care, as profound as the quality revolution in manufacturing. (See Chapter 2 in this part.)

245.6 | *Chaos theory and the science of complexity*

Science is undergoing a paradigm shift. It began in earnest when relativity and quantum mechanics replaced the mechanical, clockwork universe. Classical science is reductionist. It focuses on analysis, prediction and control. Given present positions one can calculate past and predict future positions. Classic analysis sees a world of static linear relationships and suggests that if we break down processes into their constituent elements and understand each one, we will know how the process works. However, this approach does not lead necessarily to such understanding.

The new science of complexity is integrationist. It sees ecologies, systems that comprise interactions rather than elements. The science of complexity suggests that we cannot predict a system's global properties, how it behaves dynamically, from what we know of its elements.[5] A system's global properties result from local interactions among its elements. Further, these emergent global properties feedback to influence elements' interactions and produce self-organising systems and surface order out of apparent subsurface chaos.

Chaos theory, a subset of the science of complexity, suggests that interactions among processes' elements and their environment produce outcomes that cannot be predicted by examining individual elements. Systems are non-linear. Outcomes are sensitive to initial conditions. Since we cannot know initial conditions with certainty (because measuring instruments are inherently imperfect), we cannot predict outcomes; the future is inherently uncertain. Small differences in initial conditions may produce large differences in outcomes. This idea is referred to sometimes as the butterfly effect: an Amazonian butterfly flaps its wings and produces a storm in Arkansas two weeks later.[6]

246 | The production of health

246.1 | Health production model

Patient outcomes, or patients' postintervention health status, result from the following three sets of variables and their interactions:[7]

- the patient's preintervention characteristics;
- the intervention, that is, processes brought to bear chronologically, the production systems that implement them, encompassing, for example, a doctor's ability to diagnose or categorise correctly the patient for treatment selection purposes, select appropriately the best treatment for the patient, and implement successfully the selected treatment, including recognising and managing any resultant untoward occurrences (complications), nursing and other staff;
- the environment in which the intervention takes place.

Figure II-4-1 on page 203 illustrates this basic production model, which is essential to understanding the production of health and health care quality management. It depicts the three sets of variables—and their interactions—that produce patient outcomes, for example health status improvement. They are: patient outcomes' intended producer—health care production processes; and their coproducers—patients' characteristics at the time of entering the process; and the environment in which production takes place. The relative impact of any one of these sets of variables on patient outcome will depend on the type of intervention and the era when it occurred. Moreover, the nature and importance of particular interactive effects (produced when the value of one variable affects the effect of another) may also vary dynamically.

Interactions among variables may be paramount and are often little understood. Ultimately, all effects can be viewed as resulting from interactions. The number of possible interactions rises disproportionately to the number of variables. Their effect on outcomes may be masked or indirect. For example, a certain surgical operation may generally benefit patients with a particular disease, but not a subset. The hospital in which a surgeon operates may influence his or her performance. Importantly, for quality management purposes, one must try to identify and isolate those variables and their interactions that account mostly for desired outcomes.

246.2 | Focus on outcomes

Patients seek care to improve their health status. Quality management's job is to provide patients with maximal health status improvement with as great a certainty as practical, within patients' preferences and society's resources. This goal is simple to state but difficult to accomplish. People focus naturally on patient outcomes, measured simply as whether or not the patient lived or died, or comprehensively in terms of health status improvement. Patient, intervention and environmental variables—and their interactions—produce outcomes. Outcomes can be considered only in relation to care processes, the characteristics of the patients to whom they were applied, and the environment in which they were applied.

246.3 | Measurement of patient outcomes

Appropriate and accurate measurement of patient outcomes is the key to improving the quality of care. Patient outcomes can be measured in many ways and at different times after intervention. Choosing appropriate and reliable measures and end points is the key

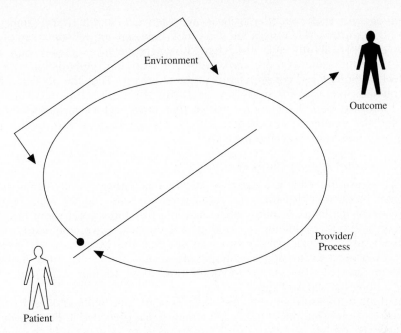

Figure II-4-1 *The production of outcome: Health care process (intended producer), patient, environment (coproducers), and their interactions*

to determining interventions' effectiveness. There are many issues in choosing what patient outcomes to measure and how to measure them. This section can only address some of the most central ones.

Ideally, patient health status is the outcome measure of choice, but its use may not always be practical. In this case, other less adequate measures must be used. They may include, for example, five-year survival, operative mortality and nosocomial infection rates. Often, investigators judge interventions' effectiveness in terms of differences in survival between experimental and control groups. Such judgments are inappropriate because they do not take into account the possibility of differences in the shape of the survival curves. Thus comparing the areas under the survival curves would be an appropriate measure of interventions' effectiveness. Usually one cannot measure health status improvement (which, as Chapter 3 in this part explains, is an integrated measure); it is best to use several patient outcome measures and to consider explicitly their relationship to health status. For example, one may find that five years after operation a greater proportion of women than men are depressed. This finding may say little about women's tendency to depression if most of the men (who might have suffered from depression) have died already.

Measuring outcomes in practice has many difficulties. Whatever outcome measures are used, they must be reliable and valid. Measurement difficulties may limit the utility of comparing outcomes achieved to those desired because of the uncertainty surrounding the measure. For example, it is hard to tell if the children in one school given daily doses of milk are taller than those in another who do not drink milk if one is using rubber bands to measure their height. The variance inherent in the outcome measures overwhelms any possible difference in the treatment's effectiveness. An imperfect measure measured perfectly may be more useful than a perfect one measured imperfectly. Trade-offs may have to be made between measures and their implementability, with selection of those that yield the best, most reliable and valid information.

An intervention's apparent effectiveness may depend on when after initiation of treatment one compares differences in outcomes between experimental and control groups. For example, shortly after discharge, treated patients' outcomes may appear better, only to be the same as the control group's a year later, perhaps because of the placebo effect or the delayed consequences of the treatment. Thus the period of follow-up (not to mention the outcome measures used) can affect apparent effectiveness. The longer the follow-up period the more chance that other factors coproduce observed outcomes, and the treatment and control groups' experience may vary in this regard, introducing both noise and bias into measurements.

246.4 | *Attribution of effect and of outcomes*

Difficulties of measuring patient outcomes pale in comparison to attributing them to preceding care processes. Measuring outcome variables tells one nothing about what produced resultant readings. A thermometer reading that indicates a room is cold, for example, may (if the thermometer is working) tell us the room's temperature but not what produced the particular temperature. To attribute the temperature to preceding factors we would need to know, for example, about the room's size, use, its heating/cooling system, and the outside temperature, and how to make the right logical connections among the states of these variables.

It is one thing to measure an outcome, such as death, and quite another to attribute its occurrence (or non-occurrence) to the intervention that preceded it. Patients may visit the doctor and recover, or they may die. Their recovery or death may have everything, nothing, or something to do with the doctor's interventions. Similarly, observation of a particular patient outcome, for example, improvement in patients' health status, does not mean that preceding processes (medical interventions) produced the improvement let alone which elements of that care were most responsible for such improvement among different types of patients.

Attribution of patient outcomes to preceding care processes is a key aspect of health care quality management. Attribution is required in two distinct circumstances:

- attribution of effect—to determine an intervention's effectiveness for particular patient populations, for purposes of formulating practice policies, for example;
- attribution of maloutcome—to determine if an observed maloutcome in an individual patient was attributable, more likely than not, to malprocess or to coproducers, for purposes of assessing care's appropriateness.

246.5 | *Attribution of effect in populations of patients*

When formulating practice policies, for example, one would like to know that proposed interventions are effective, that is, improve patients' health status. However, most often interventions' effectiveness is assumed, not known scientifically. Indeed, the lack of solid information about interventions' effectiveness (the relationship between processes and outcomes) is one of the most vexing and difficult to solve quality management problems. Quality management systems, when implemented fully, may be the key to the cost-effective provision of useful information about the relationship between processes and outcomes.

To attribute outcomes to processes with some certainty requires data derived from well-designed, well-controlled randomised clinical trials. Such trials intend to assure that patients in experimental and control groups meet study inclusion criteria and (through randomisation) are identical in every way except exposure to the intervention being tested. Under these circumstances any differences in outcomes (effectiveness) could be reasonably attributed to the interventions; under others, less reasonably. Figure II-4-2 on page 205 illustrates this comparison. At various points in time after initiation of treatment, the two groups' outcomes can be compared to determine the intervention's effectiveness.

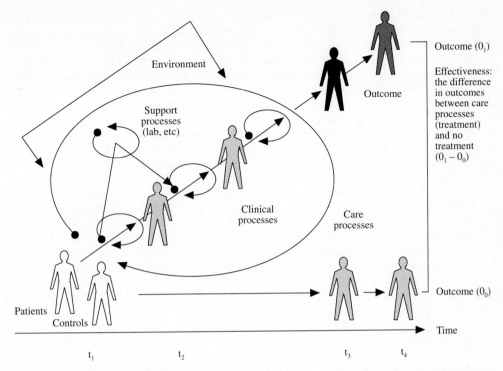

Figure II-4-2 *Processes within processes: The output of one process is the input to a subsequent process*

Patients' health status can be measured at entry into care (point 1), at various points in the production process (point 2), for treated patients, at a point in time corresponding to the completion of treatment (point 3), and at various times thereafter (point 4). Comparisons between the groups must be made based on time elapsed from the initiation of treatment, not on relative referents, for example, discharge from the hospital. Length of stay may vary for all sorts of reasons and this variance may bias comparisons between the groups.

Even well-designed, well-controlled randomised clinical trials do not prove interventions' effectiveness. Statistically (and clinically) significant differences in outcomes between experimental and control groups can arise by chance. Replicating a trial (which in the face of the results of a well-designed, well-controlled one would be hard-pressed to find the money to do) does not eliminate this problem because there is a finite probability that repeated trials will show an intervention is effective when in fact (but unknown to anyone) it is not. Confidence in inferences about interventions' effectiveness increases if one can demonstrate scientifically the mechanisms by which processes produce outcomes (which in health care is rare), or if one can at least describe plausible mechanisms. However, plausible chains of cause and effect are not necessarily valid and may depend on various assumptions. In short, the strength of the inference depends on the strength of the measurement system (e.g. randomised controlled trial, opportunity sample of cases, quality assessment, personal opinion), and the extent to which mechanisms are known or can be inferred plausibly to connect processes to outcomes.

246.6 *Attribution of outcome in individual patients*

A patient's death in the hospital may be relatively easy to attribute to medical care. The patient's death thirty days after admission may have nothing at all to do with his or her care or state at admission, but may be due to an unrelated cause. For example, the care of a patient who died in an automobile accident shortly after discharge may not be faulted by his or her assumedly unrelated death. But was the death unrelated? Delving behind the obvious one may discern that the treatment failed to cure the patient's blackouts or that the patient was not instructed properly about the side effects of the drug he or she was taking. Even for deaths during admission, the reasons the patient died may not be obvious or simple to determine.

Quality assessment—case-by-case examination of care to determine its appropriateness—depends on determining, from the patient's medical record, if he or she received all necessary care (and no other) and providers implemented it properly. Such maloutcomes as death alert quality assessors to the possibility of malprocess. They must judge, based on their knowledge of and assumptions about the relationships between processes and outcomes, whether or not the maloutcome was more likely than not the result of malprocess and, if so, which processes were deficient and therefore potential targets for quality improvement actions. Such judgments are necessary to identify processes that if changed would likely improve subsequent patients' outcomes. They will always be subjective and uncertain. There is no way to validate them scientifically because one cannot (nor would one want to) replicate the circumstances being judged. By monitoring trends in patient outcomes, quality managers can judge whether or not production system changes result in better outcomes. They face the difficulty of attributing any such improvement to production system changes.

246.7 | Outcomes for patients

One must distinguish clearly expected outcomes for populations from outcomes for specific individuals. For example, based on research one may know an intervention's expected mortality rate for a population of patients with particular characteristics. For any given category of patients, for example young women with acute cholecystitis undergoing a cholecystectomy, the hospital could calculate and display outcomes, for example death rates among treating surgeons and their variance. Given such data the hospital could tell the patient what may happen to her, even stating confidence limits. For example it could tell the patient that she has a 99.1–99.9% chance of leaving the hospital alive (with a one in twenty chance that the true estimate lies outside of this range). The patient will likely want to know whether or not she will be counted among the 99.1–99.9%, or be one of the 0.1–0.9% who are discharged dead. However, we cannot predict which individuals in a subsequent population of patients with identical characteristics to that used to derive the estimate (e.g. a stream of such patients entering the hospital) will live and which ones will die. Even if one subdivides patients ad infinitum to produce more reliable estimates (because the resultant patient groups are increasingly homogenous with respect to outcome), they will for ever remain statistical estimates. They provide expectations of outcomes for a given type of patient; in the case of the example, the probability that an individual patient will survive the procedure.

What actually happens to an individual patient depends on patient, care, environmental variables, and their interactions. That is why, for example, a young woman may enter the hospital for an elective procedure and die on the operating table, perhaps because her surgeon was impaired. To reduce the chances of such tragedies and to realise as much achievable health status improvement as possible, hospitals must devise coherent, simple, robust, stable production processes and control both inputs and processes. Working with doctors, nurses and all the other members of the hospital's staff, that is the quality manager's central function.

246.8 | Outcomes in quality management practice

Where scientifically substantiated knowledge exists, quality managers can use it to formulate practice policies and to design health care production systems and processes to maximise patient health status improvement. However, in quality management practice, one must often rely on analyses that produce uncertain results about an intervention's effectiveness (design), or be reduced to using one's judgment about the extent to which observed patient outcomes can be attributed to care processes (evaluation). One must also reconcile oneself to the fact that because of imperfect knowledge one's unaided judgment will often be wrong, reinforcing the need to measure outcomes and to use sound analytic methods applied rigorously wherever possible. One must do the best one can with available information while simultaneously identifying and taking steps to fill critical information gaps.

246.9 | Outcomes of quality improvement

For quality management purposes, the essential health production model can be applied to the production of quality improvement. Quality improvement actions, changes in practices for example, intend to improve patient outcomes. After their implementation, the quality manager must decide whether or not observed improvements (or deteriorations) were attributable to these changes. However, because it is often difficult to conduct controlled experiments in quality improvement, the quality manager must usually rely on his or her judgment. Once again, one's experience may be misleading and what is plausible is not necessarily valid. For example, a well-known industrial study showed that improved lighting increased workers' output. Years later it was realised that the investigators had drawn the wrong inference. Workers' increased production resulted from management's attention (the study) and was not attributable principally to the improved lighting. The medium was the message. Any management attention to workers would have produced the same (or at least some) increased productivity. The effect was attributable to the study (management attention), not to the specific intervention studied (the improved lighting).

247 | Health production in practice

247.1 | About health production in practice

Quality management's purpose is to improve the production of health. Improvement implies changing or redesigning production systems. All design presupposes evaluation. The health production model shown in Figure II-4-1 on page 203 provides the basis for evaluating interventions' outcomes, including their cost-effectiveness,[8] and for understanding the causes of variation in outcomes and hence reduction in variance and improvement of outcomes. Observed outcomes may exhibit substantial variation. This variation may stem from patient, intervention, or environmental variables, or interactions among these variables. Quality management's goal, and hence that of evaluating interventions' outcomes, is to identify groups of patients (with specific characteristics and preferences) who are homogeneous with respect to outcomes of specific interventions that produce maximal health status improvement for that group of patients. This information is useful for refining relevant diagnostic categories and improving selection of the most appropriate treatment corresponding to each one.

This section conceptualises the process of diagnosing and treating patients for quality management purposes. It also describes some of the patient, intervention and environmental variables that quality managers must consider in designing production systems and attributing outcomes to interventions to evaluate their effectiveness. A later section discusses the significance of variation in patient outcomes—that might result from patient, intervention, and environmental variables and their interaction—for quality management purposes.

247.2 | Diagnosis and treatment

Patients seek health care because they believe it will maintain or improve their health status, that is, alter their outcomes. This conception encompasses the worried-well who seek care. The doctor's reassurance improves their health status by calming their fears. When confronted by a patient, the provider must:

- diagnose the patient's problem, that is, assign the patient to a particular diagnostic category;
- assist the patient select among alternative interventions by providing information on each alternative, including the patient's prognosis without any intervention and that likely to result from each alternative;
- implement selected interventions;
- follow up to ensure the intervention worked as intended, to manage any side effects or other complications and, if necessary, to suggest additional diagnostic and therapeutic interventions. (See Figure II-4-3 below).

Prognosis is the doctor's prediction of the patient's future health status (or probable course of a disease), with and without intervention. Prognosis is the principal technical information for selecting among alternative interventions and courses of action (including doing nothing). The final choice of intervention depends on the patient's preferences for means and ends and his or her resources. Thus, for example, patients may select a therapy with less good prognosis because they reject the means necessary to realise the greater health benefits. Patients may not have access to some treatments, for example, because the hospital does not provide it or the patient cannot afford it.

Ideally, doctors' choices of diagnostic and therapeutic interventions would be based entirely on substantiated scientific information. Practically, however, choices must be based largely on training, experience or assumption, because of the dearth of scientific substantiation of the effectiveness of interventions.[9] Practice policies can assist doctors'

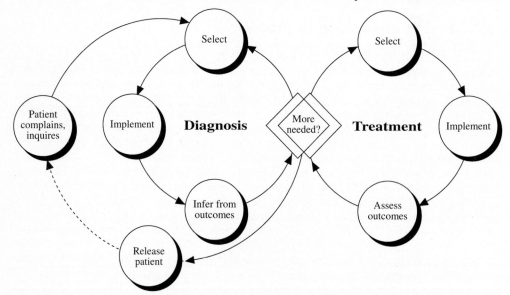

Figure II-4-3 *Diagnosis–treatment dyad*

choices. Outcomes' measurement can improve practice policies and assist patients' choices by providing objective information on expected health status improvement. Subsequent chapters in this part discuss these ideas.

Within the limits of existing technology, a patient's chances of achieving maximum health status improvement depend on his or her doctor's ability to place him or her in the correct diagnostic category (to delineate relevant therapeutic alternatives), to assist him or her select the correct therapy (that expected to produce maximal health status improvement), and to implement necessary diagnostic and therapeutic interventions properly, while avoiding unnecessary interventions and untoward outcomes. (See Figure II-4-4 below.) Populations of patients may—and usually do—exhibit considerable variation in outcomes. To improve quality one must increase average, and reduce variation in, patient outcomes. To reduce variation in outcomes one must understand their production.

247.3 │ Patient variables—diagnosis

247.31 ABOUT PATIENT VARIABLES

Patient variables are those that describe the patient and his or her health problem. With respect to the health production model, and to quality management, patients must be

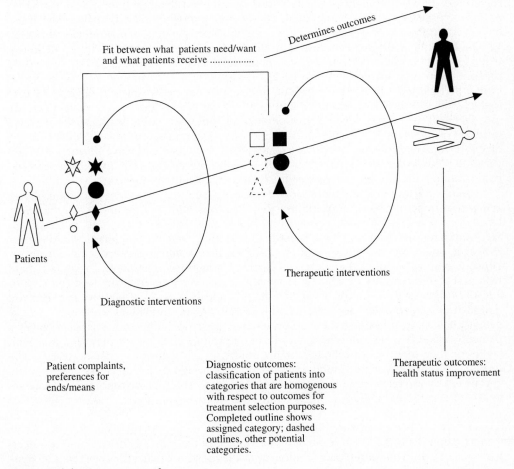

Figure II-4-4 *Patient–process fit*

classified correctly to select the therapeutic intervention that will likely provide the greatest chance of improving their health status maximally. In theory, one could fix diagnostic categories so that they are independent of treatments. However, we do not know all of the variables that could affect patients' outcomes, or how they interact with specific treatments. Further, our ability to classify patients according to relevant variables improves over time. Thus relevant diagnostic classifications change dynamically and must inherently be linked to available treatments. Since our ability to classify patients improves with advances in diagnostic interventions and we are adding constantly to our store of therapeutic interventions, we must continuously generate information about how best to categorise patients for treatment selection purposes, and about the outcomes of alternative interventions for each of the resultant categories. This challenge—of defining appropriate classification variables and delineating the best diagnostic interventions for purposes of categorising patients in relation to alternative therapeutic interventions—lies at the heart of quality management.

247.32 About diagnostic interventions

Medical care consists of two types of interventions: diagnostic—intended to categorise patients for treatment selection purposes; and therapeutic—intended to improve patients' health status. In this sense, the term 'diagnostic intervention' encompasses also those to screen individuals (to identify and categorise people with deranged physiology who may not be experiencing disease symptoms). Therapeutic intervention encompasses also those to prevent disease or its progression and to rehabilitate patients. For simplicity, it is convenient to think of diagnosis occurring at the beginning of care and leading to definitive treatment that cures the patient. This simple model does describe some portion of medical practice. However, increasingly the cycle of diagnosis and treatment may be repeated during the course of caring for a patient, and may occur many times from onset of care to the health problem's resolution or, in the case of chronic conditions, the patient's death. (See Figure II-4-3 on page 208). For example, a patient may suffer complications of initial treatment necessitating further diagnostic and therapeutic interventions. Repetition of the diagnosis–treatment cycle (or spiral) creates distinct patient pathways through the universe of possible interventions, often adding to the number of relevant diagnostic (and corresponding therapeutic) categories for quality management purposes.

Usually, doctors form an impression of what is wrong with a patient from their history and physical examination, and confirm the diagnosis with one or more specific tests. Laboratory tests, radiological, endoscopic, histological examinations, and other procedures often reveal (otherwise hidden) findings that are characteristic of particular diseases. However, sometimes a single test offers insufficient or confusing information. Diagnosis depends on conducting sufficient tests to gather enough information to classify a patient with acceptable certainty of validity. How certain is certain enough, the best (most cost-effective) strategy to reach this level of certainty, and how to best interpret the resultant information are complex and often controversial issues. Individual tests may classify patients inaccurately because they are unreliable or are not sufficiently characteristic of a particular disease or its underlying cause. For example, radiologists may disagree with others or themselves as to whether or not a radiograph exhibits a specific lesion. The given lesion may occur in a number of diseases, although it may be more common in, and hence more characteristic of, some diseases than others. Information that is characteristic of a particular disease is often referred to as pathognomonic.

247.33 Diagnostic categories

Correct diagnosis is the key to estimating the course of the patient's disease and to selecting the best treatment for the patient. Moreover, diagnostic classifications are used increasingly for administrative and other purposes, adding to their importance. Doctors face uncertainty and risk in placing patients into the correct diagnostic category. Additional tests, for example, may reduce the risk of categorising the patient incorrectly, but may cost or inconvenience the patient more than the perceived benefits that would flow from increased diagnostic certainty. Moreover, diagnostic interventions inherently possess risks to patients' health.

Diagnosis' goal is not only to label a patient's health problem but also to explain its aetiology or root cause. There are a large, but finite, number of categories into which a doctor may place a patient for prognostic or therapeutic purposes at any particular point in time. The number of, names for, and relationships among categories vary dynamically, the product of new knowledge, for example. Lack of consistent criteria results in fuzzy rather than sharp classificatory demarcations. Differences among providers regarding diagnostic classification concepts and criteria may result in variation in diagnostic outcomes (the diagnostic category to which doctors assign patients). Variation in diagnostic interventions' accuracy (in assigning correctly patients to diagnostic categories) is also a source of such variation. For any given diagnostic category, research could produce solid information on outcomes with and without specific interventions. Given the magnitude of possible diagnostic classifications and their lack of standardisation, it is not surprising that little such specific patient outcome data exists. Generating good patient outcome data requires, among other things, distinct diagnostic classifications.

Doctors diagnose patients' problems (i.e. place them into a particular diagnostic category) based on their symptoms (patient complaints or history information that doctors gather by questioning patients), signs (physical information that doctors elicit by examining patients), and signals (information that laboratory, imaging and diagnostic tests reveal about patients). Rarely is any one type or piece of information sufficient to tell what is wrong with a patient. Diagnosis is complex and results implicitly, if not preferably explicitly, in classifying the patient according to medical (e.g. disease, stage) and sociodemographic factors (e.g. age, living arrangements). The term 'medical diagnosis' refers to classification according to medical factors; patient diagnosis, to all factors, including sociodemographic variables and patient preferences.

247.34 MEDICAL FACTORS

Medical factors consist of:

- disease, classified by:
  —derangement, for example, cell mechanism, organ system;
  —producer, for example, pathogenic organism, chemical, physical force;
  —recognisable characteristic diagnostic manifestations.
- disease stage;
- previous therapies;
- comorbidities.[10]

247.341 Disease

Disease refers to any departure from health—the ability to function in society as one desires (or, more practically, as other members of one's cohort). If one considers health and normal physiology to be synonymous, disease represents deranged physiology. Physiology refers to a person's vital physical and mental processes, which are predicated on specific structures. Thus health is the outcome of normal (in contrast to deranged) physiology. Here normal is used in a static (not dynamic) sense. In one view, ageing represents an undesirable derangement of physiology since it detracts from one's ability to function as one desires. If ageing is accepted as a normal process, then the correct comparison is with persons of the same age. Thus an 85-year-old man's physiology would be compared with others in his birth cohort (most of whom would be dead) rather than with that of a

20-year-old man. Thus ultimately health is defined relatively, either by desired or expected functional abilities.

Deranged physiology may be produced by the patient's genetic make-up or such environmental factors as pathogenic organisms, chemicals, absorption of energy resulting in injury, or their interaction, and result in various characteristic diagnostic manifestations. Patients may vary in their physical, mental and emotional reactions to these manifestations. Hence the resultant symptoms, signs and signals may vary. Thus patients' ability to function and their behaviour, including decisions to seek care, are influenced not only by the deranged physiology and its producers but also by their reactions and responses to its manifestations which themselves are mediated by genetic make-up, experience and such environmental variables as culture (and the interactions among these factors).

247.342 Disease stage
Disease stage represents a recognisable place in a temporal journey from health to death along a defined route. For example, a disease's natural history may be divided into two or more stages. This concept is best known in oncology, but has now been applied to all diseases.[11] Stage also implies irreversibility: having progressed from stage I to stage II one can never again be labelled stage I.

247.343 Previous therapies
The prognosis for a treated stage II patient may be the same as an untreated stage I case, but the patient has not reverted to 'stage I'. Rather, the patient has progressed to stage II treated 'X' months ago with intervention 'A'. Thus previous therapy is another important diagnostic classification axis and includes the patient's response to therapy.

247.344 Comorbidities
So far we have discussed, implicitly, a single or 'uncomplicated' disease. Often patients have (at least what appear to be) several diseases. At any given point, for example, care episode, attention focuses on one of these disease entities; the rest are referred to as comorbidities. Each disease (focal and comorbidities) may be classified by: disease (derangement, producers, manifestations); stage; and previous therapies. Specific combinations of diseases, more precisely including their stages and previous therapies, may represent unique medical diagnostic categories for purposes of prognosis and selection of therapeutic intervention.

247.35 SOCIODEMOGRAPHIC FACTORS AND PATIENT PREFERENCES
Doctors must also classify patients by sociodemographic and any other variables that influence outcomes or treatment selection. Such variables could include, for example, age, income, living arrangements, personality type, and financial means including health insurance coverage. Clearly, patient preferences influence treatment selection and represent the ultimate factor for classifying patients into diagnostic categories. In some cases, patients' preferences for risks and benefits may affect their choice of diagnostic interventions, affecting diagnostic outcomes, the accuracy with which they can be placed into medical diagnostic categories and thus subsequently their therapeutic outcomes.

247.36 RESULTANT DIAGNOSTIC CATEGORIES
In principle, the number of categories to which a patient could be assigned is vast, even if finite. In practice, by focusing on factors affecting patient outcomes and selection among alternative treatments, their number may be quite small in some cases; more extensive in others. The number of diagnostic categories for treatment selection purposes is always less than or the same as that relevant to patient outcomes. For example, there may be only one or two treatments believed to be effective for a given disease (the major

diagnostic classification axis). For each treatment that is appropriate for a given group of patients, however, there may be—and usually are—subgroups of patients who experience different outcomes (amount of health status improvement). Thus for purposes of categorising patients with respect to outcomes (e.g. to adjust for case-mix) there are more relevant diagnostic categories than those required for treatment selection purposes. If there are many alternative treatments, each of which affects differentially distinct subgroups of patients, the outcomes for some subgroup–treatment combinations may be virtually identical.

247.37 OUTCOME OF DIAGNOSTIC INTERVENTIONS

Functionally, the outcome of diagnostic interventions, including clinicians' inferences based on them, results in patients' categorisation for treatment selection purposes. A clinician's diagnosis may be correct or it may not be. For example, the patient may be classified as having a certain disease, 'A', that requires a specific treatment, 'X', for maximal health status improvement which carries a certain risk. If the patient does not have disease 'A' (false positive), and treatment 'X' does not help his or her condition, the intervention can only prove harmful (since the patient could not possibly benefit from it). Receiving treatment 'X' precludes the patient from realising the health improvement he or she might otherwise have realised if he or she had received the appropriate treatment. Any group of patients treated for a specific disease may include those who truly have the disease and some who do not, the proportion varying by disease and by provider.

If the patient is classified as not having the disease, when in fact he or she does have it (false negative), he or she may receive no—or the wrong—treatment, impairing his or her health status. Patient outcome—health status improvement—depends not only on correct categorisation (and subsequent treatment), but also on the health risk inherent in diagnostic (and therapeutic) intervention. Patients can, and do, die while being investigated. These patients never realise whatever benefits treatment may have brought them.

All intervention carries some risk. Thus for quality management purposes the fewest, least risky (and least costly) diagnostic interventions should be applied (in the optimal order to maximise information gained while minimising risk and cost, and the time needed to reach a diagnosis) to categorise a patient correctly with some specified level of certainty. Such specification is often difficult (because of lack of the requisite information), and made more difficult if delays in diagnosis may result in health status loss. Generally, the quicker the clinician makes the diagnosis the better. However, various trade-offs may exist, for example, among speed, accuracy, risk and cost. The following section, on therapeutic interventions, assumes that the patient has the disease for which the intervention is an appropriate therapy.

247.38 ABOUT CASE-MIX

Case-mix is the proportion of patients of different diagnostic categories that a provider treats. Case-mix can affect a provider's aggregate patient outcomes or costs. Oncologists, for example, who treat only patients with advanced disease can expect more of their patients to die within one year of treatment than doctors who treat mostly patients with early-onset cancer. Obviously, comparing outcomes without adjusting for patient characteristics can lead to erroneous impressions about the quality of providers' care or its costs. Subsequent chapters in this part address this problem for purposes of assessing and measuring the quality of care.

247.4 | Intervention variables—treatment

247.41 ABOUT THERAPEUTIC INTERVENTIONS

Having assigned the patient to a specific diagnostic category, the doctor can assist the patient to select among alternative interventions. In helping patients to select among alternatives, doctors must elicit the patient's preferences for ends (e.g. adding years to life or life to years), means (e.g. surgical versus medical intervention), and their inter-relationships (e.g. distribution of benefits and risks). The alternatives may be many or few, depending on the diagnosis and the patient's preferences.

The alternatives available to a clinician may be a subset of all possible alternatives and be predicated on his or her training or such other factors as availability of equipment or services. Surgeons, for example, may favour surgery while internists may favour other interventions. Such preferences would not matter if the interventions produced the same patient outcomes. Practice style, or technically permissible practice variation, refers to favouring one set of interventions over another when patient outcomes of all sets are essentially equal. However, they may persist even if the outcomes are unequal because the doctor is skilled only in one set of alternatives. Where an alternative in which the doctor is not skilled is clearly indicated, the doctor might refer the patient to a surgeon, for example, where such referral is practical and in the patient's best interest.

247.42 THERAPEUTIC REGIMENS

A therapeutic intervention comprises two parts: a technology and its delivery mechanism. The technology is the active ingredient that produces the desired effect. In some cases, for example antibiotics, the delivery mechanism influences outcomes relatively little and is separable from it. In others, the delivery mechanism is the technology, for example psychotherapy. Interventions have general and specific effects. All interventions possess a general effect to some degree, referred to usually as the placebo effect. It is greatest when both doctor and patient believe in the intervention (whether or not it is effective), perhaps because the doctor's confidence rubs off on the patient. An intervention's specific effects (those beyond the placebo effect) define its effectiveness, the extent to which it improves patients' health status independent of doctors' and patients' beliefs and desires. Some interventions' effectiveness, for example surgery, is little or not at all influenced by external factors, for example patient behaviour. Others, for example drug regimens, are greatly influenced by such factors as the patient's willingness to take the drug as pre-scribed. Chapter 3 in this part explores these issues.

Patients' therapy may, and usually does, consist of multiple interventions, each implemented in a prescribed manner in a particular sequence, and/or repetitions of the same intervention with prescribed intervals between them. Interventions may vary in intensity and interval. Intensity is a product of dose (dose rate times duration) and number of repetitions of the dose within the intervention. Interval refers to the period between interventions' application. These concepts may be most familiar with radiation or drug therapy but also apply to psychotherapy, for example (frequency, duration and number of sessions, and their periodicity). Therapeutic regimen refers to a particular permutation of interventions and their specific implementation characteristics (referred to sometimes as a clinical pathway).

247.43 RESULTANT THERAPEUTIC CATEGORIES

For any disease there may be several alternative therapies, such as medical or surgical treatment. Further, for any therapy there may be different regimens, even if it involves only one type of intervention (e.g. radiotherapy) because what is done exactly and how it is done may vary. Thus patients' treatments may represent a vast number of therapeutic categories. Practically, one would be interested in grouping such classifications into a limited number based on their effect or outcome (for given types of patients). Nevertheless, the potentially large number of relevant therapeutic possibilities, especially when coupled with the large number of relevant diagnostic categories, makes evaluating therapeutic effectiveness quite difficult. Moreover, implementation of each regimen may produce various outcomes, the result of patient behaviour for example, which the intervention may influence in part. Some people may be disinclined to take medication, a tendency that a drug that causes nausea in a large proportion of patients might reinforce, for example.

247.44 THERAPEUTIC OUTCOMES

Given that a patient has selected the best regimen, his or her outcome—patient health status improvement—depends on the skill of the doctor and other providers (and their interaction) in implementing interventions. For example surgeons who often perform a given procedure may perform the procedure better than those performing it infrequently. Further, some hospitals may offer better support, for example nursing care, than others, or doctors may behave differently when working in different hospitals, resulting in different outcomes to seemingly similar patients, even if operated on by the same surgeon. Therapeutic outcomes observed in practice often vary substantially—the result of doctors' ability to diagnose patients, doctors' ability to assist patients select the best therapeutic regimen, providers' ability to implement properly chosen interventions, and patients' preferences for ends and means and their willingness to adhere to treatments, as well as the environment in which provider–patient interaction takes place. Sorting out these variable effects on—and hence improving—patient outcomes is very difficult, as this chapter attempts to explain.

247.5 | Environmental variables

The environment is the cultural milieu in which diagnosis and treatment take place and in which the patient lives, and may be local and largely tangible (the patient's neighbourhood environment) or national and largely intangible (*Zeitgeist*).

Environmental variables may be very important in understanding outcomes. In some cases their impact may be reflected in the patient's diagnostic classification. For example, the health outcomes of an intervention may depend on income. Thus patients may be classified according to income for purposes of selecting therapy or adjusting outcomes. In other cases their impact cannot be reflected in patient classification and some other type of adjustment is necessary. For example, if employment is an outcome of interest, an area's unemployment rate for the type of patient (e.g. diagnostic classification by occupation) may be a more important determinant of outcome than the intervention. Similarly, the type and extent of air pollution may be a determinant of the outcome of therapies for respiratory ailments. A treatment that worked in one era or area, for example for preventing drug abuse, may not work in another because it depends on the cultural milieu, for example people's beliefs and values.

In assessing interventions' effectiveness, one must either assume that environment variables have little or no effect on patient outcomes or, if they do, that they influence alternatives equally. When this is clearly not the case, adjustment must be made for the fact that interventions took place in environments that affected outcomes differentially. Such adjustments may be needed in either concurrent or historical comparisons of effectiveness. The principle of compensating for environmental variables parallels that for patient variables. For quality management purposes, one must always bear in mind the possibility that outcomes may be attributable partly to environmental variables, or more to the point, their interactions with patient and production variables.

248 | Health production systems

248.1 | The concept of a health production system

The hospital is a health production system. It intends to improve patients' health status. Production systems consist of multiple production processes linked in space-time. Figure II-4-2 on page 205 illustrates this idea. It shows that a health production system (the totality of relevant care processes) consists of a number of linked subprocesses (each depicted in Figure II-4-2 in the manner of Figure II-4-1. See pages 205 and 203.). Each production process may be a production subsystem consisting of multiple process elements. The outcome of one process is an input into the next or a subsequent process. The patient passes through the various subprocesses to emerge transformed, that is, the patient's postprocess health status is greater than it would have been otherwise and, ideally, this improvement is the maximum achievable with existing technology (referred to sometimes as achievable health status improvement or as achievable benefit).

Figure II-4-2 on page 205 shows a patient passing through three processes to illustrate simply what are often very complex production systems. The depicted processes are, in chronological order: initial consultation (a history and physical examination); diagnosis and treatment selection; and surgical operation and postsurgical care. Another process, diagnostic testing (imaging, laboratory tests), is connected to the patient's course by broken lines. This indicates that a specimen, for example, is sent to the laboratory for analysis. The resultant information enters the treatment selection process. The laboratory is a production subsystem.

The outcomes of one process affect those of others and, consequently, the system's performance, the extent to which it improves patients' health status. For example, the quality (validity) of test results affects the output of the treatment selection process. Controlling the quality of laboratory tests (and all other process elements) is obviously essential to maximise patients' health status improvement. For example, if the pathologist misreads a biopsy slide, the surgeon may misdiagnose the patient's condition and select an inappropriate treatment.

Given good information, the surgeon's diagnosis may be correct but he or she may select an inappropriate treatment. Even if he or she selects the appropriate operation, the surgeon may implement it poorly or his or her postsurgical patient management may be inadequate. The surgical team's skill in carrying out the operation and the postoperative care the patient receives obviously affect the patient's outcome. No matter how good the team and the care, if the surgeon chose an inappropriate operation the patient's health status would not be improved as much as if he or she performed the appropriate one, and may well be worsened.

While the surgeon's role is obviously important to the patient's outcome, he or she is only one of many production elements and other factors coproducing patient outcomes. A perfect surgeon working alone cannot produce perfect outcomes. The surgeon's interactions with the patient, other production elements, and their environment coproduce outcomes. For example, a surgeon operating on an important person admitted to the private patient wing of a prestigious university hospital may subconsciously pay greater attention to detail than if he or she were operating on a skid-row alcoholic admitted to a run-down city hospital, and this difference in attention itself may affect outcomes (not to mention the myriad differences in other variables).

Various eventualities may diminish the amount of achievable patient health status improvement achieved in practice. To realise achievable health status improvement, all processes must be performed within acceptable limits. These limits may be sharp boundaries, binary conditions: black or white, not shades of grey. For example, diagnosing the patient's lesion as cancerous when it is not, or vice versa, may trigger certain processes that lead to serious, not trivial, health status loss when compared to that which might have been realised if the diagnosis had been correct.

248.2 Systems' boundaries for quality management purposes

Health production systems are often conceptual rather than managed entities. One might imagine that all of the care depicted in Figure II-4-2 (see page 205) was conducted in a hospital under its manager's control. While in some instances this situation might pertain, usually it does not. The hospital admission may account for only part of the final process (surgical operation and postoperative care). The doctor might have first seen the patient in his or her surgery. An independent laboratory may have performed diagnostic tests. Once the surgeon had made the diagnosis, he or she may then have admitted the patient to hospital for an elective surgical operation. Subsequent follow-up might again have been in the doctor's surgery or in a convalescent facility. The patient's long-term outcomes—the only ones that matter in the long run—depend on picking paths among alternative interventions, and providers' performance in implementing chosen interventions. For quality management purposes, what are the appropriate boundaries of care processes?

To be held accountable for patient outcomes, managers (people whom an organisation's stakeholders or society deem accountable for outcomes) must be able to meaningfully control production systems' design and processes' implementation. A hospital, for example, must be able to decide what gets done within its walls, who does it and how, and when and where they do it. This requirement does not imply that the hospital manager dictates these decisions (most of which he or she is likely incapable of making successfully), but rather that the organisation has successfully institutionalised processes for informing, making and implementing them. Hospitals are usually only elements in health production systems, and patients' health status improvement depends on elements beyond their control. To improve quality, society must give hospitals or some other entity, for example, an accountable health plan (see Chapter 3 in this part), the responsibility and authority to manage quality, and hold it accountable for results. Alternatively, where multiple providers exist, the patient and/or his or her designated agent (e.g. primary care practitioner) may choose among them. Such choices require that society empower patients to make them, and mandate that providers disclose relevant, valid information to permit, and in a form that permits, patients or their agent to choose rationally. Patients' choices, based on providers' published performance and other relevant factors, would drive providers toward satisfying patients' desires and presumably improve the quality of care. Without one or the other, or some effective combination of both alternatives, meaningful quality improvement is simply not possible. Consider the following examples.

In the example illustrated by Figure II-4-2 (see page 205), the hospital's assessment of the quality of the patient's care—if done at all—would usually be limited to examining the documentation relating to the hospital episode. While the hospital record may indicate something of the prehospital history, physical examination and diagnostic tests, it would have told nothing about the patient's posthospital course. To improve the quality of care, hospitals must examine the continuum of care, not only isolated episodes.

Suppose that postdischarge the patient suffers wound dehiscence, for which the patient was readmitted. An examination of the two episodes individually might reveal that in each case care seemed to be excellent. In the first episode, the patient had been diagnosed correctly, the selected treatment was appropriate, and the patient's post-operative course was recorded as uneventful. In the second episode, the dehiscence was treated appropriately and the patient discharged home. Viewing each episode in isolation, the hospital may never improve the quality of its care. Only by linking episodes, examining the frequency of complications, deciding whether or not they could have been avoided, and taking the steps necessary to avoid them, can the hospital improve the quality of its care.

The hospital may be concerned only with the care given within its own walls; however, the patient's admission might have resulted from inadequate outpatient management. Further, for example, the hospital's neurosurgeon may have performed a flawless lumbar laminectomy on a patient referred to him or her for this procedure. However, if the surgeon had inquired they would have discovered that the patient had not been given an adequate course of conservative therapy, which, if he or she had received it, might have obviated the need for the operation. To discharge its responsibility to provide high quality care, hospitals should insist that their medical staffs undertake only procedures that are indicated medically and documented as such. Hospitals, and not just doctors, produce patient outcomes.

In conducting quality management activities, hospitals must be concerned with the continuum of care processes that produce ultimate health outcomes for patients, and not confine themselves to the examination of isolated episodes conducted within their walls. To improve the quality of care, quality assessment and improvement activities must include all relevant health production systems processes. The hospital, with its great concentration of resources, is the plan's logical locus for such assessment and, therefore, the centre of quality improvement efforts. Importantly, hospitals must measure long-term outcomes and relate them to prior processes. If hospitals do not undertake their responsibilities to assess quality and measure long-term outcomes, the community must create other entities to perform these tasks.

Identifying quality of care problems does not lead automatically to their resolution. Ultimately, to improve production quality—not to mention system quality—someone must be responsible for managing the health production system, even if it is not contained within a single organisational or legal entity. Historically, this role has generally gone unfilled or has been played to some extent by government, either because there was no other alternative or because government paid for patients' care. Health insurers, self-insured employers or health care purchasing agencies acting for their members, for example, could fulfil this role. They would not be passive players but active actors. They would be responsible for creating and managing health production systems fashioned from existing care facilities, for example general practitioners, hospitals and nursing homes (in the manner of an accountable health plan described in Chapter 3 of this part). Importantly, they would be responsible both for the quality of care and for its cost. Thus they, acting for their members, would be responsible for and in a position to make any trade-offs between quality and cost. These health care providers would be responsible for quality management and overseeing the quality management activities of the system's various elements. The quality management policies, plans and programs of particular health production systems would guide those of each of the system's elements, such as hospitals.

248.3 Flows of patients through health production systems

One can envision a flow of patients arriving at the hospital, or health production system, to be sorted into diagnostic categories, treated, discharged and followed-up. One can also envision one or more paths, or even a unique path, for each patient that would result in the achievement of achievable health status improvement. The term case management refers to picking paths among available alternatives. The term continuity of care refers to the surety and ease with which patients flow through the health production system during an episode or continuum of care. A patient's care may deviate from an ideal path in any number of ways for any number of reasons, reducing the patient's health status improvement from what it might otherwise have been. These flows of patients produce streams of patient outcomes, health status improvement. Longitudinal case management intends to manage patients as they flow through the health care system toward maximising patient health status improvement while minimising the cost of its attainment.

248.4 Design and evaluation of health production systems

Quality management, in its broadest sense, involves the design and evaluation of health production systems and their efficient operation. It therefore involves the design and operation of health production facilities, such as hospitals, and their interrelationships, such as patient and information flows among facilities. Further, it involves the design and evaluation of health care processes that take place within and, when relevant, outside of hospitals and other production facilities. These processes encompass specific medical interventions, for example coronary artery bypass grafts and the context (e.g. who, where and when) in which they are carried out. They are the technologies that constitute health production systems' core production processes.

Traditional quality assurance activities have focused narrowly on doctors' clinical activities. For simplicity, this manual focuses primarily on the technical quality of clinical care (provider performance). We have chosen to exclude operational aspects of health production, such as the design of hospitals and of patient flows, because until now doctors—and even hospital managers—have rarely perceived these subjects to be part of their central concern, and because the additional material would likely both detract from the manual's central purpose and overwhelm the reader.

Design presupposes evaluation. Designing new and redesigning established health care processes (practice policies and production systems to implement them) involves selecting from among available interventions and contexts those that are known or assumed to maximise patients' health status improvement (outcomes). Evaluating existing and experimental (alternative) processes involves attributing observed health status improvement (outcomes) to preceding interventions and their inputs (patients) and environment. By evaluating outcomes of alternative designs we can know their effects and select among designs to achieve desired outcomes. Only through scientific evaluation can one produce the certain knowledge necessary to (re)design health production systems to improve achievable health status improvement and to raise the level that is achievable. Increasingly, quality managers must undertake or at least supervise or participate in these endeavours if they are to improve continuously the quality of care, and must possess a working knowledge of them.

Quality managers must be concerned with both design and evaluation. They must know to what extent and with what variance existing designs produce health status improvement in comparison to what is possible, how to close any evident gap, and how to monitor the effectiveness of their (re)designs of processes. They must recognise when additional research is needed to improve medical technology, to break through current limits on what is achievable, set priorities for its conduct, evaluate the validity of results, and disseminate valid results (transfer technology) for use in practice. Quality managers must also be concerned with research to develop better ways to fund, conduct and use the results of health systems research. They must improve their access to relevant information and methods for evaluating its validity for their purposes. For the foreseeable future, quality management in hospitals is likely to be concerned mostly with improving achievable health status improvement; incidentally with raising the level of what is achievable; and peripherally with research to improve research and development.

248.5 | From design goal to design practice

Health care's purpose is to improve maximally patients' health status, using interventions consistent with their preferences, provider's circumstances and society's resources and mores. Assume the task is to restore a sick patient to health: a young woman with stage II breast cancer, for example. We might interpret our task as giving the young woman the same health status expectation as enjoyed by the average woman of her age, or as close as we can get: no mean feat. What should we do? How should we do it? What treatment modalities, for example surgery, radiotherapy, chemotherapy, would we choose? In what order? If we choose to incorporate chemotherapy in our treatment regimen, what mix of drugs would we use? In what dosages, for what durations, with what intervals between them? When should we consider high-dose chemotherapy with stem cell rescue through bone marrow transplantation, for example, with its attendant high risks and high costs. How would we monitor progress? How would adjustments be made? The questions are virtually endless, as are the therapeutic alternatives. Which regimen would produce the best outcomes, even assuming all patients were homogenous with respect to factors affecting outcomes, which they likely are not? No one possesses certain answers to these questions. What about patients' preferences for risks and benefits? They are paramount and affect the selection of diagnostic and therapeutic interventions.

Quality managers in concert with clinicians—who design practice policies—must decide these types of issues, based on knowledge or assumptions about the relationships between processes and outcomes, available resources, sociopolitical constraints, and a host of other factors, including designers' perspectives and decision makers' values. An actual production system is only one of multiple (often virtually infinite) alternative designs for improving patients' health status (its purpose). From a given perspective, alternative designs may differ in their effectiveness or efficiency in achieving the system's purpose or producing desired outcomes. As system inputs or the environment change, a different design may become the most effective or efficient. Design must be dynamic. Expected or experienced unintended negative outcomes beg ameliorative policies or system redesign.

One rarely encounters this abstract situation. Firstly, many people and groups are often involved. Coherence, and quality, may suffer. We are all familiar with the camel as a horse built by a committee. Secondly, designers rarely have the opportunity to start with a clean slate. Rather, they are usually faced with incremental redesign of processes to effect improvement in performance. There are limits to the improvement that can be achieved within such design constraints. Thirdly, products and production systems may not be the product of conscious technical designs intended to achieve maximally specified objectives. Rather, existing ways of doing things are often the product of sociopolitical evolution whose raison d'etre has been lost in antiquity or may no longer be relevant. Nevertheless, attempts to change them may invoke stiff resistance.

Where is a quality manager to start? There are two logical starting points: process and outcome. One strategy is to design the best possible process, implement and then refine it. This approach assumes that everyone involved believes that the process needs to be improved. Alternatively, one can start by measuring outcomes—variability in processes and/or patient outcomes—as a means of convincing people that improvement is needed and where it might be possible to achieve it.

248.6 | Process design

Product and production designs should prevent quality problems from arising (referred to sometimes as quality planning). Ideally, the quality manager starts by guiding medical practitioners and other health professionals to specify optimal practices in practice policies, and production systems to implement them. His or her next task is to measure

in practice. Such observed patient outcomes as mortality rates, for example, cannot be used directly (unless measured in patients known to be homogeneous with respect to this particular outcome); they must first be validly risk-adjusted, which is rarely, if ever, possible (for reasons detailed elsewhere in this part).

Quality management's principal goal is to increase average health status improvement for given types of patients and to reduce variation in this outcome. Quality managers can achieve this goal in practice by:

- measuring the extent of conformance to product and production specifications (processes)—which represents achievable benefit achieved (outcomes)—to know the shape of the curve;
- improving conformance to processes—including removing underperforming providers who prove to be incapable of improving their performance despite the hospital's best efforts to help them to do so—to shift the curve to the right;
- improving product and production specifications—to lift the curve to the right.

These concepts—no matter how complex they may appear—are simple compared to putting then into practice. Improving the quality of care is a difficult undertaking. However, by applying the principles and practices outlined in this manual, hospitals can progress toward quality maturity. Chapter 8 in this part elaborates on the ways in which quality managers can improve the quality of hospitals' care.

249.7 Variation analyses are means not ends

Health status improvement is the central measure of provider performance. Increasing average, and reducing variation in, health status improvement achieved for patients of a given type—or the fraction of achievable health benefit achieved (shifting the curve to the right) or benefit that is achievable (lifting the curve to the right) for patients generally—is quality management's central objective. Graphs such as that depicted in Figure II-4-5 show distributions of provider performance—results of production systems actions—explicit or implicit practice policies and their implementing production processes. Performance results from production processes—action and interactions. Quality managers can only change the shape of the curve (the statistical distribution of results of patient–provider interactions that comprise the relevant population of quality measurements) by encouraging, facilitating, or making changes to products and production processes—including the behaviour of individual practitioners who are instrumental in effecting them. Statistical analyses will not result in quality improvement. Showing providers graphs will not result in quality improvement. Slogans to shift the curve to the right to improve average practitioners' performance (rather than emphasis on 'weeding out bad apples') will not result in quality improvement. This essential fact seems to escape many people concerned with quality improvement.

Quality managers must institutionalise mechanisms to assess quality systematically, provide feedback to change products and production processes, and above all, provide the means to change them. The longest journey begins with the first step. Variation analysis may be that all-important first step in the long and arduous journey toward systematic quality improvement. But its completion requires many additional steps. Effective quality management requires preparation to undertake this journey and institutionalising and operationalising the means to take them. They are this manual's focus.

249.7 Priorities and strategies

Many health care quality gurus view quality management's main goal as shifting the curve to the right (motivated by evidence-based benchmarking, for example). Others think that conformance to product and production specifications is the best first step because it focuses attention on specifying quality, avoids the need for and pitfalls of interhospital performance comparisons, and leaves benchmarking until the hospital has become a quality-focused organisation that has operationalised all of the mechanisms necessary for systematic continuous quality improvement. Some would place equal emphasis on reducing variation (in conformance to product and production specification and hence expected outcomes)—at least within a given facility—to reduce patients' risk of experiencing substandard care, and promoting further quality improvement. We think that hospitals should attempt to achieve all of these objectives as expeditiously as possible. See Chapter 8 in this part and Part III.

References

1 Churchman CW. The design of inquiring systems: Basic concepts of systems and organisation. New York: Basic Books, 1971.

2 Ackoff RL, Emery FE. On purposeful systems. Chicago: Aldine-Atherton, 1972.

3 Macmahon B, Pugh TF. Epidemiology: Principles and methods. Boston, Little, Brown and Company, 1970.

4 Kuhn T. The structure of scientific revolutions. Chicago: University of Chicago Press, 1970.

5 Lewin R. Complexity: Life at the edge of chaos. New York: Macmillan Publishing Company, 1992.

6 Gleick J. Chaos: Making a new science. New York: Penguin, 1987.

7 Goldschmidt PG. Cost-effectiveness model for evaluating health care programs; application to a drug abuse treatment. Inquiry 1976;13:29–47.

8 Goldschmidt PG. A model for measuring the cost-effectiveness of treatment programs. Baltimore: Dissertation for the degree of Doctor of Public Health, The Johns Hopkins University, School of Hygiene and Public Health, 1979.

9 Williamson JW, Goldschmidt PG, Jillson IA. Medical Practice Information Demonstration Project: Final Report. Baltimore: Policy Research Incorporated, 1979.

10 Goldschmidt PG. Severity of illness: Red herring or horse of a different color? Part 1. Physician Executive 1989; 15(4):7–11.

11 Gonnella JS, Hornbrook MC, Louis DZ. Staging of disease: A case-mix measurement. JAMA 1984; 251: 637–44.

12 Wennberg JE, Mulley AG, Jr, Hanley D, et al. An assessment of prostatectomy for benign urinary tract obstruction; geographic variations and the evaluation of medical care outcomes. JAMA 1988; 259:3027–30.

13 Leape LL, Park RE, Solomon DH, et al. Does inappropriate use explain small-area variations in the use of health care services? JAMA 1990; 263(5): 669–72.

14 Restuccia, J, Schwarz M, Ash A, Payne S. An empirical analysis of the relationship between small area variation analysis in hospital admission rates and appropriateness of admission. Paper presented at the Association for Health Services Research Annual Meeting, San Diego, 1994.

Chapter 5

QUALITY AND ITS MEASUREMENT

| 251 | **Purpose of this chapter** |

Quality is an elusive concept, especially when applied to health care. Yet to improve quality one must first measure it; to measure quality one must first define it. Practically, quality is defined by how it is measured. Some people claim that health care quality cannot be defined in measurable terms. It can. Others believe that while in principle health care quality can be measured, in practice it is quite impossible—or at least impractical—to do so. It is now also practical. Recent breakthroughs in quality management concepts and technology, described in this chapter, mean that health care quality can be quantified and, for the first time, health care can be improved systematically.

Three principal developments have made the measurement of health care quality practical. They are: advances in health care quality management concepts; knowledge engineering; and computer technology. Advances in concepts provide the foundation for a breakthrough in quality management technology. Advances in knowledge engineering allow these concepts to be embodied in expert systems. Advances in computer technology provide sufficient computing power at low enough cost to implement these systems. The result is practical quality measurement and assessment systems, those capable of quantifying provider performance.

Much of people's confusion about quality—and quality improvement—stems from differences in their definition of quality. Indeed, there seem to be as many definitions of quality as there are quality gurus. Current notions of quality originated in industry and some of them have little applicability to health care, compounding health care providers' confusion. This chapter defines quality and describes how it can be measured for quality management purposes, setting the stage for subsequent chapters that describe quality assurance and improvement. This chapter describes:

- the dimensions of quality;
- the concept of health care quality;
- how health care quality can be assessed and measured for quality management purposes, a prerequisite for its improvement.

Doctors and other health care workers might be tempted to skip over the section on industrial analogies, thinking that it does not have much to do with them. In one sense they would be quite right; in another, quite wrong. Health care is different from manufacturing—the type of industry with the most experience and the most success in systematic quality improvement. The section provides important information toward understanding some of the basic concepts underlying quality improvement—in industry and in health care—and its evolution in industry, to provide a context for the rest of this part and the current debate that is raging about how industrial techniques can (or cannot) be used to improve the quality of health care.

252 | Key concepts

This chapter elaborates on the following key concepts essential to understanding quality and its measurement generally, and in health care particularly:

- To improve quality one must first measure it. To measure quality one must first define it. Quality is defined by how it is measured.
- Recent breakthroughs in quality measurement technology—described in this chapter—permit, for the first time, quantification and systematic improvement of health care quality.
- Much of people's confusion about quality—and quality improvement—stems from differences in their definition of quality. In industry, one accepted definition is fitness for use: defect-free and meeting customers' primary functional needs.
- Producing products right the first time and every time saves money. This focus gave rise to the idea that high quality costs less than poor quality. In reality, the functional quality of a defect-free product remains unchanged.
- Functional quality requires defining products' essential attributes of interest to customers, who can compare the extent to which different manufacturers' products meet them, to create an overall quality score. Products that more perfectly meet customers' needs may, but do not invariably, cost more than those with lesser functionality. This focus gave rise to the idea that high quality costs more than poor quality and that trade-offs are inevitable.
- Quality is ultimately a judgment that customers make about a product's value for money: a higher quality product provides more value for the same money or the same value for less money or, best of all, more value for less money.
- Measuring quality is a matter of statistics. Manufacturers can improve quality by producing a greater proportion of products to specifications and by

reducing variance. In industry, variance reduction is both ends and means to quality improvement.

• For any dimension of health care quality, one must distinguish between system-level quality (the quality of the health care system) and production-level quality (provider performance). Access to care, for example, which affects people's health status, must be a concern at the system level but it is irrelevant at the production level.

• For quality management purposes, health care quality (provider performance) has four dimensions:
  —technical quality (measured by patients' health status improvement);
  —resource consumption (measured by the cost of care);
  —patient satisfaction (measured by patients' perceptions of the subjective or interpersonal aspects of care);
  —values (measured by the acceptability of any trade-offs that must be made among the three previous outcomes).

• For all practical purposes, quality refers to conformance to care processes that result in maximum achievable patient health status improvement within patients' preferences and society's resources. Practice policies are the starting point for defining these processes and their expected resultant outcomes.

• Quality measurement refers to the process of quantifying the quality of a provider's entire output to produce a quality score, for example the proportion of cases treated appropriately to achieve achievable benefits (in much the same way as a factory's quality can be gauged by the proportion of its output that meets product specifications).

• Quality assessment refers to the process of examining a single episode or continuum of care, a unit of a provider's performance, to determine whether or not care was appropriate (in much the same way as a factory gauges whether or not an individual widget met product specifications), and to identify quality of care problems. Aggregating the results of individual quality assessments provides the means to quantify the quality of a provider's performance for all or particular types of patients.

• Quality assessment produces judgments about the fit between the care that patients needed to maximise their health status improvement and the care that they received. The goal is to reduce the variance in the fit between needed and implemented care processes, and in outcomes achieved consequently, and to reduce the variance in the implementation of appropriate care processes. It is not to provide to patients uniform processes irrespective of their needs and desires (which might well increase the variance in outcomes if process does not match patient).

• 'Peer review' is the traditional, but flawed, mainstay of quality of care assessment. It involves a doctor reviewing a colleague's work as documented in the patient's medical record. In Australia the term 'peer review' is ambiguous.

• Peer review's greatest strength is its central axiom: a properly qualified reviewer can review validly the appropriateness (quality) of care of any case within his or her domains of expertise. However, traditional medical peer review has a number of serious deficiencies.

• Structured quality review (SQR) overcomes the principal problems inherent in traditional peer review. Automated outcome/process assessment (OPA) screens permit cases to be reviewed objectively, comprehensively and economically for quality of care problems. Accurate screening allows care reviewers to focus on cases with potential problems and to know what those problems are that require review. Structured medical record review improves further the reliability of reviewers' judgments. Pattern (statistical) analysis of case-by-case assessments provides additional information about the distribution and nature of quality of care problems.

- Structured quality review is the most potent way to identify technical quality of care problems for purposes of quality improvement. Because it can be implemented easily, with minimal commitment of resources, structured quality review is likely to be the initial method for, and remain the mainstay of, quality assessment in Australian hospitals for the foreseeable future.

253 | Industrial analogies

253.1 | Quality management's view of quality

Quality is good; high quality is very good; low quality is, to say the least, not good. Thus the word 'quality' is often used to describe goodness. But what is it about quality that implies goodness? For quality management purposes, there is universal agreement that quality is ultimately a judgment that customers make. Further, the ultimate judgment is customers' perception of a product's value for money. Thus a higher quality product provides more value for the same money or the same value for less money or, best of all, more value for less money. The term 'product' covers any good or service and, increasingly, the distinction between a good and a service is being eroded as manufacturers strive to satisfy customers' expectations. These ideas raise several questions: Who is the customer? What is, and how do customers judge, value for money?

A customer is someone who buys a manufacturer's product. Clearly, those who buy the product believe that it will satisfy their needs or wants, whether or not experience bears out this expectation. Those who do not buy it believe that a competing product is better value for money, either in the simple sense that brand 'X' is better than brand 'Y', or that purchase of an entirely different product or service will yield greater satisfaction of needs or wants for the person's available resources. Thus no matter how high the quality of an automobile, if the person cannot afford to buy one, he or she will not become a customer. The rest of this section assumes that customers are people with some common set of needs or wants that manufacturers' products can satisfy to various extents and who can afford to buy their products, albeit to various degrees. Sometimes the person subject to the product is not the customer (i.e. does not purchase it), as in the case of a criminal incarcerated in a prison, for example.

With respect to quality, value can be conceived of as the extent to which a product meets some people's needs or wants. They are the product's potential customers. Manufacturers face the problem of discerning customers' desires and translating them into products that will delight them. Judging the extent to which a product will meet customers' expectations (needs and wants) can be tricky. Often customers rely on manufacturers' claims, in advertisements for example, or on other people's experience. However, in most cases customers can reasonably make these judgments before they buy, with the pointed exception of health care.

The term 'money' seems, but is not, self-evident. With respect to quality, it encompasses not only the price that one must pay to purchase the product, but also the cost of its acquisition and use. Thus, for example, if it costs a lot to maintain a particular automobile model, an alternative marque that is slightly more expensive to purchase but that requires far less maintenance might provide better value for money—expressed, for example, in terms of cost per transportation year or per kilometre (mile) travelled. Some readers may recognise these concepts as the essence of cost-effectiveness analysis. (See Chapter 3 in this part.)

There is a tendency to focus on the value aspect of quality at the exclusion of the cost of obtaining this value, especially in health care. Thus, for example, a new treatment that provides an incremental improvement in patients' health status at vast cost is often seen to have increased the quality of medical care. In one sense—patient health status improvement—it has. But it has also increased the cost of care, a quality-negative. Conversely, a new treatment that provides the same level of health status improvement as an existing treatment is not viewed in this same positive light. It should be. Quality management emphasises the customers' notion of value for money. Clearly, some people may value an effect so highly that they will pay virtually any price to achieve it. The reality remains, however, that the less it costs to satisfy one need the more resources are available to satisfy others. Thus quality and costs are intertwined inextricably.

253.2 | Industry's view of quality

In industry, where current notions of quality originated, there is no universal definition of quality. Quality can be viewed along different dimensions and at different levels. One accepted definition of quality is fitness for (customers') use. This idea gives rise to two distinct views of quality. One focuses on a product's defects (or more to the point, its lack thereof); the other focuses on a product's functions or its features. In reality, successful manufacturers produce products that meet specifications (without defects) and these specifications please customers. Further, they strive dynamically to perfect the fit between customers' ever-changing wants and their products.

253.3 | Focus on product defects

Early efforts to assure quality (and thus to improve it from the prevailing level) focused on producing a product to specifications—producing it right. Clearly, defective products have little hope of satisfying customers. Product inspections could identify defective subcomponents, components and final products, and thus avoid defective products being shipped to customers and engendering their dissatisfaction. However, not only did reliance on inspection increase manufacturing costs directly, but it also failed to avoid the indirect cost of rejects and rework, necessitated by repairing defective products. Further, inspection fails to detect all defectives.

Clearly, producing products right the first time and every time would save money—up to 30% or even more of manufacturing costs. With the introduction of quality control through such techniques as statistical process control, often associated with Edwards Deming, manufacturers could avoid wasted effort and increase product quality. Further, by paying attention to manufacturability when designing products, manufacturers could facilitate their error-free manufacture. Importantly, defects arise mostly from production processes—the system of manufacture—rather than from individual workers' performance. Similarly, improvements in meeting specifications came from changing production processes using the same (even if better trained)—not different—workers.

Measuring quality is a matter of statistics. The greater the proportion of products that meet specifications the better. In the recent past, reject rates of 2–3% were the norm. Manufacturers often applied statistical techniques to decide whether or not to accept entire deliveries of suppliers' components based on results of random samples of items in the shipment. Today, after the introduction of quality management methods, reject rates are measured in parts per millions and, depending on their production systems, may allow manufacturers to eliminate batch inspections.

Product specifications are often stated in statistical terms: a target product measurement, for example a widget with a length of 1 cm, and acceptable limits or tolerances, for example ± 0.02 cm. Any widget measuring 0.98–1.02 cm meets specifications. However, suppose measurement reveals that widgets meeting specifications are more or less equally distributed over this range, that is, about 25% of widgets measure 0.98–0.99 cm, 25% 0.99–1.00 cm, and so on. Widget quality could be improved by reducing this variance. If 75% (instead of 50%) of widgets measured 0.99–1.01 cm, they would be of higher quality, even if only 1% of them measured exactly 1.00 cm. Further, within limits, variance reduction is not dependent on meeting target specifications. If 90% of widgets measured 0.98–0.99 cm, they would be of still higher quality. Thus quality can be improved by producing a greater proportion of products to specifications and by reducing their variance.

This focus gave rise to the idea that quality was free, or could actually reduce manufacturing costs; that high quality was less costly than poor quality. Clearly, producing products right the first and every time could, and usually does, save money. However, while a higher proportion of products met specifications and quality increased in a statistical sense, the functional quality of a defect-free product remained unchanged. Customers would not be dissatisfied because of defects. The product met specifications; it did what its manufacturer said it would do. Whether or not it satisfied customers' needs and wants was quite another story.

253.4 | Focus on product functions and features

A product function is what a product does; its features, how it does it. Almost everyone is familiar with the development of VCRs (video cassette recorders). Early models were large, expensive and simply recorded off-the-air programs—their function. Later models added new functions such as recording from a video camera, and such features as programming recording times. These functions and features pleased customers but many people found features complex to work. The latest VCR models not only have more functions than earlier ones but their features are also much easier to use—improving their quality. Further, today's VCRs are much smaller and less expensive than the first models and their design is more appealing. Their quality has improved in all respects. They meet customers' expectations to a far greater extent and may even delight them. Of course, before SONY introduced the first VCR for home use, customers had few realistic expectations. Competition among manufacturers shaped customers' expectations for functions, features and price. Eventually, customers' preferences resulted in the VHS format becoming the standard, displacing SONY's beta format. Manufacturers shape customers' expectations and customers' preferences shape successful manufacturers' products. In competitive markets, manufacturers who refuse to listen to customers are displaced by those who do.

Manufacturers realised that the customer's voice must be heard in the product design stage and carried through to manufacturing processes on the shop floor. They achieved these ends through a process referred to sometimes as quality planning that used a variety of traditional and new techniques, such as market research and quality functional deployment (QFD). Use of such techniques enabled manufacturers to determine who were their customers and what functions and features they desired in their products, and to communicate product requirements to the people who would design and make them. Increasingly, manufacturers are realising that product price (and hence manufacturing cost) is an important design (i.e. quality) consideration.

Quality is defined operationally by how it is measured. Quality's measurement requires defining essential attributes of interest to the person who intends to use the results—the customer. One can then compare the quality—various relevant attributes— of different goods and services. One must weight the value of each attribute of a product (good or service) to derive an overall quality score. In selecting a product or service, one must compare performance on one attribute to that on others and make an integrated judgment. A person interested in an automobile, for example, may decide that appearance, comfort, engine economy, durability and ease of service are very important, while top speed, image and a host of other characteristics are less important. The customer assesses cars on the basis of these important characteristics and perhaps price, availability and financing. Admittedly, it is difficult for an individual to measure some of these important characteristics, for example durability. One has to rely on published reports of others' experience or, in the case of new models for example, extrapolate manufacturers' performance on past models. Nevertheless, with whatever information is at hand, the customer can, and does, select among alternative cars based on their actual or expected quality, and the extent to which the customer perceives the car meets his or her needs, wants and desires, given how much he or she can or is willing to spend.

The emphasis on features and functions may, but does not invariably, increase cost. Everyone will recognise that the Rolls Royce motor car is a standard of excellence. It has many fine functions and features but it also costs a great deal, far more than the average automobile. This focus gave rise to the idea that high quality costs more than poor quality and that trade-offs are inevitable. Certainly, manufacturers must make choices, for example about which customers to serve and which of their expectations to meet and at what price. There are no simple formulas that guarantee success, but manufacturers that produce products that meet or exceed customers' expectations, even at high prices, and those that offer acceptable products at low prices do better than those who produce average products at average prices (let alone unacceptable products at high prices). Clearly, winning companies produce high quality products at low prices. To achieve this level of performance with product after product—instead of producing a cheap flash in the pan—requires the self-improving structure that makes it possible on an ongoing basis to design products that more perfectly meet customers' expectations and produce them without defects. Chapter 2 in this part discusses these ideas of total quality management and continuous quality improvement.

253.5 Manufacturers' view of product quality

How do manufacturers perceive that customers gauge the quality of their products? Obviously there is no universal answer to this question. The goal is to produce a winning product, one that generates profits and/or gains significant market share by pleasing customers, meeting their needs, and offering what customers perceive to be good value for money. Among dimensions, other than price, considered important are the following: product performance; reliability; durability; serviceability; aesthetics; and image.[1]

Product performance encompasses the product's primary operating characteristics (what it does primarily that pleases the customer or satisfies his needs), secondary features (what else it does that is useful to the customer), and conformance (the degree to which performance meets established standards). Importantly, product flexibility or options—customer choices with respect to how features work—may be an important dimension of quality. Reliability is the probability of product failure occurring in a specified period; durability, the period of use before the product deteriorates beyond repair (or where failure or repair costs exceed replacement costs). Serviceability can be defined by the ease of repair if the product fails including, for the customer, time to effect and the cost of repair and experience with service people.

Aesthetics relates to how a product impacts the customer's senses—for example looks, feels, sounds—and encompasses feel-good engineering, for example the satisfaction a customer draws by the comforting substantial 'clunk' of a car door. Image refers to the status, prestige or similar satisfaction that customers draw from the product, its manufacturer or designer. Often image considerations, including the company's reputation for quality, are paramount. After all, who knows how long a timepiece you buy today will likely keep perfect time (unless the manufacturer, or better yet, independent testing laboratory, has published such data)? An expensive chronometer made by a prestigious Swiss company may be a better bet than a cheap no-name watch from a developing country. Products that rank high on all aspects of quality, the very best, are few and far between. They are also expensive: excellent quality is never cheap, but it can pay dividends for both purchaser and purveyor.

Customers can compare products on all of these dimensions as well as price, availability and other factors. Manufacturers try to influence customers' choices through advertising. While advertising can inform consumers and can even influence customers' perceptions about the product after purchase, ultimately the customers' experience with the product moulds his or her perceptions. Thus, for example, if an automobile buyer believes he or she was sold a lemon, a car that does not work properly, he or she is unlikely to want to rush out and buy another one from the same manufacturer. Swiss watch manufacturers' reputation for quality has been built over centuries by satisfied customers.

In stark contrast, patients have virtually no measurements of the quality of care to use in selecting among providers, and doctors have little information to select among interventions for their patients.

254 Health care quality

254.1 Overview

Patients seek health care in order to improve their health status and doctors may genuinely want to help them in their quest. However, until recently neither patients nor doctors could have any real idea about medical interventions' effectiveness or about the quality of their care. For most situations, doctors lacked the necessary technology even if they had the requisite desire. Only since the 1950s, with the widespread introduction of the randomised controlled trial, has it been possible to gauge an intervention's effectiveness. Only since the mid 1980s has it been possible to measure routinely at least some aspects of relevant providers' performance. Systems that are now emerging (described in this chapter) harbour the potential to bring about an order of magnitude improvement in the quality of health care through its meaningful measurement.

Health care's principal purpose is to maintain and improve patients' health status. To assure and improve health care quality, this functional product definition must be translated into product specifications. All quality assurance and improvement activities begin with quality assessment. Quality assessment begins with practice policies (or practice criteria derived from them) that state what should be done for particular types of patients to maximise achievable health status improvement within the patient's preferences and society's resources, and what should be achieved consequently. Historically, quality assessment depended on measuring individual structural, process and outcome variables and comparing results to standards or to norms. As explained in this section, an integrated—and far more sophisticated and useful—approach, to which we refer as outcome/process assessment, has replaced this simple, inadequate expedient.

Quality assessment produces judgments about the fit between the care that patients needed to maximise their health status improvement and the care that they received and how well it was rendered. The goal is to reduce firstly the variance in the fit between what is needed and implemented care processes and secondly the variance in the implementation of appropriate care processes—and hence to maximise the magnitude of, and minimise the variance in, outcome for a given type of patient. It is not to provide to patients uniform processes irrespective of their needs and desires (which might well increase the variance in outcomes if process does not match patient). By comparison, industrial quality control is far simpler. Industry's goal is to produce products to specifications with as little variation as possible. To this end, all inputs to processes and the processes themselves must be as uniform as possible. Variance reduction is both ends and means. Patients—inputs to care processes—vary inherently, and process must match patient. Further, there is considerable doubt as to which processes will maximise patients' health status improvement consistent with their preferences; not to mention the trade-offs that must be made with respect to the cost of interventions. In addition to health outcomes, patients may be interested in convenience or amenities, cost, ethics or other dimensions of providers' performance.

For any dimension of health care quality, one must distinguish between system-level quality (the quality of the health care system) and production-level quality (providers' performance consequent to provider–patient interactions). For example, access to care affects health outcomes and is a concern at the system level but is irrelevant at the production level. At this level, accessibility is not an issue: a person has become a patient. What becomes important is how well the provider performs for that patient. Again, people differ on what they consider quality to be, and weight common measures differently. The next section explores this distinction. Discussion of the relationships of performance at the different levels and their implications is beyond the manual's scope. The remainder of this chapter is concerned only with production-level quality and hence only with provider performance. It defines health care quality for quality management purposes and describes how hospitals can assess and measure its central dimension—health status improvement—for purposes of improving the quality of their care. Knowing where they stand relative to where they should be, providers can strive to improve their performance.

254.2 *System-level versus production-level quality*

When people talk of health care they may mean the quality or performance of the system or of a particular provider, for example a hospital or a doctor. When it comes to measuring quality one must make a clear distinction between these two levels. The measures one would apply to assess the quality of the system are quite different from those one would use to measure provider performance. Even if some measures were the same, for example health status improvement, their importance and implications might well be different.

Generally, at the system level people would judge the quality of health care partly on its accessibility, for example, as well as how much care improved the population's health status. A system that gave good care to 80% of the population but which was not accessible by 20% of the people might be judged inferior to one that gave slightly less good care to the average person but to which everyone had access. The population's aggregate health status might be greater in the latter than in the former, but the cost may be higher or some people may feel less satisfied. Clearly, trade-offs exist. For example, successful efforts to improve the quality of care in individual hospitals may degrade accessibility and conceivably could reduce the system's quality. Maximising the output of each system element does not necessarily maximise that of the system as a whole. The fact that improvements in hospital care may have some potential deleterious system consequences, as well as many beneficial ones, should not dissuade hospitals from trying to improve the quality of their care. Rather, national and state governments and other organisations concerned with the system as a whole should be mindful of the need to recognise the effect that their policies have on providers' performance and that providers' performance has on the system.

254.3 *Historical perspective: structure, process, outcome*

In a classic paper, Avedis Donabedian described and evaluated methods for assessing (measuring) the quality of care at the level of physician–patient interaction. He identified three approaches to assessment: outcome of care, the care process, and structure (attributes of care providers, settings and arrangements).[2]

Structural variables describe the characteristics of inputs to care processes, for example hospitals' condition, doctors' training or qualifications. If quality of care is defined in structural terms, employing only doctors with certain qualifications, for example, is sufficient to assure quality.

Process variables describe what care is provided or characteristics of its provision, for example whether or not the doctor orders or the patient receives a particular test; how long the patient has to wait before being seen by the doctor. If quality of care is defined in process terms, making sure each patient received certain tests or that tests were done within a specified period, for example, is sufficient to assure quality.

Outcome variables describe some relevant characteristic, usually of the patient, after provision of care that is presumed to be its result, for example whether or not the patient was discharged alive from the hospital. If quality of care is defined in simple outcome terms, observing the outcome (the criterion) in all or some specified fraction of patients (the standard) is sufficient to assure quality.

Measuring structural variables—inputs to care processes—is the simplest and least expensive approach. With respect to hospitals, ACHS accreditation, for example, is no guarantee that a hospital will, or did, improve a patient's health status to the maximal possible extent within the patient's preferences and its resources. Promise (the potential to perform) is quite different from performance, to which anyone who has seen an all-star, championship-winning sports team lose on an off-day can attest. Use of structural measures to assure quality makes many assumptions about the relationship between structural characteristics and intended outcomes. For example, licensure (registration) of professionals who graduate from accredited schools and pass examinations is a common quality assurance mechanism. Although intuitively appealing, such mechanisms may be necessary but insufficient to ensure quality of care, which inherently involves processes.

Measuring process variables is both more difficult and more expensive than measuring structural variables. It assumes that a given process is appropriate for all of the patients in the population; it may not be. If one does not know how processes relate to outcomes, once again they are of limited value, because the relationship between process and outcome must be assumed. Moreover, the doctor may select the appropriate intervention but may not implement it properly, impairing patient outcome.

Measuring outcome variables is the most difficult and expensive approach, but one is at least assessing the extent to which what is desired exists. Nevertheless, one may still have to assume the relationship between process and outcome—something that doctors would also have to do when treating patients. Just because the patient recovered does not mean that the doctor's care was appropriate or that his or her intervention produced the observed improvement in the patient's health status. Further, producing a given outcome for one patient may be far more difficult than for another for reasons that have little or nothing to do with the quality of the provider's performance. Care processes must fit patients and outcomes must be attributable to processes. Chapter 4 in this part explores these points in detail.

For quality management purposes, outcome/process assessment has superseded quality of care assessments based on the simple expedient of measuring one or more individual structural, process or outcome variables. Modern quality assessment—and hence quality assurance and improvement—focuses on conformance to individuated care processes (which are shaped by structures) that are believed to maximise patient health status improvement (the intended outcome), and to the achievement of expected patient outcomes. Process selection inherently involves patients' preferences regarding ends and means.

255 | Production quality—provider performance

255.1 | *Dimensions of production-level health care quality*

Production-level quality depends on providers' performance. Patients, consumers of health care, health care managers and policy makers, as well as providers themselves, have a vital interest in how providers perform. Given information on provider performance, consumers can better select the doctor of choice, for example. Health care system managers can contract with hospitals meeting performance, and not just accreditation, standards. Providers can strive to improve their performance. For quality management purposes, the following four dimensions define health care quality and, when integrated, permit a summary judgment of value for money:

- technical quality, measured by patients' health status improvement, the technical aspects of quality;
- resource consumption, measured by the cost of care;
- patient satisfaction, measured by patients' perceptions of the subjective or interpersonal aspects of care;
- Values, measured by the acceptability of any trade-offs that must be made among the three previous outcomes.

255.2 | *Technical performance—health status improvement*

The principal reason patients seek health care is to improve their health status, especially for life-threatening or serious conditions—those for which patients are often admitted to hospitals. For minor conditions, while health status improvement remains important, in judging quality of care a patient might place more importance on a doctor's interpersonal skills or the convenience of his surgery (office) hours or location than he or she might otherwise. Where there are no effective medical interventions, the interpersonal aspects of care might become paramount.

Improving patients' health status requires selecting effective interventions that are indicated by the patient's condition and circumstances and implementing them properly to provide appropriate care. For quality management purposes, practice policies define what interventions are appropriate for particular types of patients and describe what to expect consequently. Quality assessment compares what was done and achieved with what should have been done and achieved (defined in practice policies) to determine whether or not interventions were indicated and implemented properly. Subsequent sections describe in detail methods for assessing health care quality.

255.3 | *Cost*

The cost of care is a key aspect of quality. Quality cannot be considered meaningfully if cost is ignored entirely. Clearly, trade-offs exist between achievable health outcomes and the cost of their production. At first blush people may assume that measuring costs is relatively simple. It is not. While all costs are expressed simply in monetary units, for example dollars, there are many intricacies to be considered in determining the cost of care. While they may seem to be academic considerations, they can affect significantly what a treatment is said to cost and hence trade-offs involving costs. Exploration of how to measure costs for quality management purposes is beyond this manual's scope.

Costs are different from prices. A cost is what a vendor pays for the factors that go into the products it sells. A price is the amount of money a supplier accepts from a buyer for specified goods or services. The supplier's costs of producing these goods or services is not of interest to the purchaser, except possibly to the extent that they allow the supplier to perform the contract. Health policy decision makers, however, may be very concerned if a hospital, in their view, underestimates its production costs, because the deficit between revenues and costs must be made good from other sources or it will result in a budget shortfall. Further, false estimation of costs may result in hidden subsidies of some types of service by other types. Also of interest to policy makers is the effect of cost-reimbursement or revenue generation mechanisms on provider performance. These important subjects are beyond this manual's scope.

From the patient's perspective, the cost of treatment includes not only the price he or she must pay for it (which under most health care financing schemes may be little or nothing), but also the cost of lost wages, strains on family members (who might also have to take time off from work), inconvenience and other factors. Patients who do not pay for care directly may not know or be concerned about the cost of the treatment that they receive, and it may not influence their choice among alternative interventions. Lack of concern for cost on the part of patients and providers is one of the principal reasons that health care costs increase inexorably.

From the hospital's perspective, knowing the cost of different types of care is important. The hospital can determine if the payment it receives for providing a service covers the cost of its production. The hospital can also improve quality by reducing its production costs while maintaining or exceeding the level of health status improvement that the service provides. Today, few hospitals know what it costs to produce care. In Australia, for example, payments to hospitals are not linked to the services that they provide to patients (let alone the health status improvement that they produce). The idea that hospitals should try systematically to improve the quality of their care by reducing the cost of improving patients' health status—for example by changing what is done, how it is done or who does it—is quite foreign to the present culture of medicine.

255.4 Patient satisfaction

Patient satisfaction is an important aspect of the quality of care. Providers can improve the timing or location of their services or the interpersonal aspects of their care without necessarily reducing the amount of patient health status improvement they produce or increasing the cost of their care. Nonetheless, sometimes better service does cost more money and trade-offs are unavoidable. A patient, whose doctor refuses to prescribe an unnecessary medicine (thereby enhancing technical quality) but who did not explain the reasons to the patient's satisfaction, may be dissatisfied with the interpersonal aspects of care. Chapter 3 in Part IV discusses the measurement of patient satisfaction. The discussion in the remainder of this part excludes amenities, convenience and interpersonal aspects of care that do not contribute to improved health outcomes—aspects of quality that the patient can judge. However, providers' interactions with patients regarding prognosis, therapeutic compliance, drug interactions and preventive activities that are essential to maximising health outcomes in ways consistent with patients' preferences, fall clearly within the technical aspects of quality and thus must be encompassed by quality assessment, as defined here.

255.5 Values

In quality management, trade-offs among health status improvement (including provider performance), costs and satisfaction represent real choices. Unfortunately, little information is available about these choices. In part, this lack of information about choices stems from the absence of information about any aspect of quality. Sometimes no aspects of quality are measured; sometimes only one or two are measured. Even when all aspects are measured simultaneously trade-offs are not explored explicitly. Indeed, their exploration can be difficult. Actual choices, of course, depend on the values of the decision maker who may not always be the patient if, for example, a health care financing scheme must decide whether or not to pay for a particular treatment. Discussion of values, in terms of their measurement and appropriate trade-offs, is beyond this manual's scope.

256 | Measuring technical quality

256.1 | Overview of quality measurement and assessment

Quality must be measured before it can be improved. Without reliable measurement one cannot conclude improvement has occurred. One may be interested in measuring the quality of care for one or both of the following two purposes:

- to inform patients or payers, so that they can choose among providers based on their performance;
- to improve the quality of care, which is the purpose of most interest to providers.

Quality measurement and quality assessment, like so many quality management terms, are often used interchangeably. While both terms refer to a hospital's or a doctor's performance in managing (diagnosing and treating) patients, it is important to distinguish between them for quality management purposes. In this manual the terms have the following meanings:

- Quality measurement refers to the process of quantifying the quality of a provider's entire output expressed, for example, as the proportion of cases treated appropriately (in much the same way as a factory's quality can be gauged by the proportion of its output that meets product specifications).
- Quality assessment refers to the process of examining a single episode or continuum of care, a unit of a provider's performance (patient–provider interaction), to determine whether or not care was delivered appropriately (in much the same way as a factory gauges whether or not an individual widget met product specifications).

Aggregating the results of individual quality assessments provides the means to quantify the quality of a provider's performance for all or particular types of patients. Use of appropriate sampling can minimise the number of cases required to make statistically valid statements about providers' quality of care. For quality management purposes, production quality is ultimately a statistical judgment.

Quality improvement actions must rest on individual assessments of populations of cases, not on the assessment of an isolated case. One cannot make big statements on the basis of small samples, let alone an individual case. Definitive judgments about the quality of care based on a single case are best left in the hands of courts. While it is possible to assess the quality of care given to an individual patient for an episode of care, for example admission for elective hysterectomy, only when hospitals aggregate results of many such assessments can they measure provider performance, and only when they analyse these assessments can they identify systemic quality problems. Nevertheless, an individual assessment that finds a practitioner to have recklessly endangered a patient's life can appropriately lead to immediate steps to reduce that danger's recurrence.

Quality measurement or assessment requires that health care's intended product be defined explicitly, in measurable terms. Technical quality—patient health status improvement—is health care quality's principal dimension and this manual's focus. The remainder of this chapter elaborates on concepts of technical quality measurement and quality assessment, and describes the following two ways to measure health care quality:

- outcome risk adjustment (ORA)—a population-based method that relies on statistical adjustment of one or more outcome measures, for example mortality rates, for factors that affect patient outcomes and are beyond the provider's control, to produce a relative quality score, for example one hospital's performance relative to all hospitals with respect to operative mortality;

- outcome/process assessment (OPA)—a case-based method that relies on summation of individual case assessments made by comparing what was done (process) and achieved (outcome) to what should have been done and achieved, to produce an absolute quality score—the proportion of patients treated appropriately.

Outcome risk adjustment is indirect and relative; outcome/process assessment is direct and absolute. Outcome risk adjustment systems attempt to remove the influence on patient outcomes of all factors—and their interactions—other than provider performance; any residual difference in patient outcomes must be due to provider performance. Outcome/process assessment systems specify and measure provider performance directly by comparing the extent of what should have been done and achieved with what was done and achieved. With outcome/process assessment, unlike outcome risk adjustment systems, there is no need to compare providers to measure quality; but they do permit comparisons among providers based on their performance (quality scores).

For quality management purposes, outcome/process assessment is far more useful and practical than outcome risk adjustment. At best, outcome risk adjustment can measure quality of care, which would be useful for choosing among providers, for example. It is not useful for quality assessment (which inherently involves a judgment about the quality of care in an individual case). Although population-based screens employing outcome risk adjustment can identify providers whose care exhibits a high incidence of potential quality problems, such screens' utility for quality assurance or improvement purposes is limited because they do not relate care processes to outcomes—what was (or was not) done and achieved in individual cases. Because outcome/process assessment considers simultaneously both care processes and outcomes in the same patient, they can not only identify individual cases with quality problems but also shed light on the nature of those problems.

256.2 Quality measurement—quality (performance) scores

Quality measurement (referred to sometimes as quality performance measurement), provides an actual measure of a hospital's performance, either as an entity or for a particular department, service, type of patient or other pertinent parameter. Such a measure can be used directly and validly to compare providers' performance. Thus, for example, if one hospital has a quality score of 200 and the other a score of 100, one can draw the valid inference that the first hospital's quality is twice as good as that of the second hospital, for whatever dimension of quality is involved.

Quality measurement implies a comprehensive judgment of provider performance on all aspects of the technical quality of care. The resultant provider performance scores allow payers or patients to select among providers based not only on cost and convenience but also on their technical quality or performance, especially if quality scores are calculated narrowly, for a particular diagnosis or procedure for example.

256.3 Conceptual basis for measuring provider performance

Ideally, to measure the quality of care—provider performance—one would like to be able to determine, for each patient the hospital admits or the doctor treats, the health status improvement that the provider produced compared to the maximum health status improvement that the provider could have produced under the circumstances (or preferably that should have been produced technically for that patient regardless of the provider's circumstances). The resultant ratios are all one or less—unless multiplied by

100 to convert them to percentages, thus providing a more appealing score—because they relate to what is achievable, and one cannot achieve more than this amount. These ratios can be averaged to produce a mean quality score (and its variance) that truly reflects performance. Of course we cannot do this now, nor are we likely to be able to do it in the near future.

At best, we can now measure a patient's health status one or more times after treatment—itself a relatively difficult and expensive undertaking. We are still left with the problem of attributing whatever we observe to preceding interventions, and we have to calculate improvement by subtracting a consensual judgment of what would also have happened to the patient without treatment. Moreover, we would also have to use a consensual judgment of what could have been achieved technically in order to calculate the ratio of what was achieved with what could have been achieved. Lack of data, the uncertain validity of consensual judgments, and the difficulty and cost of empirical outcome measurement precludes implementing this approach to routinely measure provider performance. Nevertheless, the idea is conceptually sound and forms the basis for two emerging approaches, to which we refer as outcome risk adjustment and outcome/process assessment.

257 | Outcome risk adjustment

257.1 | Conceptual basis

Patient outcomes, such as life or death, are the basis of this approach to measuring provider performance. Outcomes are direct and intuitively appealing. However, the patient may die for reasons that have little or nothing to do with what the provider did or did not do or, at the very least, the chances of the patient dying may depend on factors beyond the provider's skills or diligence.

The essential strategy underlying outcome risk adjustment (ORA) is to measure a hospital's patient outcomes and to adjust each for factors affecting outcomes that are beyond its control in order to obtain a measure of performance. Such adjustments are statistical because outcomes are measured for the population of patients admitted to the hospital in a given period. Once such adjustments have been made, one hospital's performance can be compared validly to that of others or the average of all hospitals, assuming outcomes, patient characteristics and other outcome-influencing factors affecting outcomes are measured uniformly from one hospital to the next. Operationally, the validity of this latter assumption is often questionable. Further, various outcomes may be of interest, and the factors that affect each one may differ. Outcomes of interest include, for example, health status years, mortality and nosocomial infection rates. Factors affecting outcomes include, for example, patient case-mix, the types of patient treated and their health status at admission. Finally, because factors vary dynamically these systems must be recalibrated periodically to know by how much to adjust outcomes.

257.2 | Relationship to the ideal

Current outcome risk adjustment systems simplify the problem of measuring provider performance (achievable health status achieved) in the following ways. Firstly, they choose a simple outcome measure, for example death within thirty days of hospital admission. Death, for example, is acceptable for some conditions where it occurs commonly enough as a result of the disease—for example acute myocardial infarction—but not for others. In all cases death is an inadequate measure of health status. Secondly, they limit analysis to certain cases, for example acute myocardial infarction. Thirdly, they try to identify the non-provider, predominantly patient, factors that coproduce the selected outcome or, if there are many, the most important ones, which are obviously subject to error based on current knowledge. They calculate the probability of death within thirty days of admission among such patients in a defined population, for example all patients hospitalised for a certain condition in 1993. They use these statistically-derived weights to calculate the expected number of deaths in admissions to a particular hospital. They divide the expected number of deaths into the observed number of deaths to indicate if fewer (ratio is less than one) or more (ratio is greater than one) deaths were observed than expected. Statistical analysis can show which hospitals or doctors are 'outliers'—lie beyond two standard deviations of the mean with 95% confidence, for example.

Outcome risk adjustment has the obvious drawbacks inherent in the assumptions that are necessary to operationalise it: the relative nature of the analysis, the number of cases needed for statistical significance, and the diagnostic trap. One reason that a doctor may have few deaths among his or her patients is that some of them may never have had an acute myocardial infarction, in the case of the example, and the fraction of doctors' patients not having the diagnosis likely varies substantially. If analysis is based on diagnostic groups, the patient's diagnosis must be validated. Diagnostic errors are one of the most common quality problems. Moreover, the patient's preferences are lost to the analysis and may influence results. For example, if a patient refused treatment and died consequently, the doctor's care cannot be faulted necessarily. Assuring the integrity of data poses another set of problems which is described elsewhere.[3] Thus the apparent advantage of using this approach to compare different hospitals or doctors may be offset or lost entirely.

257.3 Present status of outcome risk adjustment

Existing attempts to adjust mortality data, for example, are both too imprecise and too crude to be a useful measure of providers' performance. The annual release of Health Care Financing Administration (HCFA) mortality data that has occurred in the United States since 1986 is the best known example of an operational outcome risk adjustment system. Each year the US HCFA, which is responsible for the nation's Medicare program (which pays for the care of people over sixty-five years of age and certain other beneficiaries), releases hospital-specific mortality data. These data are limited to the experience of Medicare beneficiaries. Critics note that these measures are simplistic and flawed because of their source (routinely collected administrative information), because of the limited adjustments that HCFA can make, and because of all of the other above-mentioned reasons. In 1993 HCFA released these data quietly to hospitals and its Peer Review Organisations rather than to the public with the fanfare that accompanied earlier releases. Industry analysts report that these data are of little help to hospitals and HCFA's administrator admits they do not provide consumers with useful information.[4] Experts continue to work to improve outcome risk adjustment and make it a practical tool for measuring and comparing hospital performance, a goal of the Cleveland project, for example.[5]

Today, lack of cost-effective outcome measurement technology and knowledge on how to adjust outcomes properly renders such systems impractical for choosing among hospitals or doctors, for example, on the basis of their quality, that is, performance. Moreover, while such systems can potentially measure a hospital's quality, the resultant measure is of more use to consumers (who can decide to avoid low scoring hospitals) than to the hospital, because by themselves such measures cannot pinpoint the reasons for low scores. For this reason some people advocate using screens that employ outcome risk adjustments to identify hospitals or doctors whose care should be examined further, for example through review of individual patient records. The sensitivity and specificity of such screens have yet to be determined. Further, the combined cost of using such screens plus medical record review may exceed that of case-based outcome/process assessment. Moreover, review of ORA-identified cases may be less reliable because automated OPA-based screens help structure subsequent review (see below).

257.4 | Severity of illness

A number of states in the United States, such as Pennsylvania, require hospitals to collect and report routinely severity of illness data as a means of adjusting outcome risk. A number of companies market such systems. Essentially, they classify hospital patients into a limited number of categories (typically five) based on the presence or absence of clinical findings, at or within twenty-four to forty-eight hours of admission, and again at specified times during the admission and at discharge. These categories are intended to reflect, for example, the probability of death or organ failure within a specified period from untreated disease.

Regulators or hospitals can use the resultant severity scores to identify hospitals or providers whose care is potentially substandard because, for example, they have a higher proportion of cases with a discharge score higher than the admission score, or to adjust for differences in patient mix when analysing hospital mortality rates or the average cost of care for patients admitted by different doctors. As explained elsewhere, such severity systems are unsound theoretically.[6] Further, their value as either a quality screening or risk adjustment tool has yet to be accepted.

The term 'severity of illness' sometimes refers also, and inappropriately, to treatment difficulty (the probability of achieving a given patient outcome) and/or resource intensity (the cost of treating appropriately a given health problem in a given type of patient).

258 | Outcome/process assessment

258.1 | Conceptual basis

Care processes are the basis for this approach to measuring provider performance. Perfect implementation of perfect processes produces maximal patient health status improvement. Outcome/process assessment (OPA) determines whether or not a surgical operation was indicated, for example, and, if so, implemented properly. Immediate patient outcomes following care processes give clues about potential malprocesses—those that were done but should not have been, those that were not done but should have been, and those that were done improperly.

Comparison of documented care processes and outcomes with practice policies or criteria (which describe what should be done for particular types of patients and expected consequently) is the essential strategy underlying outcome/process assessment. Hospitals can aggregate the results of these case-by-case assessments to produce a quality score—the proportion of cases treated appropriately. Patients and payers can use these scores to compare hospitals if assessors use uniform practice criteria relevant to each type of case as the basis for their assessments, and reliable assessment mechanisms. Invalid assessments, unwarranted generalisations from assessments based on inadequate samples of cases, and unsubstantiated claims pose a danger to consumers, if not to providers.

258.2 | Relationship to the ideal

Outcome/process assessment recognises explicitly the difficulty, if not impossibility, of measuring health status improvement directly and of risk-adjusting outcomes. Instead, it relies on specifying—in practice policies or criteria—the processes that if implemented properly would result in the maximum achievable health status improvement for the patient. Qualified assessors can check if these processes or, if very many, the most important ones (those that account for most of the improvement) have been implemented properly. Maloutcomes help to spot cases in which providers may not have implemented properly a needed process or may have omitted it entirely, or used inappropriate processes (which could also be checked directly, if their use is known or suspected). In cases exhibiting maloutcomes, assessors can determine if the maloutcome resulted more likely than not from inappropriate care (malprocesses). Ultimately, assessors can classify each case as treated appropriately or not, and can calculate the fraction of a hospital's cases treated appropriately to represent its performance.

The approach is practical to implement, can encompass all cases, avoids the diagnostic trap, and accommodates patient preferences, eliminating potential sources of bias inherent in outcome risk adjustment. But it has several disadvantages. Chief among them are the following. First and foremost is the limitation of medical practice: there may be great uncertainty about which processes or interventions would lead to maximum health status improvement. Various packets of processes would likely be regarded as appropriate. Their number and the specificity of contents would depend on the state of medical knowledge. Processes must be specified by diagnosis, and for each diagnosis practice criteria must include diagnostic validation. Many variables affect outcomes and assessors may fail to include all of the important ones.

The number and complexity of judgments about care is such that computerised screening offers the only hope of making them reliably and economically. Information for operationalising screens must be present in the patient's medical record, so the medical record must be adequate for the purpose. Computerised screens cannot yet be specified completely enough to eliminate the need for expert review of cases failing screens, although this possibility already exists for some cases. While computerised screens can be applied universally, the validity of final performance scores depends ultimately on expert reviewers' competence and their honesty.

An expert clinician must review cases, or at least those failing screens, to determine the appropriateness of care. Judgments about whether or not maloutcomes resulted more likely than not from malprocess will always be uncertain. Those regarding the fit between needed and implemented care processes may not be reliable and are certainly subjective, that is, use implicit criteria (because if they were explicit, they could have been incorporated into automated screens). Judgments' certainty and reliability can be increased, however, by structuring the expert's review of the patient's medical record and by allowing the doctor or other provider whose care reviewers criticise to respond to the criticism prior to making a final determination. This step may also compensate somewhat for possible bias and subjectivity.

Case-by-case judgments about the appropriateness of care must be supplemented by statistical analysis of the entire population of cases examined. Reviewed individually each case might squeak by as acceptable, but when all cases are examined statistically the provider's outcomes may be far inferior to the average, for example. Thus pattern analysis of processes and outcomes, as well as of quality assessment data, must be an integral part of an OPA system. Where necessary, case-by-case judgments can be re-examined based on the results of such pattern analysis.

258.3 Present status of outcome/process assessment

Existing outcome/process assessment (OPA) systems are being used to assess quality of care; not to calculate quality scores. However, in all likelihood it will be easier to develop valid OPA-based, rather than ORA-based, performance (quality) scores. Further, OPA systems are the tool of choice for hospitals because they can identify care deficiencies that hospitals can then take steps to rectify. In the near future, in the United States, payers and providers may begin to use OPA systems to measure provider performance, as well as to identify quality problems to be resolved. Accountable health plans (see Chapter 3 in this part) may use them to profile providers and to decide which ones should be included or retained in their health care networks. Hospitals may use results of structured quality review (see below) to assist recredentialling decisions, for example.

The Civilian External Peer Review Program (CEPRP) of the US Department of Defense (DOD) developed the first OPA system to assess routinely quality of care. This landmark program began in 1986 (see below), and inspired several subsequent efforts. In 1992 the US Department of Veteran Affairs decided to use the same basic approach to monitor the quality of care being delivered by its 171 medical centres. Also beginning in 1992, selected HCFA's Peer Review Organisations (PROs) began testing the UCDS (Uniform Clinical Data Set) system (see below). The only commercially available OPA system in routine use in hospitals is QSM (Quality Standards in Medicine, Boston, Massachusetts) (see Chapter 8 in this part).

Outcome/process assessment depends on the availability of detailed practice policies or practice criteria to determine for narrowly-drawn types of patients what should be done and achieved consequently (see Chapter 7 in this part). They must be computerised to make their use practical for quality assessment purposes. These two requirements exceed almost all hospitals' development resources; they must rely on commercially available systems. The sensitivity and specificity (accuracy) of paper-and-pencil screens are far too low to warrant their use in practice. Whether or not computerised screens are accurate enough is an open question. Based on both design considerations and users' informal evaluations, QSM does appear to be a useful tool for improving quality of care (see Chapter 8 in this part).

The fact remains that experts must review cases failing screens to decide if care exhibits a quality problem or not. With screens of sufficient accuracy, reviewers' workloads are manageable, but the reliability and accuracy of their judgments remains in doubt. One can improve judgments' accuracy by inviting providers to comment on reviewers' findings. However, this step involves additional work, and may generate more heat than light, unless all providers whose work is subject to review and criticism participate in a spirit conducive to rational inquiry, learning and quality improvement. This latter consideration may doom externally-driven programs from the start. Nevertheless, for motivated providers internally-driven outcome/process assessment offers a powerful way to identify quality problems—a necessary first step toward their elimination and hence quality improvement. We explore these points in detail below and in subsequent chapters in this part.

258.4 Civilian External Peer Review Program

The US Department of Defense initiated its Civilian External Peer Review Program (CEPRP) in 1986 after a number of well-publicised incidents that led the US Congress and the American public to question the quality of military patient care. The program's original purpose was to respond to, and stave off further, criticism of military patient care. In recent years it has become a quality improvement vehicle. FMAS Corporation (in Rockville, Maryland) conducts the program under contract to DOD. Originally, CEPRP focused on monitoring the quality of care in DOD's Medical Treatment Facilities (MTFs) worldwide based on computerised outcome/process assessment screens and ('peer') review of cases failing screens. In late 1994, DOD dispensed with the routine review of medical records failing screens, choosing instead to provide MTFs with statistical analyses of abstracted medical record data and to leave case-by-case judgments about care's appropriateness to individual MTFs.

Between 1986 and 1994, abstracters periodically visited each MTF and abstracted selected medical records using automated outcome/process assessment screens. They sent these data to a central processing point. Panels of civilian doctors in medical practice reviewed abstracts of cases failing screens to determine whether or not cases exhibited a quality problem. The MTF that provided the care was asked to comment on reviewers' initial judgments. Reviewers made a final determination after assessing care in light of MTFs' comments on that care. The DOD and MTFs received the results of these case-by-case assessments and statistical analyses based on them. Such analyses include, for example, the frequency of particular kinds of quality problems, and trends in and comparisons among MTFs with respect to kinds of quality problems and case improvement opportunity rates.

258.5 HCFA's Medical Quality Indicator System—MQIS

The US Health Care Financing Administration (HCFA) developed the Uniform Clinical Data Set (UCDS) for use by its Peer Review Organizations (PROs). The UCDS was primarily an outcome/process assessment system to screen hospital care provided to its Medicare beneficiaries. The system was also designed to produce an epidemiological database. The pressure for UCDS' development was the high degree of variability in rates of cases that PRO screeners (QA/UR nurses) referred to PRO physicians for peer review. Originally, PROs were to ('peer') review cases that failed UCDS system screens. But, in late 1994, HCFA replaced its UCDS system with MQIS (Medical Quality Indicator System). Instead of applying algorithms to identify cases requiring further review, this system intends only to provide PROs with statistical data pertaining to populations of Medicare cases.

With HCFA's switch from the UCDS system to MQIS, PROs will no longer assess quality of care case-by-case (hence no more 'peer review') but will instead rely on statistical analyses to effect quality improvement. Essentially, HCFA working with one or two selected PROs will develop and test 'quality indicators' for such disease specific processes as urinary tract infection, pneumonia and breast cancer.[7] Beginning in 1995, two Clinical Data Abstractions Centers (CDACs) under contract to HCFA will use MQIS software to produce abstracts of HCFA-sampled hospital medical records. One CDAC (operated by FMAS Corporation, Rockville, Maryland) will produce medical record abstracts for Medicare discharges from coastal states of the USA, and the other (operated by DynKeyPro, York, Pennsylvania) for discharges from all other states. During their first two years of operation (1995–96), HCFA expects CDACs to produce over 1.2 million abstracts. In 1995, for example, HCFA plans to have CDACs produce abstracts for 100% of Medicare-paid acute myocardial infarction cases treated in US hospitals during an eight-month period.

CDAC-produced abstracts consist of 'core data'—demographic and risk adjustment data that is common to all cases—and specific clinical information that pertains only to a certain type of case, for example acute myocardial infarctions. HCFA will provide PROs will CDAC-produced abstracts. PROs will enter into 'quality improvement partnerships' with hospitals. It is too early to tell if MQIS results are valid quality indicators, how quality improvement partnerships will evolve, and whether or not substantial and systematic quality improvement will result in US hospitals.

259 Quality of care assessment

259.1 About quality of care assessment

Quality scores are only of limited use to providers interested in improving their performance. They need to know what care processes to change and how to change them to improve their quality scores. Quality assessment (referred to sometimes as quality of care assessment) intends to identify quality of care problems and provides a judgment about the quality (i.e. appropriateness, acceptability or adequacy) of an episode or continuum of health care. If the assessment is comprehensive, that is, it involves all relevant aspects of the technical quality of care, aggregation of such judgments for a meaningful population or statistically significant sample of a provider's cases results in a quality score. Quality assessment can lead to quality improvement even if it examines only certain aspects of care, for example nosocomial infections, or if only selected cases, for example those involving surgical operations.

259.2 Conceptual basis for assessing quality of care

Quality of care assessment depends on comparing what was done and/or achieved with what should have been done and/or achieved for the patient—hence the term outcome/ process assessment. The starting point for the assessment is the implicit goal of achieving maximum achievable patient health status improvement within the patient's preference and society's resources. Until recently, such assessments were entirely subjective, and hence very variable. Peers or experts might not always agree with each other (inter-rater reliability) or even themselves (intra-rater reliability) when judging the appropriateness of care for a given case.

The availability of information about patient encounters limits quality of care assessments. Hospital records usually contain limited information about patients' pre-admission care and virtually nothing about their postseparation course. Ideally, quality assessments would use information from all relevant patient care phases, including that derived from patient followup or outcome questionnaires. Today, however, in most hospitals the patient's medical record is the only practical source of information for assessing the quality of care. Thus the adequacy of the medical record—the quality of documentation about what was done or considered, what was observed or decided, and what happened as a result—limits such assessments. The medical records must document the important facts and the first task of any quality management program must be to ensure that they do. Good medical care requires good medical records. Only care that is appropriate and documented adequately can be considered to be high quality. Hospital quality management programs, merely by delineating what must be recorded in medical records to assess adequately quality of care, can improve directly the quality of that care. Obviously, to realise such improvement hospitals need mechanisms to check the adequacy of medical records and incentives to encourage clinicians to keep adequate records.

259.3 Practical considerations in assessing quality of care

Traditionally, quality of care assessment has relied on careful case-by-case review by expert clinicians who may also have had training in quality assurance, epidemiology or research methods. Many such assessments were conducted as research studies, with all of the care and attention to detail that they imply, to show that quality of care problems existed and to illuminate their nature. For example, using a structured protocol three clinicians may have assessed independently the care provided in each case and then discussed their individual judgments to develop a consensual judgment about the quality of care. This research-based approach is quite impractical for routine quality assessment and assurance. Stated simply, it costs too much, takes too long, and trained experts are not universally available in sufficient numbers.

To be practical, quality assessment methods must economically find cases with problems in care processes that if resolved would materially improve the quality of care. In North America the traditional approach to achieve this end has been to employ 'peers' as reviewers. To reduce their workloads to manageable proportions peer reviewers usually examine samples of medical records or may target 'high-risk' cases for review. Sometimes quality assurance nurses may 'screen' cases to identify those with potential quality problems to be confirmed (or denied) subsequently by peer reviewers. Nurses may use forms that remind them what to look for, but exercise considerable discretion in deciding which cases to refer for peer review.

The incidence of quality of care problems in high-risk cases, those most likely to exhibit quality problems, may still be low, and all types of cases may exhibit quality problems albeit with even lower incidence. Traditional quality screens may be (and usually are) inaccurate, resulting in nurse screeners identifying many cases for further review that do not contain quality problems (false positives) and failing to identify others that do exhibit quality of care problems (false negatives). Clinicians' assessments of cases that screeners refer to them may be (and often are) unreliable. The entire process may be expensive and lead to little information useful for quality management purposes. The cost of identifying cases with quality of care problems, and difficulties with traditional peer review, led to the development of the quality assessment process to which we refer as structured quality review (SQR).

259.4 About peer review

In North America peer review has been and continues to be the traditional mainstay of quality of care assessment. In Australia the term 'peer review' is ambiguous. This manual uses the term peer review as it is understood generally in North America: peer review occurs when one professional reviews a colleague's (peer's) work. Medical peer review (referred to usually simply as peer review) involves a doctor reviewing a colleague's work as documented in the patient's medical record. In Australia, generally, doctors' review of colleagues' medical records to assess the quality of care has not become an accepted part of hospitals' quality management programs. In some doctors' minds, peer review has come to be associated primarily with regulatory agencies—which either conduct external peer review (HCFA's PROs, for example) or mandate internal peer review (hospital accrediting bodies, for example). They see peer review more as an instrument of the medical inspectorate than as a means for quality improvement.

Peer review's greatest strength is its central axiom: if he or she works diligently, a properly qualified reviewer can review validly the appropriateness (quality) of care of any case within his or her domains of expertise. However, traditional (North American) medical peer review has a number of deficiencies. Table II-5-1 on page 251 summarises the key aspects of traditional peer review—recognising that peer review practices vary widely, which is one of its drawbacks—in comparison with structured quality review. Traditional peer review:

- is usually conducted in isolation and rarely leads to quality improvement;
- focuses on identifying deficient care (and by implication deficient doctors), rather than on identifying patterns of care that need to be improved (e.g. by changing the system of care);
- is performed usually on (not always statistically significant) samples of medical records, few of which are likely to exhibit major quality of care problems, approximating the proverbial search for a needle in a haystack;
- involves usually the unstructured judgment of a single reviewer, and these judgments tend to be unreliable;
- may involve review of voluminous medical records, so that critical information may be missed, reducing reliability of judgments;
- is tedious, so that fatigue may set in rapidly, reducing reliability of judgments;
- is time consuming for doctors;
- involves doctors looking only at doctors' work, and sometimes surgeons looking only at surgical care, for example, rather than all medical or the totality of care;
- assumes that all doctors are equally good quality of care assessors, notwithstanding that only surgeons may review surgeons' work, for example;

Table II-5-1 *Quality of care assessment*

Comparison of traditional peer review (as understood in North America) or medical audit with structured quality review which employs automated outcome/process assessment screens

Characteristic	Traditional peer review	Structured quality review
Purpose	Identify deficient care; search for 'bad apples'	Identify quality of care problems toward their resolution, e.g. through changing policies and processes, to improve the quality of care
Scope	Doctors assess other doctors' care, usually focusing on medical aspects, e.g. surgeons examine indications for surgery or surgical technique	Doctors (and others) assess all aspects of care in the case, to identify care deficiencies whether or not they involve doctors, e.g. delays in diagnoses and/or treatment
Samples	Doctors take all or samples (random or haphazard) of cases from a defined period, or of 'high-risk' cases; review is tedious and time-consuming, like looking for needles in haystacks. Sometimes quality assurance nurses use generic or other screens to identify cases for review, but they tend to be inaccurate	Automated outcome/process screens are used on all or a valid sample of cases, to identify cases with potential quality problems, allowing reviewers to focus on these cases and the potential quality problems that the OPA screens identify; review is challenging, efficient
Criteria and standards	Usually implicit, subjective	Employs explicit, objective criteria and standards in automated OPA screens that can be refined and made more sophisticated based on review results. Reviewers of cases failing screens state the basis for their judgments, thus making explicit their implicit criteria
Assessors	A single 'peer', usually a hospital colleague	One or more qualified reviewers trained for the purpose who have demonstrated their ability to assess cases for quality problems (based on documented results of previous or test reviews); one reviewer's judgment that care exhibits a quality problem and its nature is often confirmed independently by another, to minimise reviewer misunderstandings and/or bias
Methods	Unstructured review of medical records; unreliable judgments	Structured review of medical records, focusing on potential problems identified by OPA screens; promotes accurate judgments

continues

Table II-5-1 *continued*

Characteristic	Traditional peer review	Structured quality review
Recording of findings	Unstructured; highly variable; usually minimal (judgments and reasoning remain largely implicit)	Structured; certain; defined (judgments and reasoning are made explicit)
Provider's response	May or may not allow a provider to respond	Provider is invited to comment on reviewers' findings, to eliminate further the possibility of misunderstanding of what was or was not done and why it was or was not done; the same or different reviewers complete the assessment in light of provider's comments
Statistical analysis	Usually none	Pattern analysis to identify, confirm, and illuminate quality problems, deficient processes and outcomes
Review results	Letter to care provider if reviewer finds care deficiencies	Reports to providers to show review results, including individual and patterns of care deficiencies; statistical comparisons with peers
Quality improvement potential	Little or none	When implemented as part of an integrated QM system substantial potential to improve continuously the quality of patient care and of SQR, leading to more effective and efficient quality management and further improvements in the quality of patient care

- involves implicit judgments which might vary from one reviewer to the next, about, for example:
  —which processes fit the patient's circumstances;
  —whether or not a maloutcome resulted from malprocess;
- is usually unstructured so that care problems may be missed and variable information is recorded about those quality problems that are identified;
- is usually limited to isolated case-by-case assessments without statistical analysis of findings;
- may involve bias if a doctor reviews a colleague's work;
- is usually limited to inpatient outcomes (because postdischarge information, for example, is lacking).

259.5 About structured quality review

Structured quality review (SQR) is a practical way to assess quality of care and is the most potent way to identify technical quality of care problems for purposes of quality improvement. It can provide the objective information that permits a hospital to fulfil its fiduciary responsibility to ensure that all doctors who practise within its walls are practising to standards. However, this responsibility should not overshadow SQR's main purpose—to improve the quality of care by helping doctors and other staff improve their performance through rational analysis of results and feedback of findings. Because it can be implemented easily, with minimal commitment of resources, SQR is likely to be the initial method for, and remain the mainstay of, problem identification in Australian hospitals for the foreseeable future. Structured quality review is necessary, but not sufficient, for an effective quality management program. At a minimum, hospitals must also have in place mechanisms to resolve the quality problems that SQR discovers (see Chapter 8 in this part).

Structured quality review refers to the three steps necessary to identify, confirm and illuminate quality of care problems. They are: screening, medical record review and pattern analysis. Screening refers specifically to use of automated outcome/process assessment (OPA) screens. Medical record review refers specifically to a structured process for examining medical records to assess quality of care. Pattern analysis refers to the statistical analysis of case-by-case assessments (screening data and/or structured review findings), to identify problems that can only be revealed this way or to illuminate their causes. Chapter 7 in this part details use of practice policies to develop outcome/process assessment screens. Chapter 8 in this part details structured quality review's use as the principal means for identifying quality problems toward assuring and improving the quality of care. Chapter 4 in Part IV details practical aspects of structured quality review's implementation.

Structured quality review overcomes the principal problems inherent in traditional peer review in the following ways. Automated outcome/process assessment screens permit cases to be reviewed objectively, comprehensively and economically for quality of care problems. Preliminary indications suggest that they are also more accurate than any other type of screen and more accurate than unaided medical record review. Accurate screening tools allow expert reviewers to focus on cases with potential problems, to know what those problems are that require review, and to improve the reliability of their assessments. Structured medical record review improves the reliability of reviewers' judgments. Further, pattern analysis, which automation makes practical, provides additional information about the distribution and nature of quality of care problems and permits continuous improvement in quality assessment processes.

Automated outcome/process assessment screens collect information on care processes and outcomes relevant to the care of a particular patient. Algorithms (decision rules) embedded in these screens intend to divide cases into two categories: those presumed acceptable and those requiring further review. By identifying the specific potential quality of care problems that require further review, these screens facilitate and structure subsequent medical record review.

If, after reviewing a patient's medical record, a reviewer affirms a potential quality of care problem identified by OPA screens, a second reviewer can confirm or deny its existence and nature, with a third, tie-breaking reviewer deciding the issue if the first two reviewers disagree. Presently, this degree of structure may be beyond the resources of most Australian hospitals, which might, therefore, have to rely on a single reviewer's judgment. In either case, if a reviewer identifies one or more potential quality of care problems, the quality manager should invite the responsible provider, which may be an individual clinician or the head of pharmacy, for example, to comment on the care provided and the reasoning behind it. The same, or another qualified reviewer, completes the assessment after receiving providers' comments.

Reviewers' case-by-case assessments are primarily data for subsequent pattern analysis. While in some instances findings of an individual patient's care will warrant immediate investigation or action to prevent an imminent danger to future patients, for example if reviewers suspect an operative death was due to the surgeon's impairment, in most cases proper pattern analysis is required to elucidate problems and prioritise investigation of their root causes. Through careful analysis of care processes and outcomes, doctors can learn the best way to treat patients according to current knowledge, and hospitals can improve their care systems and revise practice policies to improve patient outcomes.

259.6   Some quality assessment terms

259.61   THE NEED FOR CLEAR, COHERENT DEFINITIONS OF TERMS

We often talk here about unnecessary operations, inappropriate interventions and poor care. Clearly, all of these things diminish the quality of care. But are they all the same? The term 'appropriate' is used often in discussions about the quality of care, and mention of inappropriate care brings forth strong emotions. But what exactly does appropriate mean? Talk about the quality of care is often vague and ambiguous. Quality measurement or assessment demand precision in definitions. First we have to distinguish what is of concern. Are we trying to measure the quality or performance of the health care system or of an individual provider, for example hospital or doctor? Or are we trying to assess the quality of an episode of care? The following discussion pertains to terms that this manual uses in relation to quality assessment. Measurement of health care system performance is beyond its scope. By aggregating case-by-case assessments, hospitals can construct quality scores that measure their overall and individual provider's performance. They can use the resultant scores to monitor the extent to which their quality management program is improving the quality of their care.

259.62   QUALITY ASSESSMENT INVOLVES PROVIDER PERFORMANCE

Quality of care encompasses four dimensions: technical quality; the cost of care; patients' satisfaction (with the interpersonal aspects of care, for example); and trade-offs among the preceding three dimensions (see Chapter 5 in this part). Quality assessment focuses on technical quality: the extent that providers achieve achievable benefit for their patients. Specifically, in this manual's context, it refers to providers' conformance to care processes that if implemented properly result in maximum achievable patient health status improvement within patients' preferences and society's resources.

Practice policies are the starting point for delineating these processes and their expected resultant outcomes (see Chapter 7 in this part). Lack of knowledge limits such specifications, and hence the scientific practice of medicine. In principle, it is possible to specify all important product and production specifications (those that mostly determine technical quality) and thus to encompass all important aspects of caregiver excellence. In practice, most hospital (and external) quality assessors have failed to apply the effort necessary to maximise use of existing knowledge in quality assessment. Quality assessment is a necessary first step toward—but will only result in—systematic quality improvement if it is implemented as part of an integrated quality management system (see Chapter 6 in this part).

259.63   THE DIFFERENCE BETWEEN EFFECTIVENESS AND APPROPRIATENESS

People often confuse the terms effectiveness and appropriateness and erroneously use them interchangeably. In this manual, the term effectiveness relates to the extent to which an intervention improves the health status of a defined population of patients. The term appropriateness refers to the extent to which a provider expects an intervention to improve a particular patient's health (because he or she fits the profile of patients for whom it is an effective intervention).

Effectiveness is a statistical concept; appropriateness is a judgment. For quality management purposes, an effective intervention is one that improves the health status of a defined patient population or of the average patient in such a population—even if no, or a decrease in, health status results for some patients in the population. Clinicians, especially, usually think of effective interventions in terms of individual patients. Since medical science knowledge derives from populations of patients, they are extrapolating study findings or practice experience to a particular patient's circumstances. An appropriate intervention is one that fits the patient's circumstances and, therefore, is expected to be effective for that patient, that is, improve his or her health status beyond what it would be without the intervention.

259.64 ABOUT THE APPROPRIATENESS OF TREATMENT

Stated simply, appropriate means right for the purpose, or suitable for a particular condition, person or place. This definition is, of course, devoid of any specification of purpose or criteria for making judgments. One can only meaningfully interpret statements about the appropriateness of interventions, for example if the criteria, measurement methods, who made the judgments using the resultant measures, and how these judgments were made, are all stated clearly.

The term appropriate should be reserved for an episode or continuum of medical care (encompassing all interventions) considered as a whole. This judgment is certainly complex and includes, for example: diagnosis, treatment selection and implementation, and management of complications and such other aspects of care as patient instructions. In this context, appropriate patient care is synonymous with acceptable quality of care for that episode (referred to sometimes as adequate care or care meeting practice or clinical standards). Judging the appropriateness or quality of a patient care episode is complex and usually encompasses only one or a few aspects of the many involved. The job is simplified if concepts are kept straight and labelled (should we say it) appropriately.

Specific medical interventions can be divided into two broad classes: diagnostic and therapeutic. The adjective 'appropriate' is more often encountered in relation to therapeutic interventions, but applies to both. Use of an ineffective intervention (in the sense used here) is never appropriate. Use of an effective intervention may or may not be appropriate depending on the patient's circumstances and desires. This use of appropriate is very common. For example, one hears of 'inappropriate surgical operations'—effective interventions believed not to fit the patient's circumstances (e.g. because the clinician misdiagnosed the patient or recommended the wrong intervention for the patient's health problem). However, the non-use of an effective procedure may also be appropriate if, for example, the patient's age or frailty suggested that such intervention was contraindicated.

259.65 TREATMENT SELECTION—INDICATED, UNINDICATED INTERVENTIONS

Typically, judgments of appropriateness involve only patients who received the intervention. There may also be patients who did not receive the intervention but should have. Statements about how often an intervention is used 'appropriately' based on examining only patients who received it is obviously biased, but this flaw is often not thought about. How is one to distinguish between those who were given the intervention appropriately and those who were not given it appropriately?

When an intervention is given to those who should receive it, it should be called an indicated intervention. The same intervention given to patients who should not have received it should be referred to as an unindicated intervention (not indicated). Unindicated interventions may be subdivided into contraindicated, that is, the intervention would normally be indicated but in this particular case conditions (criteria) exist that suggest its use was contrary to the patient's interest, and non-indicated, that is, no conditions (criteria) exist to justify the intervention's use. Patients who should have received the intervention but did not, represent a missed indication; those who did not and should not have received it, a true negative indication.

259.66 TREATMENT IMPLEMENTATION

If the doctor selects the right treatment, he or she may or may not implement it properly. Implementation includes both doing the right steps in the right order (often expressed in procedural policies) and doing steps right, that is, not botching them. Proper implementation refers to following specified steps and implementing them properly. Improper implementation refers to not following specified steps and/or to botching them.

259.67 MANAGEMENT OF COMPLICATIONS

Interventions may give rise to complications, immediate maloutcomes following care processes that need to be recognised and treated to be reversed or, if irreversible, ameliorated. Proper management (of complications) refers to prompt recognition and treatment of complications; improper management (of complications), to delay in their recognition and/or their incorrect treatment. The existence of complications does not necessarily signify malprocess. Complications may be a consequence of the patient's condition or of intervention (and hence were unavoidable) or may arise from inappropriate intervention or from their improper implementation (and hence were potentially avoidable). Distinguishing avoidable from unavoidable complications may be difficult.

259.7 | *The fall of 'peer review' and rise of statistical analysis*

259.71 THE ISSUE ENGAGED

Externally-driven quality assurance efforts based on 'peer review' have generated a great deal of heat and little light; they have generally failed to improve the quality of care. Beginning in the 1990s, in the United States at least, health care regulators shifted their efforts from 'peer review' to statistical analysis of process and outcome data. The fundamental fact remains, however, that hospitals can only improve the quality of their care if they change care practices to achieve benefits not currently being achieved but are yet achievable. Traditional peer review has its flaws and its implementation has been faulty (see above). But the idea of reviewing medical records to identify quality problems is not inherently flawed; quite the contrary.

Peer review's critics focused on the tree—a way of identifying quality problems—and overlooked the forest—the need for providers to employ an integrated quality management system. Improving the quality of care requires changing care practices—practice policies and their implementing processes—which in turn requires the will and the means to change. There is significant disagreement about how best to promote quality improvement in nations' hospitals and other health care production facilities—principally external monitoring versus proper incentives for internal quality improvement efforts. As we have seen in industry, organisations—hospitals—committed to quality improvement will take the necessary steps to improve quality; the rest will not.

This manual focuses on convincing hospitals that they must commit to quality to improve the quality of their care systematically, and that modern quality management technology makes it practical to assess, assure and improve quality systematically. It remains for national governments—or such integrated delivery systems as accountable health care plans—to decide the best incentives to encourage health care providers to improve the quality of their care, thereby significantly raising the health care system's productivity, in contrast to the marginal results of the valiant but isolated efforts of the system's most committed providers.

259.72 THE HEALTH CARE SYSTEM-LEVEL PERSPECTIVE

The view that 'peer review' had failed to improve the quality of care gained currency in the United States beginning in the early 1990s; 'peer review' had become discredited as a quality assurance strategy. Traditional peer review had long been the mainstay of QA in hospitals—internal quality assurance—where it was mostly form over substance—and by regulatory agencies, principally PSROs (and later PROs)—external quality assurance—where, in deed if not design, it mostly involved protecting beneficiaries by 'weeding out bad apples'—identifying deficient providers and excluding them from the program—Medicare, in the case of HCFA's watchdogs, the PROs. They barked but did not bite. PROs review of samples of Medicare cases was highly variable and generated substantial rancor but few sanctions (actions against providers based on findings of poor quality) and precious little quality improvement.

This disillusionment with the impact of 'peer review' on the quality of care led to the implicit view that judgments about the appropriateness of care in individual cases are unnecessary—and even undesirable—because the goal is to redesign processes to improve quality—to increase patient health status improvement, reduce costs, enhance patient satisfaction, or perfect trade-offs among them.

Statistical analysis of variation has largely replaced case-by-case review as the route to the promised land, at least in US health care regulators' minds. For example, in 1992 HCFA announced its new strategy for improving Medicare beneficiaries' quality of care. Its goal is 'to move from dealing with individual clinical errors to helping providers to improve the mainstream of care'.[8] HCFA plans to:

- use uniform criteria (to overcome local variability);
- focus on persistent differences between the observed and the achievable in process and outcomes (and less on occasional unusual deficiencies in care);
- help providers identify problems and solutions by monitoring patterns of care and outcomes.

HCFA's principal thrust is to provide hospitals with statistical data on their care processes and outcomes (see MQIS above)—something that quality-focused hospitals should already be doing—and, through its PROs, to enter into forced 'quality improvement partnerships'—which would likely be unnecessary if hospitals were given proper incentives to improve the quality of their care. External agencies' statistical analysis of process and outcome variation is unlikely to be any more successful than 'peer review' unless providers are given incentives to improve the quality of their care. There is a positive danger that providing hospitals with statistical information will provide a false sense that something useful is being done and that quality must inevitably improve as a result.

External statistical comparisons of hospitals' performance on selected process and outcome variables—so-called quality or clinical indicators—certainly avoids the taint and rancor of 'peer review' but they represent a leap of faith—and a substantial commitment of scarce QA/QI resources. There is considerable doubt about indicators' validity and little evidence that providers are prepared 'to conduct the more intrusive and detailed study of who, when, and why'.[8] Further, in the case of HCFA's MQIS, being obliged to send copies of medical records to an external agency and forced to participate in 'quality improvement partnerships' is unlikely to strike many providers as 'unintrusive', especially when HCFA 'will still be responsible for imposing sanctions if education fails'.[8]

External agencies' most essential roles are clearly to set the drivers—the incentives for health care providers to engage in substantial, systematic and sustained quality improvement; to insist on mechanisms to substantiate providers' claims of quality improvement—by mandating (but not necessarily carrying out) independent audits of claims, for example; and to monitor the system's success—through providers' audited data, for example. The extent to which emphasis on the provision of statistical analyses—exemplified by HCFA's new quality improvement program, and by JCAHO or ACHS clinical indicator data (see Chapter 8 in this part)—will result in systematic and system-wide quality improvement is debatable. But in the absence of internal drive fueled by appropriate incentives, logic alone suggests that such efforts may be yet another example of hope triumphing over experience.

259.73 THE HEALTH PRODUCTION-LEVEL PERSPECTIVE

As a quality improvement strategy, traditional peer review—unstructured review of (often haphazardly selected samples of) medical records by colleagues—failed on several grounds. First, it was often cast in an adversarial context especially when conducted by external agencies—the quality police. Second, it focused on what doctors did (or did not do), as if doctors alone could improve the quality of care, and assumed that if they were apprised of the supposed errors of their ways quality would improve. Third, peer review operated in a vacuum, and, even if it identified significant quality problems, there were usually neither incentives nor mechanisms to change care processes to improve outcomes. Hospitals were not quality-focused organisations and, consequently, not organised for quality improvement.

For health care providers at least, the fundamental fact remains that conformance to processes that produce maximal patient health status improvement is essential to assure—and to improve—quality. Quality managers must inevitably decide if care is appropriate (that is, conforms to practice policies and their implementing processes) and if not, why not, to attempt to pinpoint quality problems and to redesign practices and processes to eliminate them and thus facilitate such conformance. Whenever possible one should redesign processes to produce more patient health status improvement than was possible with old designs—by introducing new practice policies or better ways of implementing existing ones. However, again the fundamental fact remains that improved quality can only be assured by conformance to new practice policies or with better ways of implementing existing ones. Assessing the extent to which conformance exists to practice policies and their implementing processes is vital to quality assurance, and hence to quality improvement. Structured quality review (see above and Chapter 8 in this part) is a practical mechanism for assessing and monitoring conformance to specified policies and processes and hence quality of care.

How can hospitals improve the quality of care? Hospitals must first commit to systematic quality improvement. Second, they must manifest their will to change—itself a major change. Third, they must demonstrate their will to change by proving the means to change. Without the will—and the necessary quality improvement structures, processes and resources—to change, no amount of case-by-case data or statistical analyses will produce systematic and sustained quality improvement.

References

1 Gavin DA. Competing on the eight dimensions of quality. Harvard Business Review 1987; Nov/Dec: 101–09.
2 Donabedian A. Evaluating the quality of medical care. Millbank Memorial Fund 1966; 44: 166–206.
3 Goldschmidt PG. The appropriate organizational locus for constructing indicators of the quality of hospitals and physicians and for evaluating the validity of those indicators. Background paper to: Office of Technology Assessment. The quality of medical care: Information for consumers. Washington, DC: US Government Printing Office, 1988.
4 HCFA distributes death rate data (quietly). Medical Utilization Review 1993; 21(17): 1–2.
5 Rosenthal GE, Harper DL. Cleveland Health Quality Choice: A model for collaborative community-based outcomes assessment. Journal on Quality Improvement 1994; 10 (8): 425-42.
6 Goldschmidt PG. Severity of illness: Red herring or horse of a different color? Part 1. Physician Executive 1989; 15(4): 7–11.
7 The quality indicator system: Description of the module development process. Baltimore, MD: Health Care Financing Administration, presentation materials, August 2, 1994.
8 Jencks SF, Wilensky GR. The health care quality improvement initiative. JAMA 1992; 268: 900–03.

Chapter 6

QUALITY MANAGEMENT, ASSURANCE AND IMPROVEMENT

---

260 | Contents

This chapter deals with quality management, quality assurance and quality improvement under the following major headings:

261. Purpose of this chapter
262. Key concepts
263. Industrial analogies
264. Quality management is a production-level tool
265. Quality management system
266. Quality control
267. Quality assurance, quality improvement and CQI
268. Utilisation review
269. Utilisation management in the United States.

261 | Purpose of this chapter

The health professions have struggled for millennia to improve the quality of care. The success of their efforts has waxed and waned, and was often isolated and sporadic. Now we are poised to place them on centre stage and make them systematic and continuous. The potential benefits are enormous. For patients, the quality revolution portends:

- guaranteed quality—true quality assurance—knowing what to expect from health care and being sure of getting it;
- enhanced quality—continuous quality improvement—more, and reduced variation in, health status improvement; contained, if not reduced, cost; and greater satisfaction with care.

Hospitals need a complete and comprehensive quality management system to guarantee and enhance the quality of their care. In Australia, externally-driven and internally-motivated quality assurance efforts have been minimal. Hospitals in Australia and elsewhere have yet to adopt successful quality management programs that take full advantage of emerging techniques for assuring and improving quality. Some hospitals have adopted some of these techniques, but have either not adopted sufficient of them, and/or have not integrated them sufficiently to create an effective quality management program. Lack of incentives to improve quality is the principal reason for lack of effective quality management programs. Feedback of results to improve practice policies, care processes and quality control elements is the principal missing link to integrate systems and to improve the quality of care.

Hospitals' quality managers must think systematically about quality control. They must decide the best mix of preproduction, intraproduction, and postproduction control mechanisms for their hospital's circumstances at both the organisational and workface levels. Hospitals are wasting their resources if they do not have in place the preproduction and intraproduction quality control mechanisms that postproduction quality control (quality assurance) activities are designed to inform, and the means to change production processes.

To succeed in the coming quest for quality, managers will have to learn how to manage information: to apply the tools of research, information science and knowledge engineering to their business, and will have to learn how to improve continuously their organisation's ability to generate efficiently and use effectively the knowledge and information it needs to be successful in improving products and operations. To date, hospitals have paid scant attention to generating quality improvement information, leaving this task to others. As part of the quality revolution, hospitals must begin to measure long-term outcomes (end results of care), and conduct or collaborate with others in the conduct of medical technology assessment and other forms of health systems research to provide the information needed to improve the effectiveness and efficiency of their care, and of their quality management programs.

This chapter summarises a quality management system's essence. It describes industrial quality control (QC) technology and techniques in reference to preproduction, intraproduction, and postproduction phases of manufacturing, and corresponding health care quality control mechanisms. In particular, this chapter describes:

- a quality management (QM) system on which hospitals can base their quality management programs;
- how a quality management system can assure and improve the quality of care (QA/QI);
- utilisation review (UR);
- risk management (RM); and
- relationships among quality management, QA/QI, UR and RM.

These are complex, extensive subjects. Moreover, hospitals' quality management programs must be based on their particular needs and circumstances. Consequently, this chapter provides an overview of concepts and approaches, not a detailed plan that they can implement.

---

262 Key concepts

This chapter elaborates on the following key concepts essential to understanding quality management (QM), quality assurance (QA), and quality improvement (QI), and to designing and implementing an effective hospital quality management program.

- Production-level quality is concerned with provider performance: the extent to which providers improve patients' health status, at what cost and with what patient satisfaction.

- Quality management is a production-level tool, useful for improving the quality of hospitals' care. It encompasses production quality control to produce products to specifications and product quality improvement, specifications that customers (patients) believe represent better value for money. Endless repetition of the conformance improvement, specifications improvement and technology improvement cycles is necessary to continuously improve products' quality.
- An effective quality management system assures and continuously improves the treatment of individual patients and the effectiveness of treatments. It encompasses mechanisms to:
  —control or assure product quality at each of production's three phases: preproduction (e.g. admissions policies, credentialling, practice policies), intraproduction (e.g. decision support technologies), and postproduction (e.g. quality assessment and quality assurance);
  —generate the information needed to validate and improve practice policies and their constituent product and process technologies (e.g. outcomes measurement, and research and development);
  —manage and improve the quality of quality management.
- Quality control takes places at two levels: the organisation and the workface. Organisations design production systems to produce products to specifications. What occurs at the workface determines products' quality. Ideally, organisational quality control mechanisms promote workface quality and workface experience shapes organisational quality control mechanisms.
- Product inspections have long been the mainstay of production quality control. At best they can identify defective products so that they are not shipped to customers. Inspections can be costly, and the cost of reworking or scrapping defective products can be very high. If a product does not meet specifications one can only reject it; one cannot inspect-in quality. Improving quality requires changing inputs to and/or production processes to prevent production of defective products.
- Classic industrial production quality control methods designed to achieve zero product defects cannot be applied easily to clinical care. Health care production quality control involves primarily ensuring that interventions match patients' health problems and desires (patient–process fit), and, secondarily, implementing them properly.
- The most cost-effective health care quality control strategy is postproduction quality of care assessment with subsequent modifications to care processes, coupled with various preproduction quality control mechanisms, including targeted preprocedure review. Eventually, intraproduction quality control will likely become routine, diminishing the need to rely on other forms of quality control.
- Health care's products are manifest principally in practice policies, pre-established clinical decision rules for treating individual patients that take into account their preferences regarding ends and means. Procedural (or process) policies operationalise elements within practice policies and thus specify them in greater, operational detail. Elemental specifications refer to the quality, cost and acceptability of elements used within production processes.
- Practice policies make explicit assumptions between health care processes (specific medical interventions) and patients' health status improvement. Conformance to practice policies will only improve patients' health status if they are effective. Conformance to effective practice policies will improve

quality, but only to the limits of the underlying technologies. Further improvement in health status requires better product and production technologies (including human factors management strategies that engender trust).

- Quality assurance (QA), utilisation review (UR) and risk management (RM) are distinct but integral parts of quality management (QM). But QM encompasses far more than QA, UR and RM.

- Quality assurance intends primarily to ensure that care conforms to specifications and to provide information to validate and improve them; utilisation review, to ensure that resources are used appropriately (a subset of QA); risk management, to reduce the hospital's exposure to financial loss.

- The cost of achieving health status improvement is an important dimension of the quality of care. Quality is improved if providers reduce the cost of achieving a given level of patient health status improvement.

- Utilisation review (UR) focuses on a provider's use of resources for the care of individual patients, and encompasses medical necessity of interventions, their timing, setting and duration. Traditionally, UR has not been concerned with questions of value achieved for money spent, nor with the efficiency with which providers deliver interventions. Utilisation review must be an integral part of any hospital quality management program.

- Quality assurance and quality improvement are important but distinct aspects of production and product quality; continuous quality improvement (CQI) is merely performing QA/QI on a continuous basis. Arguments about the superiority of CQI over QA are vacuous.

- Quality assurance, or conformance improvement (CI), refers to a cyclical process involving quality assessment—retrospective review of care outcomes and processes based on documentation in the patient's medical record—and steps to improve care processes to close any performance gaps.

- Hospitals can bring what they do and achieve in line with what they should do and achieve, and revise practice policies to reduce variation in outcomes, thereby improving their quality of care. Further quality improvement depends on changing practice policies (thereby constituting a new product), which, in turn, depends on developing better product and process technology (e.g. better diagnostic or therapeutic interventions and better ways of delivering them).

- Outcomes must be measured, not assumed. Outcomes' measurement provides information on the end results of care in relation to care processes and patient characteristics. This information can improve the design and content of practice policies, confirm or cast doubt on interventions' effectiveness, point to the need for better interventions, and help set research priorities.

- Outcomes' measurement cannot provide incontrovertible evidence about interventions' effectiveness and can never be regarded as a substitute for clinical trials or other experimental research. Patients select doctors and doctors select interventions; substantial patient–provider selection bias may exist.

- Research studies, especially controlled clinical trials (which can overcome patient–provider selection bias), provide the best information for formulating practice policies and designing medical interventions and care processes. Such studies must include the cost of practices. The often-encountered quest

for incremental effectiveness at any price must yield to the search for more cost-effective interventions.
- Given the vast deficit in knowledge and the impossibility of conducting all needed research, quality management programs that measure patients' long-term outcomes represent an untapped reservoir of potential information to improve health care quality.
- Closing the quality management gap between hospitals' current meagre quality management efforts and the structures and processes necessary to achieve quality maturity is a daunting prospect. The best approach is to create the skeleton of a complete quality management system and to develop its various elements according to the hospital's needs, circumstances and experience.

263 | Industrial analogies

263.1 | Industrial framework

Total quality management (TQM) is a management philosophy that focuses on the quality of an enterprise's products. It sees an enterprise's actions in the light of their effects on the quality of its products and services, and the productive use of its resources to produce them. Chapter 2 in this part describes the background to and the various aspects of TQM.

A quality product satisfactorily meets customers' wants or needs at a price they are willing to pay. A product's quality is determined by its design, its production and, most importantly, the relationship between the product's specifications and the processes intended to produce it. Design the right product; specify it right (so that it is manufacturable to specifications); produce it right. The tension between design creativity and manufacturing certainty must be resolved favourably to avoid designs that cannot be manufactured properly and exquisite manufactures that no one wants to buy at the offered price.

In market economies, manufacturers are free to produce and market whatever products they want, how they want, within certain legal or regulatory restrictions. Manufacturers often specialise in one or a limited number of market segments and serve only certain customers whose needs they can meet competitively. An enterprise's success depends on how well it identifies and pleases its customers. Well-designed, well-made products do well in the marketplace, especially if priced competitively. Companies making such products prosper; those who do not wither and may go out of business. Companies that offer a high quality product at a competitive or premium price, or a product of acceptable quality at a low price, are highly successful. Those that offer average products at average prices are less successful; those that offer poor products, least successful. Competition among companies for customers drives continuous improvement in product design, manufacture and distribution. Products shape customers' preferences as well as being affected by them.

Production quality can be viewed simply as conformance to specifications. Its quality goal is zero defects: producing products to specifications, the first time and every time. Rework (fixing imperfect but repairable products) and scrap (discarding irreparable products)—the results of non-conformance to specifications—are the cost of not doing it right the first time. That cost can be very substantial. The best way to do it right the first and every time is to build quality and defect-prevention into the manufacturing process, which can result in tremendous improvements in product quality, uniformity and huge reductions in production costs.

263.2 *Production quality control*

Quality control takes places at two levels: the organisation and the workface. At the organisational level, manufacturers design production systems to produce products to specifications. Production systems encompass not only production materials, machines and methods but also, for example, human factors including incentives, and quality control mechanisms such as final product inspection. Figure II-6-1 below shows these relationships in the form of a cause–effect diagram. It also equates manufacturing's 7 Ms with health care's 7 Ps. Ultimately, what occurs at the workface determines products' quality. Ideally, organisational quality control mechanisms promote workface quality and workface experience shapes organisational quality control mechanisms.

Conceptually, quality control is a production subsystem that consists of various mechanisms that production managers can select and employ to various degrees. Production quality control's goal is to produce products that meet specifications. Managers can evaluate a particular system's cost-effectiveness by comparing the extent to which alternative quality control systems result in defect-free products, or detect defective parts or products, to the cost of achieving this level of quality control (including the cost of reworking or scrapping defective products and of servicing or replacing defective products that slip through the quality control net). The most cost-effective mix of quality control strategies or mechanisms depends on circumstances and changes dynamically. The right mix depends principally on three sets of factors: technological (what is possible); economic (what is affordable); and human (what is acceptable). To the extent practical, production control mechanisms should be part of production processes or at least integrated with them.

Product inspections have long been the mainstay of production quality control. At best, they can identify defective products so that they are not shipped to customers. However, the effort required to inspect every product can be costly, and the cost of reworking or scrapping defective products can be very high. Moreover, if a product does not meet specifications one can only reject it; one cannot inspect-in quality. By itself, inspection does nothing to reduce the production of defective products, which requires changes to production processes. To the extent practical, it is best to find out immediately that manufacturing processes are producing defective products (so that they produce

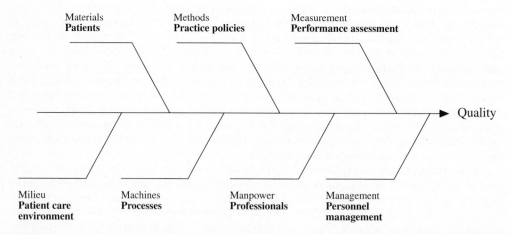

Figure II-6-1 *Factors affecting product quality—cause–effect diagram equating manufacturing's 7 Ms with health care's 7 Ps. After Ishikawa, K.* What is total quality control—the Japanese way. *Englewood Cliffs, New Jersey: Prentice Hall, 1985*

fewer defects), or, best of all, to design processes to prevent defects' manufacture. Consequently, quality control engineers have searched for ways to put quality control mechanisms at the earliest stages of production, to move inspections closer to production, and to develop production methods that promise defect-free products. Quality management methods endeavour to engage all employees in the quest to improve quality and to encourage them to collaborate toward this end.

For quality control purposes, production can be divided into three phases: preproduction, intraproduction, and postproduction. While these three phases appear to be and, in many cases, are quite distinct, in some circumstances they seem to merge, and depend on how one delineates particular production processes. Fabrication, for example of automobiles, involves adding components to an assembly of other components to produce the finished product. Individual components are usually inspected before they enter the assembly line—a preproduction mechanism for controlling the quality of the finished product. However, in some production systems (e.g. those that employ the just-in-time inventory method, explained below) components are inspected on the line. This method is usually classified as an intraproduction quality control mechanism because it takes place within production—the assembly line, in the case of this example.

This section summarises how manufacturers control the quality of the products that they produce. It describes quality control mechanisms in reference to the three phases of production: preproduction, intraproduction, and postproduction. The section intends to communicate essential concepts in industrial production control, where they originated, and to lay the groundwork for exploring the limitations of applying them to health care. It is not intended to be a manual on industrial quality control, a large and complex subject.

263.3 Preproduction quality control

Common industrial preproduction methods include materials inspection, worker selection and training, preprocess verification, and a variety of methods we label 'industrial practices'.

Products made from parts can be only as good as the parts and the way they fit together. Manufacturers who buy parts or ingredients ensure that they meet specifications before they enter production. Until recently, manufacturers relied heavily on inspecting incoming goods. Because of the sheer volume of parts, they sampled them statistically and as a result accepted or rejected batches (or entire shipments), especially if testing was destructive. While economical compared to examining every single part, batches accepted on the basis of samples could still contain quite a few defective parts that were incorporated into products and might be detected only by customers. Moreover, if defects were parts per thousand or per million, large samples would be necessary. Obviously, it might be cheaper and better to have suppliers deliver defect-free parts. Quality-focused manufacturers work with their suppliers to reduce defects to parts per million. When suppliers achieve predetermined quality levels, manufacturers can avoid the expense and time involved in inspecting incoming parts, as these costs would exceed the costs incurred from whatever defective parts remain, which, of course, may be picked up later in the manufacturing process.

Proper selection and training of workers is such an elementary idea that it hardly bears mention, except it is often forgotten or not done well. Manufacturers' ability to select among job applicants requires valid methods for determining who would and would not be a qualified employee, which is not always practical, and sufficient qualified applicants to fill all available jobs, which might not always be the case. Most people benefit from training and the ability to be trained may be the applicant's most important qualification. Obviously, employees should be trained properly before they begin work, but employers often overlook this step or have limited means of providing the necessary training. Once on the job, employee performance can be used to identify training needs (as well as other remediable problems that affect product quality). Extensive job-related training reinforces the need for proper recruitment and attention to retention, as staff turnover involves the loss of trained workers and the expense of recruiting and training replacements.

Preprocess verification involves checking that inputs and process conditions are right to produce the desired products. Industry uses a variety of preprocess verification techniques including the obvious and simple, for example checking oven temperatures before firing pottery. Two important industrial practices are proper preventive maintenance of production machines, including their calibration for example, and their proper layout to facilitate efficient production of products to specifications.

263.4 Intraproduction (in-process) quality control

In-process quality controls are those integral to production processes. They are now beginning to emerge as key quality control tools, because by checking and controlling manufacturing parameters to ensure products meet specifications they promise error-free production. With in-process quality control, postproduction inspection is only necessary to check that these controls are functioning and is less onerous than that required to weed out defects. The most promising in-process quality controls involve computer-controlled manufacturing robots. Older, simpler techniques can still be useful, such as poke-yoke, a Japanese term for fool-proofing production. For example, assemblies can be polarised so that they fit together only the one, correct way. Screws can be delivered in exactly the right quantity, to be inserted into predrilled holes until none are left.

In-process quality control can involve inspecting parts on the production line prior to incorporating them into products, for example kanban (which if done off the line would be classified as preproduction verification), and immediately inspecting products of production processes, for example statistical process control (which if done off the line would be classified as postproduction quality control). Assembly line workers often do these inspections, which enriches their jobs because they are responsible for products' quality and not just their production and they enjoy a greater variety of work activity. Inspections' proximity to production processes prevents production of defective products by avoiding incorporation of defective parts in products (kanban), or by shutting production down as soon as it begins to produce products outside of specifications (statistical process control).

Kanban, just-in-time, inventory methods were designed originally to reduce inventory costs, which they obviously do because they eliminate costs associated with parts' inventories. In addition, because assemblies are made and delivered in relatively small quantities and used immediately, in some situations kanban can quickly discover quality problems. Internal or external suppliers can rectify production processes before they produce large quantities of defective parts which have to be reworked or scrapped.

Production workers who are trained to use control charts implement statistical process control (SPC), a classic industrial quality control method. Essentially, a worker periodically measures critical parameters and plots them on the control chart. When a reading exceeds the control limits drawn on the chart the worker stops production and, alone or with help, investigates why the process went out of control and remedies underlying causes before starting it up again.

Production managers can speed up assembly lines to identify weak links in the production chain that might be strengthened. When managers speed up the line they expect the proportion of defective products will increase. By increasing the incidence of defective products, managers can investigate and remedy their underlying causes. When the retooled production line runs at normal speed, the proportion of defective products that workers produce is below that they produced previously. If after the changes workers can operate the production line faster and still produce a greater proportion of products to specifications, quality has also been enhanced by lowered production costs, creating the opportunity to provide customers with even greater value for money and workers with higher wages.

<h3>263.5   *Postproduction quality control*</h3>

Inspection or testing of final products was until recently the mainstay of industrial quality control. Until the quality revolution, some manufacturers relied on customers to perform this function, often with disastrous consequences for their bottom line. Inherently, customers will always perform the ultimate quality check. Thus customer complaints and service calls are an important source of information on product quality. Moreover, the idea that customers use products to meet some need has led some manufacturers to conclude that they are really delivering a service; the product is merely its conduit. For example, people who buy drill bits are usually interested in holes of a certain size, depth and accuracy, not in collecting shiny pieces of ironmongery.

While one cannot inspect-in quality (i.e. inspection alone cannot improve the quality of a defective product), inspection can at least weed out defective products and prevent them from being shipped to customers. Further, they can often be reworked or repaired rather than scrapped, and ultimately shipped to customers. Most importantly, identification of defective products is the first step to improving production processes to reduce the proportion of them that they produce. Quality-focused manufacturers investigate defective products' underlying causes and change products' designs, manufacturing specifications, and production systems to remove them, thereby assuring subsequent products' quality.

With a full array of upstream quality controls, final inspection may be unnecessary except to check on the adequacy with which these methods are working, which if done statistically rather than inspecting every item may yield considerable savings. Manufacturing productivity is related directly to the number and cost of defective products and the cost of quality controls This information must be integrated with that from manufacturing operations to realise maximally product quality improvement.

<h2>264   **Quality management is a production-level tool**</h2>

<h3>264.1   *Perspective*</h3>

Health care production-level quality is concerned with provider performance: the extent to which providers improve patients' health status, at what cost, and with what patient satisfaction. Production systems and, ultimately, product and process technology limit the extent to which providers can increase patients' health status improvement and reduce the cost of its achievement. Providers' performance is influenced by their organisational or operating environment, including the incentives that it contains or creates, which in turn is influenced by government policies, health care financing mechanisms, and health care's culture. This manual focuses on production-level quality and the rest of this chapter discusses a system for managing the quality of care. Subsequent chapters elaborate on this system's elements.

Quality management is a production-level tool, useful for improving the quality of hospitals' care. The twin interlocking cycles (product–production and technology–product) shown in Figure II-6-2 on page 268 (and described in Chapter 2 of this part)

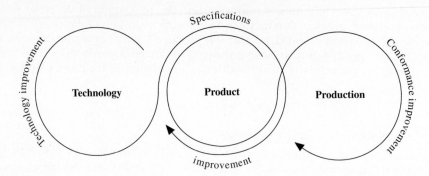

Figure II-6-2 *Quality improvement: Interlocking cycles*

determine quality. Quality management can improve health care quality through the following three quality improvement cycles:

- conformance improvement cycle, which intends to perfect the fit between what should be done and achieved (expressed product specifications or practice policies) and what is done and achieved (measured product quality or observed care processes and patient outcomes);
- specifications improvement cycle, which intends to improve product specifications or increase the amount of health status improvement that medical care can achieve with existing technology;
- technology improvement cycle, which intends to develop better product and process technology, to enhance the means for improving health status and reducing the cost of its achievement, for example.

Endless repetition of these cycles is necessary to improve continuously and perpetually products' quality. Figure II-6-3 on page 269 depicts functionally the conformance and specifications improvement cycles, modelled after the industrial PDCA (Plan-Do-Check-Act) cycle (often referred to as the quality improvement cycle and sometimes as quality control) to create the virtuous health care quality improvement spiral. As this figure indicates, traditional health care quality assurance activities involve the check and act nodes of the quality improvement cycle. Today hospitals, and even health care systems, do not manage quality through the technology improvement cycle, a major weakness in the quest for quality. If they manage quality at all, they do so rarely through the specifications improvement cycle, and mostly through the conformance improvement cycle, which they often operationalise poorly. For the foreseeable future, hospitals must depend on the interlocking conformance and specifications improvement cycles to improve their quality of care. To operationalise successfully the quality improvement spiral, hospitals must:

- design practice policies to ensure the best fit between what patients need and what they receive to produce maximal health status improvement; and standardise production processes to achieve this end;
- measure and assure conformance to process specifications (manifest in practice policies) to assure the quality of care and to reduce process variation as a source of outcome variation;
- measure first immediate and then long-term patient outcomes, and their variation; use this information to improve first conformance to process specifications and then to revise practice policies and practices to improve outcomes;

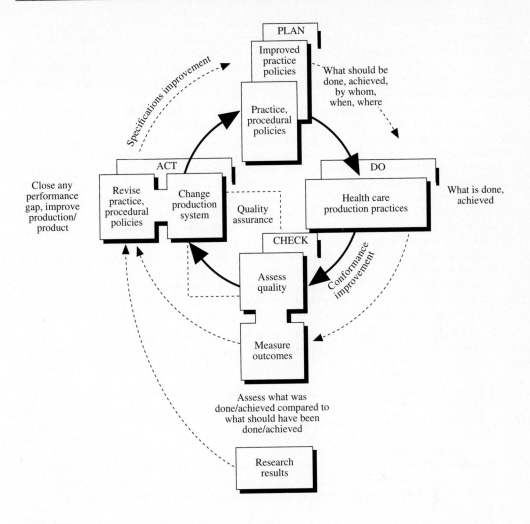

Figure II-6-3 *Health care quality improvement spiral*

- educate providers of the need for, and train them to implement properly, planned changes to processes intended to improve patient outcomes and to minimise any initial increase in their variation consequent to such changes.

264.2 | *Assuring and improving production-level quality*

Quality management has the following two principal functions:

- production quality control—controlling inputs to and the implementation of production processes to assure product quality;
- production quality improvement—generating information to improve product designs, production processes and quality control mechanisms.

The term quality control is rarely used in connection with health care. Instead, one hears the term quality assurance (QA), which encompasses only a fraction of its essential aspects. The term quality control refers to all mechanisms that intend to assure product and production quality (to produce products to specifications); traditional health care QA is one such mechanism. The broader term quality management (QM) refers to all mechanisms that intend to assure and improve product quality ad infinitum toward realising the greatest possible value for money, expressed, for example, in terms of the amount of health status improvement relative to the resources expended to achieve it. Quality management mechanisms can, and should, be subject to the same types of improvement activities to which they subject health care (QM of QM).

Some hospital managers might argue that they can exert very little direct control over what goes on in their hospitals, particularly with regard to doctors' behaviour, for example. Managers' inability to influence product quality is a failure of management, but not necessarily of managers who must function within the constraints of the system. In democratic industrialised societies, factory managers have limited powers to coerce others and must lead rather than dictate. The fact remains that market-based economic systems hold factory managers responsible for the quality of their products and, importantly, reward success. Hospital managers should be responsible for the quality of their hospitals' products. Society and hospital boards of directors should hold them accountable and reward them accordingly.

Product and process specifications are the keys to quality improvement. The combination of a health problem and the specified means for its diagnosis and treatment constitutes a health care product. For all practical purposes, assuring the quality of hospitals' care depends on conformance to these specifications. The operationalisation of quality control mechanisms depends on at least the following three types of specifications:

- product specifications—practice policies represent health care's product specifications. They state how each type of patient should be diagnosed, treated, and followed-up, for example total hip replacement for patients with painful degenerative disease;
- process specifications—procedural (or process) policies that operationalise elements within practice policies and thus specify them in greater, operational, detail, for example the way in which a given hip replacement operation should be conducted to assure the least variation in care processes (and hence patient outcomes) at the lowest possible cost;
- elemental specifications—the quality, cost and acceptability of elements used within production processes, for example in the case of a total hip replacement operation, the characteristics of the surgeon, prosthesis and radiographic images.

Workflows—the sequencing of production processes, including, for example, how the patient moves from one process to the next in or outside of the hospital—affect patient outcomes, throughput times (the period from admission to separation) and hence the cost of care and patient satisfaction. Hospitals pay scant attention to translating product specifications—practice policies—into production specifications—processes and workflows—in part because they lack explicit practice policies, for example. Once practice policies are extant, hospitals face the difficult task of translating them into optimal workflows and processes.

The first step is to produce clinical pathways or care maps that chart optimal routes through care processes. Practice policies for various diseases that the hospital manages may involve surgical procedures that take place in the operating theatre (a care process), for example. Next, the hospital must forecast time-distributed demand for the process to assure that it has the capacity, for example equipment and personnel, to meet expected demand at any given moment. All surgeons' desire to operate in the morning is an obvious example of a workflow problem. Optimal process scheduling can reduce costs associated with excess capacity and reduce patient throughput time. Various techniques exist for workflow planning and control. Their consideration and the (re)design of processes (sometimes referred to as process re-engineering) are beyond this manual's scope.

264.3 Practice policies

Hospitals' products have traditionally been amorphous. Indeed most Australian hospitals are hard-pressed to describe their output much beyond the annual number of separations. Whatever product specifications exist are implicit in doctors' minds, who likely implement them inconsistently, with great variation among ostensibly similar patients and between what the doctor says are his or her own criteria and what he or she does in practice.

Specifying products and processes to produce them is the key to improving quality. Practice policies specify health care's products: what should be done and achieved for specific types of patients. For a given type of patient, practice policies define what care is appropriate and hence what equipment and facilities are needed. The use of explicit practice policies is only now beginning. Even simple practice policies, if formulated and used consistently, can improve the quality of care. Feedback of results provides the information needed to revise practice policies toward further improving the quality of care. Quality management methods can not only improve practice policies but also improve the running of the hospital including, for example, information systems, incentives and quality management.

Quality improvement results from better conformance to practice policies—which results from quality assurance activities; better practice policies—which result from various quality management techniques; and better product and process technology—which results from research and development. Better conformance to properly implemented practice policies reduces variation in process and, for a given type of patient, variation in outcomes thereby increasing both patient health status improvement and the certainty of its attainment. For all practical purposes, practice policies define hospitals' products and are the key to assuring and improving the quality of hospital care. Consequently, practice policies are a central focus of this manual. Subsequent sections in this chapter describe practice policies' central role in quality assurance and quality improvement. Chapter 7 in this part elaborates further on practice policies and practice criteria, including their role in assessing the quality of care, the first step toward its improvement.

264.4 Procedural policies

To develop procedural policies, hospitals must examine care processes (referred to sometimes as clinical pathways, critical pathways, anticipated recovery paths, or care maps), for example operative preparation, type of prosthesis, technique of insertion, postsurgical nursing care, discharge planning and rehabilitation, in every aspect—for example what is done, the order in which it is done, who does it, how it is done—and decide exactly how and where the operation is to be done. An individual hospital, including its surgeons, may either work these details out for itself or follow someone else's blueprint. To date, we have spent virtually nothing on this type of research. Pioneering efforts by Brent James (Intermountain Health Care, Salt Lake City, Utah) have demonstrated that using these types of industrial approaches patient outcomes can be maintained or improved, while reducing costs significantly.[1] Consequently, hospitals will have to place far greater emphasis on ensuring that all of their surgeons, for example, faithfully follow specified practice and procedural policies. This manual describes procedural policies' role in quality assurance and improvement. However, their detailed consideration is beyond its scope.

264.5 Elemental specifications

The characteristics of elements in production processes are determined by training programs, device manufacturers, radiology departments (and their equipment suppliers) and so on. With respect to surgeons, for example, the hospital may identify specific performance weaknesses, guide continuing medical education efforts and monitor changes in performance. In other instances, for example radiological images, the hospital may produce the services and thus be vitally interested in improving their quality, or decide to contract out for these services if such out-sourcing will result in higher quality and/or lower cost services.

Generally the hospital is the customer for elements used in production processes and assures their quality by choosing among alternative suppliers (assuming that there is a choice and that suppliers do not produce essentially identical products). In some instances, hospitals may give suppliers feedback or other assistance to improve products, especially if the supplier practises TQM. Hospitals with quality management programs work collaboratively with their suppliers—including medical practitioners—to assure and improve the quality of inputs to health care production processes. This manual describes elemental specifications' impact on product quality; their further consideration is beyond its scope.

264.6 Quality assurance, utilisation review and risk management

Quality assurance (QA), utilisation review (UR) and risk management (RM) are distinct but integral parts of quality management (although it encompasses far more than these essential elements), which may be distinguished conceptually on the basis of their purpose.

- Quality assurance intends primarily to ensure that care conforms to practice policies (or pre-established process and outcome criteria and standards), and to provide information to validate and improve them, and hence improve quality.
- Utilisation review intends primarily to ensure that resources are used appropriately by ensuring that patients receive only needed interventions, and not unnecessary tests, procedures or days of care (and, sometimes, that all needed interventions are given, although the latter has traditionally been an aspect of quality assurance rather than UR).
- Risk management intends primarily to reduce the hospital's exposure to financial loss consequent to providing care, including that which may result from employment of care providers.

The nature of the relationships among quality assurance (QA), utilisation review (UR) and risk management (RM) often puzzles managers and doctors and even quality assurance personnel. Certainly, in Australian hospitals, as is becoming the practice in US hospitals, a single quality management department should be responsible for QA/UR/RM.

Operationally, attention to quality assurance, that is, assuring the quality of patient care, will subsume utilisation review as one aspect of health care quality and reduce risk of financial loss from its provision. For example, by adopting practice policies and, especially, by generating information on outcomes, hospitals can better inform patients about what to expect from their care, reducing the possibility of disappointments engendered by false hopes or unrealistic expectations and thereby reduce one source of malpractice suits.

264.7 Quality assurance

Traditionally, in North America at least, the term quality assurance (QA) has been associated with retrospective (postproduction) review of medical records to assess the quality of medical care (referred to sometimes as medical audit). It is largely something that regulators (the government and accrediting bodies) have imposed on hospitals and doctors. Beyond the noble motive, there are few incentives—and many disincentives—

to engage in vigorous quality assurance. In Australia, externally-driven and internally-motivated QA efforts have been minimal. Consequently, in most hospitals QA was mostly—and still is—form over substance, if it exists at all.

Traditionally, quality assurance consisted largely of isolated, episodic, sporadic or haphazard case-by-case review of medical care and, if deficiencies were found, feedback to the doctor who was as likely to argue about the so-called deficiencies as to reflect on or change his or her practices to prevent their recurrence. Almost certainly there was no follow-up to see if problems recurred or not. The lack of pattern analysis virtually precluded meaningful efforts to change practice and improve the quality of care; so did limiting quality assurance to doctors' activities with its implicit, erroneous assumption that doctors alone produce patients' health status improvement.

In this manual, the term quality assurance denotes a cyclical process involving retrospective quality assessment of, and steps toward the subsequent improvement in, the quality of clinical care. Essentially, retrospective quality assurance mechanisms must assess the quality of care and indicate whether or not changes to practices could improve it. By extension, they must encompass ways to identify appropriate improvement actions and the means to implement them. Repeated quality assessments can monitor the results of such improvement actions, including the extent to which they produce any observed improvements, and determine if additional improvement actions should be taken. An ideal system would also contain elements to ensure the quality of the quality assurance mechanism.

As used here, the term quality assurance encompasses explicitly the two elements of the PDCA (quality improvement) cycle concerned with checking (against plans) the results of doing, and with acting to ensure conformance to plans. (See Figure II-6-3 on page 269.) For all practical purposes, the health care quality assurance cycle is synonymous with the conformance improvement cycle and industrial PDCA cycle. Operationally, quality assurance requires implicit or explicit criteria and standards (specifications or plans) to assess retrospectively providers' quality of care (what providers did or did not do) toward closing any performance gaps (acting to change care systems or practices with a view to improving the quality of care). Thus in this manual we use interchangeably the terms quality assurance (QA) and conformance improvement (CI).

264.8 | Utilisation review

Utilisation review (UR) focuses on providers' use of resources for the care of individual patients. It involves the need for medical procedures, and the timing, duration and setting of medical care. While UR began in hospitals, they have had few incentives to review their utilisation of resources unless under regulatory or resource pressure. In the United States, where until relatively recently hospitals' payments were based entirely on reimbursement of their costs, UR is conducted most rigorously by payers or their agents, creating problems for providers. The last section of this chapter elaborates on various aspects of, and describes the United States' experience with, utilisation review.

In Australian hospitals, which are budget-based, there are few direct financial incentives to provide unnecessary or excessively costly care, but likewise there are few incentives for efficiency. If hospitals' resources are under pressure (evidenced by waiting lists, for example), their better use would allow hospitals to treat more patients. However, there are few if any direct incentives for such productivity improvements. Even case-based payments may not provide sufficient incentives to significantly improve hospitals' efficiency. Chapter 9 in this part discusses these points.

Utilisation review must be an integral part of any hospital quality management program. Patients must receive all appropriate, and no inappropriate, interventions. Further, they must be the lowest cost interventions that are appropriate to the patient's health problem and preferences, delivered in the least costly setting that is appropriate and in the most efficient way that is practical. Operationally, hospitals can usually subsume utilisation review under quality assurance.

264.9 Risk management

Risk management focuses on the organisation's exposure to financial losses, particularly those that would threaten its viability. The objective inherent in risk management is to reduce risk of financial loss to the lowest level commensurate with achieving the organisation's purpose—in hospitals' case, providing health care. Essentially, three strategies exist for managing risk. They are:

- risk avoidance—preventing or reducing the possibility of a loss occurring;
- damage control or loss prevention—minimising the magnitude of a loss should one occur;
- risk transfer or insurance—in which all or part of the loss is transferred by someone else in exchange for a premium.

Part V elaborates on these concepts with regard to professional liability (provision of health care in hospitals), and occupational health and safety (employment in hospitals).

265   Quality management system

265.1 Overview

Hospitals and regional health care systems require a quality management system to assure and improve the quality of care. They can either operate independently or be part of such a system. For example, a group of rural hospitals can collaborate to develop and run a quality management system. Figure II-6-4 below illustrates health production. It

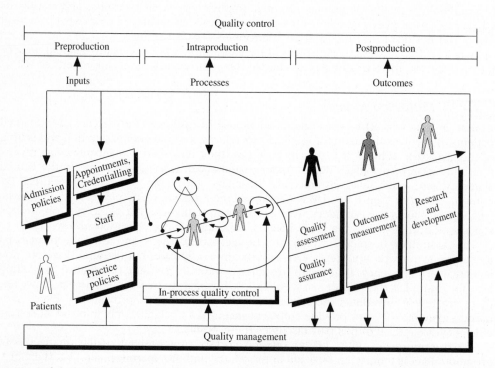

Figure II-6-4 *Health care quality management system*

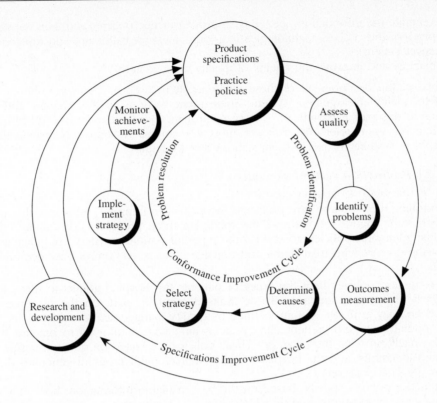

Figure II-6-5 *Continuous quality improvement through conformance and specifications improvement spirals*

depicts a conceptual health care quality management system that intends to perfect the production of health. It summarises functionally the concepts and information presented in this part. Of necessity, Figure II-6-5 simplifies a complex reality. It highlights only the essential elements of a complete health care quality management system and their essential interrelationships.

A quality management system's functional purpose is to assure and improve continuously the treatment of individual patients and the effectiveness of treatments. The system shown in Figure II-6-5 operationalises the three quality improvement cycles shown in Figure II-6-2 (see page 268): conformance improvement (through quality assurance activities); specifications' improvement (revision of practice policies based on quality assurance activities and outcomes' measurement); and technology improvement (through the development and assessment of new product and process technology). Essentially, the system's elements measure health care outcomes and processes to provide the feedback needed to control production processes and their inputs, and the information to improve production processes, practice policies and their constituent technologies.

Hospitals' care processes are quality management's central focus and this element is shown in the centre of Figure II-6-4. The system's other elements encompass mechanisms to:

- control or assure product quality at each of production's three phases: preproduction (e.g. admissions policies, credentialling, practice policies), intraproduction (e.g. decision support technologies), and postproduction (e.g. quality assessment and quality assurance);

- generate the information needed to improve practice policies and their constituent product and process technologies (e.g. outcomes' measurement and research and development);
- manage and improve the quality of quality management.

This section describes all of these elements. It focuses on their contribution to a complete quality management system. Subsequent sections in this chapter and later chapters in this part elaborate on quality control mechanisms and those other quality management system elements that are most relevant to Australian hospitals' quality management systems in their present state of development.

265.2 Production control elements

265.21 PREPRODUCTION QUALITY CONTROL

By controlling the inputs to care processes, hospitals can improve and assure the quality of patient care. Figure II-6-5 shows the following three preproduction quality control elements: admission policies, to control the types of patients treated; credentialling, to control the doctors who treat them; and practice policies, to control how doctors treat patients.

- Admission policies limit the types of patients the hospital admits to those it can treat to practice standards. These limits depend, in part, on the resources and technology available and are defined by quality management considerations.
- Appointments and credentialling policies limit who is allowed to practise in the hospital and what they may do. These policies are based on quality management considerations, and the hospital's quality management program generates data to make such decisions.
- Practice policies specify, based on the best available information, how individual patients should be treated to achieve maximal health status improvement and the amount of improvement that can be expected if policies are implemented properly. Various quality management system elements generate the information to formulate and revise practice policies.

265.22 INTRAPRODUCTION QUALITY CONTROL

Production processes are designed to yield the health status improvement specified by or inherent in practice policies at the lowest cost with greatest patient satisfaction. Various quality management functions generate this design information. Production processes may incorporate decision support technologies (DSTs) that operationalise practice policies in real-time and permit in-process quality control to assure product quality.

265.23 POSTPRODUCTION QUALITY CONTROL

The quality assessment and assurance function measures what was done and achieved, compares results to what should have been done and achieved, and through the hospital's quality management program takes steps to improve conformance to practice policies. This element can also produce information to revise practice policies and to pinpoint needed research.

265.3 Information generating elements

Outcomes' measurement provides information on the end results of care in relation to processes and patient characteristics. This element provides information to improve the design and content of practice policies, inform patients about the benefits and risks of alternative interventions, and establish research priorities (but cannot substitute for research and development).

Research and development projects, which are often beyond individual hospitals' present ability to fund or conduct, provide the best information for designing practice policies, production processes, quality improvement activities and quality management programs.

265.4 Quality management element

The final element in the quality management system depicted in Figure II-6-5 is that concerned with managing and improving the quality of quality management. In managing a quality management system, one must decide the system's boundaries, its constituent elements and their interrelationships, elements' objectives, policies for their operation, how to organise activities to achieve objectives, and how many resources to allocate to conduct them. Further, one must build an information system to track the system's performance, to assure achievement of objectives, and to gauge whether or not the system is achieving its intended purpose and at what cost.

The same principles apply to the continuous improvement of a quality management system as do to the continuous improvement of clinical care. Hospitals, for example, must be responsible for the continuous improvement of their quality management programs. Ultimately the national government must be responsible for quality management systems' performance and for their improvement. Government's essential role must be to assess what needs to be done and to provide the incentives and sanctions to promote effective quality management programs. Chapter 9 in this part examines issues related to the management of quality management.

265.5 Importance of information to improve processes and practices

Quality assessment, assurance and improvement depend on formulating, revising and improving practice policies, which represent health care's product specifications, and on improving their implementation (health care processes). This information can come from quality assurance activities (structured quality improvement), structured outcomes' measurement, structured performance benchmarking, and/or research and development.

Although hospitals may have long histories of participating in research and development (R&D), traditionally these projects have been initiated by doctors responding to their own or sponsors' (principally government's) interests. Further, while medical scientists have undertaken a wide range of research projects, they can be characterised generally as the quest to understand pathophysiological mechanisms and to find cures for disease.

Quality management requires a different, more focused, approach. The principal R&D goal must be to improve product specifications (manifest in practice policies) and production processes (manifest, for example, in procedural policies). Achieving this goal requires research into the outcomes of present practices (referred to sometimes as effectiveness research) and the evaluation of all types of existing and proposed new practices, and not just drugs and devices (referred to sometimes as medical technology assessment), and health services research to improve interventions' delivery.

Hospitals and other providers, alone or in consortia, should set priorities for funding and conducting quality management research, including effectiveness research. The results of outcomes' measurement, for example, can help guide priorities for medical technology assessments, including clinical trials and other types of R&D intended to improve the quality of health care. Research into the pathophysiological mechanisms will still be needed, of course, because such long-term investments may yield new insights into disease processes and provide new technologies that can break through performance limitations and thus improve practices and patients' health status. Such important policy considerations as how much to spend on each type of quality management research, how to co-ordinate efforts, and how to assure the integrity of data and the quality of research are all beyond this manual's scope.

265.6 Outcomes' measurement

Conformance to practice policies (QA's basic goal) will only improve patients' health status if they specify effective practices. Quality management requires measurement of long-term outcomes (end results of care) when the placebo effect inherent in a treatment has worn off and underlying pathophysiological processes unaffected by the intervention have reasserted themselves. By measuring long-term outcomes and appropriately correlating them with care processes, hospitals can improve their practice policies and practices, and identify and prioritise needed research and development activities. Structured quality review validates interventions' appropriateness; structured outcome measurement validates their, and hence practice policies', effectiveness.

In the United States the recent resurgence of interest in outcomes measurement has produced a variety of initiatives. For example, in the late 1980s, Interstudy (Minneapolis, Minnesota) launched Quality Quest to pilot the practicality and utility of collecting long-term outcomes data. Paul Ellwood was the driving force behind this initiative.[2] In the early 1990s, the Health Outcomes Institute (Bloomington, Minnesota) continued the development and dissemination of this Outcomes Management System (OMS).[2a] It intends to provide a mechanism for analysing patient outcomes as part of routine clinical practice. The Institute makes available general and condition-specific questionnaires for capturing outcomes data at nominal cost, and offers a national repository for pooling these data. While collection of patient outcomes data in ordinary health care practice can prove useful, their analysis, interpretation, and use for quality management purposes are subject to many limitations (delineated elsewhere in this part), and they can never substitute for well-designed empirical research in determining interventions' effectiveness.

Outcomes' measurement may be the only source of information, albeit imperfect, to validate practice policies and to guide quality improvement efforts. For example, it may show that medical and surgical interventions produce about the same poor or good results for seemingly similar patients. Such a result does not mean necessarily that both interventions are equally effective for all types of patients, nor that either is in fact effective for any type of patient. Outcomes' measurement can never overcome the inherent biases in patient–provider selection, for example, which can only be overcome by random assignment of patients in the manner of a controlled clinical trial. While, if designed and implemented properly, such trials can produce solid information to validate and improve practices they are not—but are sometimes praised as if they were—a panacea. Even with the most efficient designs, there is neither enough time nor money to do all the randomised controlled trials that could or should be done. Sometimes trials are impractical for social or ethical reasons.

Finally, results of clinical trials are subject to the laws of chance. Interventions that they indicate are effective may, in abstract reality, not be effective.

265.7 Research and development

To manage quality, we must determine interventions' cost-effectiveness and improve medical technology. To improve medical technology, research and development must focus on developing both better interventions, for example drugs, devices, surgical operations (product technology), and better ways of delivering or implementing them (process technology). The results of assessing existing and developing new technologies (driven in part by the demonstrated inadequacies of existing technologies) form the basis of improved products (practice policies) and practices. Medical technology assessments must focus on the cost of care (including the cost of provision, costs to patients) as well as their traditional focus on effectiveness (or efficacy and safety). The quest for incremental effectiveness at any price must yield to the search for more cost-effective interventions. In an era of constrained resources, cheaper interventions with the same effectiveness may be at least, if not more, socially valuable than those that offer incremental improvements in effectiveness at vast increases in cost.

To improve quality management, R&D must focus on its various aspects—all of the activities described in this part. They include, for example: synthesising the best available information for use in practice, making such information available for use in medical practice, and evaluating the results of its use; the continuing education of health professionals; conducting quality management programs; and prioritising and funding research needed to improve quality management. Today this type of research receives scant attention and little funding. Medical technology assessments too are woefully underfunded. To improve quality and its management, we must spend much more money on these types of research. Moreover providers, such as hospitals, must be in charge of such increased funding to focus research on what is most needed to improve the quality of care.

266 | Quality control

266.1 | An expanded view of traditional quality assurance

Early efforts to improve quality focused on the training and qualifications of doctors and other health professionals. Certainly, proper training is necessary to assure the quality of care but it is not sufficient. Subsequent efforts to improve quality focused on hospitals' structures and, to a limited extent at the organisational level, on care processes. While they may indicate a capacity to provide high quality care, the present reliance on meeting accreditation standards does not assure hospitals' quality of care. Recent efforts to improve quality, for example, in the United States the JCAHO's clinical indicators initiative and a similar initiative, in Australia, by the ACHS, focus on care processes and their immediate outcomes. However, to be truly successful in improving quality, hospitals must focus to a far greater extent than do these initial initiatives on performance rather than promise. Only by assessing conformance to practice policies and measuring immediate and long-term outcomes and relating them to care processes can hospitals improve health care production processes and hence the quality of their care. These initiatives' effectiveness depends on hospitals putting in place mechanisms to use productively this feedback to control production processes.

Quality assurance activities intend to ensure conformance to specifications. Where they have existed, they have tended to be implicit review criteria, not practice policies, which are required for an effective management program. In principle, quality assurance activities, through serious attention to correcting whatever quality problems they identify, can lead to some improvement in the quality of care. However, such improvement is likely only to be realised if quality assurance activities are part of a complete and comprehensive quality management program, which, for example, includes elements that control inputs to and the implementation of production processes. Further, because of their limited nature, quality assurance activities can go only so far in improving the quality of care. For example, outcomes' measurement is essential to shed light on the relationships between patient outcomes and care processes. Thus, to be effective, traditional quality assurance activities—retrospective review of the quality of care based on medical records—must be part of, and not a hospital's entire, quality management program.

Hospitals need a complete and comprehensive quality management system to guarantee and enhance the quality of their care. The program's goal is to design—and through evaluation to redesign—production systems to ensure that patients receive all appropriate interventions (and no others), in the right order, in the right setting, implemented properly with minimum total duration, at the lowest possible long-term cost. The program must include mechanisms to improve conformance to practice policies—production quality control mechanisms—and those to provide the information and technology for improving practice policies and care processes—product and production quality improvement mechanisms.

Quality control mechanisms can ensure products' technical quality in three fundamentally different ways, related to the three phases of production. Hospitals must employ all of these mechanisms to the maximum extent practical to have an effective quality management program. They are:

- preproduction quality control—verification of inputs (structures) and processes;
- intraproduction (in-process) quality control—real-time control of product-producing processes;
- postproduction quality control—product assessment to identify changes to production processes and their inputs and/or the production system needed to produce products that conform to specifications.

266.2 | Quality control in practice

Classic industrial production quality control methods designed to achieve zero defects cannot be applied easily to clinical care. Health care production quality control involves primarily ensuring that interventions match patients' health problems and desires (patient–process fit) and, secondarily, implementing practices properly. The most cost-effective health care quality control strategy—now and in the foreseeable future—is postproduction quality of care assessment, with subsequent modifications to care processes, coupled with various preproduction quality control mechanisms including targeted preprocedure review. Eventually, in-process quality control will likely become routine, diminishing the need to rely on other forms of quality control.

Production quality control is a new concept for most hospital managers and medical practitioners. While hospitals have embraced quality control procedures in their laboratories, for example, they lack integrated quality control systems to guarantee the quality of patient care. Most hospitals would be hard-pressed to point to anyone who was responsible for the quality of care, let alone integrated mechanisms to guarantee quality. Since hospitals do not presently measure the quality of their care, they can neither assure nor improve it. By conceiving of hospitals as health-producing facilities, quality managers can think systematically about quality control.

Quality managers must decide the best mix of preproduction, intraproduction, and postproduction control mechanisms for their hospital's circumstances at both the organisational and workface levels. Clearly, preproduction quality control is an excellent way to assure quality because the factors are known and are controllable and hence can be adjusted to produce the desired product. In-process quality controls are desirable because they permit error-free production. However, preprocess and intraprocess quality controls may be technically difficult to design and expensive to implement, especially in health care. Hence reliance on postproduction quality control that assesses products' quality toward changing inputs and production process to increased conformance to practice policies. It is also essential to provide information toward improving specifications, manifest principally in practice policies. They permit creation of a learning organisation, one that learns through feedback of its own performance and from others' results and the way that they produce them (e.g. benchmarking) to improve product and production quality.

Practically, quality control takes places at two levels: the organisation and the workface. At the organisational level, quality control mechanisms ensure that production systems are organised to produce products to specifications. Such mechanisms include, for example, credentialling of medical practitioners to certify that they are qualified to perform specified procedures. However, what occurs at the workface determines products' quality. On any given day a medical practitioner's performance may be impaired (e.g. because of excessive tiredness), even though he or she is credentialled to perform the planned procedure. To date, preproduction quality control has focused on credentialling surgeons but not assessing their fitness to operate prior to each operation, for example. Credentialling is relatively easy, inexpensive and acceptable (if not always accepted) and represents a prudent and cost-effective preproduction quality control mechanism. On the other hand, a preoperative fitness test is difficult to design, would be costly to administer routinely, would likely be unacceptable to surgeons, and would likely not improve quality commensurate with its costs. In this circumstance, the best that hospitals can do is to encourage staff to report a surgeon's impairment as an incident to be investigated subsequently. See incident reporting in Chapter 8 of this part.

Health care's production processes principally involve professionals working on or interacting with patients. Thus they are somewhat intangible. If one defines production processes in terms of professionals' actions and interactions, one can regard all of the following factors as inputs to production processes: professionals' qualifications, experience and preparedness to undertake processes; information provided by practice policies, medical records and laboratory tests; and patients. Quality control mechanisms may act directly, for example, guiding surgeons in their selection of interventions or controlling who may operate on patients, or indirectly, for example providing surgeons with the training necessary to successfully perform an operation or, more indirectly, improving the quality of the training.

Preprocess verification (often referred to as preprocedure review) is an increasingly important aspect of production control. An effective intervention may not be appropriate for a particular patient and thus would not improve maximally the recipient patient's health status. Ensuring that a surgical operation is appropriate for a particular patient before its conduct has obvious advantages. One could assume that qualified surgeons could be entrusted to perform only indicated operations. However, medicine is fraught with uncertainty and replete with conflicting incentives. Further, the harm from and cost of unnecessary operations can be substantial. But the cost of preprocedure review— verifying each operation's appropriateness prior to conducting it—can also be substantial unless built into the process of care. Nonetheless, targeted preprocedure review is a cost-effective quality control mechanism if, for example, the patient has a high chance of dying from the procedure, it is very expensive, or indications for its use are controversial. The section on utilisation review in this chapter explores these points.

Eventually, in-process quality controls, manifest in decision support technology, will likely play very important roles in health care production control. They will check an operation's appropriateness before it is conducted or guide doctors in their selection of interventions to assure their appropriateness and, eventually, with the use of robots, help to assure that operations are conducted according to specifications.

Postproduction quality control mechanisms—traditional quality assurance activities— have been, and for the foreseeable future will remain, the primary means of assuring and improving the quality of health care. However, a hospital is wasting its resources if it does not have in place the preproduction and intraproduction quality control mechanisms that quality assurance activities are designed to inform, and the means to change production processes to resolve quality problems.

Effective quality assurance depends on the existence of such preproduction quality control mechanisms as practice policies that specify what should be done and achieved for particular types of patients and, to the extent practical, intraproduction quality control mechanisms that ensure specified policies are implemented properly. If quality assurance activities reveal that certain policies are not adhered to, hospitals must change inputs to and/or production processes to increase compliance and/or they must redesign the production system to utilise practice policies and practices to which adherence is easier to achieve (with little or no loss in patient health status improvement). Such changes may involve, for example, inputs (e.g. retraining personnel) and production processes (e.g. the use of checklists and computerised reminders to ensure patients receive needed interventions in a timely fashion and to document clearly when they occurred).

266.3 Preproduction quality control in practice

266.31 OVERVIEW

Preproduction quality control involves assuring that inputs to care process conform to specifications and that proposed care processes are appropriate to improve maximally an individual patient's health status. Ordinarily, inputs are assured at the organisational level, for example through credentialling, rather than at the workface. Practice policies may guide practitioners in their selection of procedures or be used in preprocess verification (preprocedure review). Subsequent paragraphs describe the following eight preproduction quality control mechanisms:

- Patient admission policies
- Hospital service policies
- Provider credentialling
- Provider training, incentives
- Practice policies
- Clinical information
- Preprocess verification
- Industrial practices.

266.32 PATIENT ADMISSION POLICIES

Hospitals should admit only those patients that they are equipped and resourced to treat to quality standards. Quality management activities provide information to inform decisions about admissions policies. If patients have no alternative source of care, less than optimal health status improvement may be preferable to none at all, a point covered elsewhere. Nevertheless, in principle health-producing facilities should try to assure the quality of their care no matter what standards they adopt. There is no implication that these standards must be universal, but they should be stated.

266.33 HOSPITAL SERVICE POLICIES

Hospitals should carefully assess their capabilities to continue or to add new technologies and services. They would be well-advised to continue or to add only those services that they can deliver to standards and, for those services they do provide, to accept only those patients that they can treat adequately, referring others, after medical stabilisation if required. Clearly, a hospital's quality management program plays a vital part in such determinations.

Quality management demands that hospitals pay more attention than they do now to the introduction of new medical technology and its integration with existing production systems and clinical practices. In particular, those staff who will use or be most affected by the new technology should have a hand in planning for its introduction and indeed in deciding whether or not it should be acquired at all. When hospitals acquire new equipment, for example for use in neonatal intensive care, the nurses who will use it must be properly trained in its use to realise potential patient outcomes. On-the-job training after the equipment has been put in use is no longer acceptable. Further, hospitals must educate doctors or staff in the correct indications for using the technology. To prepare fully for its use, hospitals must also make arrangements for service and repair of equipment, backup arrangements if it fails to perform as expected and, if acquired on a trial or approval basis, mechanisms to evaluate the technology.

266.34 PROVIDER CREDENTIALLING

Through a properly structured credentialling process, the hospital can control who practises in the hospital and what medical practitioners are permitted to do within its walls. These policies relate not only to the practitioner's ability to perform procedures but also to the hospital's capability to support their performance. Credentialling policies and decisions can be informed through standards published by professional bodies (e.g. criteria that practitioners must meet in order to be credentialled to perform specified procedures) and through its own quality management activities (e.g. practitioners' procedure-specific performance).

266.35 PROVIDER TRAINING, INCENTIVES

For their particular production systems hospitals can, and should, determine appropriate staffing levels, for example number of nurses per bed, and employ sufficient qualified staff to meet them. By employing only qualified staff in sufficient numbers to treat patients, hospitals can increase the probability of achieving desired patient outcomes. However, proper personnel inputs are necessary but not sufficient to assure quality. Hospitals must compare promise to performance to inform providers how they are performing, to maintain skills, for example through continuing medical education programs, and to reward success and give providers incentives to perform excellently.

Adequate training of staff to keep up with advances in practice, quality assurance methods and so on is essential to maintain and improve the quality of care. Hospitals in Australia spend very little on this activity and few professional organisations in Australia demand formal continuing education to keep current membership, credentials or licensure. In the United States, where billions of dollars are spent annually on continuing medical education (CME) for example, the problem is any plausible connection between CME activities and performance. Hospitals need mechanisms, which are virtually non-existent presently, to identify valid CME needs, that is, documented practice performance deficiencies. Whether or not a particular CME activity would alleviate the deficiency is an empirical question. Structured quality review (SQR) offers one way to identify performance-based CME needs and to monitor quality of care, which should improve after effective CME designed to remedy performance deficiencies.

Structured quality review also offers a way to inform certifying and licensing bodies that providers are performing to the standards required to maintain certification or licensure. In the United States, speciality boards are increasingly giving only time-limited certification and are experimenting with performance-based recertification in place of or as a supplement to re-examination. Eventually one could envision a situation in which doctors whose performance fails to meet minimum standards despite targeted CME would be permitted to practise only in areas of demonstrated competence, or if substandard in all areas of practice to lose their license to practise.

266.36 PRACTICE POLICIES

Practice policies (pre-established decision rules for diagnosing and treating individual patients) specify how care should be provided with what results and, by extension, who should provide it; the latter being reinforced through credentialling. Practice policies make explicit assumptions between health care processes (specific medical interventions) and patient health status improvement. Practice policies specify medicine's product; for most hospitals, assuring conformance to them may be the only practical way to improve the quality of care.

266.37 CLINICAL INFORMATION

Clinical care depends on clinical information. Often providers elicit such information directly, by history and physical examination for example. They must also rely on medical records for some information—for example details of past illnesses and treatments—hence their importance to quality of care. Moreover, clinicians must rely on information from laboratory, radiology and other types of tests to arrive at a correct diagnosis, assist the patient choose the appropriate treatment, monitor medical management, chart the patient's progress and assess prognosis. The quality, accuracy, precision and timeliness of such information obviously affects the quality of care. Detailed consideration of assuring and improving the quality of laboratory, medical record, and other ancillary services that provide information for clinical decision-making is beyond this manual's scope.

266.38 PREPROCESS VERIFICATION

When production errors result in irreversible consequences or costly losses, as they can in health care, it may be prudent to verify the appropriateness of planned processes, settings, or procedures prior to their implementation, because postproduction repair is not possible or not practical. Input verification may involve, for example:

- preprocedure review—verifying that a planned admission or surgical operation is medically necessary, or double-checking a medication dose prior to its administration;
- operator preparedness—checking that a surgeon is credentialled to perform the operation for which he or she has booked the operating theatre, and is in a fit state to conduct it;
- patient preparation—checking that the patient is the one on whom the operation is to be conducted and that the proper part is operated on, for example, amputation of the right and not the left—wrong—leg.

266.39 INDUSTRIAL PRACTICES

There are numerous industrial practices that qualify as preproduction quality control mechanisms, although they are rarely considered as such. These quality control mechanisms include, for example, proper preventive maintenance and calibration of equipment so that, for example, test results are accurate and ventilators work correctly, and good housekeeping practices to reduce all kinds of possible accidents and errors.

266.4 Intraproduction (in-process) quality control in practice

266.41 OVERVIEW

Preproduction verification intends to affect outcomes by setting up processes to assure the correct conditions for their production. In-process quality controls are systems or techniques that are an integral part of production. They intend to assure the quality of the product (outcomes) by controlling production processes as they are occurring. The extent of control can be quite limited (e.g. aide-memoires, if one remembers to use them) or controlling (e.g. fully-automated systems designed for error-free production). In health care, systematic in-process quality control is presently quite limited.

Traditional in-process quality control mechanisms include, for example, check lists to ensure procedures are followed precisely, and in-process inspection of interventions' results. Newer forms of in-process quality control mechanisms include, for example: real-time computerised decision support technologies (DSTs) that assist doctors diagnose patients; medication delivery systems that monitor blood levels and automatically adjust infusions to maintain a predetermined level; and use of robots in surgical operations. Use of artificial intelligence offers the best example of in-process quality control in medicine and the best hope for improving the quality of care. Chapter 7 in this part describes this emerging technology.

266.42 IN-PROCESS INSPECTION

In-process inspection occurs after a process that is an integral part of the entire production process has taken place. In health care it serves two potential purposes: to identify production problems toward remedying them and/or to determine whether or not desired outcomes were achieved so that, if not, additional interventions can be implemented without delay to achieve intended outcomes or remedy maloutcomes. Postproduction review, after care has been delivered, is a far more efficient way to identify production (quality of care) problems, because in-process inspection depends on reviewing process-by-process results immediately after the process.

In-process inspection to monitor for and manage complications has long been an important aspect of health care, even if it has not always been systematic. For example, if a patient suffers an adverse drug reaction, its prompt treatment may result in no long-term health status loss; ignoring it may result in the patient's death. Traditionally the hospital's nursing staff has always been alert to such possibilities and has taken prompt action including notifying the patient's doctor, who may change the patient's therapy or order additional specific therapeutic interventions. Well-articulated production systems, well-established practice policies and properly trained staff may obviate the need for special systems such as so-called concurrent review.

As practised presently, concurrent review usually involves specially trained nurses reviewing patients' medical records during the hospital stay (hence the term 'concurrent'). These reviews may be conducted every three days, so that a reviewer may handle a patient's medical record multiple times during the admission. Joyce Craddick, Medical Management Analysis (which is no longer an independent business), developed the quintessential concurrent review system (often referred to simply as MMA). The experience of one Australian hospital, the Royal North Shore Hospital, Sydney, points to disappointing results. This type of concurrent review requires tremendous effort to implement. The same resources deployed in other ways would likely yield greater improvements in health care quality.

Conceived originally as a utilisation review technique, so-called concurrent review can also shape the quality of care, for example by expediting processes and picking up complications early rather than late (or complications that might have been missed entirely) when something might be done to minimise the patient's resultant health status loss. In addition, reviewers can note the presence or absence of events, for example renal failure not present on admission, that may bear on the quality of care received. Results of these so-called concurrent occurrence screens can be used to identify cases for subsequent structured quality review or analysed statistically. Their use for this purpose constitutes early retrospective review of care because they merely record outcomes and do not affect them (although their use may affect subsequent care processes and outcomes).

266.43 DECISION SUPPORT TECHNOLOGY, ROBOTS

Decision support technologies (DSTs) and, eventually, robots that assist the conduct of procedures will increasingly provide the means to assist doctors and other health care providers to select the most appropriate diagnostic and therapeutic interventions for patients' circumstances and to implement them properly. Consequently, the quality of care should improve immensely. The information necessary to operationalise DSTs must come, preferably, from empirical research or otherwise from experts' structured group judgments—the same sources that should inform practice policies. DSTs have already been introduced into practice in some hospitals in the United States. Chapter 7 in this part elaborates on the use of DSTs. Use of robots is already beginning to improve interventions' implementation, for example hip joint replacement, and their use can be expected to grow substantially. Consideration of the use of robots to improve the quality of care is beyond this manual's scope.

266.5 Postproduction quality control in practice

266.51 OVERVIEW

Inspecting products at the end of the assembly line to determine if the desired product was produced is the classic example of postproduction quality control. This postproduction examination permits reworking (repair of defective products) or their outright rejection. It can also provide the information needed to identify defective production processes and to change them so that they produce future products to specifications. In health care, postproduction quality control—quality assessment to monitor production processes and provider performance—is presently the key to quality improvement in hospitals. Through this mechanism hospitals can compare what they are doing and achieving to what they should be doing and achieving, and take steps to close any performance gaps. Moreover, quality assessment results can inform admissions policies, credentialling decisions and practice policies, for example.

266.52 REWORK, READMISSIONS

Because health care is a state-transforming process, there is no product that can be reworked to remedy the effects of defective production processes, and patients that suffer maloutcomes cannot be scrapped, although some may die. Instead, for patients that survive malprocess, providers must apply additional interventions to improve patients' resultant health status after the application of defective care processes. Often these additional interventions cannot restore patients' health status to what it would have been if original interventions had been appropriate and/or implemented properly. These considerations underlie the logic of preproduction quality control, especially preprocess verification, to avoid the occurrence of defective production processes, and of postproduction quality control to identify and solve production problems to avoid their future occurrence.

In health care, the closest activity to rework is the extra care that hospitals must provide to patients whose outcomes necessitate additional interventions or days in the hospital to manage complications that better production systems or practices could have avoided. Such rework may occur during an admission or in a subsequent admission. Rework that occurs during an admission can be identified during the patient's stay (see in-process inspection above) or, more efficiently, postdischarge, using structured quality review, for example, toward its reduction.

Readmissions to the hospital because of inadequate prior care are comparable to customers returning defective products to the manufacturer for repair. Monitoring readmissions suffers from a number of drawbacks, including the following. Firstly, not all readmissions result from inadequate prior care and so some mechanism must exist to determine this fact. Secondly, inadequate prior care does not always result in readmission to the same hospital. For example, patients may die, be admitted to another hospital, or be cared for in a nursing home, outpatient clinic or doctor's surgery. These cases are lost to view unless hospitals track cases and measure long-term outcomes.

266.53 QUALITY ASSESSMENT

Postproduction (retrospective) review of care outcomes and processes and outcomes based on documentation in the patient's medical record is the key to improving hospitals' quality of care. In this context, the term outcomes includes such process outcomes as length of time from induction of anaesthesia to beginning operation, as well as such patient outcomes as death. Chapter 8 in this part describes a practical approach for assessing hospitals' quality of care: structured quality review (SQR). In addition, there are many other postproduction sources of information that can reveal care deficiencies or quality problems, opportunities for improvement. They include, for example, analysis of immediate outcomes (such as nosocomial infections) and practice patterns (such as diagnostic test use), outcomes' measurement, and comparison of a hospital's processes and performance on various parameters with those of other hospitals (benchmarking).

Quality assessment intends to identify problems in the delivery of care. Subsequently, hospitals can investigate problems' root causes and change production processes to eliminate them. If implemented successfully, these changes would improve the quality of care, assuming that the hospital had correctly identified problems' root causes and had selected effective solutions. Hospitals must monitor changes to production processes to ensure that they do improve care, attribute observed changes to action, and determine if any additional actions are warranted. This cycle of problem identification and resolution has virtually defined traditional quality assurance.

267 | Quality assurance, quality improvement and CQI

267.1 | Quality assurance or quality improvement

Recently it has become fashionable to talk about quality improvement (QI) rather than quality assurance (QA), for any number of reasons. Two reasons stand out, however. The first is to break with the past and differentiate new approaches from old programs. The second is to promote improvement, which sounds better than mere assurance. Continuous quality improvement (CQI) sounds even better. In health care, some CQI advocates disparage QA as merely an attempt to fix problems, not to improve operations. Arguments about the superiority of CQI over QA are vacuous. Quality assurance is an essential mechanism for continuous quality improvement.

No one can deny that a business bent on continuous improvement in products and operations—never being satisfied that its present way of doing business is necessarily the best way—is likely to be better than one that is satisfied to turn out the same products in the same way, merely fixing a faulty production process when one is found. The quality revolution focused business managers' attention on the importance of product quality (and hence production quality) in winning, and continuous quality improvement in keeping, customers. Competition among manufacturers or producers for customers often does more to bring forth 'improvements' than exhortations to do better, as economists and others have known for a long time. The quality revolution has come to health care only recently, for various reasons, not the least of which was the inability until recently to assess practically the quality of care. (See Table II-6-1 on page 288.)

267.2 | Continuous quality improvement

Quality management is a production-level tool for continuous quality improvement, and consists of various technologies and techniques for managing continuous quality improvement efforts, designing quality into products, controlling production quality and assessing product quality. Most of these technologies and techniques are the outgrowth of various disciplines, for example organisational development and production engineering, and in industry have been well known—if not well applied—for quite some time.

Table II-6-1 *Assuring and improving quality in manufacturing and health care*

Aspect	Manufacturer	Hospital
Product		
Product specifications	Manufacturing specifications for materials, processes, finished products	Practice (and procedural) policies
Preproduction		
Preproduction quality control	Materials inspection; worker selection, training; industrial practices, e.g. equipment preventive maintenance; process layout, lighting, housekeeping, etc.	Patient admission, service policies; credentialling; training clinical information, e.g. medical records, imaging laboratory, other diagnostic tests; industrial practices
Intraproduction		
In-process quality control	Poke-yoke, computer-controlled machine tools, robots	Decision support technology, robots
In-process inspection	Kanban, statistical process control	So-called concurrent review
Postproduction		
Postproduction quality control	Inspection of final product, scrapping or reworking defects; service calls	Readmissions, additional interventions, from poor quality care
Quality assurance, improvement	Inspection results, service calls, customer complaints feedback to improve products, production processes	Structured quality review, other structured problem identification mechanisms to find, and structured problem resolution mechanisms to fix, quality problems

Manufacturing procedures are well established; their equivalents in hospitals are described in this manual, but for the most part have yet to be implemented.

Health care quality management's central purpose is to produce greater and greater health status improvement for patients. Since resources are limited, such improvement should ideally be accomplished without any significant increase and preferably a decrease in cost. Further, since such improvements may affect the interpersonal aspects of care, they should not result in any appreciable diminution of and preferably an increase in patient satisfaction. To effect continuous quality improvement, hospitals must measure simultaneously health status improvement, cost and patient satisfaction.

Health care quality management improves quality by:

• producing products to specifications (expressed in practice policies), thereby increasing aggregate patient health status improvement beyond that being realised now;

• improving product specifications and production systems (practice policies and their implementation) to realise even more patient health status improvement.

Producing products to specifications requires establishing practice policies, putting in place the quality control mechanisms described in this chapter, and operationalising the conformance improvement spiral. Improving practice policies and production systems requires operationalising the specifications improvement and technology improvement cycles. (See Figure II-6-2 on page 268.) Continuous quality improvement in hospitals (the virtuous spiral shown in Figure II-6-3 on page 269) principally involves operationalising the interlocking conformance improvement and specifications improvement spirals shown in Figure II-6-5 on page 275.

- The conformance improvement spiral perfects the fit between what should be done (expressed essentially in practice policies) and what and how well it was done (measured through structured quality review, for example) by changing production systems to close any performance gaps.
- The specifications improvement spiral improves practice policies.

Continuous quality improvement is the cumulative result of multiple discrete changes. Continuity and discreteness are a matter of scale. Inherently, the conformance and specifications improvement spirals operate on two different time scales. Conformance improvement represents mostly small, incremental, frequent improvements; specifications improvement, mostly significant, discontinuous, infrequent changes. Moreover, sufficient time must elapse between an action and gauging its effect to determine if it improved quality. Introducing frequent changes without properly gauging their effects on quality will likely not result in improvement and may lead to chaos—unpredictable oscillations in product quality.

Better practice policies—new policies that produce more health status improvement or the same health status improvement at less cost and/or with greater patient satisfaction than old ones—constitute a new, better product—one that more perfectly meets customers' (patients') needs or wants. Existing technology limits the new or better products that can be designed and produced. New or better technology can enhance the elucidation of customers' needs, relax the constraints on designs to meet them, and improve production processes, organisational forms, quality management, and the generation and appropriate application of useful technology for all the foregoing.

Road construction, something at which the Romans excelled, reduced the time it took to travel between one point and the next. The horse and carriage was a great advance on existing means of overland transportation for the nobility (who could afford it). Within the limits of the technologies that were available to them, coachmakers could, and likely did, go to great lengths to please their wealthy customers with whom they could interact directly. The horseless carriage, the automobile, improved overland transportation and mass production extended the possibility to more people. The aeroplane reduced still further the time needed to travel between distant points and air travel largely replaced laggardly sea travel for voyages over water.

No matter how diligently he laboured, no matter how clever his CQI program, the coachmaker could not compete with the new forms of transportation if customers wanted to travel between distant points in the shortest possible time using any means that was safe and affordable. The coachmaker had to switch products, not merely improve the old one or its production, and, consequently, learn about entirely new technologies and production, marketing and business methods. At some, often imperceptible, point, CQI gives way to strategic business development and quality management merges with general business management.

267.3 *Product specifications are the key to quality improvement*

Product specifications inherently limit end product quality and are the starting point for its measurement. Explicit consideration of production processes (including their inputs) when specifying products improves end product quality. Thus, for example, practice policies—which specify how patients should be treated and what they can expect as a result—must take into account hospitals' facilities and other resources (and doctors' and other providers' skills) for treating patients. Practice policies are the starting point for conformance improvement (quality assurance). (See Figure II-6-5 on page 275.) They are also the basis for developing quality assessment screens that anchor structured quality review. (See Chapter 7 in this part.) Practice policies must state explicitly what outcomes to expect from their proper implementation to facilitate their validation and improvement.

Disappointment with actual outcomes may stem from exaggerated expectations or from inadequate performance. Disentangling one from the other through structured quality improvement, structured outcome measurement, structured performance benchmarking, and research studies is the key to successful health care quality management. (See Chapter 8 in this part.)

There are two schools of thought about initial specifications. One school emphasises the need for any reasonable set of specifications to start the virtuous quality improvement spiral; the other suggests starting with the 'best' set. In principle, we prefer starting with the best set that can be developed reasonably and, in practice, not being overly concerned that it is the best because there is no practical way to make this determination.

The best set of practice policies leads to greatest patient health status improvement (at the lowest practical cost), given patients' preferences (for ends and means) and society's resources. Because there is little scientific evidence about interventions' effectiveness for particular diseases, types of patients and so on, because patients' preferences for particular interventions vary, and because of differences in available resources, multiple acceptable alternatives are likely to characterise initial practice policies. For example, conservative medical therapy and surgical intervention may be considered equivalent because there is no acceptable scientific evidence or professional consensus of opinion that one is superior to the other in improving patients' health status. As a result of quality management activities, one intervention may emerge as clearly superior to the other for some types of patients and hospitals can revise their practice policies accordingly.

Some practice policies may be more robust than others, that is, lead to less variability in processes (and/or in outcomes for given types of patients). Thus expectations about practice policies' effects on performance variability (and hence on patient outcomes) may be an important consideration in their specification. By reducing variability in processes, hospitals can improve outcomes. Stated simply, if providers follow valid practice policies and implement them properly, they would, by definition, produce maximal health status improvement given present knowledge and technology. Were this happy state to exist, further improvement would require better practice policies, that is, those that if implemented properly would produce more patient health status improvement. Clearly, health status improvement may be limited by patients' preferences and resource constraints as well as by knowledge and technology.

267.4 *Conformance improvement leads to quality improvement*

In a practical sense, quality management's goal is to guarantee quality: patients can be sure that hospitals will provide care in a certain way (defined in practice policies) and with certain results (those specified in practice policies, with as little variance as practical). To make this guarantee, hospitals must ensure that practices conform to policies, and measure results to ensure that they are those that were expected. For quality assurance purposes, health care's quality is defined essentially by adherence to process specifications, expressed in practice, procedural and elemental policies. The conformance improvement (quality assurance) spiral continuously reduces variation in patient–process fit (between what patients need and prefer and what they receive), subsequent production processes and consequent patient outcomes. Ideally, observed outcomes approximate those stated in practice policies—the starting point for quality assurance and improvement. Variation in outcomes for given types of patients and the occurrence of maloutcomes alerts one to potential malprocesses that if changed would improve patient outcomes.

If one has a definite notion of what should be done or what should occur (product and/or process specifications) a deviation from those specifications is a quality problem that if rectified would improve quality. For example, repair of a malfunctioning machine will fix a problem (the broken machine) and improve the quality of the machine's product and the factory's performance. In the same vein, removal of an aberrant practitioner will prevent recurrence of the problems he or she was causing and improve the hospital's performance. Fixing one machine will obviously have no effect on others, although paradoxically, removing an aberrant practitioner might cause others to pay closer attention to detail or, more likely, to act defensively devoid of the context of an effective quality management program. There is, however, no implication that quality assurance, defined here as assuring conformance to specifications, is limited to simple fixes of such obvious problems as broken machines.

Through the conformance improvement spiral, hospitals can identify quality problems (deviations from specifications or expectations), investigate their root causes, and change practice policies, care processes and other aspects of care delivery in order to resolve them and eliminate their root causes. Quality assurance mechanisms compare what is done and achieved against what should have been done and achieved, and provide the means to close any performance gaps. If quality assurance activities find and close performance gaps, they result in quality improvement—increased mean, and/or reduced variance in, health status improvement. Sometimes quality may be improved best by redesigning production processes or products. The creation of new or better products (and their design including manufacturing specifications) has not been part of traditional health care quality assurance but it is a vital part of quality management.

267.5 | Specifications improvement leads to quality improvement

Given specified practice policies, quality can be improved basically so far and no further. Using feedback from quality assurance activities, hospitals can bring practices in line with policies and may modify practice policies to reduce variation in outcomes, for example, improving further the quality of care. However, at some point further improvement in quality—increased patient health status improvement—depends on changing discontinuously (rather than incrementally) practice policies (thereby constituting a new product).

Structured quality improvement, with its focus of finding and fixing quality problems, provides limited information to improve practice policies. By comparing results of different practice policies (and production systems), structured performance benchmarking can provide information to align one's own with those of the best performers. Structured outcome measurement provides information about long-term outcomes to validate and improve practice policies, but the link between process and outcomes may be weak. The best information for improving practice policies comes from research studies because, if designed and implemented properly, they can provide strong evidence that (improved) effectiveness is attributable to interventions. Unfortunately, today few studies result in scientifically substantiated findings.[3] Further, one must recognise that even in well-designed well-controlled clinical trials that demonstrate a statistically and clinically significant difference in outcomes between experimentals and controls, these findings may arise purely by chance and produce false facts: instead of being effective the intervention is, in reality, ineffective.

Changing practice policies to align them with research results in order to realise a tested intervention's supposed benefits will not lead to any improvement in patient health status if they stem from inadequate studies or pure chance. In the absence of quality management programs that characterises health care today, the resultant lack of patient health status improvement may go unnoticed for decades. For example, in the United States over 80% of heart attack patients now receive nitrates and magnesium, the result of inferences drawn from multiple clinical trials conducted over several years. However, the latest study involving over 50 000 patients suggests these interventions are ineffective. According to Richard Peto, who oversaw this study, earlier studies' results must have been due to 'the play of chance'.[4] To avoid erroneous inferences, science generally insists that results be replicated, preferably many times, before they are accepted as facts. Because full-scale clinical trials can cost hundreds of millions of dollars and take decades to complete, their replication is virtually impossible given competing uses for resources, even when they are done at all.

267.6 | Improving technology leads to quality improvement

Knowledge and technology (as well as economic and sociopolitical considerations) limit health care product and production specifications—and our ability to improve them— just as much as technology and manufacturing know-how limit what manufacturers can produce effectively and efficiently. Historically, we have emphasised the development of product technology—cures for diseases. Once discovered or developed, we assumed simply that providers would learn of, be able to assess, use appropriately and deliver efficiently such knowledge and technology. Variation in practices and growth in costs suggests these assumptions were unwarranted. Quality managers must assist providers to exploit maximally existing technology (by formulating the right practice policies) and to improve the technology that is available to them (by focusing research and development where it is most needed and will produce the most useful information). The acceptance and extent of quality management technology and its diffusion (e.g. trained quality managers) limit accomplishment of these objectives.

Improving the treatment of colon cancer—that is, specifying what should be done by whom and how, and seeing that it is done properly—would, by at least one account, produce a huge improvement in patients' health status. So huge, in fact, as to overshadow any improvement that could reasonably be expected with any set of better specifications that can be envisioned to result in the near future from the ongoing search for better treatments.[5] A cure for cancer—some set of different processes for treating (if not preferably preventing) colon cancer—would offer a vast improvement in practice policies, if it were to exist. However, we cannot allow quixotic quests for such cures to impede our efforts to improve patients' health status through better use of existing technology.

Quality management may not be as glamorous as the search for cures but its benefits are likely larger and far more certain. Cost-effective health status improvement depends as much on better quality management and process technology as it does on better product technology, a point we often overlook in our quest to discover cures for diseases. Moreover, by measuring outcomes, the effects and costs of care, we can better prioritise research and development efforts to produce the technology that we need but do not have, to improve people's health most cost-effectively. Finally, to create a virtuous spiral we need to establish mechanisms to assess new technologies' cost-effectiveness as a prelude to their incorporation into practice policies.

267.7 | Improving R&D leads to quality improvement

Research and development (R&D) generates the knowledge and creates the technology that is the key to improving product and production specifications. The knowledge revolution is based on an idea that most people fail to grasp sufficiently: it is possible to mass generate scientifically and apply systematically useful knowledge and information to achieve practical ends. To succeed in the coming quest for quality, managers will have to learn how to manage information—to apply the tools of research, information science and knowledge engineering to their business—and how to improve continuously their organisation's ability to generate efficiently and use effectively the knowledge and information it needs to be successful in improving products and operations. Success will go to those companies and nations that spend sufficient money on the right research and development, organise the production of knowledge in the right way to ensure the utility of results, and apply results in the right way to effect systematic improvement in products and production processes, including health care.

The United States has generally led the way in health research, spending far more than other countries and producing more scientific papers. However, the United States is vulnerable not only to increased spending by other countries but also, and more significantly, to improved quality of research elsewhere. By some measures, Australia's biomedical research establishment, for example, can be considered more efficient than that of the United States, that is, it produces more research papers per dollar expended.[6] Volume of papers, of course, is a poor proxy of the quality or value of the information they contain. Again, the very limited evidence that exists may suggest that the United States is slipping here too.[7] The United States spends relatively very little on the types of health systems research that would improve medical practice and its technology. In Australia, spending on such research is minimal, severely limiting information useful for improving the quality of care. Ways to improve the quality of research and development (encompassing, for example, how much is spent, on what it is spent, and with what effect) and how R&D's fruits can be applied systematically to improve patient care are topics beyond this manual's scope.

267.8 | Quality management's challenge

Everything is capable of being 'improved', ad infinitum. Continuous quality improvement represents quality management's central challenge. Stated simply, to improve something one must have a vision of what constitutes improvement and the means to realise it. Practically, one must have sufficiently valid and reliable ways of measuring performance (quality) to know what one is achieving, know that there is a way to improve performance, and possess the know-how, resources and authority to effect the changes that are expected to result in the desired improvement. Having made these changes one must again measure performance to show that it did improve as expected. Suppose that there was no improvement. What could have gone wrong?

Quality may fail to improve for any number of reasons. Perhaps the measure was not reliable. Repeated measurement might show an improvement, compounding the problem of achieving real improvement, of course. Perhaps the measure was not sensitive enough: improvement did occur but it was too slight to register. If so, the improvement was insignificant or, if significant, a more sensitive measure must be employed. Perhaps improvement occurred in areas not being measured. Certainly this result is possible but, if important, the performance of these other areas should also be measured. Perhaps the changes were not implemented properly or, if implemented properly, not effective, or if effective, produced additional effects that resulted in no net increase in performance. Even if the changes did result in increased performance, was the increase due to the substance of the changes, the fact that changes were made (virtually any change would have done the trick), or factors beyond the changes? Sorting all this out is never simple, and in the production of health it often proves extremely difficult.

267.9 | Closing the quality management gap

Quality management is far easier said than done. Meeting the quality revolution's challenges will both require changes to and produce changes in health care's culture. Quality management focuses on the product, drives the entire organisation, and involves measurement and use of resultant information to improve products and production processes thereby improving the extent to which products conform to specifications (reducing variance and lowering costs). Quality management works to improve product specifications, redesign processes to improve their production, improve methods for developing new product and production technologies, and set priorities among these activities. Improvement suggestions reflect implicit (usually unstated) problems (that the suggestions are intended to solve). Finding and fixing problems (deviations from specifications)—QA's essence—is necessary to improve processes and products. However, finding problems should not be equated with finding fault with individual workers or doctors. Problems usually arise in production systems. Fixing problems or implementing improvements mostly involves changing production processes. Chapter 8 in this part elaborates on these points.

How do hospitals close the quality management gap between their meagre quality management efforts and the structures and processes necessary to achieve quality maturity? Closing this gap can be a daunting prospect for even the most energised quality manager. There is no single or simple answer. Once the hospital's management has committed to quality management, created the structure and provided the resources that are the manifestation of such commitment, the hospital can take its first steps to assess, assure and improve the quality of care. The best approach is to create all of the elements required for a complete quality management system, at least in skeleton form. Thus, for example, if the hospital identifies quality problems, it can determine their root causes and take steps to eliminate them. The hospital can then control the development of the system's various elements according to its needs, circumstances and experience. Chapter 6 in Part III describes the practical aspects of getting started on and progressing along the long and arduous journey toward quality maturity for which this chapter provides a map.

268 | Utilisation review

268.1 | Cost as a dimension of quality

The cost of achieving health status improvement is an important dimension of the quality of care. Quality is improved if providers reduce the cost of achieving a given level of patient health status improvement. Not only is the same benefit achieved at less cost, but the savings can be used to pay for other interventions that could well further improve the same or other patients' health status, or for other efforts to improve their welfare. In contrast, incremental improvements in a patient's health status using more costly interventions requires either additional resource inputs into health care or shifting resources from some people or patients to others or, for a given person or patient, denying them some other interventions. The net effect of costly incremental improvements in some individual patients' health status may be reduced population health status or welfare if the value of the resultant health benefits is less than those forgone to pay for the specific medical interventions.

Whenever payers, often government, have attempted to control rising health care expenditures, providers and patients have, quite rightly, been concerned with proposed measures' effect on the quality of care—despite the lack of objective measures to support this concern. However, providers have generally eschewed any interest in systematically finding ways to reduce the cost of care, thereby increasing value for money spent on health care. Government's or people's health care expenditures are providers' incomes. In competitive industries, suppliers strive to offer greater value for money, often by finding cheaper ways to satisfy customers' needs, because they know that, if they do their profits may increase, and if they do not, competitors' innovations may drive them out of business. This quality improvement mechanism is absent in health care because of the lack of a practical way to measure the value of its products (amount of health status improvement from providers' specific medical interventions) as well as the lack of incentives born of its tradition and the culture of which it is part. Quality management focuses as much on production costs as it does on products.

The cost of care may represent:

- unnecessary or useless interventions—a waste of money with a detrimental effect on health status because they either harm the patient directly, preclude useful interventions, or consume resources that could be better spent on other patients;
- useful but expensive interventions which represent funds that if applied elsewhere would yield greater health status improvement, albeit to someone else;
- useful, cost-effective interventions delivered inefficiently, so that they cost more than the same services offered elsewhere, reducing overall population health status improvement potential (because the wasted money could be better spent elsewhere);
- useful, cost-effective interventions at the lowest possible long-run price.

One may gravitate naturally to the latter interventions as socially most desirable. Apart from the difficulty of ensuring that only useful cost-effective interventions were applied as efficiently as possible, this situation would require, at a minimum, detailed knowledge about the cost-effectiveness of interventions and providers' performance, and incentives to avoid of use of interventions and services that are not considered cost-effective. Whether or not government should prohibit people using their own money for interventions it considers not cost-effective in an attempt to limit national health care expenditures to maintain international economic competitiveness, for example, is itself a contentious sociopolitical issue. Government's decision to pay only for cost-effective interventions would likely result in explicit recognition that only the rich can get certain treatments (e.g. those with little effect and large cost) even if everyone received basic health care, thereby having a profound effect on the social fabric. These social policy considerations are beyond this manual's scope.

This manual focuses on the technical dimension of quality—health status improvement—for two principal reasons. Firstly, it is the most salient, the least examined, and the most difficult to improve systematically. Secondly, we want to avoid introducing other—and to most readers what would be even more foreign—new concepts necessary to understand the paradigm shift needed to improve the quality of care, including reducing or containing its cost. Nevertheless, the manual would be incomplete if it entirely omitted attention to resource use. This section focuses on utilisation review, mechanisms to control costs through the review of health services' use. However, as explained below, utilisation review covers only a fraction of the determinants of the cost of care. This section describes how utilisation review fits into a hospital's quality management program. The last section in this chapter summarises how utilisation review has evolved in the United States, where most of the experience to date resides.

268.2 Scope of traditional utilisation review

268.21 ABOUT UTILISATION REVIEW

Utilisation review (UR) focuses on a provider's use of resources for the care of individual patients. Clearly, patients' and providers' decisions about appropriate responses to health problems result in observed aggregate national health care expenditures. In most industrialised countries, they have increased at alarming rates. Generally, utilisation review is limited to technical questions of resource use:

- medical necessity (which traditionally has often been considered a quality of care issue)—whether or not use of a specific medical intervention (e.g. surgical operation) is necessary or appropriate, that is, could plausibly provide information toward improving or improve a patient's health status;

- timing—whether or not the intervention is needed now even if it might be needed in the future, for example, a planned lumbar laminectomy might be deferred pending the results of conservative therapy;
- setting—whether or not the patient needs to be hospitalised, or a specific medical intervention requires hospitalisation or could be done in an outpatient setting;
- duration—usually the appropriate length of hospital stay (hospitalisation) for the patient's condition or for a planned procedure.

Traditional utilisation review is not concerned with questions of value achieved for money spent (e.g. whether or not an 85-year-old man should receive a kidney transplant even if his health status were expected to improve as a result) nor with the efficiency with which providers deliver interventions (e.g. the cost of a necessary X-ray). Utilisation review must be distinguished from rationing, choices, production-level technology assessment, and the efficiency of care provision.

268.22 RATIONING—WHAT OTHERS CHOOSE FOR PATIENTS
Rationing is concerned with the competing use or allocation of resources among different patients each of whom's health status is expected to be improved by specific health care interventions. Thus hospitals may have mechanisms (e.g. committees, practice policies) to determine who gets into an intensive care unit (ICU) for example. Obviously, people who do not need to be in an ICU, that is, their health outcomes are not improved as a result, should be excluded from the ICU. This concern is utilisation review's classic focus. However, others who would benefit may also be excluded, that is, care rationed, because the expected health benefits are not sufficient to justify use of the resource, either because another patient who is waiting for or expected to require such care would benefit more, or because the cost of the treatment does not justify the expenditure (even if no one else is waiting or expected to arrive momentarily who would require the resource).

268.23 CHOICE—WHAT PATIENTS CHOOSE FOR THEMSELVES
Rationing is a decision made by others that affects patients' consumption of health care resources. In contrast, patient choices are concerned with the competing use of the patient's own or his or her entitlement to resources. Such choice occurs, for example, when the patient chooses surgery (which may be an expensive choice) over conservative therapy (which may be an inexpensive choice). In practice, many decisions have elements of rationing and choice. For example, a patient may prefer the surgical operation but it is excluded from his or her insurance policy and he or she is unable or unwilling to bear the cost, limiting his or her choice among alternative therapies.

268.24 PRODUCTION-LEVEL TECHNOLOGY ASSESSMENT
The wisdom of purchasing new equipment or providing additional services, for example, falls within the purview of production-level technology assessment, not utilisation review. Production-level technology assessment is concerned with hospitals' decisions to acquire or to use technology or to provide certain interventions or services, not the actual use of resources for individual patients' care. By extension, practice policies are constrained by the technologies and services that hospitals make available for patient care. They may prescribe explicitly or implicitly what resources should be used to treat patients and thus may explicitly ration care or constrain patients' choices.

268.25 EFFICIENCY OF CARE PROVISION
Inefficiency of care provision takes many forms. For example, tests may be done in the hospital that could just as well have been done prior to admission. Patients may languish on wards because their doctor has not discharged them. The social worker may start

looking for a nursing home bed at the end of the patient's stay instead of on the first day (which may be possible by using a model to predict nursing home need, for example). The clinical laboratory performs a test for $50 that could be performed for $45 if its volume were higher or its operation were more efficient. The ways the same (or better) care can be produced at less cost are literally endless. Traditionally, those concerned with interventions for individual patients (e.g. proper site for tests, prompt action by doctors, early discharge planning) have fallen within utilisation review's scope; those concerned with providers' operations (e.g. efficiency of laboratories, laundry), have not.

268.3 | Evolution of utilisation review

In the United States, utilisation review began in hospitals but, beginning in the mid 1960s, payers rapidly took up the charge. Originally, utilisation review was an initial attempt to control, limit or prevent use of ineffective or inappropriate care, specifically to challenge and document the medical necessity of care. In the 1970s utilisation review meant concurrent (during the hospital stay) or retrospective (postdischarge) review. Wanting to lock stable doors before horses had bolted, beginning in the 1980s payers began prospective utilisation review programs. Their objective was to prevent unnecessary interventions, to make sure interventions took place in the most appropriate setting, and to reduce the duration of interventions to the minimum. With this emphasis, utilisation management (UM, sometimes called managed care) began to replace or subsume traditional concurrent and retrospective utilisation review. In the 1980s UM's primary goal was cost cutting; that of quality assurance (QA), improving health care outcomes. Increasingly, in the 1990s UM is being subsumed under quality management or quality improvement. After all, resources are applied to improve patients' health status; focusing on health outcomes makes the most sense. The last section in this chapter chronicles the evolution, present nature and likely future direction of utilisation management in the United States.

268.4 | The impetus for utilisation review (utilisation management)

The impetus to manage resource use and thus for utilisation review (UR) stems from two principal factors: the increasing amount of third party, for example government, payment for health care, and the rising cost of that care. Thus, from the payer's perspective, UR's central purpose is cost containment. However, payers have several other potential cost-containment strategies in their armoury, including the following, further discussion of which is beyond the manual's scope:

- supply design or restriction (various techniques for limiting the supply or availability of resources, e.g. doctors, hospital beds);
- benefit design or rationing (various techniques for shaping patients' effective demand for care, e.g. coverage exclusions, cost-sharing or patient payments, consumer education);
- delivery design and control of patient's access (e.g. restricting patients' choice of provider, using gatekeepers or triage to control patients' access to specialists and expensive services);
- payment of care strategies and financial incentives for providers (e.g. prospective payment through DRGs, capitation, shared savings).

As the term suggests, cost containment, or limiting expenditures for health care is of most interest to those who pay, particularly third party payers who bear the majority of health care costs, such as the federal government. Generally, hospitals have only been interested in utilisation review if pressed by payers or regulators, or if they faced serious resource constraints. In the United States, where most utilisation review experience resides, hospitals' lack of response to payers' concerns led to external utilisation management programs designed to control providers' use of resources. However, success has been elusive, to which the soaring cost of care attests. Moreover, utilisation management programs may now be adding to rather than saving on health care costs. Emerging strategies of returning financial risk to hospitals while holding them accountable for quality may give them the incentive to engage in utilisation review as an integral part of quality management to minimise costs while assuring quality.

The medical profession's principal concern about utilisation management is that cost cutting (e.g. restrictions on length of stay) impairs quality, for example by causing patients to be discharged from the hospital too soon, that is, at a point that results in poorer outcomes. Recent evidence from the United States suggests that as a result of Medicare DRGs patients were discharged sooner, that is, length of stay was reduced, but that outcomes were not worsened. Instead, hospitals shifted the cost of patient care elsewhere, principally to relatives at home.[8] Paradoxically, as lengths of stay decrease, the average cost of a hospital day (and conceivably of a hospital stay) increases, because if occupancy rates remain unchanged the hospital's use of resources intensifies, or if days of care decrease (because there are insufficient replacement bed days) relatively high fixed costs must be spread over fewer bed days.

268.5 Utilisation review in hospitals

Hospitals that receive fees for services have a positive financial disincentive against utilisation review since it can only reduce revenues. Its use at such hospitals depends on the desire to deliver high quality medical care, or regulatory or payer pressure. To be most effective, this pressure must include being at risk for the financial consequences of unnecessary tests and treatments and other forms of inefficient care. In budget-based systems, such as those experienced by Australian public hospitals, there are presently fewer direct financial incentives to render unnecessary care, because revenues do not flow as a result. However, there are also few incentives to reduce unnecessary care (such as unnecessary use of diagnostic tests, inappropriate hospital admissions, or unnecessary lengths of stay) or to improve efficiency in any other way. If patient throughput increased through eliminating unnecessary days of care, for example, the intensity of care would also likely increase, requiring additional resources (beyond those budgeted presently) and/or increasing workloads. If there were no patients in need of care presently, occupancy rates or workloads would decrease which might prompt disliked budget reductions or work might expand to consume all available resources. Utilisation review works best when the hospital's resources are under pressure and/or providers have tangible incentives to improve the efficiency of their use.

268.6 Role of UR in an integrated quality management program

Resource utilisation—the use of tests and other interventions to treat individual patients—is an important aspect of quality. Clearly, doctors should use only needed interventions; all interventions used should be needed. Utilisation review—the examination of use of interventions with a view to reducing their unnecessary or inappropriate use—was one of the first quality assurance and improvement strategies, although it is now associated mostly with payers' concern to contain care costs. A hospital's quality management program can employ utilisation review techniques to improve the efficiency and effectiveness of care. To date, lack of incentives has resulted in lack of use. Hospitals need to use different mechanisms to improve operational efficiency, for example to reduce the cost of an X-ray. Their consideration is beyond this manual's scope.

The remainder of this section describes various utilisation review techniques that hospitals can apply as part of a quality management program. They are often classified as prospective (preproduction), concurrent (intraproduction), or retrospective (postproduction). Not only does the time of review vary but so does its purpose and character. Utilisation review is case-based at all production stages. Postproduction utilisation review can be population-based, for example examining statistically doctors' cost in treating given types of patients. Generally, hospitals will find retrospective utilisation review to be most efficient—at least early on in implementing a quality management program. Utilisation review is best integrated into the quality management program via the process of structured quality review.

268.7 Preproduction—prospective utilisation review

Prospective review occurs before resources are used to treat individual patients; it is inherently case-based. At this production stage, utilisation review's purpose is:

- to ensure interventions' medical necessity including, for example, elective admissions to the hospital (emergency admissions can be reviewed retrospectively), and that the care setting is appropriate, for example inpatient versus outpatient surgery;
- to review the appropriateness of care plans, for example discharge planning—before the patient's admission to hospital, explicit consideration of what is likely to be necessary to discharge the patient from the hospital, for example placement in a nursing home.

Discharge planning should be routine with any hospital admission and a hospital should set up a mechanism to ensure that it is carried out. The idea of reviewing prospectively all elective hospital admissions or care plans is quite foreign and likely to be quite repugnant to Australian medical staff. Moreover, unless part of a computerised clinical decision support system, the cost of reviews would likely outweigh savings from avoiding interventions considered medically unnecessary or reducing lengths of stay. Nevertheless, hospitals should consider making targeted prospective utilisation review part of their quality management program. Targeting may be based on:

- risk to the patient—a patient's risk of dying from the procedure may be high and assurance is needed that the potential benefits outweigh these risks;
- cost of the intervention—preprocedure review may be cost-effective for high cost interventions or if structured quality review had found that a procedure is often used inappropriately;
- provider performance—structured quality review may have found that some providers perform unnecessary procedures so that preprocedure review is warranted to assist the doctor improve his or her practice (to avoid the need to withdraw privileges).

268.8 Intraproduction—so-called concurrent utilisation review

Intraproduction utilisation review involves either use of decision support systems or so-called concurrent utilisation review. Use of computerised test ordering or decision support systems are a form of in-process quality control. For example, they can advise on the most cost-effective diagnostic strategy for the patient's condition, or prevent ordering of tests not in conformance with practice policies or require approval for exceptions to practice policies, especially if the proposed test poses substantial risk to the patient or is very costly. Further, such systems can facilitate retrospective utilisation review because they track who orders which tests for what patients.

During an admission, (specially trained) nurses may review the patient's progress and expedite care, for example make sure the doctor writes separation orders, or explains why the patient still needs to be in the hospital. This kind of so-called concurrent utilisation review aims to improve the efficiency of care, specifically the care delivery process. Only by weighing the cost of such expediting systems against resource savings can hospitals estimate its value. Further, even if savings outweigh costs, one must consider opportunity costs—the cost of achieving these or greater savings in other ways, for example, new practice policies, better production systems or incentives for doctors to be more efficient or cost conscious.

268.9 | Postproduction—retrospective utilisation review

Retrospective utilisation review was the first and is still likely the most commonly used strategy. It may be case-based (review of resource use case-by-case) or population-based (statistical analysis of resources used for populations of cases). In general, hospitals will find it most cost-effective to integrate utilisation review into structured quality review rather than consider retrospective utilisation review as a separate set of activities. Results of such reviews and analyses may well point to problems in use of resources that should be subject to investigation and to improvement actions.

The highest quality is attained if the desired product is produced at the lowest cost. Specifying the processes needed to improve patients' health status maximally permits one to calculate the resources necessary to provide them, either in terms of money or resource units, for example days of care. Practice policies can encompass resource use. Quality of care review criteria encompass such utilisation measures as length of stay, blood usage and medical necessity of interventions. They also encompass the locus of care, for example necessity for hospital admission, and whether or not ambulatory surgery was indicated. In this latter regard it is important to recognise that surgeons can be criticised for conducting an operation in an outpatient setting that should have been performed in the hospital (which may well use more resources) as well as vice versa (which likely would use fewer).

Currently, case-by-case structured quality review is not concerned generally with details of resource use, for example determining whether or not each and every diagnostic test should have been ordered or examining the order of tests with a view to determining if another diagnostic strategy would have been more cost-effective and should have been employed. Indubitably, such reviews will occur with the increased sophistication of outcome/process assessment screens.

Retrospective review can look not only at the care given to individual patients but also at patterns of resource use, specifically by an individual doctor. Obviously, many factors affect resource use including the patient's health problems and characteristics. Thus simple comparisons of average cost of admission by doctor or his or her use of a particular intervention may be misleading. However, comparisons of cost or use of specific tests or treatments for like patients may serve to pinpoint causes of concern. Statistical analysis of resource use may be a useful screening tool to focus structured quality review, especially if the data are already available in electronic (computerised) form and some type of risk adjustment is possible to avoid large numbers of false positives. Its effectiveness in relation to other screening techniques is largely unknown.

269 | Utilisation management in the United States

269.1 | About utilisation management in the United States

In the United States, health insurance companies and other third party payers, including self-insured employers (here referred to collectively as payers) embraced utilisation review programs in the 1960s, and their use has grown steadily ever since and is still expanding. Their goal was to save money. The key question then—and still today—is whether or not they do. With so much money at stake, payers and providers are engaged in a dynamic game to conserve or corner resources. For example, payers' push to move care from costly—but highly-reviewed—inpatient hospitals to presumed less-costly—but unreviewed—outpatient settings has set off an increase in outpatient costs with the inevitable call to review use of these services. In some cases, hospitals may now charge more for the same operation performed on an outpatient than on an inpatient basis. Ominously, some observers believe that all of the easy savings have been realised and that health care costs are poised to increase even more rapidly.[9]

In the United States, utilisation management (payers' use of utilisation review, especially prospective utilisation review) has become extensive, almost all-pervasive for inpatient care. Payers still put much faith in such programs, perhaps because they are relatively simple to implement and give the illusion that they are doing something to retard the growth of health care costs. Paradoxically, the more payers use these programs, the more they question their benefits. The view is now emerging that present utilisation management (UM) programs may cost more than they save. Payers are reluctant to discontinue their programs, however, because they are uncertain what would replace them and fear a cost explosion if they relaxed their vigilance. They continue to search for ways to manage utilisation cost-effectively.

This section summarises the evolution and the present nature of utilisation management in the United States. Given utilisation review's long history and the diversity of existing utilisation management programs, the section intends only to provide an overview of salient points relevant to quality management in hospitals; not a definitive history or complete description of the current state of affairs. The section also describes commonly used utilisation review tools. It ends with a brief review of some of the future directions that utilisation management is likely to take in the United States.

269.2   *Evolution of utilisation review in the United States*

Gradually, utilisation review's focus has shifted from expediting care to examining the timing, duration and place of care, to confirming its medical necessity. Consequently, utilisation review's scope has expanded from resource use to encompass some aspects of the technical quality of care. At the same time there has been a parallel shift from emphasis on retrospective review, to concurrent review, to prospective review. Presently, prospective utilisation review predominates, and is referred to often as utilisation management or managed care; the generic term utilisation review is now often taken to mean retrospective utilisation review.

Initially, utilisation review was retrospective. While hospitals could, at least in theory, change their practices if they discovered inappropriate utilisation of resources, payers could only deny claims for inappropriate care. Payment denials upset providers and patients who, for example, found that their payer would not pay for a procedure that their doctor had already performed. Increasingly, retrospective review was seen as locking stable doors after horses had bolted. Focus shifted to preprocedure review: money would be saved by not expending it on, and patients would be shielded from, unnecessary or inappropriate care. Payers could point to savings and to patients with still-intact uteri, for example. While intuitively appealing, universal preprocedure review—all cases all of the time—is likely not cost-effective.

With retrospective review some unnecessary surgical operations, for example, may be done initially. However, if providers were not paid in such cases they might be expected to be more judicious in their future use of surgical interventions. This result would be cold comfort to the patients who had already undergone unnecessary surgery. For obvious reasons, in allocating resources, specific benefits and harms to identified individuals often take precedence over larger, but anonymous, benefits or harms to society. Universal preprocedure review lives on, despite having outlived its utility.

When advocates first convinced payers to introduce utilisation management programs, claims of substantial savings quickly followed. Their introduction does seem to result in one-time savings but, after they have been realised, the aggregate cost of care continues its inexorable upward climb. More concerningly, after whatever initial savings it may provide, universal preprocedure review likely costs more than it saves. Moreover, patients see payers' intrusion into the doctor–patient relationship as a barrier to receiving the care that their doctor said they needed. Doctors view the need to obtain prior approval for specific medical interventions as a nuisance and an additional cost. Some want to be reimbursed for the time they spent discussing cases with payers' utilisation review staff.

From a system's perspective it is far more cost-effective to place the financial risk for unnecessary or inappropriate care where it belongs: with the provider. However, retrospective review coupled with incentives linked to necessary and appropriate care requires both the will and the means to forge the link, and holding providers accountable, which has proven politically difficult to do. Trends toward care by vertically integrated health care systems (referred to sometimes as managed care networks) and other health care reforms—which emphasise managed competition among health plans that are accountable for results—promise to shift more of the financial risk to providers and, consequently, alter the nature of utilisation management programs. If providers are at-risk for payments and continuation of their contracts, they are expected to be more inclined to manage care to increase its value for money. In the future, providers—not payers—may become the primary users of utilisation management programs, because payers will give them financial and other incentives to reduce unnecessary and inappropriate care. Ironically, providers may then use desktop decision support technology to perform universal preprocedure review.

269.3 | The present nature of utilisation management in the United States

In a recent report the Institute of Medicine in the United States defined utilisation management as:

> a set of techniques used by or on behalf of purchasers of health care benefits to manage health care costs by influencing patient care decision-making through case-by-case assessments of the appropriateness of care prior to its provision.[10]

Utilisation management may be divided simply into prior review and high-cost case management. Prior review includes a variety of techniques including preprocedure (or preadmission/admission review), second opinions, continued-stay review and discharge planning. High-cost care management focuses on those patients whose care is proving or is likely to be very expensive. In 1980, for example, in the United States 1% of the population accounted for 29% of total health care expenditures.[11] This type of utilisation management may involve remodelling a patient's house if this intervention would allow him to be cared for at home rather than requiring him to be institutionalised, which would be the more expensive alternative. Further discussion of high-cost case management and its social policy implications is beyond this manual's scope.

269.4 | Preprocedure (preadmission) review

In the United States, before the introduction of prospective payment (DRGs), hospitals' costs were simply reimbursed. Denial of reimbursement after care had been provided upset both provider and patient, hence the shift to prior review. Prior review eliminates the patient's financial exposure but increases the nuisance and irritation level for providers. In both cases the payer accepts the financial risk, which he tries to limit by spending money (e.g. on prior review) to save money (by reducing unnecessary or inappropriate care). Since costs may now be exceeding benefits, payers are again interested in shifting or sharing the financial risk with providers. Providers are now interested in accepting this risk—which in any other business would normally rest with the supplier—to reduce problems and to share in the rewards of improved, more efficient care.

Payers may require patients, or their doctors, to obtain prior approval for interventions for non-emergent problems, for example elective surgical operations, if they want the payer to meet their full cost (within policy limits). Generally, the patient's doctor calls the payer (or a contracted utilisation review company) to obtain approval for the operation. The preprocedure utilisation reviewer, usually a UR nurse, approves the operation if criteria suggest that it is indicated. Otherwise the reviewer passes the case on to a staff or contracted medical doctor who discusses the proposed treatment with the patient's doctor and decides whether or not to approve it for payment purposes.

Present concerns with this type of preadmission review include the following. Doctors are unhappy with the nuisance involved in obtaining approvals. They are also concerned that reviewers are reluctant to disclose the criteria they use to approve or deny payment for care, so-called black box review systems. Payers may counter that if doctors knew the criteria, they would game the system, that is, tell the reviewer what he or she wanted to hear to obtain approval. From the payers' perspective, while doctors may not make up symptoms that the patient does not have, for example, they may be willing to interpret the patient's symptoms as being present for three months if they know this duration is the minimum cut-off for approval. Patients could be denied operations they need, especially if payers impose very strict criteria, or give reviewers incentives to deny requests for specific interventions, with serious consequences.

Early on, payers pointed to savings from prior review. However, now the belief is growing that universal preprocedure review costs more money than it saves. Every case that is reviewed incurs an expense to the payer and to the doctor, which would likely be made up subsequently through increased fees which would be paid ultimately by the payer. Payers must weigh the cost of reviewing proposed procedures against resultant savings from refusing to pay for interventions that they consider to be medically unnecessary. Such refusal saves only the difference in cost between the requested care and what the patient actually receives. The difference in payers' costs between the proposed procedure and its alternative may not always be substantial and conceivably the patient's treatment could end up costing more.

For example, in some cases a criterion for surgical operation is failed medical treatment. If the payer tells the doctor this precondition at the time of the original request for approval of the operation, he will dutifully give the patient the medical treatment unless he believes it would harm the patient either directly or indirectly through the consequences of delaying the operation (in which case the patient may have to pay for the operation himself or herself and/or sue the payer). The success or failure of such treatments is often in the mind of the beholder. The patient told by the doctor that he or she needs the operation may be predisposed to judge the medical therapy a failure, and the doctor who believes an operation is indicated may also be predisposed to this interpretation. In this case, the payer ends up paying for both the conservative therapy and the operation; not just for the operation.

Preprocedure review intends to reduce payment for unnecessary interventions. Clearly, it may result in patients being denied payment for needed medical care. How often payers refuse to pay for proposed procedures and how often such denials are warranted is unknown. Also unknown is how often payers knowingly pay for procedures that they consider unnecessary, for whatever reasons, and how often preprocedure review systems fail to detect unnecessary care. Tightening criteria (the rules used to assess an intervention's appropriateness) may increase savings but may also increase the risk of denying patients payment for needed care. Denial of needed treatment is just as much a quality of care problem as doing unindicated treatments. The issue boils down to the best way to manage patients. Validated practice policies are the key to assuring the quality of care and to preprocedure utilisation review.

Closing stable doors before horses have bolted (prior review to prevent unnecessary surgical operations) is intuitively more appealing than rounding up horses after they have bolted (identifying retrospectively unnecessary operations). But, unlike horses, providers may be educated and given incentives not to bolt (perform unnecessary operations). Thus continuous surveillance of the quality of care, including resource utilisation, with proper incentives for improvement and sanctions for abuses may—in the long run—yield more health benefits and result in better use of resources at less cost.

269.5 | Second opinions

Once a popular utilisation management technique, second opinions for surgical operations have now been largely displaced by preprocedure review. Such review may still call for a second opinion if there is disagreement on whether or not an operation is indicated. Second opinions as a utilisation management technique originated in the 1950s but met with much resistance from organised medicine. Only in the 1970s did they gain widespread support, after wider acceptance of the idea that a substantial number of operations were being performed unnecessarily.

Generally, second opinion programs are confined to certain surgical operations. Second opinion programs are of two types: voluntary and mandatory. By checking whether or not an operation is indicated, they serve two purposes: conserving payers' funds and informing patients. At times, these two purposes do not coincide. For example, a patient in two minds about an operation may decide to go ahead if a second surgeon confirms the first's opinion. Under some programs, a third opinion is required if the second one disagrees with the first. As might be expected, in voluntary programs patients do not always seek second opinions. Mandatory programs show much higher rates of confirmation of the need for surgery than voluntary programs, perhaps because in voluntary programs patients with doubts tend to be those who seek a second opinion. The fact that payers will pay for a second opinion is of benefit to patients. However, the cost of second opinions must be balanced by savings from avoiding unnecessary operations if they are to be successful as a utilisation management strategy. The evidence about the utility of second opinions as a cost-containing measure is equivocal, but the technique is generally regarded to have failed to save money.

269.6 | Continued stay review and discharge planning

Payers' principal strategies to shorten lengths of stay are continued stay review and discharge planning. Use of prospective payment (DRGs) obviates this need for payers (but reinforces it for providers) because providers are paid a fixed amount for a given hospital episode, regardless of length of stay.

When the patient is admitted to the hospital, the payer's case reviewer grants the patient's doctor an expected number of days of stay. On the day before the granted number of days has elapsed, the reviewer calls the doctor to see if the patient has been or will be discharged as planned. If not, the reviewer ascertains the problem, for example complications, and grants additional covered days of stay. Clearly, the existence of such systems keeps doctors on their toes and thus may reduce utilisation below that which it might otherwise have been. However, the extent to which such systems save money, let alone improve the quality of care, is an open question.

Working with the patient's doctor and hospital staff, insurance company utilisation reviewers, who are usually nurses, try to reduce the patient's stay to a minimum by planning the patient's discharge before he or she enters the hospital.

269.7 | Retrospective utilisation review

Payers may conduct retrospective utilisation review for one of four purposes: to audit preprocedure (preadmission) review, to review an emergency admission, to monitor types of cases that are not considered problems, or to profile providers. If it appears that inappropriate utilisation is becoming a problem, the payer may (re)institute preprocedure or preadmission review for that type of care.

Payers may profile doctors' use of resources and compare them to their colleagues (norms) or to standards. Differences in patients can account for some of the variance in resource use, of course. Payers may recognise this problem even if they make no adjustments to account for it. Analysts could use various data to adjust for difference in patients, for example severity of illness scores, although their validity is questionable. Feedback of utilisation information may be used in an attempt to change providers' behaviour, especially if coupled with sanctions for continued consumption of resources past some acceptable upper limit. Of course, being at the low end of utilisation may make one a model of efficiency, or a quality problem because one was not doing all that one should be doing, underservicing rather than overservicing patients.

269.8 | Utilisation review instruments

A variety of instruments is used to assess the need for hospital inpatient care. They are based mostly on criteria that were developed originally in the 1970s for retrospective review of care by Professional Standards Review Organisations (PSROs). Today, the most widely used instruments are the Appropriateness Evaluation Protocol (AEP) and the ISD-A criteria set (intensity of services, severity of illness, discharge and appropriateness) screens, both of which were developed originally to gauge retrospectively the extent of inappropriate hospital use. They have since been adapted for prospective use and are available in paper and computer form. Various companies market such instruments. For example, Utilisation Management Associates (Wellesley, Massachusetts) has developed MCAP (Managed Care Appropriateness Protocol) a successor to the AEP, and MPAP (Psychiatric Appropriateness Protocol). Inter-Qual (Worcester, Massachusetts) markets ISD-A criteria. Value Health Sciences (Santa Monica, California) and Medical Intelligence (Brookline, Massachusetts) market computerised systems to assess prospectively the medical necessity of about thirty specific procedures.

Statistical norms are used to assess the appropriateness of lengths of stay. They are derived either from published data, for example those compiled by CPHA (Commission on Professional and Hospital Activities in Ann Arbor, Michigan) or from those compiled by the payer.

269.9 | Some prospects for utilisation management in the United States

Payers are beginning to focus preprocedure review programs on particular cases where the patient is at high risk from the planned intervention or where the expected savings from avoided inappropriate care are greater than the cost of reviewing cases in order to improve value for money (savings in health care costs that result from UM expenditures). The increasing use of high technology, high risk, high cost medical care interventions—such as high-dose chemotherapy with stem cell rescue for the treatment of breast cancer—is arousing payers' concerns about their proven effectiveness (in contrast to their experimental or investigational nature) and their appropriateness for the individual patient whose doctor has recommended the treatment (even if effective for some type of patients), often suggesting it represents the patient's last chance to live. Such recommended interventions can shorten (rather than lengthen) lives and reduce (rather than increase) the quality of the patient's remaining life, cost US$500 000 or more, and result in litigation that costs millions of dollars. Medical Care Management Corporation

(Bethesda, Maryland) provides expert panels to assess high technology intervention's appropriateness—a unique service to payers, providers and patients throughout the world.

Increasingly, payers will use sophisticated, computerised systems to perform preprocedure review. Their use is expected to increase and to expand, even as preprocedure review becomes increasingly focused. Review criteria will become more specific and have better documented validity. These systems will be integrated with administrative systems and will be transparent to the user. Their use will spread from inpatient care to all settings, especially ambulatory care, including provision of services in patients' homes. The most sophisticated systems will provide automated authorisation at the point of service, except in those instances that fall outside of its capabilities or that very likely represent inappropriate care. They will reduce significantly or eliminate entirely the need for UR nurses to screen cases and also reduce the number of cases requiring review by doctors working for payers. These systems are likely to move from the utilisation reviewer's desk to the patient's bedside and may become the first widespread use of clinical decision support technology (DST).

Utilisation management's focus is expected to shift from episodes to continuums of care, and result in longitudinal case management. Continued facilitation and oversight characterise longitudinal case management. It begins with patients' entry into the care system and may involve preprocedure review, for example. However, rather than ending when patients are discharged from the hospital, longitudinal case management continues, for example, to prevent recurrence of illness or inappropriate use of such services as emergency room care. As well as providing educational and preventive interventions, the longitudinal case manager can collect long-term outcomes data. When patients require additional interventions, they can be channelled quickly to the most appropriate and least costly settings. Effective longitudinal case management is expected to result in greater patient health status improvement and lower total costs—even after accounting for the increased cost of case management. Primary care doctors may be the longitudinal case managers of the future. They would be responsible for both patients' health status and the cost of their care, and they would be paid accordingly.

Provider profiling will become increasingly important as managed care networks seek to credential providers based on their quality and cost performance. Once credentialled, providers' performance can be monitored retrospectively and unobtrusively, greatly decreasing the need for case-by-case preprocedure review. Provider profiling is heavily dependent on collection of performance data and its proper interpretation. Existing claims processing systems may be expanded to meet this need, although presently they contain too little clinical data to be truly useful for this purpose. Retrospective quality assessment systems (e.g. QSM, marketed by Quality Standards in Medicine in Boston, Massachusetts) are likely to become an increasingly important source of information for provider profiling. Where done, preprocedure reviews will be added to profiling databases. Provider profiling will enable payers to focus on preprocedure review on particular patients, providers or procedures. It will require development of criteria and standards, norms, and statistical models to analyse data automatically, with expert system interpretation to identify providers on whom health care network managers need to focus their attention.

References

1 Kosha MT. Using CQI methods to lower postsurgical wound infection rate. Hospitals 1992; May 5: 62–3.
2 Ellwood PM. Shattuck lecture—outcomes management. A technology of patient experience. N Eng J Med 1988; 318(23): 1549–56.

2(a) An introduction to the Health Outcomes Institute's Outcomes Management System. Bloomington, Minnesota: Outcomes Management Institute, 1993.

3 Williamson JW, Goldschmidt PG, Colton TC. The quality of the medical literature: an analysis of validation assessments. In Bailer JC, Mosteller F (eds). Medical use of statistics. Boston: NEJM Books, 1986.

4 Weiss R. Dazzled by 'tortured data': faulty number crunching comes back to bite some medical studies. Washington Post Health 1993; Nov 23: 6.

5 McArdle CS, Hole D. Impact of variability among surgeons on postoperative morbidity and mortality and ultimate survival. BMJ 1991; 302(6791): 1501–5.

6 Goldschmidt PG. Declining American representation in leading clinical-research journals (letter). N Eng J Med 1990; 323(9): 610.

7 Smith R. International comparisons of funding and output of research: bye bye Britain. BMJ 1988; 296: 409–12.

8 Rogers WH, Draper D, Kahn KL, et al. Quality of care before and after implementation of the DRG-based prospective payment system: a summary of effects. JAMA 1990: 264(15): 1989–94.

9 Schwartz WB, Mendelson MPP. Hospital cost containment in the 1980s: hard lessons learned and prospects for the 1990s. N Eng J Med 1991; 324: 1037–42.

10 Institute of Medicine. Controlling costs and changing patient care? Washington, DC: National Academy Press, 1989, p.17.

11 Berk ML, Monhelt AC, Hagen MM. How the US spent its health care dollar, 1929–1980. Health Affairs 1988; 4: 46–60.

Chapter 7

PRACTICE POLICIES AND CRITERIA

| 271 | **Purpose of this chapter** |

Product specifications are the key to quality improvement. They must be the right specifications and they must be implemented right. Quality can be assessed and assured only in reference to product specifications, and improved only by closing the gap between what is done and achieved (practice) and what should be done and achieved (specifications), and improving those specifications to provide customers with greater value for money. This chapter focuses on specifying health care's product for quality management purposes.

The idea that product specifications can be formulated for health care is quite novel and even somewhat disturbing to many medical practitioners who regard the practice of medicine as an art rather than a science. Health care is a production function. To improve production processes requires specification of products. In industry, product specifications inform production workers and, increasingly, production machines what the product is supposed to look like and how to make it so that it turns out the way it is supposed to look. In health care, practice policies prescribe the interventions that maximise health status improvement consistent with patients' preferences and society's resources. Health care is a state transforming process. Practice policies inform doctors and other professionals how to change patients' state from poor health to better health, that is, to improve their health status. They focus on interventions. Procedural (or process) policies focus on how to implement the interventions specified in practice policies. Process engineering focuses on how best to implement practice policies and procedures to realise achievable health benefits, minimise the cost of their attainment, and ensure greatest patient satisfaction; workflow engineering on how patients should flow among processes. However, detailed consideration of procedural policies and process and workflow engineering is beyond this manual's scope.

Health care's product is seemingly amorphous and intangible, and, if defined as maximal achievement of a patient's health status, apparently fixed at any given amount. These characteristics complicate quality management efforts and confuse practitioners. Unlike manufactured goods, health care's product (improved health) cannot be measured directly in any meaningful fashion. It is not that health status cannot be measured. It can. The problem is the difficulty of attributing any change (or its lack) to preceding interventions (rather than other factors); structured outcome measurement not withstanding (see Chapter 8 in this part).

Health care's ultimate product—improvement in patient health status—must be defined operationally in terms of practices and processes intended to produce this product. Practice policies—and, by extension, the working of systems, procedures, machines, people, etc., that implement them—specify these practices and processes. Thus, for all practical quality management purposes, conformance to product specifications (practice policies)—and, by extension, production specifications (implementing processes)—is health care's product. Further, materially different practice policies (which may result in greater patient health status improvement) represent a different product.

Practice policies differ from practice guidelines. Practice guidelines are principles that guide action. Practice policies are standing answers to patient care questions—specifications regarding who should do what and how, and when and where it should be done—that take into account patients' preferences and society's resources and thus may involve socioeconomic as well as technical considerations. Lack of facts limits the development of science-based practice policies. Practitioners must often select among interventions based on experience and intuition rather than research results.

This chapter:

- explains the need to establish product specifications (practice policies and criteria) for quality assessment and improvement purposes;
- defines, and differentiates between, practice policies and practice criteria;
- describes how the best available information can be synthesised to develop practice policies for quality management purposes;
- describes the use of practice criteria in quality assessment;
- discusses the incorporation of practice policies in decision support technology (DST) to assure prospectively the quality of health care.

The development of valid practice policies or criteria requires substantial effort. Further, once developed they must be reviewed periodically (if not continuously) and, if warranted, updated to maintain their currency and hence utility. This manual introduces and explains concepts. Detailed discussion of how to formulate practice policies or criteria and update them is beyond its scope. Similarly, how to incorporate practice policies in decision support technologies is also beyond this manual's scope. In the long run, as knowledge explodes and interventions become more numerous and powerful, DSTs may offer the best hope for operationalising practice policies and hence building quality into health care's product.

272 | Key concepts

This chapter elaborates on the following key concepts essential to understanding how health care's products can be defined for quality management purposes in practice policies (and criteria):

- Manufacturers design products that satisfy customers. Product (manufacturing) specifications flow from these designs which take into account manufacturability. Manufacturers produce products to specifications with as little variance in processes (and hence products) as practical.
- Product (and process) specifications are limited by technology.
- Patients' health status would be improved maximally if existing technology were used appropriately and implemented properly. The health benefits to be derived from delivering existing treatment to specifications may be far greater than those that could be expected from the introduction of new treatments under development or that could be developed plausibly in the near future.
- In health care (unlike manufacturing), process specifications define the product because in practice it is impractical to routinely measure patients' health status improvement and virtually impossible to attribute reliably any measured improvement to specific interventions.
- Health care's product is defined by practice specifications, which may take the form of practice policies (sometimes referred to as guidelines or parameters) or practice criteria (sometimes referred to as criteria and standards).
- Practice policies are the basis for practice, providing direct guidance or instructions to providers about how patients should be managed, including who should manage them and where they should be managed.
- Practice criteria are the basis for quality assessment, guidance or instructions to quality assurance personnel, including medical record reviewers, about judging how patients should have been managed, and which provide indirect guidance or instruction to providers about how patients should be managed.
- Practice policies represent the best way to manage individual patients. They must take into account patients' preferences and may encompass sociopolitical constraints.
- Synthesising knowledge to determine best practice (which involves only technical issues) must be distinguished clearly from formulating policies (what should be done in specific circumstances, which is influenced by non-technical issues, e.g. an intervention's cost-benefit).
- If available, which usually they are not, fully-elaborated practice policies can be translated easily into practice criteria to assess retrospectively the quality of care.
- Practice criteria state how particular cases should be treated and care documented; specifically, for purposes of screening medical records for potential quality of care problems. When used directly to review medical records, practice criteria serve as an aide-memoire to guide the review.
- For screening purposes, criteria must be clear and unambiguous. Their utility is proportional to their complexity: the more that criteria parallel the complexity of medical practice, the greater their utility. If criteria are met, care is presumed appropriate and, if not, reviewed further. Cases may fail screens: if specified, needed process elements were not applied; if specified, inappropriate processes were applied; and if process or patient outcomes

suggest that a needed or inappropriate process was implemented improperly or an inappropriate process was applied.

- Developing practice policies and criteria requires specific expertise and is expensive. Their widespread use, however, may save many times their development and revision costs as well as improve health outcomes.
- Because of the complexity inherent in useful practice policies and criteria, they must be computerised and embodied in expert systems, a type of decision support technology (DST).
- Expert systems are already available to screen cases for potential quality of care problems and in the next thirty years we can expect to see greater use of DSTs in all phases of medical practice.
- Continuous quality improvement results from greater and greater conformance to specifications (practice policies), but must rest ultimately on improving practice policies, which in turn depend on better information about best practice and better technology.

273 | Industrial analogies

Successful manufacturers produce high quality products, those that meet product specifications (fall within pre-established limits with as little variation as practical on all parameters), that meet customers' needs, and that customers perceive represent best value for money when compared to similar products produced by other manufacturers and to other, different products that compete to satisfy customers' needs. Both manufacturers' capabilities and customers' needs change dynamically. Stimulated by competition, manufacturers must strive constantly to improve their products' specifications to ensure they continue to meet customers' needs—or, better yet, delight customers—to improve conformance to specifications and to lower manufacturing costs. The interplay between product specifications and manufacturability is an important determinant of a product's quality. An appealing design that cannot be manufactured reliably may not be as pleasing to customers as an acceptable design that works as specified for many years without breaking down.

Given products of equal manufacturability, design is determinant. Automobiles replaced the horse and carriage because of their superior specifications, not because they were produced more exactly to specifications (although they may have been as well). Manufacturers use various techniques to determine customers' present and perceived future needs—for example, focus groups to find out consumers' preferences and test marketing of prototypes to find out their reactions to proposed products; customers' suggestions; sales persons' perceptions; sales information; and social trends. Most product innovations originate with customers. But customers do not produce products. Hence success goes to producers who listen to customers and strive to improve their products' quality. Successful manufacturers innovate: they anticipate or generate customers' needs and produce products that customers cannot conceive of or did not know could be produced until the manufacturer shows them. Successful development and introduction of new products demands a careful interplay between manufacturers' visions and capabilities and customers' latent or actual needs and willingness to pay to satisfy them.

As part of finalising a product's design, the manufacturer produces detailed specifications for all materials, parts and processes necessary to manufacture it. Once these specifications have been finalised, emphasis shifts to quality control to ensure that the product is produced within specifications with as little variation in materials, parts and processes, and hence product, as practical, and at the lowest practical cost.

With manufactured goods, customers and manufacturers can usually readily appreciate the extent to which the product meets the most important quality characteristics. If a manufacturer finds a product does not meet specifications, the manufacturing process is obviously at fault. With services, the product—for example massage—is often inseparable from the producer—the masseur. Excellent interpersonal aspects can more than make up for any slight imperfections in technique, if indeed they can be defined or appreciated reliably by anyone.

Health care is one service in which technical considerations, the extent to which it improves patients' health status, are of overriding importance. While it is possible to measure health status and, through health systems' research, the extent to which improvement is attributable to specific health care intervention, in routine practice it is difficult to measure health status improvement and virtually impossible to attribute reliably any measured improvement to specific interventions. Customers' (patients') and producers' (providers') inability to assess product quality directly reinforces the importance of specifying production processes and ensuring conformance to them. In health care, for all practical quality management purposes, process specifications define the product. These specifications are the basis for health care quality assurance and quality improvement.

274 | Practice specifications: from guidelines to policies

274.1 | Historical context

Efforts to codify medical knowledge are virtually as old as the practice of medicine. Some of the most ancient writings—Mesopotamian clay tablets and Egyptian papyri—are treatises on how to treat different diseases. These early writings are most likely the works of individual authors drawing on the conventional wisdom of their day. The idea of systematically reviewing medical writings to discern best practices existed even in ancient times. Soranus of Ehesus, a Roman physician of the second century AD, epitomised a school of thought known as the methodisers. His influence dominated the practice of medicine during the early Middles Ages.

> No matter what trend (previous physicians) had represented, he studied their writings to learn from their experience. . . . (He) made extensive use of the medical knowledge handed down from the past . . . and was scrupulous in giving chapter and verse for whatever he quoted. . . . His writings are clear, simple, and impressive, being devoid of superfluous rhetoric. Soranus wrote a number of books intended to guide practice . . . (including his famous) textbook on midwifery and gynaecology . . . (that was) illustrated . . . (and included) diagrams of the uterus and the various positions of the child.[1]

The advent of practical printing with movable type, in the fifteenth century, facilitated the widespread dissemination of information including medical writings. Even today medical textbooks represent the principal distillations of medical knowledge and prescriptions for recognising and treating different diseases. They still represent the opinions of individual practitioners who have little time (even if they have the inclination and skill needed) to review systematically the world's medical literature, and whose experience is inevitably limited.

Since 1977 the Office of Medical Applications of Research of the US National Institutes of Health (in Bethesda, Maryland) has been publishing consensus development statements. This program has been a model for many practice guidelines formulation efforts, even though its assessments pertain primarily to new technologies rather than accepted clinical practices.[2] This approach has also been adopted in other countries.[3] In 1977 the US Public Health Service funded a project to demonstrate a method 'to elicit, validate, and summarise the most authoritative data and information on a health problem'.

The result was three 'state-of-the-science' reports.[4] In 1988 the American Medical Association established its Office of Quality Assurance.

Medical professional organisations have been developing practice guidelines or issuing assessments of medical practices on and off for well over fifty years. In the United States, the number of organisations involved in developing practice guidelines or conducting medical technology assessments, and the number of resultant products, has exploded in the last ten years. Prior to 1980 eight medical professional organisations were developing practice guidelines according to a 1991 report of the American Medical Association; that year, fifty of them reported such activity.[5] This report lists over 1300 practice guidelines. In 1989 the US Congress established the Agency for Health Care Policy and Research as part of the US Public Health Service, on the same level as the National Institutes of Health. One of the Agency's mandates is to develop practice guidelines. Many other players have entered the field, including health insurers, hospitals, managed care plans and their trade associations. Hospitals' interest in practice guidelines or policies is relatively new. It began to emerge in the 1990s, well after hospitals had begun to embrace the idea of continuous quality improvement, beginning in the mid 1980s.

Several important characteristics differentiate the best of today's from earlier guidelines' development efforts. They include: a concern for the proper process to formulate practice guidelines, including who should formulate them; an attempt to assess formally and systematically the scientific evidence and practice experience for and against specific medical interventions; and an interest in encouraging the use of resultant guidelines in practice.

274.2 Present guidelines' formulation efforts

Today the medical profession, payers of care and others are paying increased attention to how patients are and should be treated. This interest stems from a desire to improve the quality of care and to contain its cost. Thus, at least in the United States, the principal factors propelling the development of practice guidelines are rising health care costs and the belief that billions of dollars are wasted on inappropriate interventions and that practice guidelines can eliminate this waste and hence stem the rise in costs.[6,7,8] Expectations have risen so high that practice policies are in danger of being seen as a panacea for solving all of the health care system's problems. Whether or not quality management generally or practice guidelines specifically can save money is an open question. They certainly harbour the potential to improve the quality of care, if developed appropriately and used properly in practice.

Pluralism best characterises the variety of efforts that the renewed interest in practice guidelines has spawned. These efforts vary in their purpose, scope, methods and the quality of resultant guidelines. There is little consensus on what the term practice guidelines encompasses, what constitutes a set of valid guidelines or what is a valid approach to producing them. Essentially, all guidelines formulation efforts involve the synthesis of information from the literature or from experts, or a combination of both sources, often involving iteration. The extent of such procedures and the rigour with which they are carried out varies tremendously. Most guidelines produced to date are generally inadequate.[9]

Most practice guidelines that medical professional societies and others had developed to date are the products of less than rigorous assessment of the scientific literature and of limited professional input. For the most part, they are still too general, fail to state expected outcomes, do not take patients' preferences into account explicitly, and avoid social issues inherent in cost-effectiveness and cost-benefit considerations. However, the Herculean task of practice guidelines formulation must start somewhere. The pursuit of perfection often precludes performing the possible. Ultimately, however, to be used, practice guidelines must be useful and address all of these points.

In Australia government and some professional colleges are beginning to recognise the need for, or importance of, practice policies (guidelines). In some hospitals, circumstances have pressured medical staff to lay down rules concerning who should conduct certain procedures and, to a very limited extent, how doctors should manage some conditions. Most hospital medical practitioners would think of themselves as practising scientific medicine, yet the concept of practice policies has barely filtered through to consciousness.

The inadequacy of present guidelines' formulation efforts is more than offset by the enthusiasm for guidelines, or at least the hope that they can solve some, if not all, of the health care system's problems. For the time being at least, this enthusiasm has given much needed credibility to the idea that practice guidelines should be formulated. Apart from lack of attention to quality management principles, present efforts suffer from limited resources exacerbated by difficulties in setting priorities.

Inevitable resource limitations have prompted the view that the government should formulate practice guidelines to avoid duplication of effort.[10] While a limitless number of inadequate efforts can lead to nothing useful, the idea of a single purveyor of the truth raises more troubling questions than it answers, especially given the dismal state of medical knowledge. Given the uncertainty of how best to treat patients, competition among adequately funded efforts, which inherently involves duplication of effort and may seem wasteful in the short run, is likely to be most efficient in the long run.[11]

Clinical practice guidelines are useful only if they are used in practice and are valid. Once formulated, guidelines must be updated, that is, reviewed at least annually and, if necessary, revised, to remain relevant to clinical practice. The cost of formulating and updating guidelines is considerable, especially if they are to be acceptable to intended users, as they must be if they are to be used (and therefore useful), to achieve their intended purpose of improving clinical practice.

To be accepted, intended users must accept the methods used to formulate and update guidelines and the guidelines developed using these methods. To ensure acceptance, intended users (or at least their legitimate representatives) must be able to review and comment on methods and guidelines. Such review and comment procedures incur considerable cost, beyond that needed to develop the guidelines' formulation process and formulate and update guidelines. In the ultimate analysis, guidelines' formulation is a political process and the validity of resultant guidelines depends on the acceptability of the process used to develop them. The essential characteristics of valid guidelines and hence processes to produce them, and of methods to validate and improve guidelines, are subjects beyond this manual's scope.

274.3 Cost of present efforts

The estimated costs of developing practice guidelines varies from a low of US$5000 to a high of over US$1 000 000 per formulated guideline. Three principal factors account for this extraordinary variation in costs: scope (what is attempted); methods (how it is undertaken); and what costs are (and are not) counted. Most organisations that formulate guidelines do not account fully for the cost of their production. Most organisations count only out-of-pocket expenses, for example contracted costs, consultants' fees, travel, mailing. Costs for program staff are often not included in estimates. Experts who formulate guidelines are mostly volunteers, usually members of the organisation formulating them; the value of the time they spend on the effort is not reflected in cost estimates.

The RAND Corporation (Santa Monica, California) is said to spend an average of US$750 000 per guideline, with a range between US$500 000 and US$1 000 000. The

AHCPR estimates the average cost of producing a guideline to be US$500 000; others have put its costs as high as US$800 000. The American College of Physicians (a professional association of internists in Philadelphia, Pennsylvania) which runs the Clinical Efficacy Assessment Project (CEAP) estimates the cost of an assessment (i.e. guideline) to be US$50 000. According to a US General Accounting Office survey of medical speciality societies, their guidelines cost between US$5000 and US$130 000 to formulate.[12] By building on others' guidelines, for example those that AHCPR has already developed, the Healthcare Education & Research Foundation (Minneapolis, Minnesota) estimates that it costs US$40 000 to develop one of its guidelines. The Foundation's biggest cost is mailing guidelines to physicians for feedback; the experts who formulate the guidelines are volunteers. To date, most guideline formulation efforts have been voluntary and, as RAND's Robert Brook has said, 'you get what you pay for'.[13]

We estimate the cost of developing and updating practice guidelines for the 100 most important health problems to be about US$40–60 million per year, if their development were divided among a few organisations devoted to this purpose. The cost of 3000 practice guidelines, about all that would be cost-effective, is about US$600–700 million per year, given proven methods and economies of scale. This sum, while not insignificant, represents only a small fraction of US health care expenditures. It would take less than a one-tenth of a per cent improvement in resource use to recoup this entire investment, not to mention the economic value and other benefits of the resultant health status improvement.

Given the increasing globalisation of medical practice, there is no reason to suppose that any one country must meet the entire burden of formulating practice guidelines for all of medicine. Clearly, an effort this large may be beyond the resources of a low-population country such as Australia. However, there is no reason that Australia could not become the world's leader in formulating practice guidelines for the rational treatment of a small number of disease categories such as heart disease and breast cancer, for example. In reality, we are still a long way from realising this vision of international competition and co-operation in the quest for quality improvement. In 1993 the National Health and Medical Research Council (NHMRC) initiated the first attempt in Australia to develop a national practice policy (guidelines). The expert committee is charged with the task of developing a national policy for the diagnosis and treatment of breast cancer. Compared with the United States, very much smaller resources will be available for this effort.

274.4 Some relevant terms

The plethora of practice guidelines' formulation efforts has spawned new terminology which has yet to be defined precisely. Indeed, there is no agreement on the term practice guideline. To some it is an encompassing term; to others, a narrow one. This section defines and differentiates among relevant terms for quality management purposes. Necessarily, this discussion is limited to the most common terms and their most common usages.

- *Practice specifications*—encompasses generally all of the following terms and others with similar meanings that are intended or used to aid clinical or administrative decision-making related to health care practice, including certification of practitioners, insurance coverage and indemnification, and quality assurance. Practice specifications are explicit statements about the processes that providers should follow for individual patients. For quality management purposes they can be divided into practice policies for use in preproduction and intraproduction quality assurance, and practice criteria for use in postproduction quality assurance.

- *Practice protocols*—are research tools to ensure that only patients meeting certain diagnostic criteria are included in studies, that these patients receive the treatments being tested appropriate to their diagnostic classification, and that these treatments are implemented in the prescribed manner. They are beyond this manual's scope.
- *Practice policies*—are the basis for practice, direct guidance or instructions to providers about how patients should be managed, including who should manage them and where they should be managed, and what to expect consequently. In its widest context the term also encompasses procedural (process) policies (sometimes referred to as clinical protocols).
- *Practice criteria and standards (practice criteria)*—are the basis for quality assurance, guidance or instructions to quality assurance personnel about judging how patients should have been managed, which provide indirect guidance or instruction to providers about how patients should be managed. They can be derived from practice policies, if existent, or, if not, must be formulated de novo.

In the United States, the term (clinical) practice guidelines is used in much the same way as we use practice specifications. The American Medical Association prefers the term practice parameters. We prefer the term practice specifications to reinforce the notion that we are talking about what should be or should have been done in a certain set of circumstances, rather than statements of principles to determine a course of action, which is implied by a guideline, for example. Professional societies may issue practice guidelines; providers follow practice policies for quality management purposes. When a hospital, for example, adopts or adapts someone's guidelines for treating given types of patients, they become its practice policies—statements about how its patients should be treated and who should treat them.

We use the term policy in health care with the same sense that it is used in business. Business policy encompasses the business' objectives and policies. The term health care policy encompasses the objectives and policies of the entire health care system, that of a region, an ownership grouping or another entity to which it applies; medical policy, the objectives and policies of medicine; hospital policy, the objectives and policy of the hospital. Objectives describe what is to be accomplished; policies, how objectives are to be accomplished. Policy statements describe an organisation's objectives and policies. Policies embody a principle, plan or course of action. They provide standing answers to questions that are raised during the course of conducting business (or practising medicine). Because the singular term, policy, is sometimes confused with the word's broader use—health care policy, for example—in this manual we use the plural term practice policies and avoid its singular.

274.5 *About practice policies*

Practice policies state who should do what and how, and when and where it should be done. Fully elaborated practice policies must take into account patients' preferences and society's resources. To be most useful, valid practice policies relevant to the patient must be readily accessible at the time the doctor is seeing the patient, for example. Computerised decision support technology (DST) is needed ultimately to achieve this end and is now beginning to emerge. Once fully developed, DSTs will make possible inprocess quality control, and result in an order of magnitude improvement in quality and reduction in cost.[14] Nevertheless, formulation and use of even such rudimentary practice policies as deciding who can treat certain cases, through credentialling for example, can improve quality and reduce risk. Figure II-7-1 on page 317 shows the relationship of practice policies (and practice criteria) to production.

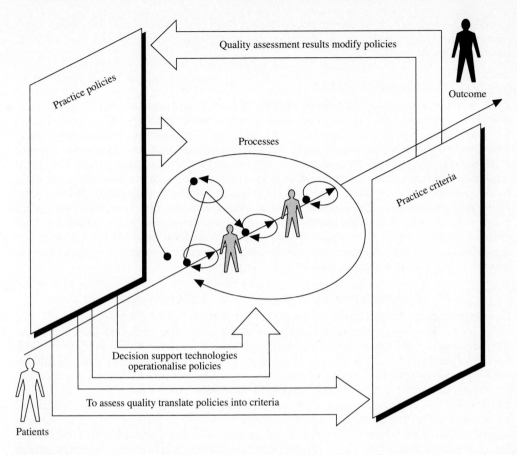

Figure II-7-1 *The nature of and relationships between practice policies and practice criteria*

Practice policies pertain to individual patients, or at least narrowly drawn types of patient (e.g. white women with stage II previously untreated breast cancer, aged thirty-five to fifty-five years). Patient types are delineated by factors that affect outcome (health status improvement), for example health problem, disease stage, age. In these regards, practice policies are closer to treatment protocols than the general advice offered in textbooks or treatment guidelines. Practice policies are more than treatment protocols because they take into account patients' preferences and society's resources. Practice policies are more than practice guidelines because they state how patients should be treated and who should treat them rather than espousing principles. Moreover, practice policies state explicitly expected outcomes, thereby informing patients and permitting them to choose among alternatives, as well as permitting comparison with observed outcomes for quality management purposes.

Given the present state-of-the-art, practice policies cannot take into account every contingency that could be encountered in practice. Doctors and other health professionals must exercise considerable judgment both in applying practice policies and treating patients whose circumstances are beyond those described in practice policies. Nevertheless, for the circumstances that they encompass, practice policies serve the critical function of defining heath care's product: those interventions (processes) believed to maximise patients' health status improvement (outcome). Use of and experience with practice criteria for quality assessment purposes is often the starting point for establishing practice policies.

274.6 About practice criteria

Practice criteria are used to assess quality of care retrospectively. They should be consistent with, and can be derived easily from, practice policies, if existent. If not, practice criteria must be developed de novo. Practice criteria are much easier to develop than practice policies because they are used to assess care that has been rendered and consequently they need to encompass fewer considerations. Since care has been rendered, practice criteria need check only on the soundness of a clinician's judgments, while practice policies must help the clinician make those judgments. While fully-elaborated practice policies should state what outcomes to expect, historically statements about outcomes (which might signify malprocess) are associated more commonly with practice criteria, which must not only assess what was done but also how well it was done. Today, practice criteria are usually limited to the clinical aspects of care and rarely involve costs or cost-benefit considerations, for example.

274.7 Use of practice policies and criteria in quality management

Meaningful quality management requires practice policies or at least practice criteria. For all practical purposes, quality assurance is conformance to practice policies, those interventions that are known or believed to maximise patients' health status improvement. Reducing variation between what is done (documented processes) and what should be done (processes specified in practice policies or criteria) improves quality. Quality can be improved further by comparing expected outcomes (stated in practice policies) to those achieved in practice. Such comparisons can help to determine if any observed variation results from failure to implement policies, a failure in their proper implementation, or failure of properly implemented policies to produce expected results. Standardisation of practices, in accepted practice policies, simplifies the interpretation of variation in outcomes because proper implementation of practice policies eliminates one of the greatest sources of variation in outcomes: variation in care processes. Comparisons of outcomes achieved at hospitals with different practice policies may shed light on their validity.

If observed outcomes fall short of expectations, clinicians can review their care to check whether or not they are following practice policies and, if so, implementing them properly. If practice policies are being implemented properly, expected outcomes can be revised downwards to reflect reality. If observed outcomes exceed expectations, expected outcomes stated in practice policies can also be revised upwards to reflect this reality. Expected outcomes stated in practice policies inform patients' choices among alternative interventions. Further, they indicate what can be expected realistically from medical care. This information is useful for prioritising research to improve practice policies, and hence quality, thereby realising greater patient health status improvement.

Practice criteria are the starting point for assessing quality of care and hence its improvement. Explicit criteria are useful for the structured review of medical records intended to identify quality of care problems. They are essential to the development of manual or automated screens to identify cases with potential quality of care problems that expert clinicians can then confirm or deny. Use of practice criteria is facilitated if practitioners who are to be subjected to review agree on the criteria before the review begins. In these regards, practice criteria are prototypical practice policies.

As hospitals progress along the road to quality maturity they must decide who can treat what cases within the hospital (credentialling), assess the quality of their care (practice criteria for structured quality review), put in place practice policies that state how patients are to be treated to maximise health status improvement within patients' preferences and society's resources and what they can expect consequentially (practice policies), measure long-term outcomes to improve practice policies (structured outcomes measurement), and, eventually, conduct research to improve medical technology and health care processes (health systems research).

275   Need for practice policies

275.1   Perspective on practice policies

Properly formulated practice policies can improve the quality of care by improving patients' outcomes, reducing the costs of care and promoting patient satisfaction. Practice policies, and by extension practice criteria, often evoke ambivalent feelings in medical practitioners. On the one hand they represent the best distillation of knowledge and experience to guide (or assess) practice, the epitome of scientific medicine. On the other hand they present constraints on what practitioners may do in what they perceive to be the patient's best interest without raising questions about the so-called 'art' of medicine. This tension that springs from the inseparable interplay between the reality of knowledge and the self-expression inherent in art is as old as civilisation and extends to all facets of life. In medicine, it may be the patient's life which is at stake. This section looks at the fundamental problem that practice policies intend to solve, their essential use in quality management and some of the advantages of their use, including practising scientific medicine, facilitating improvement, spurring innovation and limiting risk.

275.2   Nature of the problem

Decisions must be made in practice whether or not solid information exists. The principal reason to develop practice policies is the need to make the best information available to practitioners to help them make decisions in practice to improve patient management and hence the quality of care. Practitioners face tremendous uncertainty, made worse by the increasingly rapid introduction of technology, expanding volume of published research reports (often with contradictory results) and by rising demands for them to be held accountable for their decisions, manifest by rising malpractice suits for example.

Doctors may be uncertain about which diagnostic interventions to use, the order in which to use them, or how to interpret the resultant information. Nevertheless, they must diagnose the patient's health problem in order to treat it. Doctors may be uncertain about the patient's treatment goals or which treatment would best accomplish them. If complications occur, doctors may be uncertain as to why they occurred or how best to manage them. Patients are unique individuals. Interventions must be matched to patients. Under these circumstances, improving medical practice would seem to be a problem that defies comprehension, let alone solution.

Traditionally, doctors have learned how to treat patients through education, which has become longer and more rigorous; continuing medical education, which has become more formal; and practice experience, which may be subject to misinterpretation. It is one thing to learn something at one point in time and quite another to apply it correctly in practice at another. At the moment one may forget, or misremember, or misjudge the circumstance. Practice is increasingly difficult because of patients' heightened expectations, the explosion of medical information, the bewildering array of interventions and the complexity of the health system. Paradoxically, concerns about the quality of care have increased as resource consumption has grown. Rising costs and increasing complexity have driven these concerns.

Today for the most part practitioners are still dependent on essentially fifteenth century technology—the printed word—for medical practice information. While the contents of textbooks have improved over the years, each still represents a few individuals' distillation of their understanding of research results and their inherently limited experience. Textbooks offer general advice but are not very helpful in selecting among interventions for individual patients' circumstances. They are often out of date, left behind by advances in practice published in medical journals, or those yet to be published but announced on television or in the daily press. Moreover, none of the information stored in textbooks is readily accessible in real-time, when the doctor is treating the patient.

The contents of medical journals have become more erudite and scientific, although their utility to medical practitioners still leaves much to be desired. Facts, generated by medical technology assessment for example, must be translated into information for use by health care practitioners and quality assurance personnel. Today this translation is often done by the practitioner who, for example, reads about a new surgical operation and then tries it out. If the operation's originator merely suggests its adoption one would be concerned about use of an unproven treatment. If the research report claims the operation's superiority over existing treatments, one would be concerned about the practitioner's ability to assess their validity. If the practitioner simply tried the operation, depending on its complexity and his or her preparedness, one would be concerned about his or her competence.

Increasingly, professionals and others are calling for explicit consideration of evidence for interventions' effectiveness, the formulation of recommendations for their use in practice based on such evidence, and the dissemination to practitioners of resultant recommendations with encouragement to adopt them. For the twenty-first century, practice policies must represent the structured synthesis of the best available evidence from research and practice, and must be disseminated through computerised decision support technology. The results of such efforts define health care's product for quality management purposes.

275.3 | Managing health care quality

Health care's product is seemingly amorphous and intangible and, if defined in terms of health status improvement, apparently unchanging. Health care's principal product may be defined as maximal improvement in patients' health status using interventions consistent with their preferences and society's resources, at least cost and with greatest patient satisfaction. For simplicity, this section focuses only on the technical aspects of care, health status improvement, and the resources necessary for its achievement. The same principles apply to all dimensions of quality, including trade-offs among health status improvement, costs and patient satisfaction.

Maximal health status improvement is achieved if a practitioner classifies (diagnoses) the patient's health problem correctly as quickly as possible, if he or she selects the best (most effective) treatment for the patient's problem that is consistent with the patient's preferences, and if he or she implements it properly, without delay. Resource constraints may limit such achievement. Given any set of patient symptoms and signs, one can envision the most cost-effective strategy to diagnose and treat the patient's health problem, that is, the strategy that will yield the maximal health status improvement at the least cost (within established constraints) and with the greatest degree of patient satisfaction. The requisite diagnostic and therapeutic interventions and their proper implementation specify the processes that represent the highest quality health care. The greatest problem we face today is not knowing scientifically which processes would produce this desired product, nor much about the cost-effectiveness of most health care interventions—points that other chapters in this part cover in detail.

Practice specifications represent the cornerstone of clinical quality management. Because of the difficulty of measuring health status in individual patients and the near impossibility of attributing changes to interventions, case by case, health care quality can be judged and assured only in relation to process. Ironically, for all practical quality assurance purposes an emphasis on outcome—health status improvement—boils down to conformance to processes believed necessary for its production. Further, improving the quality of care (more health status at lower cost and with greater patient satisfaction) requires improving care processes. Normally one can change process, measure outcome, and assume plausibly the linkage between cause (process change) and effect (outcome change). In this respect, medicine faces three seemingly insurmountable obstacles that make some people despair of ever improving the practice of medicine, despite human-kind's best intentions.

- Process (how doctors treat patients) exhibits great variation, the magnitude of which is usually unknown. Variation in process is likely to produce variation in outcome that may exacerbate or dampen variation from other coproducers of outcome, unless the process is largely ineffective, that is, unable to influence outcome (in which case only variation caused by other coproducers will be evident).
- Measuring outcome in terms of health status improvement is difficult and expensive and virtually never done routinely.
- It is virtually impossible in ordinary practice to attribute unequivocally any observed outcome to process, or change in outcomes to change in processes. For various reasons it is even difficult to achieve such attribution in research studies, and they usually involve so few variables that even if done well they inform practice only to a limited extent.

Health care can be improved systematically and cost-effectively if its products are defined directly and pragmatically, namely:

- focus clearly on the desired principal outcome—patient health status improvement;
- specify (based on the best available knowledge and experience) in practice specifications the process (for each type of patient) that is believed to produce the desired outcome (maximal health status improvement) and expected immediate outcomes (to facilitate quality assurance);
- assure that specified processes are implemented properly (e.g. structured quality review);
- collect data about long-term outcomes in relation to process (e.g. structured outcome measurement) and conduct health systems research to improve practice specifications.

Practically, quality assurance can be conceived of as assuring that specified processes (and no others) are implemented properly (not botched). Surveillance of immediate outcomes, for example nosocomial infection, is essential to alert one to the actual or possible existence of malprocess, that is, deviations from specifications (which if reduced would improve outcomes). Clearly, quality assurance can only improve desired outcomes by ensuring conformance to specifications. But reduction in process variation may result in both immense improvement and reduction of variation in desired outcome, reducing uncertainty for the patient. Further quality improvement requires better specifications— those that produce more health status improvement, and/or that cost less, and/or result in greater patient satisfaction. When co-ordinated, structured quality review, structured outcome measurement and health systems research can produce better practice policies and a vast and continuous improvement in the quality of care. Quality management is synonymous with formulating product specifications, measuring and improving conformance to these specifications, and establishing mechanisms to improve specifications. This chapter focuses on product specifications. Chapter 8 describes mechanisms to assure conformance to specifications and mechanisms to improve them.

275.4 Practising scientific medicine

Practice criteria are essential to measure and hence improve quality of care, a seemingly obvious point that one cannot overemphasise. They are used in the retrospective assessment of quality of care. To define products and hence to assure quality prospectively, one must formulate practice policies. To doctors, practice policies smack of 'cookbook' medicine, the slavish following of recipes to manage patients' problems with minimal, if any, need to think. The current state of medical knowledge does not allow the degree of specificity needed to write this type of recipe, even if desired. This situation is not likely to change in the near future. Even if detailed specifications did exist and were embodied and used routinely in decision support technology, doctors would continue to play a vital and pivotal, albeit somewhat altered, role in patient care.

Practice policies represent the epitome of scientific medicine: experts' carefully considered opinions of how patients with certain signs, symptoms and signals should be managed on the basis of evidence gathered from research studies and systematic evaluation of experience. Research studies are concerned, for example, with interventions' effectiveness for patients of the type and with the disease being studied. They can be designed to examine the effect of variations in patients' characteristics or practitioners' skills for example, on interventions' effectiveness or such knowledge may emerge from results of analyses (but possess lesser certainty of validity). Ideally, as a result patients can be classified according to factors affecting outcomes, including best practices to achieve them. Consequently, for a given class of patients who chose best practices, variation in outcomes would be expected to be small. Any residual variation in outcomes might be due to unknown factors that affect them, the adequacy of implementation of specified interventions, or chance variation.

A clinician following the results of such valid research, embodied in practice policies, is practising scientific medicine. The clinician who prescribes a dose of medication that varies from what research indicates is optimal is venturing into terra incognita. Here the art of medicine is transformed into an art form with patient as canvas. By definition, there is nothing to say that the prescribed dose would not produce better health outcomes for the patient than the dose that research indicates is optimal. Statistically, however, the chance of such a beneficial result would be vanishingly small. The fact that it might be observed in a single case would only serve to obfuscate the fact that in 1000 other cases the outcome would be less than optimal.

If a doctor believes his or her treatment is truly superior, he or she should submit it to a properly designed clinical trial. Given the choice, patients may be more inclined to go for the experts' recommendation than the lone practitioner's hunch. Admittedly, a patient in dire straits, with an incurable disease may gravitate to any practitioner holding out the hope of a cure. Such cures, however, would be best submitted to scientific test lest they engender false hopes. The placebo effect is powerful but it is no substitute for scientific medicine, especially in an age when the magic has passed from the medicine man to the medical machine.

Some doctors may argue correctly that valid research results exist to substantiate only a fraction of the decisions they must make in practice every day, and that their decisions are likely as good, if not better than, anyone else's (or any other doctor's at least). This latter justification is likely only to be true at the margin of circumstances not considered by practice policies. Even if research results are lacking, in the long run the considered opinions of experts using whatever research information is available are likely to outperform the choices of individual clinicians. Waiting for researchers to demonstrate unequivocally that practice policies make sense is an unwise delaying tactic. If practitioners insisted that they use only scientifically-proven interventions, they would have little to do. Logic alone supports, and rising costs may force, practice policies' use. Where fully-elaborated practice policies are silent, insufficient information exists to recommend a course of action. In this case, structured outcomes measurement can monitor patients' long-term outcomes to determine if some do better than others and, if so, what patient characteristics or care processes might be responsible for these observed differences in outcomes. If need be, these findings could be confirmed through appropriate research studies.

275.5 │ *Facilitating improvement*

Practice policies (criteria) are essential to assess, and hence improve, health care. Moreover, the uniformity in process that accepted policies promote facilitates the interpretation of outcomes. Stated simply, observed variation in outcomes cannot arise from variation in process (because it is uniform). Thus, given proper implementation of practice policies, variation in outcomes stems either from coproducers (patient or environmental variables) or is inherent in the process, in which case it must be changed to reduce variation in outcomes and thus improve quality. Structured outcome measurement and, to a lesser extent, structured quality improvement can monitor effects on patient outcomes, costs etc., of changes to practice policies. (See Chapter 8 in this part.)

275.6 │ *Spurring innovation*

Medicine has made great advances in the last fifty years, although, as pointed out elsewhere, perhaps on reflection these advances have not provided as much improvement in patients' health status as might have been expected. Critics of practice policies suggest that they would stifle innovation and increase costs. They might cite the increasing time and cost it takes to bring drugs to market as a case in point. Without commenting on the efficiency of the pharmaceutical industry, it is possible to respond to this vacuous criticism. Certainly patients should receive the benefits of useful innovations as soon as possible. However, patients, and society, which foots all or most of the bill, must protect itself as well as patients from the introduction of useless or harmful diagnostic and therapeutic innovations. The balance in benefits and risks is dynamic and, ultimately, is a social decision. Assessing an intervention's effectiveness is difficult, and enthusiastic practitioners who believe they have found a better way can be easily misled by their uncritical interpretation of inadequate assessments.

Some practitioners fear that practice policies will become rigid and once formulated hard to change. Certainly this risk exists. However, it can be minimised by establishing at the outset the mechanisms necessary to review periodically and, if necessary, to revise practice policies. While conceding this possibility critics suggest the mechanisms might be slow and cumbersome. But there is no reason to believe that they must inevitably be so. Finally, they suggest that the rules of evidence might be too strict so that change is slowed to status quo. These rules must be established as part of the policy formulating mechanism. The evidence for the superior effectiveness of new treatments must be at least as good as that for the effectiveness of existing treatments. Given the costs of change, and those of being wrong, one could argue that the superiority of innovations must be demonstrated convincingly before they are put into widespread use.

Practice policies could spur genuinely useful innovation in a number of ways. Firstly, their formulation would draw attention to the inadequacy of existing scientific knowledge and to the need for more and better research. Secondly, they would give impetus to the search for sorely needed cost-reducing technologies. Thirdly, they would encourage practitioners to test innovations. Tremendous controversy surrounds medical interventions and their introduction into practice. Practice policies provide a framework for dividing accepted from investigational interventions. Different rules apply appropriately to investigational interventions, for example, for research protocols, informed consent. The use in widespread practice of unproven or inadequately assessed technologies and techniques likely harms more patients than it helps and certainly drives the cost of care ever higher. Appropriate mechanisms to formulate, review and revise practice policies can avoid some of these pitfalls and spur useful innovation.

275.7 | Limiting risk

Medical practice is dominated by uncertainty. Things can and sometimes do go wrong. Increasingly there is a tendency to think that if the outcome is faulty, someone must have been at fault. The result is defensive medicine, for example doing tests not genuinely indicated but the absence of which might lead to one being faulted in a court of law. The existence of well-accepted practice policies holds out the hope at least that courts will eventually make it much harder for plaintiffs to win cases where practice policies were followed demonstrably and indicated interventions were implemented properly, and hence reduce the number of suits. In the absence of specific legislation, there is no guarantee that the courts will find this way, of course. Most importantly, such legal acceptance of practice policies would permit them to state, and the practitioner to use, only interventions presumably considered necessary in the circumstances saving, in the United States at least, 10–15% of the nation's health care costs and improving the quality of care.

Paradoxically, the number of malpractice suits may rise initially because patients who suffer a perceptible maloutcome, and more to the point their lawyers, will have a handy frame of reference with which to judge the doctor's performance. Such suits, especially if successful, would reinforce doctors' adherence to practice policies. Adherence to practice policies reduces variation in outcomes and makes risks more known. For this reason alone, insurance companies offering medical professional liability insurance may want to foster their adoption and offer reduced premiums as an incentive. Again, were this idea to be adopted, adherence to practice policies could be expected to increase markedly. Incentives and other pressures to adopt and adhere to practice policies make it all the more important that the policies be scientifically valid and acceptable to doctors, to patients and to society.

276 | Practice policies

276.1 | Introduction to practice policies

Practice policies are explicit statements intended to give providers direct guidance or instructions on how to diagnose, treat and otherwise manage patients, and what to expect consequently. They may vary from simple statements about what doctors can do in the hospital—which support credentialling decisions and determine, for example, whether general practitioners, internists or cardiologists may treat patients with myocardial infarction—to those that result from sophisticated synthesis of knowledge and experience and are intended to guide every facet of patient management.

Policies may be classified in a number of ways. In the hospital, for example, policies may be divided into facility policies and practice policies. Facility policies describe how the hospital is to be organised, staffed and run. Hospital facility policy may specify, for example, that a minimum of three nurses be on duty in each ward at all times, or that deliveries will be accepted only between 8.00 am and 11.00 am, or that practice policies will be used by the hospital's visiting medical staff. Practice policies describe how doctors, nurses and other providers are to conduct their clinical work. Medical practice policies (which we refer to simply as practice policies) describe how doctors are to manage patients. Procedural policies describe how to implement interventions specified in practice policies and thus provide practice specifications in operational detail. This section discusses only practice policies and focuses on those concerned with guiding doctors on how to manage patients.

For quality management purposes, practice policies are embodied in credentialling (which we discuss elsewhere) and in explicit statements about how a patient should be treated. To formulate the latter, a hospital must usually start by collecting relevant practice guidelines produced by professional societies and others. Their medical staffs must evaluate these guidelines in light of their members' experience and either adopt or adapt them to their circumstances. Today it is very unlikely that a hospital will find sufficient guidelines or policies in use by other hospitals to prepare easily the fully-elaborated practice policies that this section describes. Further, considerable effort and expertise is needed even to collect and adapt existing guidelines, a subject which is beyond this manual's scope. This section's principal purpose is to give the reader a vision of what fully-elaborated practice policies would look like, and thus serve as a goal toward which to work.

276.2 Purpose and nature of practice policies

Practice policies' purpose is to improve patients' health outcomes. They intend to improve patient care by informing practitioners about the best course to follow given the patient's specific circumstances. Practice policies must state the objectives they intend to achieve, the steps to be followed to achieve these objectives, and the limits under which specified steps will achieve objectives. The best course to follow depends on the exact outcomes that a patient prefers and the nature of any needed trade-offs that he or she makes. Considering outcomes in health status terms (a concept described in detail elsewhere in this part) simplifies specification of practice policies somewhat, because it standardises outcomes and ways patients can express their preferences. Nevertheless, it is as well to remember that the best course to pursue depends on the exact outcome to be achieved. For example, a different course may be required if the patient wants to live as long as possible irrespective of the state in which his or her life will be lived. For example, does he or she want to be able to play sports while alive even if this means lower life expectancy?

Practice policies are not cookbooks whose authors tell doctors exactly what to do without the need to exercise their judgment. Doctors' objection to practice policies may result from the one-size-fits-all approach that has often characterised practice guidelines and similar initiatives to date. Practitioners believe rightly that interventions must be tailored to an individual's circumstances and preferences. While practitioners must treat individuals, knowledge is derived inherently from studies of populations of patients. The key is placing one's patient in the correct diagnostic classification, the doorway to correct treatment selection.

Practice policies must reflect the complexity of medical practice and improve patient outcomes beyond those that would have been achieved in their absence, otherwise they are not useful. They aid, and do not replace, the doctor's judgment. Practice policies' guiding principle is to maintain and improve maximally the health status of the patients to whom they apply. These statements may be national, regional or local (applying within a single hospital). They pertain to patients with specific symptoms, signs, signals, diagnoses, preferences, circumstances or other characteristics. Ideally, they should offer specific guidance of the type 'if this ... , then that ... , except if ... , then ... '. Because of medicine's inherent complexity, these types of practice policies must be computerised to be used in practice. Practice policies are the information base for decision support technology (DST). Further, they must state who is qualified to implement specified interventions, in terms of training experience and other relevant parameters. Present practice policies, if they exist at all, are often less instructive, limiting their utility.

276.3 Contents of practice policies

Fully-elaborated practice policies would describe:

- the policies' purpose—why they were produced and their intended function;
- what the policies cover—their scope, depth and limitations;
- how they were developed;
- who sponsored (paid for, supported, or organised the effort) and who developed (authored) them, identifying any actual or apparent conflicts of interest;
- who authorised the policies' use, their force and when they apply (policies about policies).

The main body of the policies—what the policies cover—would describe how to manage patients and the expected results (outcomes) of following them. The inclusion of these data are critical to subsequent verification and improvement of the policies, by structured outcome measurement for example. The policies would represent the thinking and experience of their authors, substantiated by whatever knowledge and information they drew on. Specific policies might actually refer to the relevant supporting literature or other information and explain why it should be done, a type of substantiation useful in teaching people about or convincing them to use the policies. Further, practice policies may address what practitioners might expect to be done, especially if it had been embodied in previous policies but is omitted from the present policies, and explain why it should not be done. Conflicts with other practice policies would also be obvious candidates for such mention and explanation.

276.4 Scope of practice policies

276.41 Technical and other considerations

Practice policies may involve only technical considerations or involve such other considerations as cost-effectiveness, net social benefit and social impacts. To date, most practice policies have been concerned only with technical considerations. Technically, quality of care can be defined as maximal improvement in health status using interventions consistent with the patient's preferences. Consequently, practice policies specify how to achieve this goal for different types of patients.

Patients who do not want a surgical operation, even though it may produce a better outcome, should not be forced to undergo the operation. Payment schemes can offer incentives, whether intended or not, favouring one intervention over another, usually to reduce cost. Thus practice policies must explicitly address patient preferences where they are known or can be envisioned to exist. Clearly, practice policies cannot address every nuance of patients' choices any more than they can deal with every possible detail of practice. Which patient preferences are legitimate—that is, recognised by law or ethical principles—is beyond this manual's scope. Similarly beyond this manual's scope are questions of a provider's rights, for example, not to carry out a procedure he or she objects to on moral grounds, even if legal—for example a patient's demand to abort a foetus of the 'wrong' sex and his or her responsibilities to the patient in such circumstances.

The line between technical and social considerations is often blurred. For example, the idea that renal dialysis for old people is not justifiable medically may be no more than a doctor's informal cost-worth calculation. Increasingly, practice policies will have to address economic, ethical, legal and social considerations. These areas are foreign to most doctors and they are unfamiliar with them. Moreover, doctors fear others' intrusion into clinical practice. In reality, doctors' clinical freedoms are being challenged increasingly. Practice policies not only formalise these limits but also hold out the hope of removing the fear inherent in the uncertainty of not knowing what is viewed as acceptable.

276.42 PATIENT PREFERENCES—RISKS AND BENEFITS

Practice policies must take patient preferences into account explicitly. If a surgical operation is generally the preferred way to treat a particular health problem, practice policies must specify what to do for those patients who do not want (or who are not fit enough) to undergo a surgical operation. These kinds of decision points are clear-cut. Other assessments or risks and benefits are less so. They depend on patients' preferences for outcomes as well as the means for and the certainty of their attainment. Take the following hypothetical example—hypothetical because today the requisite data to inform patient's choices do not, but should, exist.

For a population the effectiveness stream of the best practice may be apparent, for example 12% die in the hospital, 40% lead a miserable life for one year, 45% live a reasonable life for two years, and 3% lead a good life for two years. Without the intervention all patients live a reasonable life for one year. Without discounting outcomes, the intervention is clearly superior 238 hsy versus 200 hsy (hsy—health status year—is an integrated measure of health state weighted by its value to the patient, a concept described elsewhere in this part). However, some patients may not want to risk dying in the hospital. They discount the distant health status improvement to such an extent that no treatment is the preferred option. In this sense, risk focuses on a specific outcome that is a negative component of the total stream of like benefits. The rationality of such choices is an issue that is beyond this manual's scope. However, there is a growing body of evidence that properly informed patients make different choices than they would otherwise make, and that patients differ in their choices depending on their age, sex and other factors.[15,16]

276.43 SOCIOECONOMIC CONSIDERATIONS

Generally, while practice policies have recognised variation in the resources available to providers, they have usually been developed without regard to socioeconomic factors. For example, if computed tomography is available, one set of diagnostic interventions would be appropriate; if not, another would apply. Rarely are practice policies developed with explicit consideration of whether or not a surgical operation, for example, is ever justified. Increasingly, people believe that for pragmatic and equity reasons economic factors and the attendant social choices must be considered in formulating practice policies.

The principal concern is an intervention's value relative to its cost. Should an 85-year-old person with multiple-system disease have a renal transplant, paid for by government or other social financing scheme, even if this intervention provides only a little additional health status improvement over an alternative, and much less expensive, treatment? Doctors are used to weighing the risks and benefits to the patient of alternative medical interventions but not their social value. Understandably, few people like making such judgments but they are inevitable if demands outstrip resources, as they do increasingly with respect to health care. The process of formulating practice policies involving such considerations must include representatives of those affected by them, for example policy decision makers responsible for financing schemes and patients.

A health care financing scheme might conclude, for example, that an expensive operation is not worthwhile for certain patients: the extra health status improvement is small, the cost very high. In this circumstance one can envision that practice policies might mention the operation's inadvisability for certain patients but the doctor could carry it out. However, practice policies might proscribe the operation for certain types of patients in which case the doctor might not be paid (reimbursed) for carrying it out (and, depending on legal circumstances, might be prohibited from asking the patient to pay for it). An extension of this approach might suggest that certain conditions not be treated aggressively; only supportive care provided. The legitimacy of such choices depends ultimately on their acceptance by those who are subject to them. In the case of the example, the decision's legitimacy might be greatest if the individual subscribers to the payment scheme made this choice collectively.

Quality of care, and hence quality management, cannot be oblivious to cost. While some would hold that everyone should be entitled to everything that might improve health status, others believe that this ideal can never be attained in practice, especially with the present proliferation of ever more costly medical interventions. They argue that explicit recognition of resource limitations will prevent the pursuit of the impossible from precluding attainment of the practical. Today these unpleasant social choices are often made implicitly rather than expressed in practice policies. Such policies may be set by economists, not doctors, unless doctors choose to participate in the process. Doctors should recognise that resource allocation decisions are social, not medical, choices, and that practice policies can alleviate them of this burden.

276.44 INITIAL PRACTICE POLICIES

To begin with, practice policies should likely be limited to technical considerations. Socioeconomic and other considerations can be added later after the initial policies have been adopted lest the entire effort be stymied at the outset because of irreconcilable value conflicts. Practice policies should describe the best way to treat patients given the state of medical science knowledge (from research), information (from quality management systems), and experience (from practice). Today practice policies are most likely to incorporate a number of equally acceptable alternative interventions and rarely venture into great specificity. Policies professing one true way must be based on solid scientific information about health improvement lest their use in practice preclude use of better alternatives or cause harm. Policies' force must be proportional to the strength of the scientific evidence that supports them. Incontrovertible evidence can cause a thousand opinions to conversion on a single fact.

276.5 Depth of practice policies

At one level, practice policies can give very general guidance; at another, they can be highly specific. General guidance might say that if a certain condition is suspected, an antibiotic should be administered immediately. Specific guidance might list all of the acceptable antibiotics, their routes of administration, doses, for example in the form of amount per kilogram, other details of administration, and specific caveats or other treatment implementation considerations. At the outset, developers must decide the depth to which they want to formulate practice policies. These design decisions might be made section-by-section, as it may be appropriate to vary policies' depth depending on quality management considerations for example, as well as knowledge.

276.6 Force of practice policies

276.61 LIMITS OF DISCRETION

Generally, practice policies describe how patients should be managed, leaving practitioners with considerable latitude to decide when they apply. However, the policies' force may vary from advice to the force of law. On this basis, practice policies can be divided into the following four classes. A set of policies may contain some or all four types: mandatory, optimal, acceptable and open.

276.62 MANDATORY PRACTICE POLICIES

Mandatory policies, sometimes referred to as mandatory standards or standards, are enshrined in legislation or issued by government, professional societies or other regulatory bodies and dictate what must be done (or not done). Deviations from these standards can result in explicit sanctions being applied against the practitioner, for example decertification, monetary fines. There are few, if any, examples of mandatory policies in clinical medicine. This type of policy is rarely warranted and the uncertain validity of clinical knowledge makes them inadvisable, at best. However, the legal standards of practice established by courts in adjudicating malpractice suits constitute an amorphous set of practice policies. Further, as practice policies come to be accepted, legislatures or regulatory bodies may make some policies mandatory or court decisions may have this same effect. In these circumstances failure to follow policies when indicated would constitute malpractice.

276.63 OPTIMAL PRACTICE POLICIES

Like mandatory policies, optimal practice policies are intended to be followed except there are no explicit or implied sanctions for not following them. However, practitioners may be asked to explain why they deviated from the policies and may be in jeopardy of malpractice actions. Optimal practice policies should be confined to those situations for which solid scientific knowledge suggests one practice is clearly superior to any other. One could expect few such policies to be formulated today. Optimal practice policies are sometimes referred to as best practices.

276.64 ACCEPTABLE PRACTICE POLICIES

Acceptable practice policies describe what should be done, but leave open the possibility of pursuing alternatives and may describe two or more equally acceptable policies. Deviation from one of the alternative policies may still leave the practitioner's clinical judgment open to questioning but it can be defended, for example, by reference to the uncertainty of knowledge or the patient's special circumstances. Today most practice policies would be limited to acceptable practices because of the lack of scientifically substantiated results of medical interventions.

276.65 OPEN PRACTICE POLICIES

In some circumstances medical science and experience may be so lacking that no policy beyond prudent use of experience and judgment is warranted. In such cases, fully-elaborated practice policies would state those instances when no particular technical guidance can be given, while, for example, describing the ways in which practitioners usually treat the problem (sometimes referred to as options). Today many practice policies would be open; again due to lack of scientific medical knowledge. Nevertheless, merely describing how practitioners are managing patients and noting lack of knowledge of effectiveness does add value. Such statements inform practitioners of the limits of their discretion, and patients of the uncertainty of interventions' outcomes.

276.7 | *Practice policies' development*

The level at which practice policies should be developed and who should develop them are two related questions without clear answers. Some people would argue that fully-elaborated practice policies should be developed at the national level with government sponsorship. They cite the high cost of their development, the small number of experts in policies development, and the desire for unambiguous, uniform, national practice standards. Certainly, policies' development costs money and expertise is limited now. However, the number of experts required is relatively modest and they can be trained over the next several decades.

The scientific underpinnings of medicine are very limited, leading to different opinions about optimal or even adequate practices. Competing practice policies development efforts, at any level (national, regional or local), would be advantageous at this stage of their development, at least in the United States which could afford to sustain them. Competing efforts would spur improvements in practice policies' formulation and yield better elaborated policies at lower long-run cost. At the national level, for example, medical speciality societies or colleges might assess the scientific evidence supporting interventions used in practice or develop practice guidelines based on such assessments. Regional health authorities or individual hospitals might assess this evidence or guidance in relation to their resources to formulate their practice policies.

More might be accomplished by insisting that all hospitals adopt practice policies that meet some set of minimal criteria of adequacy than by trying to force doctors to adhere to national practice policies. A hospital group, for example, would be free to adopt or adapt policies formulated elsewhere or to develop its own. Over time, with structured outcome measurement, the results of policies' variations can be evaluated. Ultimately, policies' improvement may lead to their convergence. Differences in policies may remain, however, especially if there are no demonstrable differences in outcomes. Thus, for example, hospitals may follow the 'NSW policies' for one condition and 'AMA policies' or 'Mayo clinic policies' for another. But at least how they treat patients would be known to patients, and these practice policies could be the subject of quality improvement efforts.

277 | Formulating practice policies

277.1 | Programmatic considerations

There are no accepted ways of formulating practice policies. To date, even in the United States, little effort has been devoted to the systematic development of practice policies. Most efforts have been limited to the formulation of practice guidelines by US medical speciality societies and, most recently, the US Agency for Health Care Policy and Research. The methods used in or suggested for these efforts have been documented in varying degrees of detail.[4,9,17-20] Although experience and expertise in guidelines' formulation, dissemination and use in practice is somewhat limited, one can draw productively on existing principles and experience to date. Figure II-7-2 on page 331 shows interlocking cycles for establishing and revising mechanisms for formulating practice policies and for their formulation and revision (depicted in the form of quality improvement spirals).

The same quality management principles described in this manual in relation to clinical care apply—and should be applied—to the formulation of practice policies. This process begins with determining what would be most useful to their intended users and ends (and begins again) with evaluating policies' use in practice and how they can be improved to help practitioners further to improve the quality of their care. Before policy decision makers encourage, or more concerningly mandate, use of particular practice policies, they must be reasonably certain that if the proposed policies are followed, in the aggregate they would yield more benefits to patients than does whatever variation exists in current practices.

Government, professional bodies, payers or other entities may formulate practice guidelines and each may have a different purpose in mind. Only health care providers can establish practice policies (which may mean adopting others' guidelines). Practice guidelines' or policies' legitimacy depends on their acceptance by those who must use

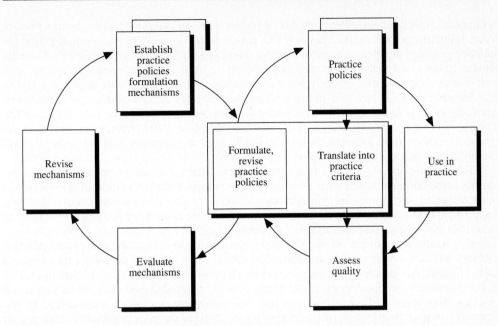

Figure II-7-2 *The practice policies formulation and revision spiral interlocked with that for improving formulation mechanisms. (The same interlocking spirals apply to developing practice criteria.)*

them, which, in turn, depends on the credibility of their formulators and the process they used to formulate guidelines or policies. The process used to formulate practice policies must be published, and to the extent practical should be open to all affected and interested parties and not exclusive. It is all too easy for practice policies formulation mechanisms to decay into forums for protecting vested intellectual, ideological or economic interests. The process must be structured to make best use of existing scientific information, to permit pro- and contra-positions to be discussed and decided rationally, and to make decisions. It must involve the best medical scientists and clinicians. Their role is to produce the facts. Policy decision makers, patients and others must have a role in deciding what should be done when other than purely clinical considerations are involved, as they are almost inevitably.

Well-resourced groups with the expertise and experience necessary to formulate acceptable practice guidelines or policies are most likely to exist at the national level. However, local practice policies have the distinct advantage that they have to be acceptable to a much smaller audience, usually the practitioners who formulate them. To formulate practice guidelines, national governments and medical speciality societies, for example, must begin with existing facts, whereas to formulate practice policies, hospitals can begin with existing practice guidelines or others' practice policies, if they exist. This essential difference in scale becomes a difference in kind, and makes hospitals' task manageable. Nevertheless, in adopting or adapting practice policies, hospitals must establish a program and put in place mechanisms to achieve this end. In this regard they must solve the same types of problems, albeit on a smaller scale, that medical speciality societies and others face in formulating practice guidelines. We recognise that in the absence of others' practice guidelines or practice policies, individual hospitals—in Australia or elsewhere—likely do not possess the resources needed to formulate their own practice policies to acceptable specifications.

Formulating and updating practice policies requires the commitment to begin, to establish sound processes, and to provide the resources necessary to formulate practice policies according to specifications, to complete them in a timely fashion, and to revise them regularly ad infinitum. The need to revise practice policies means that funds for practice policies' development must expand continuously until policies exist for all worthy subjects and need only be revised periodically. Nothing is as deadening to the little enthusiasm that practitioners may have for practice policies as a process that is so slow that resultant policies are out of date when they appear or one that never reconsiders them. Practice policies age, become useless, if not an encumbrance, and may leave the impression that practice policies formulation is a complete waste of time. To remain useful practice policies must be reviewed periodically and, if necessary revised promptly and disseminated quickly to practitioners.

This section focuses on the formulation of practice guidelines or policies for use by medical practitioners to improve patients' health status. It outlines some of the steps for, approaches to, and issues in, formulating and revising practice policies, many of which have been examined elsewhere in the context of consensus development.[2] This section describes key points relevant to quality management. It is not intended to be a how-to manual. Readers interested in establishing mechanisms to formulate and revise practice policies would be well advised to consult with experts before undertaking this arduous task. Ultimately, practice policies' success depends on their use in practice. The determinants of use are complex, but likely rest more on the environment in which the policies exist than in their intrinsic merits. The following discussion is restricted to the formulation and revision of practice policies, including their dissemination and use in decision support technology. It does not attempt to examine the competing incentives and sanctions that determine the extent to which policies are used in practice.

277.2 Steps in formulating practice policies

Figure II-7-3 on page 333 illustrates the steps involved in formulating and updating practice policies. Figure II-7-4 on page 334 details those involved in their development. Formulating practice policies involves:

- setting priorities among health problems, and between updating existing and formulating new practice policies;
- defining the subject of the practice policies and identifying relevant, valid facts;
- drafting practice policies, sending them for review to those whom they will affect, for example the clinicians intended to use them, and reformulating practice policies on the basis of reviewers' comments;
- testing practice policies (by translating them into practice criteria and using these resultant criteria to assess the quality of care of cases of the type for which the practice policies are intended), and finalising them on the basis of test results;
- disseminating and using practice policies, including their incorporation into decision support technologies (and evaluating their use in practice and policies formulation mechanisms);
- updating practice policies to accommodate experience in their use, changes in practice, and advances in technology.

277.3 Setting priorities

One of the most difficult problems is knowing where to start, what to do first. Early on, quality managers must decide what are the most urgent or the most needed practice policies. They must establish an explicit mechanism for this purpose. Further, the priority-setting mechanism must weigh the value of revising existing policies (and thereby permitting their continued use) or formulating them for other health problems, for example. Priorities can be set using any number of criteria. However, the most appropriate calculus is likely to be net health status improvement. Thus priority setting

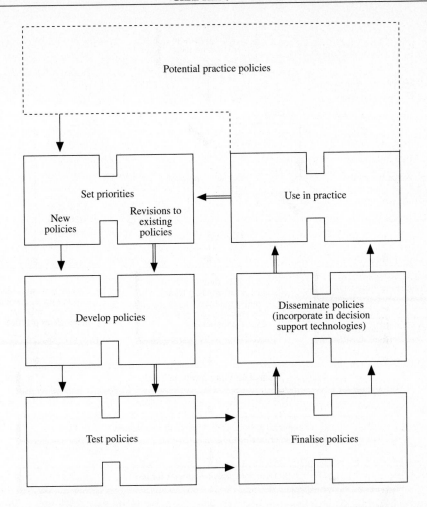

Figure II-7-3 *Steps in formulating practice policies. (The same steps apply to the development and revision of practice criteria.)*

may involve considerable effort, for example to determine the number of patients with the health problem and estimate how much the policies would improve patients' health status. These estimates are likely to be derived from experts' estimates rather than empirical studies because of the present lack of relevant data.

277.4 | Defining subjects and identifying relevant, valid facts

277.41 DEFINING THE SUBJECT OF PRACTICE POLICIES

The first step in formulating practice policies is to decide their focus, purpose, scope, depth and force. For ease of comprehension, we limit the following discussion to the clinical aspects of practice, but it applies generally to other considerations as well. The next step is to define in detail the health problem that the policies are to address and the knowledge needed to formulate them. If practice policies already exist, this step involves their review to determine the adequacy of the existing definition of the health problem and of knowledge needs.

Health problems are the most appropriate focus for formulating practice policies. Today they are often expressed in terms of medical diagnoses. This approach often

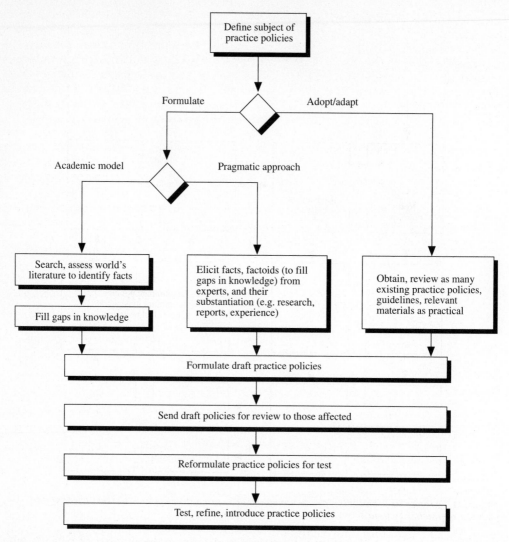

Figure II-7-4 *Process for developing practice policies (or practice criteria)*

assumes the practitioner can diagnose the subject health problem. Diagnosis-based practice policies must contain medical criteria for arriving at or validating the diagnosis. Preferably, practice policies are based on symptoms and signs, guiding the practitioner through the diagnostic process, including the selection and interpretation of tests. To date, symptom/sign-based practice policies have been limited to simple algorithms, such as those advocated for use in developing countries, which are of limited utility to doctors, or have been incorporated into expert systems because of the complexity of using them in practice.

277.42 SOURCES OF RELEVANT, VALID FACTS

The scientific basis for medicine is extremely limited, especially with respect to the most needed facts—the extent to which alternative interventions improve health status. To formulate practice policies representing the best information for treating patients requires identifying gaps in knowledge and filling them with expert judgments until more solid information becomes available. Expert judgment is used not because experts are right but because there is no better alternative. Relying on the limited, uncritical judgment of individual practitioners would assume that there are no experts and that careful evaluation of evidence and experience is useless. Decisions must be made in practice whether or not research-based information exists. Practitioners cannot wait until all of the needed research has been done, because the wait would be interminable and the benefits of using imperfect but useful practice policies would be lost. Practice policies' purposes are to improve practitioners' decisions and to permit quality of care assessment and improvement. Practitioners draw on their store of knowledge, experience and intuition to make decisions. These decisions can be improved if all valid, relevant information can be presented to clinicians when needed. Thus the formulation of practice policies for a health problem must start by:

- synthesising knowledge (research findings) to establish what is known (natural facts) and what is not (gaps in knowledge) and to generate additional knowledge from research findings, for example through meta-analysis (artificial facts);
- filling knowledge gaps through structured expert opinion (creating factoids).

277.43 IDENTIFYING FACTS

A review of the world's literature is often a first step toward developing practice policies. However, because of the literature's inadequacy it may be appropriate to proceed directly to compiling practice policies or other information for decision-making, citing whatever research information experts know about in support of facts or recommended policies. Essentially, two approaches exist for compiling facts to formulate practice policies. They are the academic model and the pragmatic approach.

277.44 ACADEMIC MODEL

The academic model involves formal review of all or a specified subset of the world's literature preparatory to asking experts to interpret it for policy decision-making purposes. This review must involve both the identification and validation of relevant facts. Several publications exist to guide this task. This approach is favoured by RAND researchers and has been adopted, implicitly at least, by the US Agency for Health Care Policy and Research (Bethesda, Maryland).[20]

In theory this approach has much to commend it, because the experts would start from a firm knowledge base (knowing what is known and how certainly it is known), even though it is time-consuming and expensive. In addition, meta-analysis can be performed on research findings pertaining to the same fact. Further, once done the synthesis can be updated by reviewing literature published since the last synthesis, or expanded by searching a greater fraction of the literature than was done previously. In practice, there are often so few scientifically provable research findings relevant to the subject of the synthesis that this step can be safely omitted. For example, a recent RAND report on appropriateness of acute care for the elderly noted 'When we began this work ... we knew that the literature was sparse. However, we were not adequately prepared for both the lack of information and the relatively low quality of the studies that we found'.[21] The only criticism that could be levelled at someone for searching the world's literature for known facts is that the money would be better spent on an alternative approach.

277.45 PRAGMATIC APPROACH

The pragmatic approach assumes that what is worth knowing is known to experts and that in any case little is known scientifically. Thus, while searching the literature will produce interesting data, it is unlikely to contribute much to the development of a fact base for, or formulation of, practice policies. The pragmatic approach is manifest by the Medical Practice Information Demonstration Project.[4] Here, experts on the subject in question (content experts) were asked to give their best estimate of a relevant fact, and its substantiation: research finding, extrapolation from research or assumption. Cited research reports were examined by biostatisticians (methods experts) to determine the extent to which findings were substantiated by the methods used to produce them. In this project, content experts provided estimates for 872 data points. Only six were (facts) substantiated by research findings; the rest were experts' best estimates (factoids). Experts can also be asked to rate the certainty of validity of facts and factoids to estimate the extent to which they believe them to be true. These ratings can be used in sensitivity analyses, for example, as well as to describe confidence in estimates.

277.46 FILLING GAPS IN KNOWLEDGE

Given that knowledge needs have been defined and existing knowledge has been synthesised, gaps in knowledge can be identified. These gaps must be filled by expert opinion through the creation of factoids. Various approaches have been used to fill knowledge gaps, most involving group judgment techniques.[4] Factoids often emerge from meetings of experts, although one can use computer-mediated communications and other techniques.

As mentioned above, the pragmatic approach elicits facts and fills gaps simultaneously. In the academic model knowledge gaps must be filled after facts have been identified. Meta-analysis can be performed if there are different research findings for a given fact. Mathematical models can be used to extrapolate from known facts needed but missing facts. Finally, one might simply generalise findings from one group, place or time to all patients who suffer from the health problem.

277.47 GATHERING EXISTING PRACTICE POLICIES

Individual hospitals likely do not have the resources to develop practice policies de novo. They must depend on adopting or adapting practice guidelines developed by medical speciality societies or professional colleges for example, either in their own country or abroad. Hospitals' greatest difficulty in this regard is identifying existing practice guidelines. They may be published in the medical literature or compiled in special publications such as that of the American Medical Association.[22] In the absence of any existing practice guidelines or others' practice policies, hospitals may wish to form consortia or work collaboratively with medical speciality societies to develop them.

Paradoxically, hospitals with well-developed quality management programs may be better able to revise practice policies than the professional body that formulated them. Hospitals may want to share their results with such bodies to aid in the interpretation of the results of quality management outcomes and suggest legitimate changes that may stem from such results. Individual hospitals may find themselves in an awkward position if their practice policies are at odds with those of a national professional body's guidelines, even if the latter are inferior in some way.

277.5 Drafting practice policies

Technical information is the heart of practice policies. Cost-effectiveness, net social benefits, and social and other impacts are considerations that depend on, but are separable from, effectiveness. One cannot overestimate the importance of differentiating clearly the identification of relevant, valid facts from the formulation of policies. Policies translate facts and factoids into information for use in practice and, thus, incorporate policy makers' value judgments. These judgments may be limited to considering which medical interventions are appropriate based on their potential to improve or harm the patient, or they may involve considering net social benefits and their ethical, legal and social implications. These latter considerations are usually beyond the expertise, and certainly the exclusive purview, of medical practitioners, who, nevertheless, may be bound by the resultant practice policies.

Policies formulators must consider explicitly the certainty of interventions' effectiveness. Where a high degree of uncertainty exists, the utility of one intervention may be virtually indistinguishable from that of another. Policies formulators must go beyond population studies which show, for example, that treatment 'A' is better than treatment 'B', and deal with individual cases. They must be practitioners' surrogates and develop the information that they can use in practice (and that can be entered into a clinical decision support system). For any given health problem this requires, at a minimum, that formulators:

- select critical patient outcomes, principally those related directly to health status improvement or maintenance;
- identify relevant patient preferences, those most likely to be encountered in practice. For example, a surgical operation may be the best treatment technically but some patients may not want the operation. What should be done for them?
- classify patients into groups homogeneous with respect to outcomes and preferences;
- distil knowledge and experience about alternative interventions relevant to each patient type, including practitioners' characteristics, for example qualifications, and other practice considerations, for example the availability of certain equipment;
- provide guidelines for trade-offs, when needed;
- present all of this information in ways that can be used in practice.

Practice policies must be specific to patients and reflect the complexities of medical practice. Practice policies that are too general are of little or no help to medical practitioners. The more specific, the more helpful they are. Ultimately, computerised decision support systems will likely be needed to implement practice policies with the required specificity necessary to improve practice certainly and substantially. To facilitate the evaluation of practice policies and to encourage their use in practice, they should not only describe what should be done, but also why it should be done and what can be expected to occur as a result (making them useful for quality assessment and improvement purposes). Further, they document the evidence for all of these statements and grade its certainty of validity.

Policies formulators should ask practitioners for whose use they drafted the practice policies to review them, and incorporate any relevant feedback into the policies prior to testing them. Ideally, all intended users should be allowed to review the proposed practice policies. If there are many, the views of large samples rather than token representatives should be solicited. Such solicitation can be made in the form of a public notice, for example an announcement in a medical journal. However, a direct mailing to samples of practitioners might be more beneficial.

277.6 Testing and finalising practice policies

Practice policies can—and should—be tested prior to their widespread dissemination by developing practice criteria based on them and using the resultant criteria to assess the quality of care being provided presently. Use of such assessments to test proposed practice policies permits the juxtaposition of abstract formulations and practice realities. There is no implication that practice policies must reflect all existing practices (only the acceptable ones). However, such tests permit practice policies to be refined prior to their use in practice. It also permits the simultaneous development (and refinement) of practice criteria necessary to assess quality of care subsequent to policies' introduction into practice.

After policies formulators have revised practice policies on the basis of test results, if changes are extensive they may wish to again submit them to review by the same groups who reviewed them initially and retest the revised policies. Because this process can substantially lengthen the policies' formulation period, policies formulators may wish to test draft practice policies and revise them based on test results before submitting policies to review by outside groups. If outside groups have already reviewed draft policies and test results dictate substantial revision, policies formulators would be ill-advised to omit the subsequent review round to save time or money, because practice policies' use depends on their acceptance by their intended users. Some people advocate 'validating' practice policies prior to their use in practice. A later section discusses the meaning of and considerations inherent in validating practice policies.

277.7 Disseminating and evaluating policies' use in practice

Practice policies must be used to be useful. This aspect of their formulation is often neglected or even forgotten entirely. Careful consideration of what is useful may affect what policies one attempts to formulate. A perfectly correct technical policy that would narrow the indications for a particular surgical operation may not be adopted, for example, because it would reduce practitioners' incomes substantially, or be hard for the public to believe after so much publicity about the operation's supposed benefits. In this case, imperfect practice policies that would likely lead to a reduction in the number of unindicated operations may be more useful. After their successful adoption, they can be revised periodically to restrict indications until they conform to prevailing technical information.

Dissemination of practice policies does not guarantee their adoption. The diffusion and adoption of medical technologies and practice policies is little studied and little understood. There is little doubt, however, that environmental variables, including the incentives and sanctions that impinge on practitioners, play a key role. To foster the adoption of practice policies, hospitals should: involve clinicians who will be subject to practice policies in their formulation; actively disseminate the resultant policies (e.g. by holding seminars to educate clinicians about use of policies); monitor compliance with and the effects of using practice policies including resultant patient outcomes; feedback results to practitioners; revise policies when indicated; and, above all, provide incentives to conform to practice policies.

277.8 Updating or revising practice policies

To date, one of the biggest problems has been the lack of or inadequate provision for revising whatever practice policies have been issued. This problem has doomed almost all practice policies to the scrap heap shortly after they were formulated, because of the cost of keeping them up to date and competition for resources between updates and formulating policies for additional health problems. Not surprisingly, practices have tended to escape from practice policies, diminishing if not eliminating their utility. To remain useful practice policies must be revised periodically, for example as medical practice advances.

Quality managers must maintain mechanisms to review practice policies and, if advisable, to revise them immediately to accommodate technological breakthroughs or other urgent matters. These mechanisms must be capable of acting expeditiously, otherwise practice policies will be outmoded and health benefits will be lost needlessly. Clearly, trade-offs may have to be made between the thoroughness of mechanisms to revise policies and the timeliness of revisions. Paradoxically, use of rational policies may inhibit their revision if complacency sets in. Practitioners must resist this tendency if health care is to be improved continuously. They must also resist pressures to change practice policies frequently for no good reason, assuming that they were set originally in a rational and reasonable way. At least annually, hospitals must gather accumulated evidence relevant to their practice policies.

Prior to revising practice policies, hospitals must evaluate carefully the evidence that proposed changes will increase patient health status. Such evidence may come from practitioners (who may point out study results or other evidence that the developers may have overlooked initially or provide the benefit of their experience in using policies); feedback from structured quality improvement mechanisms (e.g. structured quality review); structured performance benchmarking; structured outcome measurement; or research reports. Clinicians may want to consult with biostatisticians, epidemiologists, health systems researchers, or other relevant experts who can better assess studies' validity or better interpret the meaning of research reports and statistical data. Once revised, practice policies must be subjected to the same review and test procedures described above for newly-formulated practice policies.

Revising practice policies implies that in the long run the revised practice policies will result in more patient health status improvement than the original ones are capable of producing. The idea of the long run, whatever its period, is important for two reasons. Firstly, early results may be disappointing if, for example, the revised practice policies involve a new procedure (which raises questions of appropriate credentialling). With perseverance surgeons may climb the learning curve and, after sufficient practise, results may improve, often significantly. Ultimately, the new procedure produces better results than the old one, even though patients subjected to it early on may experience fewer health benefits than if they had received the old one (which may raise tricky issues of informed consent). Secondly, revised practice policies may result initially in an increase in process variability and, in the short run, result in less aggregate health status improvement. The conformance improvement cycle can subsequently reduce process variability and realise revised policies' potential to produce greater aggregate patient health status improvement.

To know that revised practice policies produce more patient health status improvement, hospitals must know the results of the original practice policies and of the new ones after a specified interval during which conformance to processes stabilises. Original (and revised) practice policies produce a given level of health status improvement, with certain variability, if performed as specified (which defines what is achievable) and given frequency of deviations in processes and outcomes among the provider population (which determines what level of health status improvement is achieved). Differences in results may stem from a change in what is achievable or that fraction of the achievable achieved, or both reasons. Hospitals may pilot test revised practice policies prior to their widespread adoption to ensure they in fact produce an improvement. On the one hand, such a deliberate process may slow innovation and deprive people of health benefits they might otherwise have enjoyed. On the other hand, speedy introduction of untested changes may not lead to increased health status improvement and could waste a lot of resources. For example, implementing new policies may be more expensive than old ones and there is an inherent cost in disseminating and making changes, including retraining costs for example. Hospitals must strike a balance between petrifying practice in the tried and true and unbridled use of inadequately tested innovations.

277.9 | Validating practice policies

The more actively one disseminates and encourages the use of practice policies, the more one must ensure their validity prior to dissemination. It is one thing for a misguided practitioner to follow his own policies and quite another matter, for example, for the government to insist that practitioners follow national practice policies. How can one validate practice policies? The issues are the same as those encountered in assessing the quality of care, as is their resolution. One can validate practice policies in one or more of the following three ways:

- evaluate the methods used to produce them;
- compare expected patient outcomes, especially long-term outcomes (specified in policies) with those observed in practice;
- conduct clinical trials to determine patients' outcomes in the hands of practitioners following practice policies and those treating patients without the benefit of practice policies (or of following old rather than new policies).

For all practical purposes, validating practice policies depends on evaluating the methods used to produce them (in the same way that assessing the quality of care depends on examining the extent of conformance to processes believed to produce maximal patient health status improvement). Policies formulators must establish a set of criteria for judging the acceptability of methods used to formulate practice policies and hence the acceptability (validity) of the resultant policies (assuming that they were produced according to specified methods, which would be one of the criteria). They can then adhere to these criteria in formulating practice policies or use them to judge the validity of those produced by others. Only practice policies meeting such criteria should be considered for use in practice. This chapter (and the works it references) form a sound basis for developing such criteria.

Meeting process criteria, of course, does not mean inherently that practice policies are valid, that is, result in expected patient outcomes, improve patients' health status maximally, or produce greater aggregate patient health status improvement. However, demonstrating empirically any of these facets of policies' validity before their use in practice is too onerous a standard (and virtually assures that they will never be used, in the same way that insisting that practitioners use only validated interventions would virtually assure that no one would ever receive medical care). The health benefits to be gained from use of practice policies versus no policies is likely so large that logic alone dictates the use of acceptable policies (those meeting process criteria). The argument is simple. Experts' properly considered judgments about how best to treat given types of patients supported by whatever empirical evidence exists (including that from quality management information systems) likely produce superior patient outcomes compared to those of lone practitioners' practices. Further, practice policies are the foundation for all health care quality management. Provisions must exist to assess practice policies' outcomes, both to validate them and to improve the quality of care.

Beyond adherence to processes believed to produce valid practice policies, their validation depends on comparing immediate and long-term patient outcomes with the expectations of the experts who formulated them (e.g. by structured outcome measurement) or by comparing the outcomes of different practice policies (e.g. structured performance benchmarking). In setting practice policies it is essential that experts state explicitly what outcomes they expect to result in order to facilitate comparison of expectations with experience. Disappointment with actual outcomes may stem from exaggerated expectations or from inadequate performance in implementing practice policies. Structured quality review can assist hospitals measure and improve conformance with practice policies. Hospitals may change practice policies based on such feedback. They must assess revised practice policies' validity first according to process criteria and subsequently based on results of using the revised practice policies compared to those achieved with the original ones, to demonstrate that they improve patient outcomes.

Comparing patient outcomes of different practice policies is a useful strategy for their assessment and improvement. (See Chapter 8 in this part.)

In principle, practice policies could be validated empirically in the manner of a randomised clinical trial. For example, practitioners could be assigned randomly to treat patients according to practice policies or to treat them as usual. Key outcome measures would be patients' health status improvement and the cost of its attainment. Such experiments must be reserved for critical demonstrations, rather than routine use, because of their complexity and expense. The quest for empirically-validated practice policies represents an unattainable ideal. In practice, to validate practice policies hospitals must rely initially on assessing the process used to formulate them and subsequently on comparing expected patient outcomes with those experienced in practice.

To ensure practice policies' validity, hospitals must assess and improve continuously their mechanisms and methods for formulating and revising them. The same general quality management principles apply here as apply to clinical care. In principle, the cost-effectiveness of alternative practice policies' formulation processes could be subjected to empirical research. In practice, the usual method is likely to be the evaluation of mechanisms and methods in comparison to experts' opinions of their appropriateness (process criteria), supplemented when necessary by studies of such individual process elements as the identification of relevant facts. As with clinical care, processes and their inherent structures determine outcomes—practice policies' validity and hence their utility.

278 | Practice criteria

278.1 | Historical context

For quality assurance purposes, quality of care assessments have rested on 'peers' reviewing practitioners' care, as documented in the patient's medical record. Peer has been defined variously, but usually means an experienced practitioner in the same speciality as the patient's medical practitioner or an expert clinician who is familiar with the circumstances of the doctor's practice. In conducting such assessments, reviewers have relied traditionally on implicit criteria and standards about what should have been done for the patient and what should have been achieved consequently, especially to determine if a maloutcome was attributable to malprocess—the selection of inappropriate, or malperformance of appropriate, interventions.

In the United States, widespread interest in explicit review criteria predates that in practice guidelines by about fifteen to twenty years. Their development was spurred by the passage of legislation in the early 1970s that set up PSROs to monitor utilisation and the quality of care. We describe these organisations elsewhere in this part. Professional Standards Review Organisations (PSROs) were expected to develop their own regional review criteria based on model criteria sets which it published in 1976. The American Medical Association, for example, led an effort to develop such model criteria sets. A key issue in the development of review criteria was the availability of scientifically supportable information. This concern led the US Public Health Service to fund the Medical Practice Information Demonstration Project in 1977.[4]

Peer Review Organisations (PROs), successors to PSROs, were granted considerable latitude to use national or to develop their own criteria based on local practices for both prospective utilisation review and retrospective quality of care assessment.[23] Not surprisingly, PRO review criteria exhibit considerable variation,[24] and their precision, specificity and documentation have also been criticised.[9] Several organisations have inventoried existing review criteria. For example, to assist PROs the American Medical Peer Review Association compiled review criteria for some 3000 surgical procedures. In 1991 the US AHCPR began a pilot project to develop review criteria from some of the practice guidelines that it has developed. Many private companies have developed review criteria, used mostly for preprocedure utilisation management, that are proprietary. Use of these 'black box' criteria has been criticised because practitioners to whom they apply are not told what they are (to prevent gaming, according to their developers, as well as to preserve competitive advantage) and because they vary from company to company.

Early review criteria were merely lists of symptoms, signs and signals (test results) that justified a particular intervention, for example appendectomy. They applied to all cases and there was little or no attempt to tailor them to individual patients' circumstances. As conceived originally, review criteria were lists of elements, for example urinalysis, urine culture. In these instances it was necessary to specify when the criterion applied (acceptable variation from a criterion), for example urinalysis in 100% of cases; urine culture in previously untreated cases.

Reviewers used these criteria to review medical records in one of two ways. The first way was to decide if the care rendered to each individual case was appropriate. The second way was to determine the number of cases (in the population being reviewed) that met the criterion—for example in 85% of visits examined, paediatricians recorded the infant's head circumference. While one could concede that a paediatrician should measure periodically the infant's head circumference, it may not be necessary to do so on every visit. For example, if head circumference had been measured a week ago at a routine visit, it would not be necessary to do so when the baby was brought back with severe diarrhoea. Sometimes results of reviews using multiple criteria were expressed simply in terms of the percentage all of the case/criteria met, making them even more difficult to interpret.

Even today the term review criteria encompasses criteria for utilisation review—preadmission, continued stay, as well as retrospective review—and those for quality of care assessment, and their use for both case-based and population-based reviews and assessments. This undifferentiated use causes considerable confusion. This manual focuses on criteria for quality assessment and describes elsewhere the relationship between utilisation review and quality assessment. For quality management purposes, quality assessment has evolved into two distinct approaches: one based on case-by-case assessments (derived directly from traditional peer review), for example structured quality review; the other based on statistical assessments of populations of cases, for example outcome risk-adjustment. Increasingly, case-by-case assessment involves manual or automated screening of cases and further review of those failing screens, that is, cases that screens identify as exhibiting potential quality of care problems. The term (medical) review criteria refers specifically to the decision rules that operationalise such screens for purposes of either utilisation review or quality of care assessment.

278.2 About criteria and standards

Considerable confusion exists about terminology and concepts that have evolved over time. For purposes of this manual, practice criteria and standards (referred to here usually as practice criteria, or criteria) are explicit practice specifications necessary to assess retrospectively quality of care case-by-case. Practice criteria can be used to guide quality of care assessments or to screen cases for potential quality of care problems. While practice criteria may usefully represent a quality assessor's aide-memoire, the term applies here principally to the starting point for the development of quality of care screens, particularly automated screens.

A criterion is a means of judging and in common usage is often synonymous with standard, although criterion connotes a rule for measuring quality whereas standard suggests some measure of quality. This manual uses these terms in this sense. A criterion refers to the parameter or variable that is measured. A standard is the value (level) of that parameter or variable used for assessment purposes. For example, the length of a surgical operation may be a criterion, and its duration (two hours) the standard, that is, how long it should take (and no longer). Thus for purposes of developing quality of care screens:

- *Criteria* define processes of care necessary and sufficient to diagnose and treat the patient, including prevention and rehabilitation. They are predetermined interventions or elements of care. For example, blood culture is a criterion for the treatment of septicemia. Taken as a whole, criteria define operationally the quality of care for screening purposes.
- *Standards* refer to performance relative to a criterion (care process), either the outcome of a specific care process, for example the time from the induction of anaesthesia to the beginning of the surgical operation must be thirty minutes or less, or to a patient outcome (of one or more or all care processes), for example the patient died during admission. Importantly, as used here standards pertain to individual cases, not to populations of cases in the manner of thresholds for clinical indicators, for example.

Criteria apply to processes and standards to outcomes (e.g. of processes or to patients). As this manual emphasises, for all practical purposes the quality of care is defined by and can only be assessed in reference to processes. The occurrence of maloutcomes alerts one to the possibility of malprocess—process that if improved would result in better outcomes.

Further clouding the prevailing picture, the term standard sometimes means best or optimal clinical practice, defines the boundaries of acceptable practice, or refers to the legal minimum. In this sense, criteria are elements of practice on which to base such judgments. Standards may refer to professional standards—those established by consensus among experienced practitioners; normative standards—those established empirically (what most doctors do); or legal standards—those established as acceptable care, which if not met constitute malpractice. In the United States the term 'standard of care' is:

A term used in the legal definition of medical malpractice. A physician is required to adhere to the standards of practice of reasonably competent physicians, in the same or similar circumstances, with comparable training and experience.[25]

In Australia, while the terminology relating to 'standard of care' varies somewhat from the American, the same principles apply.

278.3 Need for practice criteria

Judgments about quality of care are complex. Traditionally, reviewers have made such assessments using implicit criteria. Implicit criteria are those in the judge's mind, which may or may not be articulated in the judgment. Implicit criteria have the distinct advantage that they can be applied to all types of care that a reviewer is competent to assess. However, they are inherently unreliable because different clinicians may apply different criteria. For example, reviewers may disagree about whether or not a given diagnostic test is necessary. Moreover, reviewers may not only disagree with each other but, on multiple reviews of the same medical record, with themselves.

Judges may reach different conclusions based not only on differences in criteria, for example whether or not a test was necessary, but also based on different readings of facts, for example whether or not the test was done. Although explicit criteria do not help overcome the latter source of error directly, their use in screens to identify potential quality of care problems can help to reduce such errors by focusing reviewers' attention on potential quality of care problems. Later chapters in this part describe ways to improve the reliability of quality of care assessments.

Leaving aside such mechanical problems as misreading or misinterpreting the medical record (which may stem in part from recordkeeping inadequacies), interreviewer variability boils down to differences in practice policies. Making reviewers' implicit criteria explicit is clearly a step forward. Explicit criteria permit discussion of and agreement on what constitutes acceptable practice for quality of care assessment purposes.

278.4   Purpose of practice criteria

Practice criteria are essential for screening medical records for potential quality of care problems and hence for assessing the quality of care provided to individual patients to identify improvement opportunities. They state how particular cases should be treated and care documented for purposes of screening medical records for potential quality of care problems. When used directly in case-by-case assessments of the quality of care, practice criteria serve as an aide-memoire to guide an assessor. The assessor's interpretation of criteria is subjective and to determine the quality of care for the particular case the assessor must usually go beyond them.

Practice criteria, in use today to screen cases for potential quality of care problems, are usually but not necessarily limited to the technical or clinical aspects of care (but not necessarily only those aspects of care for which medical doctors are responsible). Resource use or utilisation review is usually limited to aspects that bear directly on quality of care—for example length of stay as an outcome which if exceeded might signify malprocess—rather than extended to cost considerations—for example the fact that repeat tests were done when one would have been sufficient.

278.5   Relationship between practice policies and criteria

Practice policies state what should be done and achieved consequently. Practice criteria operationalise policies for quality assessment purposes. If practice policies exist, they can be translated relatively easily into practice criteria. Ideally, practice policies and criteria should be developed simultaneously. Using practice criteria, assessors can review samples of medical records to identify quality of care problems relative to policies. Based on these review results policies can be tested and refined prior to their introduction into practice. This step permits policies formulators to gauge the effect of proposed policies on clinical practices. The theoretical considerations that often dominate policies' formulation meet practical realities. Clinicians are often poor at conceptualising policies in the abstract but good at judging whether or not care was appropriate in an individual case, because such judgments reflect practice.

Today practice policies are usually lacking. Consequently, practice criteria development is one of the daunting tasks that confronts quality managers. However, once developed and used in quality assessment, appropriate policies can emerge iteratively from the cycle consisting of practice policies/criteria development and case-by-case assessment that leads to the (re)formulation of practice policies/criteria for future use, ad infinitum. Clearly, practice policies must be consistent with practice criteria.

278.6   Nature and contents of practice criteria

278.61 FOCUS OF PRACTICE CRITERIA

Practice criteria usually pertain to an episode of care, for example, hospitalisation for chronic cholecystitis, or to a continuum, for example management of diabetes. They may focus on diagnoses or procedures, for example surgical operations, drugs, or other discrete diagnostic or therapeutic interventions. For a given diagnosis, the criteria must address appropriate interventions. For a given therapeutic intervention, they must taken into account the diagnosis; for a diagnostic intervention, the patient's symptoms, signs and signals (test results to date). While in principle one could envision a matrix of diagnoses and interventions that would encompass all of medicine, in practice, criteria are needed or can be set only for a limited number of diagnoses and/or interventions. This section focuses on diagnosis-specific criteria as the most useful. The same general considerations apply to both diagnosis- and intervention-specific criteria, although there are some specific differences.

287.62 VALIDATING THE DIAGNOSIS

Quality assurance efforts may focus on a population or sample of cases discharged from the hospital with a diagnosis of acute myocardial infarction (AMI), for example. Diagnosis or procedure, usually in the form of International Classification of Diseases (ICD) coding, is most often the point of entry for quality of care assessments because cases can be classified and identified by using this parameter. However, medical record coding may be erroneous. In screening cases for potential quality of care problems, the first step must be to validate the diagnosis using findings present in the patient's medical record. Obviously, a case of congestive cardiac failure can be expected to fail a screen for AMI. More importantly, diagnostic errors are among the most common and often the most serious quality of care problems. The doctor may have failed to investigate adequately the patient's symptoms, signs and signals or he or she may have drawn the wrong diagnostic inference from the information available about the patient's condition. One must validate the patient's diagnosis to avoid falling into the diagnostic trap: assuming the diagnosis is correct when in fact it is not.

278.63 OPTIMAL VERSUS ADEQUATE PRACTICE

Practice criteria can be formulated to reflect any desired quality of care level provided that one level can be distinguished from another. Generally one can distinguish between optimal and adequate care. As used here:

- *Optimal care* refers to best practices for a given type of patient, a consensus judgment of experts in treating that type of patient (supported by whatever valid scientific literature exists). Any other care is less than optimal and, by extension, unacceptable. Optimal care produces maximal health status improvement and lowest variance in health outcomes for a given patient type.
- *Adequate care* refers to that care for a given type of patient that all or almost all practitioners qualified to judge the quality of care consider appropriate. Care that falls outside of these boundaries is thus not appropriate. Adequate care improves health status, but not necessarily maximally, and health outcomes may exhibit substantial variation.

Practice criteria designed to screen cases for potential quality of care problems usually employ the adequate care concept. Here, all practices consistent with adequate quality of care would be acceptable. For example, a surgical operation and a medical intervention might be equally acceptable treatments. The task is reduced to identifying cases that fall beyond the boundaries established by practice criteria for further review of the quality of care. Expert clinicians determine if the patient's circumstances were beyond those that the screen was designed to assess (and care was appropriate) or if care was inappropriate.

278.64 FROM PROCESS TO OUTCOME

Practice criteria consist of process elements and immediate process and patient outcomes useful to screen for or identify, case-by-case, imperfect process. For quality assurance (QA) purposes, medical care can be conceived of as a series of processes intended to improve patients' health status. Perfect process (the right interventions for the patient's circumstances implemented properly) produces maximal health status improvement. QA's central goal is to identify less than perfect process so that it can be improved.

Imperfections in process can be identified by assessing processes and outcomes. Process assessment intends to see that appropriate (and no inappropriate) processes were used and their implementation was correct procedurally. Outcome assessment intends to identify outcomes that may signify malprocess, either selection of inappropriate process or improper (botched) implementation of process (whether or not the process was appropriate to the patient's circumstances).

278.65 FROM CRITERIA TO SCREENING CASES

Explicit criteria cannot be used directly for screening. They must first be translated into questions (sometimes referred to as the defined data set) that generate the data to which the criteria can be applied, and the decision rules (sometimes referred to as algorithms) for their application. This step is essential for computerised systems and involves considerable skill. Computerised systems are essential to operationalise fully-elaborated practice criteria. Further, because considerable translation is involved, their performance (sensitivity and specificity) cannot be predicted easily from the criteria so that extensive testing and refinement of screens is essential.

278.7 Use of criteria to screen cases

Cases may fail screens:
- if specified, needed process elements were not conducted;
- if specified, inappropriate processes were applied;
- if process or patient outcomes suggest that needed or inappropriate process was implemented improperly or inappropriate process was applied.

Quality of care screening criteria are binary. They are answered either 'yes' or 'no'. For example a stool culture—a process element—may usually be required for all patients suffering from diarrhoea. Either the patient's stool was cultured or it was not. Any patient whose stool was not cultured would fail the screen and it would require further review to determine if his or her care was appropriate or not. However, if stool culture was indicated usually only in patients under five years of age, then the case would fail the screen only if the patient's stool was not cultured and the patient was under five years of age.

Criteria may also contain process and patient outcomes that may signify inappropriate process or appropriate process implemented improperly. For example, criteria may refer to processes known to be carried out relatively often that are usually not appropriate for the type of case being reviewed. Documentation of such a process in the patient's medical record would lead to its further review. Additionally, suppose competent surgeons can usually conduct a given operation in about one and a half hours; it is quite unusual for an uncomplicated case to take more than two hours. An operation taking more than two hours may signify a quality of care problem, and this process outcome can be used as a screening criterion. Similarly, the care of any patient who dies in the hospital may be reviewed further, that is, the patient outcome 'death in the hospital' is a screening criterion.

Logically, if one specifies all practices and outcomes that are appropriate it follows that all of those not mentioned might be inappropriate. However, for processes, negative criteria of the form 'care is presumed appropriate if . . . was not performed', draw attention to common (or at least not rare) interventions that are considered generally to be inappropriate. For outcomes, they permit a short list of potential problems to be substituted for a long list of non-problems (expected and therefore appropriate outcomes).

If all screening criteria are met, care is presumed appropriate and therefore acceptable and is not reviewed further. If all of the criteria are not met, care must be reviewed further to determine its appropriateness. Clearly, depending on their sophistication, the greater the number of criteria in the screen, the more chances a case has to fail the screen. There is no implication that if a case fails to meet screening criteria that care was unacceptable. The case may have been unusual and the care provided may have been appropriate. The case failed the screen because its circumstances were beyond those that the screen was designed to assess; hence the provision for further review of cases failing screens. Expert clinicians conduct this further review using implicit criteria (because, inherently, if explicit criteria existed they could be incorporated into automated screens to reduce the number of cases that reviewers would have to review). Even if the reviewer finds that care could have been better than that rendered, it does not follow necessarily that medical malpractice was involved, which is a legal judgment, as explained elsewhere.

278.8 *Complexity of practice criteria for screening cases*

Simple criteria sets, such as generic screens (see Chapter 8), involve few criteria and are prone to low sensitivity and low specificity. Diagnosis-specific screens which may involve thousands of criteria tend to have high sensitivity but relatively lower specificity. Improving specificity requires increasing screens' sophistication, which in turn requires more sophisticated computer systems. Presently the sensitivity and specificity of screens is largely unknown and untested. Ideally, only screens of known high sensitivity should be used otherwise quality problems remain undetected. Further, specificity should be as high as possible given achievement of the first objective to reduce the volume of cases failing screens that reviewers determine subsequently do not have quality problems. Clearly, there is a trade-off between sensitivity and specificity. In outcome/process assessment systems, the validity of quality assessments depends on using screens of high sensitivity and further review mechanisms that produce reliable judgments to classify accurately cases failing screens as exhibiting a quality problem or not. Chapter 8 describes the use of such systems in quality assessment and improvement.

For screening purposes, the more that criteria parallel the complexity of practice, the greater their utility. Simple criteria can be used to identify care that falls outside of normal boundaries of appropriate practice; sophisticated criteria, to match what was done and achieved in a case against what should have been done and achieved. While simple criteria are useful to demonstrate the approach, sophisticated criteria are far more useful for quality assurance purposes. Sophisticated criteria offer a highly reliable way to identify potential quality of care problems. They can take into account most, if not all, of the individual circumstances that are usually encountered in medical practice. Their complexity, however, demands computerisation because of the inherent limits on conditional logic that can be expressed on a printed form.

Initially, screens' utility grows exponentially with increasing sophistication. At a certain point, however, the costs of increased sophistication outweigh its benefits. Gathering the data to operationalise screens that encompass all eventualities may cost more than losses associated with missing one or two quality problems and/or the cost of reviewing further the extra cases that the screen fails inappropriately. Of course, over time this point is pushed further and further in the direction of increased sophistication as the cost of elaborating and operationalising screens diminishes. Nevertheless, one need specify only how most cases should be treated most of the time. Cases exhibiting circumstances not covered by the screen will likely fail, that is, not meet screening criteria, and be sent for further review (where clinicians can apply implicit criteria).

By analysing samples of cases passing screens, criteria can be refined to reduce the number of cases that the screen misses (those that have a quality problem that the screen does not find). By analysing review results of cases failing screens, criteria can be refined to reduce the number of cases that fail inappropriately (do not have a quality problem).

So far, automated screens have been used exclusively to identify cases that should be reviewed further. There has always been a clear reluctance to judge the quality of care without referring it first to a qualified clinician to confirm the screen's findings. Now the technology may have reached the point where automated screens can be used to designated cases as exhibiting certain quality of care problems without the need for further review by a clinician. Nevertheless, for the near future further review will be required for most cases failing automated screens. While the sophistication of automated screens will doubtless increase rapidly, it may neither be technically feasible nor cost-effective to elaborate them to the point that they encompass virtually all practice circumstances so that they do not miss problems and only identify cases with problems, and thus obviate the need for further review by expert clinicians.

278.9 Developing and revising practice criteria

If fully-elaborated practice policies exist, they can be translated directly into practice criteria for quality of care assessment purposes. Today, however, few such policies exist, and the first time that clinicians think systematically about the boundaries of acceptable practice is when they are confronted with the task of developing practice criteria for quality assurance purposes. The same considerations apply to developing and revising practice criteria as apply to formulating and updating practice policies. Since we cover them above, we do not repeat them here. Describing all of the steps involved in developing, testing, refining and revising practice criteria is beyond this manual's scope. This section is necessarily limited to a few key points.

Explicit practice criteria are stated, and thus objective. They must be clear and unambiguous. When coupled with a computer they can be used reliably and relatively inexpensively to screen cases for potential quality of care problems. Explicit criteria state exactly what should be done (and, if warranted, not done) to diagnose and treat patients and what to expect (and, if appropriate, to avoid) consequentially. They represent a synthesis of knowledge, from research and experience, and may express policy choices and social values.

Developing practice criteria is inherently easier than formulating practice policies because they examine providers' judgments and actions rather than assist doctors make them. Diagnosis illustrates this point the best. Practice criteria can simply list the symptoms, signs and signals that validate, that is, are minimally consistent with, the diagnosis. For example, results of enzyme or ECG studies can be used to validate a diagnosis of acute myocardial infarction (AMI). This job is a far easier one than assisting a clinician to decide when enzyme or ECG studies should be ordered, which would be the situation in formulating practice policies.

While the task of developing practice criteria is somewhat simpler than that of formulating practice policies it can, nonetheless, still be quite difficult and expensive. Developing and testing practice criteria requires specific expertise and is time consuming. If available, existing practice policies or criteria developed by others constitute a convenient starting point. There is no need to reinvent the wheel. Clinicians are well advised to guard against rejecting others' work products simply because they did not produce them and thus they cannot possibly apply to them. As is the case with practice policies, criteria must be revised periodically to account for advances in medical knowledge and changes in practices. Finally, criteria developers must evaluate periodically their methods for developing and revising practice criteria to improve their cost-effectiveness.

279 Decision support technology

279.1 About decision support technology

In its ultimate form, decision support technology (DST) guides clinicians' patient management, building quality into the health care delivery process, and relieves them of all separate test ordering, recordkeeping and other administrative requirements. Further, such DSTs can gather data useful for quality assessment and improvement, medical technology assessment, practice policies formulation and health policy decision-making. For the foreseeable future, DSTs will not replace doctors. Moreover, it is doubtful that they will ever do so, except perhaps in science fiction stories. There is more to medical practice than information processing. However, DSTs can unburden doctors, permitting renewed emphasis on the human aspects of care, while reaping even more of the benefits of scientific medicine. By making the latest, best information immediately available to doctors, they can speed diagnostic classification, improve treatment selection and enhance patient management.

Decision support technology (DST) refers to decision aids for clinical practice and administration. While DSTs range from such simple, printed aids as decision-trees, the term refers usually to sophisticated, computerised expert systems and other forms of artificial intelligence (AI). Decision support technology helps providers to make decisions about the diagnosis and treatment of individual patients, and quality managers to assess the quality of care. An expert system is a computer program that can process information to solve a problem at, near, or exceeding the level of a human expert. Expert systems consist of two principal parts: a knowledge base that contains rules and an inference engine that applies these rules to patients' circumstances, and may suggest additional information that would allow completion of an inference to its logical conclusion.

Expert systems solve problems. They usually operate in very narrow domains, for example diagnosis of infections. If asked to consult on a case inappropriately, unlike a human expert the expert system will act as if the consultation were appropriate (but nevertheless may arrive at a correct answer within its domain). Within their limited domains, expert systems can be highly effective. The expert system MYCIN, for example, was developed at Stanford University in the 1970s to assist determine if the patient had bacteraemia or meningitis. In blind tests, MYCIN proved to be as effective as Stanford's medical experts.[26] MYCIN, and its shell (an empty expert system that can be used for different applications), EMYCIN (E stands for empty), proved to be landmarks in expert systems' development. MYCIN is often regarded as the first true expert system (with separation of knowledge base from inference engine); EMYCIN, as the first expert system building tool.

279.2 Need for decision support technology

Worldwide, people and their governments spend trillions of dollars on health care each year. Much of this money is simply wasted; it does not improve health. Some of the money is spent inefficiently on unneeded tests or ineffective treatments, because the best knowledge is not used to diagnose and treat patients. Consequently, proper diagnosis and treatment may be delayed or missed entirely. Effective DSTs harbour the potential to save billions of dollars annually and to improve health care at the same time.[14] While this seems too good to be true, the logic is compelling: DSTs allow the best knowledge and information to be brought immediately to bear on the patient's problem. There is no implication that less money will be spent on health care; that is a social choice. What it can mean is that better value will be obtained for dollars expended.

279.3 | Past decision support technology

Use of computers in medicine has developed over the past thirty years. Their application to clinical practice to date has been very limited—even though medicine has been at the forefront of AI applications—because of three principal factors. Firstly, needed computing power was too expensive. Secondly, relatively few resources were devoted to exploring computer applications, in part because of lack of credible leadership. Thirdly, applications were neither relevant to the types of decisions clinicians had difficulty making, nor user-friendly. Consequently there were no demonstrated benefits to spur development. The increasing complexity of medical practice, advances in computer technology and knowledge engineering, and doctors' increasing familiarity with computers may now be sufficient for a new generation of systems to succeed where others failed. Lack of resources devoted to this effort and lack of validated medical knowledge are still formidable barriers. Exploding health care costs may spur DST development if decision makers exhaust plausible alternatives or see DSTs as a credible means to control costs and improve quality.

279.4 | Present decision support technology in quality management

Throughout the world, developers are working to perfect expert systems' application to health care. This section describes a few examples to illustrate use of DST in the different phases of production that can be the focus of quality management in hospitals. In the next several decades we can expect many more sophisticated systems to emerge that will improve the scientific practice of medicine. However, examples of present applications in routine use are quite limited.

279.5 | Preproduction decision support technology

In the United States, much time and attention is being paid to utilisation management (UM). (See Chapter 6 in this part.) One aspect of utilisation management is preprocedure review, where a doctor must obtain authorisation to operate on the patient, for example. Typically, the doctor calls a company (often referred to as a utilisation manager) to obtain the needed authorisation. The third party responsible for paying for the operation (the patient's employer or employer's insurance company) retains the utilisation manager (who is thus sometimes referred to as the fourth party; the patient being the first and the provider the second party). The utilisation manager employs reviewers who, on the basis of information supplied by the doctor, and sometimes the patient, decides whether or not the operation is justified (often referred to as medical necessity or appropriateness). Reviewers, who may be specially trained nurses, may use an expert system to screen these requests for authorisation. Cases failing this screen are then referred to a medical doctor who discusses the case with the patient's doctor and decides whether or not to authorise the operation. In the United States, several companies, including, for example, Medical Intelligence (Boston, Massachusetts) and Value Health Sciences (Santa Monica, California), market such systems. Essentially, such systems use prospectively practice criteria, which must be limited inherently to symptoms, signs and signals known preoperatively.

Another system—Certify!—marketed by Huron Systems (Ann Arbor, Michigan) permits hospitals to manage payment-related certification, and clinical and operational support activities. The system identifies activities that the hospital must perform for a patient encounter by comparing patient-specific information to hospital-specific rules (requirements or policies). It automatically communicates requirements (and solutions) to affected hospital areas, and can track their completion. In the United States, the system emphasises checking that the patient has met all of the requirements of his or her health insurance policy prior to admission to maximise the hospital's chances of full and timely payment for care.[27] However, if the hospital builds the requisite rules, the system can check for any requirements, including those related to quality, utilisation and risk management. For example, for a patient to be admitted under Dr Jones' care, the system can check if he is credentialled to do the elective procedure for which the patient is to be admitted. If Dr Jones has had his privileges withdrawn temporarily because of medical recordkeeping deficiencies, the system will not allow any patient to be admitted under his care. If certain tests should be done prior to admission (or surgical operation), the system will check that they were in fact done. When the patient is admitted, the system can notify social work service that the patient must be discharged to a nursing home after an expected length of stay of seven days, so that discharge planning can begin immediately. In these regards, the system is a vehicle that allows the hospital to operationalise its administrative and practice policies.

279.6 Intraproduction (in-process) decision support technology

279.61 BENEFITS OF IN-PROCESS DECISION SUPPORT TECHNOLOGY

The greatest potential for DSTs, and for quality improvement, is in the phase of in-process quality control. Here, DSTs can aid doctors diagnose and treat patients and document care. They embody practice policies and assure their application. The very best DSTs are quite transparent to the user, being integrated totally in the way doctors work. For example, PUFF (used at the Pacific Medical Center, San Francisco) interprets pulmonary function data. It is coupled with the measuring instrument, processes the measurements and prints out a recommendation.[26] Two systems in use presently show DSTs' potential to improve clinical care. Both systems are the product of over twenty years of development work by Homer Warner (University of Utah, Salt Lake City, Utah).

279.62 HELP

The HELP patient care system, marketed by 3M Healthcare (Salt Lake City, Utah), is designed to satisfy a hospital's complete clinical information needs. The system is integrated, avoiding the need to duplicate data entry (and its associated errors), and employs expert logic to provide alert and decision support capabilities.[28] At LDS Hospital (Salt Lake City, Utah), HELP runs on a ten-processor Tandem Non-Stop Computer system, which has more than 600 terminals and 100 printers attached and sixty offsite access points via a dial-up-network. The Tandem system interfaces with the hospital's other computer systems. Annually, LDS Hospital (LDSH) admits approximately 25 000 patients and has 22 000 outpatient visits. Three HELP functions illustrate how the system assists providers improve the quality of care.

> In a study at LDSH, the system revealed that patients who were given prophylactic antibiotics before surgery developed infections only half as often as those given antibiotics after the start of surgery. As a result, the system now automatically alerts doctors to start giving antibiotics at least two hours before a patient scheduled for surgery gets to the operating room. Prophylactic antibiotics can be safely discontinued forty-eight hours after surgery if the patient exhibits no sign of infection. However, busy physicians sometimes forget to rescind the order. Now, if a patient's postoperative culture is negative and there is no evidence of infection, the HELP system reminds the doctor to discontinue the antibiotic, thereby saving patients as much as US$50 a day.
>
> LDS Hospital fills about 2000 prescriptions a day . . . The HELP software automatically checks that the drug is not contraindicated by a patient allergy or by interaction with other medications. The system also checks that appropriate companion lab tests have been ordered for certain drugs . . . LDS pharmacists no longer have to decipher illegible handwritten prescriptions. The on-line prescription orders are clear and easy to read, eliminating confusion or potential error.
>
> Each year LDS Hospital performs approximately 500 000 laboratory tests . . . orders are entered into the Tandem system and instantly relayed to a terminal in the hospital's

clinical lab. (Test) results are reviewed by the HELP software, then transmitted back to the nursing station and the patient's record within seconds . . . The HELP system generates an alert if the patient's results exceed the normal accepted range or indicate a life-threatening condition . . . physicians (prefer) receiving the real-time computer alerts.[29]

279.63 ILIAD

Iliad represents the culmination of over twenty years of research at the University of Utah, and is an outgrowth of HELP. It is supported commercially by Applied Medical Informatics (Salt Lake City, Utah). Iliad's knowledge base covers almost 1000 diseases. The system makes use of almost 12 000 disease manifestations (signs, symptoms, signals) that have diagnostic significance.

Iliad is designed to teach and supplement the problem-solving skills required of a good clinician. Iliad operates as an expert consultant to provide a differential diagnosis, and as a second opinion to critique a presumptive diagnosis. In consultation mode, Iliad allows free-text entry of observations made by the clinician during a patient workup, can provide consultation to the clinician at any stage of the diagnostic process, and can assist the clinician on the most appropriate observation to make next. Iliad can also generate any number and variety of simulated patients' cases. In simulation mode, Iliad permits a physician to evaluate his or her performance by comparing his or her problem-solving approach to an optimal strategy derived from Iliad's knowledge base.[30] Most recently, Applied Medical Informatics has extended Iliad's technology to consumers in a product called 'Medical HouseCall', that provides consumers with an interactive home medical guide. It analyses symptoms and their causes, helps organise information to take to the doctor, and keeps track of medical history information.

To date, Iliad has been used mostly to teach medical students:

The Iliad patient simulator provides students with a structured opportunity to practice working up patients while receiving feedback about the appropriateness of their diagnostic problem solving. . . . Iliad is designed to make students aware of the relative cost and information gain for various procedures. Each query by the student during the test case can be evaluated in terms of the cost of a procedure relative to the information gain by the procedure.[31]

279.7 | Postproduction decision support technology

For the foreseeable future, postproduction quality management—traditional quality assurance—will be the mainstay of broad quality improvement. Practice criteria (which embody what should have been done and achieved) are compared to what was done and achieved. Review usually involves a two-step process if all or significant samples of cases are to be reviewed: case-by-case screening followed by further (expert clinician) review of cases failing screens. Screening may involve use of an expert (outcome/process assessment) system to improve its objectivity and accuracy. The US Department of Defense uses such an expert system as the first step in assessing the quality of care being delivered by its hospitals. Quality Standards in Medicine (Boston, Massachusetts) markets a similar system to private hospitals. Other chapters in this part describe both of these systems. Computerisation supports further review of cases failing screens but as yet these systems do not employ an expert system for this purpose, because of doctors' reluctance to interact with computers rather than technical limits. Pattern analysis can also be automated with expert systems. They can identify quality problems or patterns of care that the hospital should investigate to determine if a quality problem exists. Such expert systems are beginning to emerge as data for their operationalisation become available.

| 279.8 | *Future decision support technology*

During the next thirty years we are likely to see a tremendous growth in the use of DSTs. Mostly likely, initial DSTs will be stand-alone systems, such as those that focus on specific health care problems (e.g. rheumatology), phases (e.g. diagnosis), issues (e.g. drug interactions), or functions (e.g. structured quality review). Integration of DSTs with existing computer systems and with each other is likely to result from standardisation of variables and their computer representations or automatic translation from one set to another, rather than development of all-encompassing, unitary systems. Such standardisation or automatic translators (sometimes referred to as connectware) will permit linking the best elements into a complete system, much in the same way as one can now build a stereo system from separate components to suit one's individual needs and tastes. Advances in or additions to particular elements can be accommodated easily without the need to redesign or replace the entire system. The key to widespread use of DSTs is the availability of machine-intelligent medical records (in which data are represented in a way that computers can manipulate) to overcome enormous data entry costs, and of a user-friendly interface to capture data to create machine-intelligent medical records.

Use of DSTs is essential to realise major improvement in the quality of care. They make possible a second wave of improvements beyond those realisable from structured quality improvement. (See Chapter 8 in this part.) This wave of the future will improve the fit between an individual patient's needs and the interventions he or she receives. Improved needs–interventions fit will reduce in-process variation and improve health care quality. Expected benefits will include: quicker diagnosis; more appropriate treatment selection; better treatment implementation, including fewer complications; less defensive medicine or unnecessary tests and treatments; and, quite possibly, improved patient satisfaction. Use of DSTs for in-process production control will likely render obsolete the need for utilisation review and most other forms of quality control, and permit structured quality improvement efforts to focus on monitoring their effectiveness and improving knowledge, which in turn will improve DSTs. The extent of DST use depends ultimately on sociopolitical considerations as well as technical factors and their cost.

References

1 Sigerest HE. The great doctors. Garden City, NY: Doubleday & Company, 1958, pp. 41–7.

2 Institute of Medicine. Consensus development at the NIH: Improving the program. Washington, DC: National Academy Press, 1990.

3 Institute of Medicine. Improving consensus development for health technology assessment: An international perspective. Washington, DC: National Academy Press, 1990.

4 Williamson JW, Goldschmidt PG, Jillson IA. The medical practice demonstration project: Final report. Baltimore: Policy Research Incorporated, 1979.

5 American Medical Association. Directory of practice parameters. Chicago: AMA, 1991.

6 Leape LL. Practice guidelines and standards: an overview. QRB 1990; Feb: 42–49.

7 Eddy DM. Clinical decision making: from theory to practice. Practice policies—what are they? JAMA 1990; 263(6): 877–8.

8 Nash DB. Practice guidelines and outcomes. Where are we headed? Arch Pathol Lab Med 1990; 114: 1122–5.

9 Field MJ, Lohr KN (eds). Guidelines for clinical practice. Washington, DC: National Academy Press, 1992.

10 Brook RH. Practice guidelines and practicing medicine: Are they compatible? JAMA 1989; 262:3027–30.

11 Goldschmidt PG. Practice guidelines (letter). JAMA 1990; 263:3021–2.

12 (U.S.) General Accounting Office. Practice guidelines: The experience of medical specialty societies. Washington, DC: GAO, PEMD-91-11, 1991.

13 Tracking guideline costs proves confounding. Report on Medical Guidelines and Outcomes Research 1992; 3(7):1.

14 Decision support technology: Will VA spark wider agenda? Computers & Medicine 1986; 15(3):1–3.

15 Kaplan AK (ed). The future of the patient in emerging approaches to quality assurance. Washington, DC: American Association of Retired Persons, 1992: 17–18.

16 Goldschmidt PG, Bertram D. The influence of certainty of outcome on choice between treatments. Managed Care Medicine 1995; 2(5): 14–21, 47.

17 Institute of Medicine. Medical Technology Assessment Directory. Washington, DC: National Academy Press, 1988.

18 Eddy DM. A manual for assessing health practices and designing practice policies: the explicit approach. Philadelphia: American College of Physicians, 1992.

19 Attributes to guide the development of practice parameters. Chicago: American Medical Association, 1990.

20 Wolf SH. AHCPR interim manual for clinical practice guideline development. Rockville, Maryland: Agency for Health Care Policy and Research (publication no. 91-0018, 1991.

21 Brooke R. Appropriateness of acute medical care for the elderly: An analysis of the literature. In Crouch JB (ed). Health care quality management for the 21st century. Tampa, Florida: American College of Physician Executives, 1991.

22 Toepp MC, Kuznets N (eds). Directory of practice parameters. Chicago: American Medical Association, 1994.

23 Field MJ, Lohr KN (eds). Clinical practice guidelines: directions for a new program. Washington, DC: National Academy Press, 1990.

24 Kellie SE, Kelly JT. Medicare Peer Review Organization preprocedure criteria: an analysis of criteria for three procedures. JAMA 1991; 265(10): 1265–70.

25 Campion F (ed). Grand rounds on medical malpractice. Chicago: American Medical Association, 1990.

26 Harmon P, Maus R, Morrissey W. Expert systems tools & applications. New York: John Wiley & Sons, Inc, 1988, page 6/200.

27 CERTIFY! Ann Arbor, Michigan: Huron Systems, Inc, 1994.

28 HELP patient care system software architecture. Salt Lake City, Utah: 3M Company, 1990.

29 HELP system supports physicians and manages medical data at LDS Hospital. Cupertino, California: Tandem Computers, Inc, 1988.

30 Iliad 4.2: physician diagnostic and treatment software. Salt Lake City, Utah: Applied Medical Information, 1994.

31 Turner CW, Williamson JW, Lincoln MJ, et al. The effects of Iliad on medical student problem solving. In: Miller RA (ed). Fourteenth annual symposium on computer applications in medical care. Los Alamitos, California: IEEE Computer Society Press, 1990.

Chapter 8

STRUCTURED QUALITY IMPROVEMENT

---

280 | Contents

This chapter sets the context for and describes the concept of structured quality improvement under the following headings:

281 | Purpose of this chapter

Prevention is the key to good health and to effective quality assurance and improvement. Hospitals must design their production systems to produce quality products to prevent known threats to quality, and institutionalise mechanisms to assess routinely their products' quality, to find and fix quality problems, and to redesign their products and production systems. Beyond quality planning (design of products and production systems to produce them to specifications), quality improvement depends primarily on identifying and resolving quality problems and eliminating their root causes to prevent problems' recurrence. Eliminating quality problems' root causes requires feedback—information and action—to reinvent the organisation, redesign production systems, re-engineer processes and change practices to improve quality. Change neither begins nor ends at the workface—be it shop floor or bedside—but must involve the entire organisation. Hospitals must design and deploy quality management structures and processes to collect and evaluate information on quality and to plan and implement change. Only if hospitals' management culture supports useful workface change can they improve the quality of their products and production systems.

This chapter:
- explains that all quality improvement depends on analysing variation in production performance, particularly deviations from what should have been done and achieved;
- describes three essential quality improvement strategies:
  - —structured performance benchmarking—to learn what performance is possible, where one stands in relation to the best, and how to achieve superior performance;
  - —structured quality improvement—to find and fix quality problems (this chapter's focus);
  - —structured outcome measurement—to measure long-term outcomes and determine their relationship to processes.
- elaborates on the virtuous conformance (quality assurance) and specifications improvement spirals (see Chapter 6 in this part) that begin and end with practice policies (see Chapter 7 in this part);
- details the essence of structured problem identification, particularly structured quality review and structured problem resolution.

If implemented successfully, these three quality improvement strategies likely have greater potential to improve health care's cost-effectiveness in the next twenty years than any other technology, even 'cures' for such specific diseases as cancer. This chapter provides the basis for a practical system to improve continuously the quality of hospitals' care. Already elements of this system are in use in the United States and elsewhere. Their integration into a complete system is the challenge facing Australian hospitals. Necessarily, this chapter focuses on concepts and cannot provide blueprints for their implementation.

---

282 | Key concepts

This chapter elaborates on the following key concepts essential to understanding the context of and methods for structured quality improvement, the basic strategy for effecting quality improvement in hospitals.

- Quality management's central goal is to improve product quality and to reduce production variance. Variation in patient outcomes or deviations from specified processes may signify a quality problem.
- A quality problem (an overt or covert improvement opportunity) is a health care process or practice, including its documentation, that if changed (or done when omitted) or implemented differently (or properly when done improperly) would improve outcomes, that is, provide additional patient health status improvement, reduce cost, increase patient satisfaction, or perfect any trade-offs among outcomes. An improvement suggestion implies a quality problem—one that the suggestion intends to resolve.
- All strategies for improving the quality of care depend ultimately on analysing variation in production performance and resultant outcomes, to generating information (feedback) to improve products (practice policies) and production processes (their implementation);
  - —structured performance benchmarking is based on variation in performance, usually among, but also within quality-immature hospitals;
  - —structured quality improvement is based on variance (deviation) from what should have been done and achieved, or from expectations;
  - —structured outcome measurement is based on such variation and variance in long-term outcomes.

- Structured performance benchmarking (SPB) refers to the strategy of measuring competitors' (colleagues') performance to identify the best performers, to discern what processes, patient flows and organisation seem to produce this performance, and to establish where one's performance stands in relation to the best. Consequently, one can align one's production system with that of the best performers toward improving one's performance. Today structured performance benchmarking is beyond the means of all but large-scale hospital systems and those hospitals participating in such efforts.
- Structured quality improvement (SQI) refers to a hospital-wide strategy to systematically identify quality problems, discover their root causes and routinely eliminate these causes. Quality-focused hospitals must design and deploy mechanisms for these purposes. It is the basic strategy for improving hospitals' quality of care and it is now practical.
- Structured outcome measurement (SOM) refers to the strategy of measuring the long-term outcomes (end results) of health care interventions. It examines the extent to which conformance to specifications actually improves patient health status and produces information to improve them. It is not a substitute for, but may help prioritise, needed research. Only the largest hospitals are likely to have the resources necessary to launch a structured outcome measurement program or conduct the clinical trials that its results suggest.
- Structured quality improvement operationalises the quality improvement spiral. It pertains mostly to conformance improvement (getting done what needs to be done in the way it should be done each and every time), but also informs specifications improvement. Structured performance benchmarking and structured outcome measurement provide information mostly for specifications improvement (what to do and how to do it).
- Structured quality improvement involves a hospital-wide system for:
  —structured problem identification—to identify systematically priority quality problems and their root causes;
  —structured problem resolution—to resolve routinely priority quality problems and eliminate their root causes, to improve conformance to and/ or practice and procedural policies, patient flows, and the hospital's organisation and its management.
- Structured problem identification (SPI) involves:
  —defining and measuring or assessing quality;
  —identifying priority quality problems;
  —determining priority quality problems' root causes.
- Structured problem resolution (SPR) involves:
  —evaluating and selecting among alternative improvement actions to remedy priority quality problems and eliminate their root causes;
  —planning and implementing chosen improvement actions;
  —measuring quality to ascertain if it has improved, to attribute any observed improvement (or its lack) to improvement actions, and to identify any other problems that they may have created.
- Hospitals can employ the following problem identification mechanisms:
  —systematic review of care or cases (patient records that document care processes and outcomes);
  —systematic surveys of people's perceptions and suggestions;
  —incident reports, including patient complaints and allegations of malpractice, and compliments;
  —quality assurance studies;

—group problem-solving techniques, for example quality circles.
- At a minimum, hospitals must perform hospital-wide systematic surveillance of care or cases, using either, or preferably both, of the following methods:
    —structured quality assessment—reviewing care case-by-case—for example structured quality review or unaided structured medical record review to identify and characterise quality problems;
    —structured quality monitoring—population based screening—watching rates of events in populations of cases to trigger review of providers' care if rates exceed pre-established limits.
- Structured quality review (SQR) refers to case-by-case quality assessments to reveal patterns of care. It involves three steps:
    —screening—systematic case-by-case assessment using automated outcome/process assessment screens to identify potential quality problems;
    —review—structured medical record review to confirm potential quality problems and to characterise them;
    —analysis—statistical (pattern) analysis of screening information and medical record review results to reveal patterns of care.
- Structured quality review is a tool for comprehensive structured quality assessment and intends to identify all of the important quality problems in a case. By aggregating results, hospitals can create a quality score to monitor quality improvement. Because it can be implemented easily, with minimal commitment of resources, structured quality review is likely to be the initial method for, and remain the mainstay of, systematic problem identification in Australian hospitals for some time to come.
- Screening's central purpose is to focus expert clinician reviewers' attention on cases likely exhibiting quality problems, thereby reducing their workload to a manageable level and improving their productivity. Outcome/process assessment screens match what was done and achieved with what should have been done and achieved to identify cases with potential quality problems, and thus that require further review. Screening offers objectivity (because it uses explicit practice criteria) and economy (because it can be done by specially trained nurses or medical records technicians).
- Structured medical record review (SMR) refers to a systematic process in which expert clinicians examine medical records to:
    —confirm quality problems identified by outcome/process assessment screens;
    —identify quality problems if the hospital uses unaided review (i.e. does not employ such screens).
- Pattern analysis refers to the statistical analysis of screening data and/or structured medical record review findings to reveal patterns of care. It may identify trends in, and reveal the distribution of, quality problems, discover additional quality problems, illuminate their causes and guide subsequent investigations.
- Population-based screening depends on the statistical analysis of case process or outcome variables. It intends to identify providers whose cases should be reviewed further to determine if they exhibit exceptional rates of quality problems and to elucidate their nature. Ultimately, quality assessment depends on expert clinician review of medical records.
- Clinical indicators are population-(rate-)based screens. They are not quality scores and do not measure hospitals' quality of care; they are not quality indicators.

- Systematic surveillance of staff and patient perceptions and improvement suggestions are a valuable adjunct to—but cannot be a substitute for— systematic quality assessment as a source of quality problems and improvement suggestions. Periodic staff surveys may reveal morale and other problems that affect the quality of care and may be a useful source of suggestions for improving the hospital's operational efficiency and its personnel management.
- Patient perceptions and suggestions are the only source of information on the interpersonal aspects of the quality of care and on the acceptability of any trade-offs among quality's various attributes. Patient satisfaction surveys are likely to be the principal instrument for collecting patients' perceptions, including satisfaction ratings, and their suggestions. Other instruments include question-naires administered in waiting areas, clinics and wards, and focus groups.
- All hospitals must have in place mechanisms that permit staff to report and the hospital to analyse incidents—something that happened as a result of or in connection with patient care—and to record and analyse patient complaints (including threats of or actual malpractice suits) and compliments.
- Identifying a quality problem is only the first of several steps toward its resolution. Hospitals may identify many problems, necessitating their prioritisation for purposes of investigating their root causes, if not obvious. To fix problems and ensure they remain fixed, one must establish problems' root causes, those that if eliminated would prevent the problem's recurrence; not only their apparent causes, which are merely the problem's antecedent manifestations.
- Investigation of a quality problem should result in a brief report that summarises why it was undertaken, how it was done, what was found and, if appropriate, what options exist for remedying the apparent quality problem and, preferably, eliminating its root causes.
- Hospitals must put in place a system for fixing quality problems and checking that they stay fixed. Hospitals' structured problem resolution mechanisms should involve actively all relevant organisational levels in the process and devolve decisions to operational units to the greatest extent possible. Usually, existing organisational units can plan change and implement quality improvement actions. Exceptions include changes in organisation and the redesign of hospital-wide care systems or processes or those that transcend organisational units.
- Resolving quality problems may require changes in one or more of the following three areas:
  —care processes—how doctors and other health care providers treat or manage patients (encompassing practice and procedural policies and their implementation);
  —patient flows—how patients are routed into and from clinical processes, how the hospital manages care delivery, and the interrelationships among care processes;
  —organisational management—how the hospital structures the production system or enterprise and how it manages people and processes.
- Hospitals should describe each practical option for resolving the immediate quality problem and eliminating its root causes, including the steps necessary to effect the option, and its chances of success, costs and implications. This report should also recommend which option the hospital should implement, if any, and the rationale for the choice.

- Resource and other constraints likely mean that not all problems can be resolved at the same time; priorities must be set. Further, the cost of solving a quality problem may outweigh that of its continuance, or problems may be reduced rather than eliminated because beyond a certain point marginal costs exceed marginal benefits.
- Hospitals should pilot test solutions before widespread introduction if their implementability or cost-effectiveness is in doubt, or concern exists that a solution might generate other, even worse, quality problems.
- Planning is required to co-ordinate and effect operational changes. Planned changes may be small, affecting specific practices for example, or sweeping, affecting everyone in the hospital. All planning should result in an implementation plan, which should be a simple but formal document that describes what is to be done, how it is to be done, who is responsible for doing it according to what timetable, with what resources and, if relevant, under what policy or other constraints. Most importantly, the plan must specify expected results according to a time line, if relevant, and expected implementation costs and operational costs or savings. The plan must also specify the means to measure results and costs (or savings), and to attribute them to the chosen improvement actions (or other factors).
- Frequent changes to operations can lead to confusion and quality degradation rather than its improvement. Thus the introduction of changes (e.g. too many, too rapidly, too poorly planned) may be a root cause of quality problems—one to be avoided if at all possible.
- Hospitals should monitor solutions' implementation and their effects and report progress in accordance with the implementation plan. At the conclusion of the planned reporting period, hospitals should prepare a brief, structured quality problem completion report that documents the extent to which the quality problem diminished after planned changes, and evaluates changes' costs and effects. This evaluation should include improvement actions' implementation and recurring costs (or savings) and the extent to which any observed diminution of the quality problem can be attributed to these changes.
- Hospitals must set up a structured quality improvement (SQI) tracking and reporting system, to track progress in resolving problems, to evaluate the results of improvement actions, to assess their quality management program's cost-effectiveness and to improve future quality improvement efforts.

283 | Industrial analogies

We have come finally to the point where we have run out of ready-made industrial analogies. While some manufacturers have built extensive TQM programs, none face medicine's inherent complexity and uncertainty. Manufactures are the products of human conceptions. They can be made because they are makeable. The manufacturer's central goal is to produce a specified, saleable product as uniformly and cheaply as possible. Doctors must manage patients and their diseases whether or not they understand their causes, using whatever knowledge they possess about existing interventions and their consequences. The doctor must fit the patient's needs to available interventions, faced with a variety of often competing incentives. To achieve a perfect fit scientifically requires an unimaginable amount of knowledge or information, which we have yet to produce, and its certain delivery to the doctor when needed, mechanisms for which we have yet to devise. Doctors' fallibilities and desires, for example for income and prestige, professionalism notwithstanding, and the social milieu shape the care that they deliver and its outcomes.

Nevertheless, industry has shown that quality can be improved systematically. In the pursuit of quality improvement, industry has also shown the importance of defining and measuring quality and of using this information, and of developing the will and the means to improve quality. Measuring and improving the quality of clinical care requires different, more complex, techniques than those used by manufacturers. Industrial techniques such as SPC (statistical process control) and quality circles can play a useful, but minor, part in improving quality in hospitals, especially operational efficiency and the personnel aspects of management.

284 | Quality improvement strategies

284.1 | Classifying quality improvement strategies

Quality management's central goal is to improve product quality and to reduce product variance. In health care, this goal translates into improving patient health status to the maximum extent possible within patients' preferences and society's resources, at the lowest practical costs, with the greatest patient satisfaction and the most acceptable trade-offs among these three types of outcomes. For any given patient population, this formulation begs the following two central questions:

- What is the maximum amount of health status improvement that providers can (or should) produce for any given type of patient?
- What is the minimum amount of variation that one can expect with respect to this outcome?

The same type of questions applies to the other aspects of quality (cost, patient satisfaction and trade-offs). However, for simplicity, health status improvement serves to illustrate all of these aspects. Practice policies serve to specify health care's product. (See Chapter 7 in this part.) However, specifications are production intentions, not production performance.

There are any number of ways to rationally improve production performance—the quality of care—and no simple way to classify them. Ultimately, they all rest on analysing variation in production performance: either on measuring outcomes and determining what processes produced especially good performance or on identifying quality problems that if resolved would improve the quality of care. Further, one can measure immediate or long-term outcomes (end results of care). On these bases, one can identify the following three quality improvement strategies, ways to measure care outcomes and/or to assess care processes in order to improve products (practice policies) and production (their implementation in practice) to produce more, and reduce variation in, patient health status improvement. (See Figure II-8-1 on page 362.)

- Structured performance benchmarking—focuses on interventions' delivery—the extent to which what is being done and achieved for patients is in line with what others do and achieve.
- Structured quality improvement—focuses on interventions' appropriateness—the extent to which what should be done and achieved for patients is being done and achieved.
- Structured outcome measurement—focuses on interventions' effectiveness—the extent to which presumed appropriate care processes improve patients' health status.

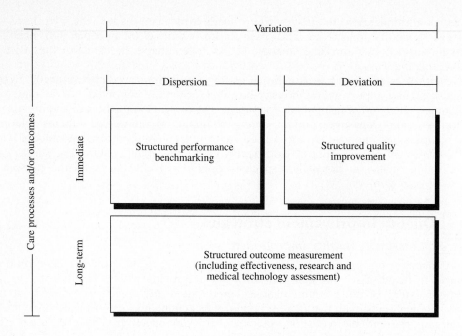

Figure II-8-1 *Types of quality improvement strategies*

Structured performance benchmarking refers to the strategy of measuring competitors' (colleagues') performance to determine the best performance at present (to set a target for one's own performance), what processes, patient flows and organisation seem to produce this performance, and where one's performance stands in relation to the best. This comparison implies that if a hospital's performance is much inferior, it should change its processes (encompassing practice and procedural policies and their implementation), patient flows and organisation to align them with those of the best performer toward improving its performance (and check that such changes resulted in performance improvement).

Structured quality improvement refers to an organisation-wide strategy to systematically identify quality problems, discover their root causes and eliminate these causes, thereby resolving or preventing the recurrence of the identified and any related quality of care problems.

Structured outcome measurement refers to the strategy of measuring the long-term outcome (end-results) of health care interventions—to determine their effectiveness and, by extension, which processes produce the best outcomes—with a view to changing practice policies and implementation processes, patient flows, and organisation toward realising superior patient outcomes.

The rest of this section describes some relevant aspects of variance analysis and these three quality improvement strategies. The rest of this chapter details structured quality improvement, the strategy most likely to be useful to and within the means of Australian hospitals in their present stage of quality maturity. Complete descriptions of each of these strategies and ways to implement them are beyond this manual's scope.

| 284.2 | *About variation in production performance*

Variation in production performance may arise from one or more of the following production factors and their interactions. It may, but because of the influence of other coproducers (discussed later in this section and elsewhere in this part) need not invariably, lead to variation in health care outcomes, complicating the interpretation of measured or observed outcomes. It may arise from:

- failure to implement specified processes properly—improper implementation of appropriate (and/or inappropriate interventions);
- failure to implement specified processes at all (and/or the implementation of unspecified or unnecessary processes)—errors of omission and commission, use of inappropriate or unnecessary interventions;
- failure of specifications (e.g. poor practice policies)—specified use of ineffective interventions or effective interventions in inefficient ways;
- failure of technology—lack of effective interventions;
- random events and their interactions with production factors and outcome coproducers.

| 284.3 | *About quality of care problems or improvement opportunities*

For quality management purposes, a quality of care problem (sometimes referred to as, and differentiated from, an improvement opportunity) is a health care process or practice, including its documentation, that if changed (or done when omitted) or implemented differently (or properly when done improperly) would improve outcomes, that is, provide additional patient health status improvement, reduce cost, increase patient satisfaction or perfect any trade-offs among outcomes. An improvement suggestion implies a quality problem—one that the suggestion intends to resolve.

Identifying quality of care problems or improvement opportunities often depends on one or both of the following two forms of variance or variation analysis. (See Figure II-8-1 on page 362.)

- Variation in performance (usually such central patient outcomes as health status improvement and the cost of its production) among health care providers, for example hospitals and/or individual doctors in hospitals (sometimes referred to as dispersion analysis)—the basis of structured performance benchmarking;
- Variance from what should have been done and achieved (sometimes referred to as deviation or discrepancy analysis), either product and/or production specifications, for example failure to follow practice policies or achieve an expected patient outcome or expectations, for example a patient complaint arising from a discrepancy between what the patient expected and what he or she experienced— the basis of structured quality improvement.

| 284.4 | *About performance variation analysis*

Variation analysis refers to examining the performance of populations of providers with a view to reducing the observed variation (without reducing, and preferably simultaneously increasing, average performance) thereby improving quality of care. Selecting appropriate performance measures and correctly interpreting results are critical to deciding what quality improvement actions to take. Specific difficulties relate to the need to risk adjust validly patient outcomes. Chapter 4 in this part discusses these points. This section illustrates these difficulties with examples based on hypothetical data.

For quality management purposes, from an organisational, for example hospital, perspective, there are two types of variation analysis:

- Interhospital performance: the organisation compares its performance (e.g. measured in terms of patient health status improvement and the cost of its attainment) in treating particular patient populations to that of its competitors (other hospitals that treat patients with the same health problem, for example).

- Intrahospital performance: the hospital compares the results of the various ways in which it treats particular patient populations, which may involve analysing individual doctors' performance in treating patients with a given health problem, for example.

Interhospital variation analysis depends on the availability of relevant performance data. Since hospitals do not usually generate these data, such analysis is rarely possible now. When such data become available, one could identify the best and the worst performers. (See Figure II-8-1 on page 362.) The best performing hospitals could serve as benchmark providers, to determine what level of performance is possible and to examine how these hospitals achieve their excellent performance. Hospitals with lesser performance could then change their practices accordingly, and expect their performance to improve, if benchmarking had successfully identified the difference (in processes) that make a difference (in outcomes). As a safeguard, one can also examine the production systems of the worst performers to try to understand why they perform so poorly. In this way one can avoid instances when one thinks one has isolated a production factor or method that makes a difference (exists at the best performers) when, in fact, it does not (exists also at the worst performers).

This discussion assumes no or low intrahospital variation in performance. Today, because hospitals are not quality-focused organisations, there is usually substantial variation in care processes, and hence doctors' performance, which confounds interhospital comparisons. If there are large differences in individual doctors' performance, interhospital differences may overpower intrahospital differences so that there is little difference in hospitals' performance. In such situations, individual providers rather than hospitals are the appropriate focus for the variation analysis. Today the most common circumstance is likely large interhospital variation (among institutions) and large intrahospital variation (in providers within a given institution).

Quality-mature hospitals perform production processes according to specifications (with no or very little process or patient–process fit variation). Consequently they have eliminated one of the greatest sources of outcome variation: variation in production processes applied and their implementation. Such quality-focused providers must rely on interhospital comparisons to check their performance, as well as on controlled changes to their own production systems (discussed later in this chapter) to identify additional improvement opportunities. In hospitals at the initial stages of a quality management program, analysis of variation in their providers' performance may serve the same purpose that interhospital comparisons serve for quality-mature hospitals. However, quality-immature hospitals may lack the means to conduct such analyses and to make such comparisons and may be best advised to begin with structured quality improvement through the adoption of practice policies, the use of structured quality review to identify quality of care problems, and the institutionalisation of structured problem resolution mechanisms.

284.5 *Accounting for patient types and other outcome coproducers*

Comparison of providers' performance is often problematical because health care outcomes may vary for reasons other than the goodness of their providers' production processes and hence performance. Some performance measures, such as quality scores derived from structured quality review, do not exhibit this problem because the method used to generate them takes into account differences in patients. With respect to such patient outcomes as health status improvement and such patient-dependent outcomes as the cost of its production, providers' observed or apparent performance depends on the following factors and their interactions:

- patients—the types of patient treated;
- production processes—the central factor of interest in performance variation analysis—interventions applied, how they are applied, and the hospital environment in which they are applied;
- period—the era or macroenvironment in which the hospital operates, which is especially important when comparing historical to present-day data.

Whenever quality managers show doctors their observed performance the poor performers' first retort is usually 'but my patients are different'. Indeed, they may be, and one must have some way of accounting for differences in patients (and, if relevant, periods) when making comparisons among providers' performance. Accounting for differences in periods is very difficult (and hence the preference for concurrent rather than historical controls in clinical trials). The rest of this section examines the omnipresent and pressing problem of accounting for differences in providers' patients. There are three ways to account for such differences and, ideally, use of any one of them should result in the same decision, that is, identify the same providers as being the best and the worst performers. They are:

- risk adjustment, which depends on the statistical analysis of a large population of providers and their cases;
- grouping patients into categories or groups that are homogeneous with respect to outcomes (sometimes referred to as risk stratification), based on the best available scientific knowledge and clinical experience;
- case-by-case assessment (specifically, structured quality review) which takes into account each patient's individual circumstances.

284.6 | Alternative ways to account for patient types

While health status is the most appropriate quality measure, mortality data and rates will serve to illustrate the principles involved in the alternative methods of accounting for differences among providers' patients, because they are likely more familiar to readers and simplify explanations. Suppose that we are interested in hospitals' performance in treating patients with coronary artery disease and confine our analysis to patients with proven disease who receive a coronary artery bypass graft (CABG) when such intervention is indicated. This example is a gross simplification of the usual state of affairs, of course. Usually one does not know if all of the patients who receive a CABG have proven disease for which the operation is appropriate, which complicates the analysis of mortality outcomes. Operating on patients who have little or no disease may obviously produce better outcomes (a point discussed elsewhere in this part).

Comparing mortality rates, for example, assumes inherently that any observed differences are both statistically and clinically significant and hence meaningful. Statistical significance refers to the probability that observed differences may have arisen by chance. Such probability depends, for example, on the magnitude of the difference and the size of the samples or populations observed. Clinical significance refers to the magnitude of the difference. In very large samples, small observed differences may be statistically significant but have no clinical significance because patients, for example, would not differentiate among providers based on such a small difference in their performance.

Risk adjustment, described elsewhere in this part, produces a ratio of expected versus observed mortality among a hospital's cases. If there are more deaths than expected, the ratio is larger than one; if fewer, less than one. These ratios are distributed approximately normally so that, for example, one can use the critical value of two standard deviations to identify high and low outliers. Risk adjustment depends on the specific outcome of interest and the data set in use. For example, risk adjustment factors for this year's mortality analysis may differ from those for last year. Risk adjustment is a statistical method for accounting for patient differences on those variables that have been measured and is devoid of cause and effect considerations.

For purposes of illustration, hospital A has fifty deaths among 200 patients in 1995 (a mortality rate of 25%) and hospital B had sixty deaths among 250 patients (a mortality rate of 24%). Hospital A's mortality ratio (expected divided by observed mortality) was 0.89 and hospital B's was 1.25. Thus, while hospital A had fewer deaths, its mortality rate was about the same as hospital B. But after risk adjustment one would infer that hospital A's performance was better than hospital B's, because hospital A's expected to actual mortality ratio was less, and hospital B's was greater than 1.0. Hospital A may treat a greater proportion of 'difficult' patients (those that are sicker, i.e. at higher risk of operative or immediate postoperative death).

Based on risk factors known from research studies or assumed from practice experience, one can group patients according to expected outcomes. For example, one might divide patients into 'difficult' cases and 'easy' cases, based on certain characteristics—for example, age, physiological functioning and disease stage—that are known to influence significantly care outcomes (mortality in this illustration). Such groups would likely endure from year to year, but are not immutable because of changes in knowledge and technology, for example. Today we have little reliable information to form such groupings. Were they to exist, we might find that 75% of hospital A's and 40% of hospital B's patients were 'difficult' cases. The mortality rates were as follows: for hospital A, 29% for 'difficult' and 12% for 'easy' cases; for hospital B, 42% for 'difficult' and 8% for 'easy' cases. Thus we can see that hospital A did a better job of treating 'difficult' patients and hospital B a better job of treating 'easy' patients—information we did not get from risk adjustment. We could risk adjust separately the data for 'difficult' and 'easy' patients, of course. However, while risk stratification can be used for small populations, risk adjustment requires large populations. In this illustration, which compares two hospitals' performance (and involves 250 cases), risk stratification, but not risk adjustment, is possible.

Given sufficient resources, we could employ structure quality review to assess case-by-case hospital A's and hospital B's performance. Reviewers could decide, in each case in which the patient died, whether provider performance rather than other factors was more likely than not responsible for patients' deaths. These judgments are often difficult to make and therefore tend to be unreliable. They also may be invalid because no one really knows the critical reasons patients die, because of a lack of research and quality management. Reviewers could also assess the care of patients who did not die. They may find cases in which poor care increased patients' risk of death, but in which patients survived such threats to their lives. Because structured quality review assesses both care outcomes and processes, it provides far more useful information than risk adjustment or risk stratification (neither of which directly assess care processes).

For purposes of illustration, assume reviewers can determine reliably and validly whether or not better care would likely have avoided a patient's death. Reviewers found that thirteen of hospital A's deaths and twenty of hospital B's deaths could have been prevented—avoidable mortality rates of 26% and 33% respectively. They found further that at hospital A 63% and at hospital B 46% of cases received appropriate care. Thus one might infer that care at hospital A is better than that at hospital B. Applying this same analysis to 'difficult' and to 'easy' cases at the two hospitals showed that for 'difficult' cases, at hospital A 63% and at hospital B 15% of cases were treated appropriately. The corresponding figures for 'easy' cases were at hospital A 63% and at hospital B 67%. Thus again one might infer that hospital A did a better job of treating 'difficult' cases than hospital B and vice versa for 'easy' cases. With structured quality review, we learn also the nature and distribution of quality problems, the first step toward their resolution. This simple illustration ignores the statistical significance of differences in hospital A's and hospital B's rates—a critical issue in drawing inferences about their performance.

In theory, and in this illustration, the various methods lead to the same conclusions. Whether or not they would do so in practice is unknown because variation analysis is employed infrequently and, to the best of our knowledge, no one has ever compared the results of using the various methods on the same patient population. Further, in many instances hospitals treat few cases and one cannot measure their performance in terms of such simple and stark outcomes as deaths and mortality rates. These circumstances complicate comparisons, but their consideration is beyond this manual's scope.

284.7 *Structured performance benchmarking*

Structured performance benchmarking intends to measure competitors' performance so that one can know what outcomes are possible at present for particular patient populations, and where one stands in relation to the best performers. It refers to a systematic process for collecting outcome data on all or significant samples of providers (or using such data collected by others) to identify the best present performance and hence best present performers. While the best performers offer a benchmark against which to assess and set targets for one's own performance, they do not necessarily represent the best possible performance. Even the best performers can usually improve their performance. After one had identified the best (and the worst) performers, one can attempt to identify the care practices, processes and organisation that seem to produce this performance. Consequently, one can align one's own practices, processes and organisation with those of the best performers and/or make other changes toward improving one's performance and possibly even exceeding that of the current best performers.

Today, structured performance benchmarking is beyond the means of all but large-scale hospital systems or hospitals that participate voluntarily in arrangements that facilitate benchmarking, such as that exemplified by QSM users. It requires the collaboration of all or many hospitals to generate comparable performance data, involves substantial expertise to analyse and interpret the resultant data, and requires substantial resources to examine, analyse and evaluate the best and the worst performers' production processes, not to mention the will to act to change practices. For these reasons, in Australia and elsewhere, structured quality benchmarking is likely to be practical only at the national, state, regional, or system levels, and represents a late, rather than initial, phase quality improvement strategy. Further, intrahospital structure performance benchmarking works best if hospitals have standardised their production systems to eliminate, or at least reduce, the influence of intrahospital variation. Further, hospitals can reap the benefits of structured quality improvement without the need to compare their performance to that of their competitors (other hospitals).

Structured quality benchmarking depends on the existence of variation—by choice or by chance—in providers' production processes, patient flows and organisation, and hence their care outcomes. Thus, as the health care quality movement progresses and hospitals adopt practice policies and take other steps to reduce product (and hence outcome) variation, its utility will probably shift from individual institutions to hospital systems to national and international comparisons. This evolution will likely take thirty to fifty years or longer.

284.8 Structured quality improvement

284.81 ABOUT STRUCTURED QUALITY IMPROVEMENT

Structured quality improvement operationalises the quality improvement spiral. (See Figure II-8-2 below and also Chapter 6 in this part.) Structured quality improvement encompasses:

- structured conformance improvement—via the conformance improvement (or quality assurance) cycle—to improve the extent to which production conforms to product and production specifications (quality control or quality assurance);
- structured specification improvement—via the specifications improvement cycle—to improve product and production specifications (quality planning/improvement).

Structured quality improvement pertains mostly to conformance improvement (getting done what needs to be done in the way it should be done each and every time), but also informs specifications improvement. (See Figure II-8-3 on page 369.) In contrast,

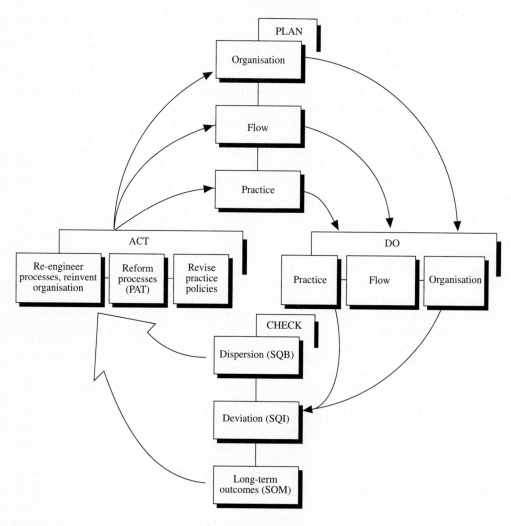

Figure II-8-2 *Organisation-wide quality improvement cycle*

structured performance benchmarking and structured outcome measurement provide information mostly for specifications improvement (what to do and how to do it).

The conformance improvement (CI) or quality assurance (QA) cycle intends to improve conformance to specifications (practice policies)—and thus to reduce variability in patient–processes fit, practices, and hence outcomes—illuminate their validity (the extent to which practice policies improve patient health status), and provide information toward their improvement. This cycle starts with specific practice policies or criteria (i.e. specifying what should be done and achieved), involves assessing the extent to which it was done and achieved and efforts to close any performance gaps, and ends with assessing the extent to which improvement actions produced greater conformance to practice policies. (See Figure II-8-4 on page 370.)

The specifications improvement (SI) cycle intends to improve product specifications (practice policies). Structured specification improvement is the process for determining that set of care specifications which if implemented properly would result in maximal outcomes, for example patient health status improvement. It involves revising practice policies in light of careful consideration of evidence about which interventions maximise patient health status improvement within patients' preferences and society's resources. Information to set or revise specifications can be derived from clinicians' experience, structured quality improvement, structure performance benchmarking, structured outcomes measurement and research reports.

Structured quality improvement is essentially about identifying quality problems (deviations from specifications) and their causes, and resolving them (remedying apparent problems and eliminating their root causes). For effective quality management, hospitals must have in place systems to identify and resolve quality problems (deviations or deficiencies) that if resolved would improve the quality of care. Structured quality improvement involves:

- identifying quality problems—structured problem identification—which involves a hospital-wide system comprising structured quality assessment and various other methods for identifying quality problems and their root causes;
- resolving them—structured problem resolution—which may involve changes to care processes (practice and procedural policies and their implementation), patient flows, and the hospital's organisation and management, to improve conformance to and/or practice policies.

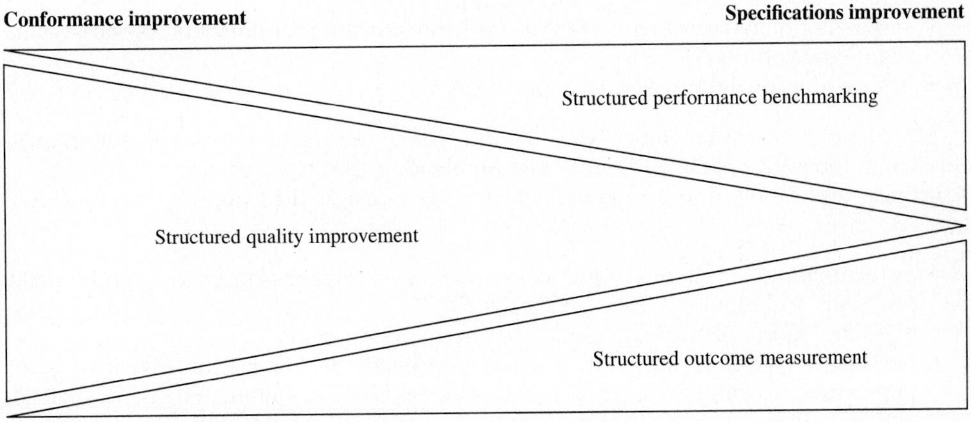

Conformance improvement   **Specifications improvement**

Structured performance benchmarking

Structured quality improvement

Structured outcome measurement

Figure II-8-3 *Quality improvement strategies' relative contributions toward conformance and specifications improvement*

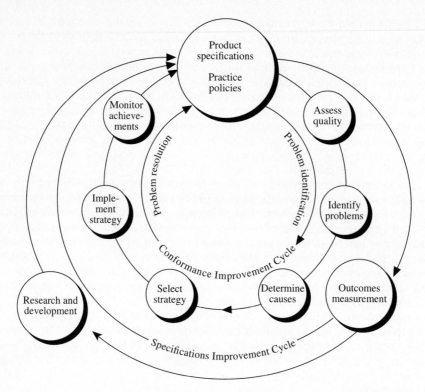

Figure II-8-4 *Continuous quality improvement through conformance and specifications improvement cycles*

Structured problem identification (the first half of the quality improvement spiral)—finding potential and confirming actual quality problems and determining their root causes—involves:

- defining operationally and measuring quality;
- identifying quality problems (deviations from specified, or deficient, processes, and from expected outcomes);
- determining quality problems' root causes.

Structured problem resolution (the second half of the quality improvement spiral)—remedying apparent quality problems and eliminating their root causes to prevent their recurrence, and monitoring and evaluating changes designed to improve the quality of care—involves:

- evaluating and selecting among alternative improvement actions to remedy quality problems and eliminate their root causes;
- planning and implementing chosen improvement actions;
- measuring quality to ascertain if it has improved (evaluating the extent to which improvement actions remedied the quality problem or eliminated its root causes, and whether or not further action is required); attributing any observed improvement (or its lack) or changes to improvement actions; and identifying any other problems that improvement actions may have created.

284.82 ORGANISING FOR QUALITY IMPROVEMENT

Structured quality improvement requires that hospitals institutionalise structures and systems to identify and resolve quality problems. The quality manager's principal role is to design (and when necessary redesign) them. The hospital manager, supported by the board of directors, must establish the structures and provide the means to operationalise quality improvement systems. The quality management committee's role is to establish the policies necessary to operationalise them. The quality management department conducts, and guides line units (e.g. clinical departments) in the conduct of, quality improvement efforts.

284.83 STRUCTURED PROBLEM IDENTIFICATION

Problem and solution are complementary parts of a whole. Improvement suggestions are solutions to implicit problems; explicit problems beg solutions. The first step in improving quality is to define it for purposes of measuring it. Quality problems are deviations from expectations. Various mechanisms exist to identify quality problems. They can be classified according to whether or not one searches for quality problems, and when and how one conducts these searches, or whether or not one waits for problems to surface serendipitously. (See Figure II-8-5 on page 372.) For quality improvement purposes, hospitals can employ the following problem identification mechanisms:

- Systematic review of care or cases (patient records that document care processes and outcomes):
  —case-based mechanisms (quality assessment), for example structured quality review;
  —population-based mechanisms, for example clinical indicators.
- Systematic surveys of people's perceptions and suggestions:
  —staff surveys;
  —patient satisfaction surveys.
- Incident reports:
  —staff incidents;
  —patient complaints (including allegations of malpractice) and compliments.
- Quality assurance studies
- Group problem-solving techniques, for example, quality circles.

Quality-focused hospitals must quantify the quality of their products and put in place systems to identify (and resolve) quality problems. At a minimum, hospitals must perform hospital-wide systematic review of care or cases. They must employ such structured quality assessment methods as structured quality review, and/or clinical indicators with such appropriate follow-up as structured medical record review to confirm quality problems. When tracked systematically, staff incident reports and patient complaints (including the results of investigating individual incidents and complaints) form an important supplemental way to identify quality problems and improvement suggestions. Eliciting improvement suggestions is both simple and cheap, but may be misleading or imprecise and thus important problems may be missed entirely.

For quality improvement and risk management purposes, hospitals must systematically collect and analyse incident reports. Quality assurance studies may play a useful role in identifying quality problems (but cannot substitute for other methods). Group problem solving may be a useful adjunct to (but cannot substitute for) other methods. In group problem-solving techniques the same people both identify and resolve, or at least suggest a solution to, the identified quality problem. All other problem identification mechanisms employ different people to identify problems from those who resolve them.

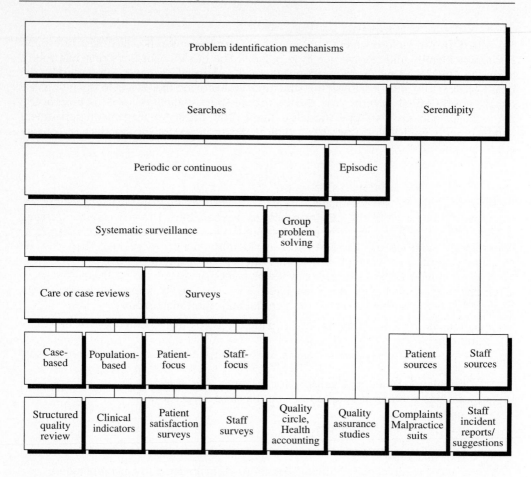

Figure II-8-5 *Mechanisms to identify quality of care problems*

284.84 STRUCTURED PROBLEM RESOLUTION

Once a solution (or improvement action) has been implemented the focus shifts to evaluating the extent to which the improvement action resolved the problem (or realised the expected improvement). Such evaluation is needed to determine if further action is required or not, attribute observed improvement (or its lack) to the solution, and identify any other problems that improvement actions may have created. Improvement actions may not resolve a quality problem (either because they were ineffective in eliminating its root cause or because quality managers did not identify all of them). Conversely, the problem may have resolved despite (rather than because of) the solution. Further, improvement actions may have created new quality problems and they may be worse than the problems they solved.

Resolving quality problems may require changes in one or more of the following three areas. There are no clear boundaries between them and one may influence another.

- Care processes (practices)—how doctors and other health care providers treat or manage patients (what providers actually do and how they do it, who does it, in what circumstances), including, for example:
  —practice policies—what interventions they should apply;
  —procedural policies—how they should apply them.

- Patient flows—how patients are routed into and from clinical processes, how the hospital manages care delivery, and the interrelationships among care processes.
- Organisational management—how the hospital structures the production system or enterprise, for example in departments, including mechanisms to assess and improve quality, how it functions, and how it manages people and processes (which may be influenced by such environmental variables as medical care payment schemes, for example).

284.9 Structured outcome measurement

284.91 ABOUT STRUCTURED OUTCOME MEASUREMENT

Structured outcome measurement (SOM) examines the relationships between long-term outcomes and care processes. Structured outcome measurement examines the extent to which conformance to specifications actually improves patient health status. Such validation of practice policies requires their consistent and continuous use for an adequate period to stabilise processes. Structured outcome measurement is not a substitute for research but may help prioritise needed research. The resultant information can be used to improve specifications and to determine research priorities.

Health care product specifications (practice policies) tend to be process specifications. (See Chapter 7 in this part.) Generally, practice policies state what should be done, for example surgical operation; and detail process policies, how it should be done, for example the correct way to carry out the surgical operation. High postoperative mortality, for example, may result from lack of conformance to process policies or from their poor implementation; little health status improvement, for example, may result from lack of conformance to practice policies or specification of the wrong treatment (which implies an alternative treatment would yield greater health status improvement).

284.92 THE NEED FOR STRUCTURED OUTCOME MEASUREMENT

Structured quality improvement involves assessing care processes and resultant outcomes that occurred during the hospital admission (or immediately afterwards). However, patients may be discharged alive but die a few months later as the result of poor care, for example. Ideally, hospitals must measure the end results of care to judge the extent to which they actually improved patients' health status. Practically, it is difficult and expensive to measure routinely long-term outcomes. Nevertheless, ultimately hospitals must incorporate structured outcome measurement (SOM)—the routine measurement of long-term outcomes in comparison to care processes (sometimes referred to as effectiveness research)—into their quality management programs if they are to be truly effective.

There are two reasons for measuring long-term outcomes. Firstly, measuring and assuring the quality of some products, for example CABG (coronary artery bypass grafts), virtually requires measurement of long-term outcomes to be able to differentiate providers based on performance and to identify quality problems that hospitals can correct. Secondly, measurement of long-term outcomes provides valuable information to judge the validity and appropriateness of clinical practice policies (product specifications), and to suggest where additional research might be needed. In both cases one must decide the appropriate length of time to follow patients, which will vary as a function of diagnosis and its associated treatments.

Measuring long-term outcomes for quality improvement purposes is merely an extension of the ideas embodied in the use of practice criteria to operationalise product specifications (practice policies). Thus, for example, if a hospital's two-year patient survival rate is much lower than expected (i.e. as stated in practice policies) or than achieved by others, the hospital can investigate this quality problem's root causes and might even benchmark the best performers, for example.

284.93 VALIDATING AND IMPROVING PRACTICE POLICIES

Measuring long-term outcomes to validate practice policies is difficult and involves attributing outcomes to care processes. Care processes might not have produced observed outcomes. Patient and environmental variables, as well as postprocess events, may have produced—and almost inevitably coproduced—observed outcomes. Attributing outcomes to interventions is one of the most difficult and challenging quality management tasks. Use of structured outcome measurement to validate practice policies is facilitated by, and useful only if, clear-cut practice product and process policies have been established and implemented continuously and consistently by all providers for an adequate period with little variation in outcomes (an indication of stable processes), and if careful attention has been paid to relevant data collection requirements. To the extent practical, all data necessary to interpret long-term outcomes must be specified prior to implementing structured outcome measurement and collected concurrently, that is, when the patient is treated. Inherently, practice-generated data may exhibit bias, if for no other reason than patients select providers and vice versa (often referred to as patient–provider selection bias or simply as selection bias).

Use of structured outcome measurement data may reveal that cases treated medically experience the same or better outcomes than those treated surgically, at less cost. In this case, medical management of the health problem may be preferable and practice policies changed accordingly, reserving surgery for certain types of cases or special circumstances, for example, patients unable or unlikely to comply with medication regimens. In some cases, structured outcome measurement data may be ambiguous or controversial, necessitating clinical trials or other methods capable of providing unequivocal results, if designed and implemented properly.

284.94 ORGANISING FOR STRUCTURED OUTCOME MEASUREMENT

In Australia, and elsewhere, only the largest hospitals or entire hospital systems are likely to be able to have the resources necessary to launch a structured outcome measurement system or conduct the clinical trials that its results suggest. Moreover, they would be well advised to do so only after implementing structured quality improvement, at least in rudimentary form. Smaller hospitals can participate in structured outcome measurement and clinical trials under the leadership of a large hospital or research institute by using common protocols and pooling data, for example. The correct interpretation of data that result from structured outcome measurement is crucial but tricky. Errors in interpreting resultant data may lead quality managers to take actions that they believe will improve patient outcomes but that instead will actually degrade them. While such errors, if they were to occur, could theoretically be detected by SQI/SOM systems, the treatment of many cases could well have occurred prior to their detection.

285 | Structured problem identification: systematic surveillance

285.1 | About systematic surveillance

285.11 TYPOLOGY OF METHODS

Hospital-wide, systematic surveillance of care or cases is essential to identify quality problems. Hospitals can employ either, or preferably both, of the following methods:
- structured quality assessment—reviewing care case-by-case, for example, using structured quality review to identify and characterise quality problems;

• structured quality monitoring—watching case population rates, either to screen care to identify cases or circumstances that require further review (population-based screens) or to identify quality problems (if rates are quality measures, which they are rarely).

This section summarises these methods and the systematic surveillance (surveys) of staff and patients' perceptions and suggestions. It also describes the limited role that periodic quality assurance studies can play as part of hospitals' quality management program. Later sections focus and elaborate on the various facets of structured quality assessment, particularly structured quality review and its constituent elements—case-based screening, structured medical record review, pattern analysis—and the construction of quality scores. They also describe in detail population-based screening, including JCAHO (and ACHS) clinical indicators and surveys of staff and patient perceptions and suggestions.

285.12 ORGANISING FOR SYSTEMATIC SURVEILLANCE

Quality assurance efforts to date have tended to emphasise the identification of quality problems (deviations or deficiencies) to the point that clinicians often think of quality assessment or quality monitoring as synonymous with quality assurance. Clearly, identification of genuine problems is necessary, but not sufficient, to improve quality. Both the will and the means to resolve problems must exist if the quality of care is to be improved. The ideal surveillance system would identify continuously all important quality problems so that they could be examined and, if warranted, be subjected to improvement action. The present state-of-the-art makes it possible to approach this ideal. However, systematic care or case review requires a sophisticated structure for its successful implementation and most hospitals in Australia and elsewhere may find it impractical to implement it hospital-wide in the near future. But they should start now.

Structured quality assessment, preferably structured quality review or, otherwise, unaided structured medical record review, must be the mainstay of hospitals' quality management programs. Structured quality monitoring, specifically population-based screening, may supplement these efforts to identify systematically potential quality problems to be confirmed by subsequent structured medical record review, for example. Population-based (and case-based) screens use process or patient outcomes to identify potential problems in care processes. Only by identifying and rectifying malprocesses can hospitals assure and improve patient outcomes.

285.13 STRUCTURED QUALITY ASSESSMENT: CASE-BASED SURVEILLANCE

Systematic quality assessment refers to the routine examination (often referred to as retrospective review) of medical records (sometimes referred to as patient records or care documentation) to identify quality of care problems (often referred to as quality problems or improvement opportunities). Hospitals may use these case-by-case assessments to quantify quality (if they assess all or statistical samples of cases) and to determine the existence, nature, extent and distribution of quality problems and illuminate their causes (if they aggregate and analyse them subsequently).

The term medical record refers to any documentation pertaining to an individual patient's health care that the patient or a health care provider generates from information elicited during health care encounters, patient–provider interactions, including utilisation and/or cost data. Medical records are still mostly paper but increasingly they are electronic or computer-based. The term medical record encompasses abstracts and indexes of patient record information and other derivative records, for example, billing or insurance claims (sometimes referred to collectively as secondary patient records, their sources being referred to as primary patient records).

To improve the effectiveness and efficiency of structured quality assessment, hospitals should use quality of care screens (sometimes referred to as quality assessment screens, or simply quality screens) to identify cases with potential quality of care problems. The preferred method—structured quality review—employs outcome/process assessment screens, with expert clinician review of cases failing screens and pattern analysis of results. Such screening permits reviewers to concentrate on cases with potential problems and to focus their attention on specified quality problems to confirm or deny their existence. Traditional peer review (unstructured review of medical records by clinical colleagues as conducted in North America) is far too unreliable, and unaided structured medical record review is too expensive, to warrant their use for the systematic surveillance of the quality of care.

285.14 STRUCTURED QUALITY MONITORING: POPULATION-BASED SURVEILLANCE

Structured quality monitoring refers to watching continually one or more monitors (population parameters), with the implication that some action will follow in some pre-established circumstances. For example, parameters being watched may trigger action if one or more of them falls below or goes above a threshold value, or if specified parameters values taken in combination (e.g. in the form of decision rules or mathematical models) indicate the need for such action. With respect to clinical indicators, subsequent action involves first confirming (or denying) a quality problem's existence and, if confirmed, determining its root causes. Usually, confirming a quality problem's existence involves case review. If the monitor is a quality measure, subsequent action involves determining the problem's root causes, as the monitor establishes the quality problem's existence.

Monitors are rates of events in populations. They may be, and usually are, the basis for population-based quality of care screens (often referred to as rate-based or clinical indicators), and may be quality measures. Some monitors are sentinel events, for example maternal deaths, rate-based indicators with 0% threshold, so that if the event occurs it triggers review of the case (and possibly all of a provider's similar cases for a given period) because it indicates a potential or actual quality of care problem. Quality monitoring is not synonymous with population-based screening, even though it uses monitors. Most poignantly, population-based screens may trigger review of providers' cases simply because they lie at the extreme of a statistical distribution (sometimes referred to as a critical or cut-off value).

Population-based screening depends on comparing the rate of an event (often process or patient outcomes) in an individual provider's population of cases with a standard (absolute) or norm (relative comparison). For example, hospitals may examine condition-specific nosocomial infection rates by doctor or by department. Standards may be experts' judgment about what should be achieved (and hence is achievable) or rates observed among best providers (e.g. derived from structured performance benchmarking). Norms are what practitioners achieve usually. For example, for a certain procedure the standard or expected mortality rate may be 0.5%. If a practitioner exceeds this rate it signals that a quality problem may (but does not necessarily) exist. Examination of the practitioner's cases—for example to check if he or she followed appropriately and implemented properly specified practice policies—is necessary to confirm a problem's existence. Population-based screening can only identify providers who seem to be experiencing problems and may miss those who are delivering substandard care but who do not exceed screening thresholds or cut-offs. Ultimately, quality assessment depends on expert clinician review of medical records.

285.15 SURVEYS OF STAFF AND PATIENTS

Systematic surveillance of staff and patient perceptions and suggestions is a useful adjunct to structured quality assessment and, if employed, structured quality monitoring. Patient satisfaction surveys are essential to assess the interpersonal aspects of the quality of care. Their analysis can pinpoint quality problems that hospitals can investigate and resolve. Hospitals can also use such surveys as a sounding-board for new services and for gathering other information on community beliefs and attitudes that bear on the quality of care.

Systematic staff surveys offer a useful way to surface quality problems and gauge workers' morale. Managers should encourage and facilitate employee suggestions for improving the quality of care. They are particularly useful in improving operational efficiency, management, the human aspects of work and the quality of worklife. Suggestions represent people's perceptions of problems. Prior to their implementation, the quality management department must validate the implicit problem, either empirically (data confirm them) or consensually (people agree that they are problems), and confirm that the suggestion addresses the problem's root causes.

285.16 QUALITY ASSURANCE STUDIES

The quality assurance literature is replete with reports of 'studies'. They probably represent the tip of hospitals' quality assurance iceberg. Studies, by definition, are of finite duration. They may be undertaken out of personal interest or in response to a perceived problem. They may involve a single individual or be the work of a group in one or more hospital departments. They may merely try to identify problems or to effect their resolution. While well-designed studies may be illuminating and serve their designers' interests, they hardly constitute a systematic means of improving hospitals' quality of care and may accomplish nothing useful. Useful quality assurance activities must identify problems, resolve them and demonstrate their long-term resolution. Studies, indicating that potentially avoidable or remedial quality problems do exist, may convince doubters that quality improvement efforts are needed and worthwhile. However, this spur to action must be followed by co-ordinated action if quality is to be improved.

Continuous quality improvement requires continuous quality assessment and routine follow-up to fix quality problems and to ensure that they remain fixed. Quality assurance studies do not constitute, and cannot substitute for, an effective quality management program based on structured quality improvement, systematic quality assessment and structured problem resolution. However, from time to time hospitals may need to conduct focused quality assurance studies as part of their quality management program. Such studies should begin life as a brief protocol that describes the study's purpose, why it is necessary, and what use will be made of resultant findings, and how the study will be accomplished, including sources of data methods for their analysis. They should end in a well-documented report that is the basis for quality improvement action. If a quality assurance study is worth doing, it is worth doing well and in a context that can lead to documented quality improvement.

285.2 │ *Structured quality assessment*

285.21 ABOUT STRUCTURED QUALITY ASSESSMENT

Structured quality assessment is the essential mainstay of structured problem identification. It refers to the routine retrospective review of patients' records—after care has been rendered, whether or not the patient is still in the hospital at the time of review—to assess the adequacy of their care and to identify quality problems. It encompasses the review of medical records and such focused methods to identify quality problems as nosocomial infection reporting. Hospitals' quality management programs must integrate their various problem identification mechanisms into a coherent whole. If hospitals assess routinely all aspects of patient care for all, or statistical samples of discharges—for example using structured quality review—they can construct quality scores to measure quality and to monitor their performance and the extent to which they are improving the quality of their care.

With respect to identifying quality problems, hospitals' quality management committees must answer the following five related questions:

- What to look for?—all or some quality problems.
- Where to look?—the types of cases and how many of them to examine.
- How often to look?—continuous or periodic assessment.
- In what depth to look?—searching for boulders or sifting for pebbles.
- How to look?—what methods to employ.

This section describes and answers these questions. It also describes two automated systems: QSM (marketed by Quality Standards in Medicine, Inc, Boston, Massachusetts), which operationalises structured quality review (provides a completed outcome/process assessment system, supports review of cases failing screens, and reports results), and provides some illustrative data from QSM hospitals in the USA and UK. Later sections describe structured quality review and the operationalisation of its various facets.

285.22 COMPREHENSIVE VERSUS PROBLEM-BASED ASSESSMENT

Hospitals can review cases and identify all of the quality of care problems they exhibit (comprehensive assessment) or select particular problems, for example nosocomial infection, and identify all of the cases that exhibit them (problem-based assessment), or they can use a combination of both approaches and integrate the resultant mechanisms.

Traditionally, hospital quality assurance activities have been fragmented and haphazard, if they have existed at all. To date, quality assurance has involved predominantly some aspect of, or problem in, care across all or a large fraction of cases, for example nosocomial infections, blood usage, antibiotic prescribing. Most hospitals have institutionalised such problem-based activities as the surveillance of nosocomial infections. Where hospitals have applied quality assurance to many, if not all, aspects of care, it has usually been haphazard or sporadic; predominantly some form of 'peer review'. Hospitals' use of structured quality review permits them to conduct comprehensive quality assessments.

285.23 UNIVERSAL VERSUS FOCUSED ASSESSMENT

Ideally, hospitals should subject all cases to systematic surveillance to identify quality problems. For the foreseeable future, resource limitations will likely make this ideal difficult to approach, and its attainment may only be cost-effective with computerised medical records. Some types of cases are seen more frequently than others; some likely harbour more important quality problems amenable to solution than others; and resolving some problems will likely yield more health status improvement or cost less to resolve than others.

The types of cases that might be subjected to structured quality assessment review, for example, include those meeting the following criteria:

- high volume;
- high cost per episode (aggregate cost is the number of cases times cost per episode);
- high gain—proper medical care makes a large difference in health status improvement;
- high risk—improper medical care can be very detrimental to the patient;

- high concern—it is believed that a substantial number of soluble quality problems may be found;
- high profile—people are concerned particularly about this type of case, for whatever reason;
- high impact—action will demonstrate quality management's utility or permit evaluation of a particular quality management technique.

The types of cases that may meet one or more of these criteria include, for example, such diagnoses as acute myocardial infarction, breast cancer, ectopic pregnancy, and such procedures as coronary artery bypass graft, hysterectomy and high dose chemotherapy. Hospitals can rely either on expert judgments of where to look, with all of the weaknesses it implies, and/or use a targeting system to help focus quality of care assessments. Targeting systems use the results of initial assessments to focus later efforts. This strategy is explained later and elaborated further in Part IV.

Usually hospitals must review all cases of these types to assess the quality of their care and to track medical staff's performance. However, sampling providers' caseloads may be adequate for this purpose. Sampling reduces the number of cases that need to be reviewed and therefore improves the efficiency of the hospital's quality management program. However, sampling has a cost and introduces the risk that estimates do not reflect reality. Hospitals contemplating sampling caseloads would be well advised to consult with biostatisticians about these risks and appropriate sampling strategies. Their consideration is beyond this manual's scope.

285.24 CONTINUOUS VERSUS PERIODIC ASSESSMENT

Continuous assessment is obviously the ideal and usually the norm for the surveillance of such problems as nosocomial infections. With respect to structured quality review, for example, continuous assessment of all cases may prove difficult if not impossible, especially initially, because of limited resources. In this circumstance, assessment efforts may have to involve sampling cases by period, for example, all cases every other month, or in the first quarter of each year. Sampling by period may be problematical if there is seasonal variation in cases (or performance). Further, period sampling reduces one's ability to examine variability in trends. Sampling discharges on a given number of days each month is a possible strategy that conserves resources, if hospitals' caseloads are sufficient to permit sampling them. Alternatively, hospitals might choose to conduct systematic surveillance on a given type of case for a period in order to identify quality problems, then focus on another type, and return to the first type after an appropriate interval to check on improvement actions' effectiveness.

285.25 DEPTH OF ASSESSMENT

The finer the sieve, the greater the effort. If hospitals employ quality of care screens, the depth at which hospitals choose to assess the quality of care is an important determinant of resource use because their operationalisation requires the abstraction of information from patients' medical records (unless they are computerised). The most sophisticated outcome/process assessment systems, like QSM, allow hospitals to control the screen's sieve size (often referred to as their granularity). If hospitals find that certain quality problems occur frequently they can focus their attention on them in all cases, restricting in-depth screening for statistical samples, to ensure that new quality problems are surfaced and resolved.

285.26 STRUCTURED QUALITY ASSESSMENT METHODS

Hospitals can use one of two principal methods to assess comprehensively the quality of care. They can identify quality problems by using structured medical record review alone (referred to as unaided structured medical record review), or by first employing quality screens to identify cases with potential quality problems that can be confirmed (or denied) by subsequent medical record review.

Screening offers several advantages. Chief among them are objectivity—because they use explicit review criteria; and economy—because they can be used by specially trained nurses or medical records technicians, depending on the system. Advanced automated quality assessment screens can identify well-specified quality problems without the need to resort to structured medical record review to confirm them. Thus cases exhibiting only such quality problems can bypass the step of structured medical record review. However, for the foreseeable future hospitals will likely want to review all cases failing screens to confirm the potential quality problems that they identify.

Structured medical record review (SMR) refers to a systematic process of examining medical records to assess the quality of care. Inherently, the assessment is limited to those specific aspects of quality that medical care documentation permits one to judge. Structured medical record review may involve all or samples of cases (if used alone to identify quality of care problems), or it may involve only those failing quality assessment screens. It can be used to assess the quality of care in cases identified by any means, including case-based and population-based quality assessment screens. This chapter describes structured medical record review in the context of structured quality review.

Hospitals can analyse statistically the results of case-by-case assessments (screening data and/or structured medical record review findings) to identify trends in or patterns of quality problems, to identify problems that can only be revealed this way, or to illuminate their causes. This chapter describes pattern analysis in the context of structured quality review.

Structured quality review refers to case-by-case quality assessments to reveal patterns of care. It involves outcome/process assessment screens, structured medical record review of cases failing screens, and pattern analysis. Structured medical record review refers to the structured expert review of cases failing screens. Pattern analysis refers to the statistical analysis of screening data and/or structured medical record review findings. If a hospital reviews all or statistical samples of cases, structured quality review can also measure quality in terms of the proportion of cases treated appropriately (to the hospital's quality standards). A later section describes some of the requirements for, advantages of and practical considerations in conducting structured quality review. Part IV elaborates on these points. Necessarily, a blueprint for implementing structured quality review in hospitals is beyond this manual's scope.

285.27 QUALITY STANDARDS IN MEDICINE—QSM

The QSM system (marketed by Quality Standards in Medicine, Inc, Boston, Massachusetts) is the only structured quality review system (using automated outcome/process assessment screens) available commercially to hospitals. It employs sophisticated screens (that hospitals can tailor to their practice policies), provides automated support for further review of cases failing screens, and integrates the results of both screening and structured medical record review for reporting purposes. Further, because QSM clients agree to provide their data to Quality Standards in Medicine, they can compare their performance against one another. At QSM's annual users' meeting, QSM clients discuss these results (see next section).

> The QSM System is designed to support each step necessary for the assessment of clinical quality in acute-care hospitals. It is the first and only system which defines and assesses the quality of care based on medical science and clinical practice experience.

The medical content of the system is provided by the QSM Medical Advisory Panel, comprised of well-known practicing physicians (medical practitioners) representing major clinical specialties . . .

The system employs explicit medical criteria to screen cases for potential problems; automates the process of physician peer review of cases failing screens; integrates the results of computerised screening with peer review; and reports the quality findings.

The system is easy to install and easy to use. Data collection is efficient, through use of an expert system, and the time required for peer review is minimised through computer analysis, reserving for physicians the complex judgements which are beyond the scope of the computer.

Detailed reports produced by the QSM System serve as a concrete foundation for a total quality improvement program and provide the basis for compliance with the JCAHO and other regulatory agencies.[1]

Hospitals using QSM provide their results to a central database. QSM is thus able to provide client hospitals with feedback on how their performance compares with that of other, similar hospitals. These comparisons, especially with respect to screening results, are extremely useful because they point out what is possible and where one stands. Because hospitals can also use QSM to capture long-term outcome information, they can link the end results of care to care processes. Thus QSM is also a potentially useful tool for both structured performance benchmarking and structured outcome measurement.

285.28 SOME ILLUSTRATIVE DATA FROM QSM HOSPITALS

In 1990, QSM (Quality Standards in Medicine, Boston, Massachusetts) began installing its outcome/process assessment system in hospitals. In October 1994, at its third users' group meeting, QSM was able to compare users' performance, and to share their success in improving quality for the first time. QSM users include teaching and non-teaching hospitals in the United States and the UK. QSM provides a uniform data collection mechanism and most QSM hospitals review 100% of their discharges (with the rest reviewing probability samples), at least for the topics present here. This uniformity eliminates possible data collection and sampling biases that plague many comparisons. Nevertheless, there may be some residual variation in data integrity among QSM hospitals, for example with respect to abstractors' accuracy. QSM does not audit users' data.

QSM users' results are both striking and important. First, hospital data reported to QSM—covering over 130 000 cases—are informative. For example, they indicate that 5.6% of adult medical/surgical patients at QSM hospitals suffer a nosocomial infection and that two in a thousand of them fall while in the hospital and half of these falls result in a fracture. Second, there is considerable variation among hospitals in terms of the quality of care—and no hospital is best overall [QSM, personal communication, 1995].

A given hospital may do well in diagnosing acute myocardial infarction, for example, but poorly in treatment implementation for the same disease. Even the best hospitals for any given phase of disease care exhibit room for improvement. Figure II-8-6 on page 382 shows hospitals' quality of care with respect to medical record documentation. We chose to present the results of this outcome/process screen because its items generally represent quality of care directly, and thus do not have to be confirmed by review of cases failing screens. As explained elsewhere in this chapter (see structured quality review) cases may fail screens' clinical criteria but care may be appropriate because their circumstances were beyond those encompassed by screens.

Clearly, some types of documentation may be more important clinically than others. For example, UK hospitals do not always record time of admission or patients' weight, which they readily acknowledge they should do. UK hospitals do a better job with respect to recording patients' history of allergies and sensitivities, for example. See Figure II-8-6. The results of QSM outcome/process assessment screens involving such clinical criteria

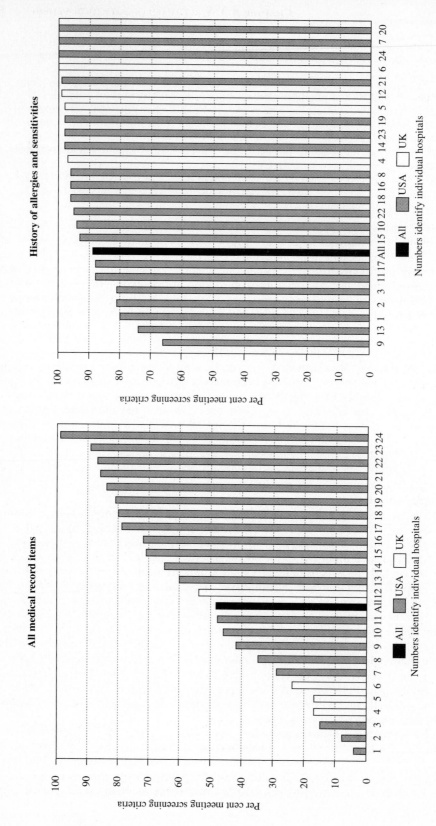

Figure II-8-6 *Medical record documentation of adult medical surgical cases at Quality Standards in Medicine hospitals. Source: Quality Standards in Medicine, Inc (Boston, Massachusetts), 1995*

as indications for surgical operations paint a similar picture of substantial variation among hospitals and room for improvement even at best performers. Can hospitals improve the quality of their care?

Initial QSM results indicate that hospitals committed to quality can improve the quality of care—without relying on statistics generated by external agencies (like government, or JCAHO or ACHS) or recourse to comparisons with other hospitals. Deciding what practice policies are appropriate—for example, those manifest in QSM outcome/process assessment screening criteria—and improving conformance to them when appropriate is quality improvement—and it is achievable. For example, Figure II-8-7 below shows one hospital's caesarean section rate from 1987 to 1993, the latest year for which data were available at the time of the analysis. The result of introducing QSM in 1991 was a dramatic downturn in what had been a rising caesarean section rate. The hospital's medical director attributes this downturn to a change in obstetricians' practices subsequent to feedback. The result was an important improvement in the quality of care. Further, avoiding inappropriate caesarean sections saved patients—or their health care financing schemes—over US$120 000 per year.

QSM outcome/process assessment screens also cover complicated medical diagnoses such as care for acute myocardial infarction (heart attack). Here too they provide useful information for motivated hospitals to improve the quality of their care. For example, in the third quarter of 1992 one hospital was giving thrombolytics within two hours of arrival to only half of its patients who should have received the drug within this period. Concerns over this quality problem motivated the hospital's clinicians to remedy it. One year later, over 80% of patients were receiving thrombolytics within two hours of arrival—a dramatic change, as Figure II-8-8 shows—but one that still leaves room for additional improvement. QSM also revealed another change. Whereas in the third quarter of 1993, 90% of patients

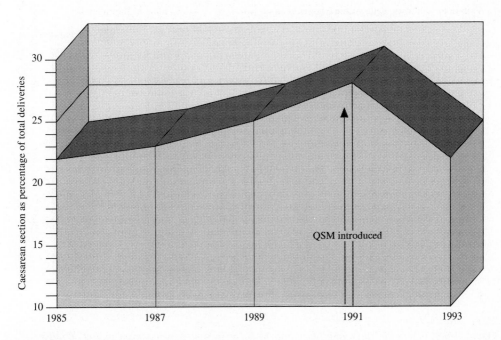

Figure II-8-7 *Quality Standards in Medicine's impact on the caesarean section rate at a US community hospital. Source: Quality Standards in Medicine, Inc (Boston, Massachusetts), 1995*

who received a thrombolytic received streptokinase, one year later this proportion had shrunk to 42%; tissue Plasminogen Activator (t-PA) had become predominant. See Figure II-8-8. However, t-PA costs far more—but seems only marginally more effective—than streptokinase. QSM provides data for looking at the quality of care and its cost to illuminate potential trade-offs between quality and cost.

The extent to which better conformance to practice policies (which specify best practices, those believed to provide maximal health status improvement within patients' desires and society's resources) actually translates into increased patient's health status is an important—but open—question that lies at the heart of doubts about medical care's effectiveness. This central question lies beyond individual hospitals' resources to answer. We must measure long-term outcomes and conduct more and better research to improve practice policies. Systems like QSM can help point to where we might need to focus our initial attention. Other chapters in this part elaborate on these points.

285.3 Structured quality review

Structured quality review (SQR) is a tool for comprehensive structured quality assessment and intends to identify all of the important quality problems in a case. It is a practical way to identify quality of care problems using patients' medical records. Because it can be implemented easily, with minimal commitment of resources, structured quality review is likely to be the initial method for, and remain the mainstay of, systematic problem identification in Australian hospitals for some time to come. Although straightforward, structured quality review must be applied thoroughly and rigorously to realise its benefits. In the United States, computer software exists to assist hospitals implement all aspects of SQR: screening, review of cases failing screens and pattern analysis. (See QSM above.)

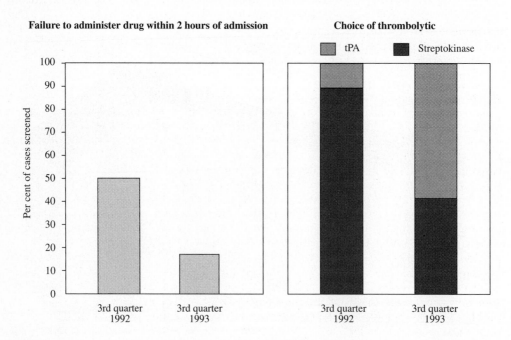

Figure II-8-8 *Two results in Quality Standards in Medicine's acute myocardial infarction outcome/ process assessment screen at a US hospital. Source: Quality Standards in Medicine, Inc (Boston, Massachusetts), 1995*

If designed and implemented properly, structured quality review is a powerful learning tool as well as a potent way to identify quality problems. Hospitals and doctors should approach and engender an environment for its use in this spirit, rather than as a means to identify bad apples. Most quality problems result from poorly-designed processes; not individuals' malfeasance.

Structured quality review is a three-step process:

- screening—systematic case-by-case assessment using automated outcome/process assessment screens to identify potential quality problems based on abstracted (or, with electronic medical records, extracted) medical record information;
- review—structured medical record review to confirm potential quality problems in cases identified by outcome/process screens (often referred to as cases failing screens), and to characterise such problems;
- analysis—statistical analysis of screening information and medical record review results to reveal patterns (often referred to as pattern analysis).

The following sections describe each of these three steps generally and in relation to structured quality review specifically.

285.4 | Quality assessment (case-based) screens

285.41 ABOUT SCREENING

Screening's central purpose is to focus expert clinician reviewers' attention on cases likely to exhibit quality problems, thereby reducing their workload to a manageable level and improving their productivity. It substitutes data analysis (population-based screens) or less expensive medical abstracter or nurse reviewer personnel (case-based screening) for very expensive expert clinician reviewers. This section discusses case-based screens (often referred to as quality assessment screens, quality of care screens, or quality screens). It describes the concept of sensitivity and specificity applied to quality assessment systems and quality screens, generic and smart screens, and focuses on automated outcome/process assessment screens used in structured quality review. A later section discusses the use of population-based screens to identify quality problems.

285.42 SCREENING OUTCOMES

Case-based screening depends on examining individual patients' medical records to identify cases with quality of care problems. As understood commonly, it involves comprehensive quality assessment, but may be limited to a quest to identify certain types of quality problems, for example nosocomial infections. Quality assessment screens divide cases into two: those in which care can be presumed acceptable (based on the screen's scope); and those that exhibit potential quality of care problems and thus require further review. Cases with potential quality problems are said to have failed the screen. They require further review to confirm or deny the quality problem's existence. Customarily, the term potential quality problem refers to screens' findings because expert clinician review of cases failing screens is necessary to confirm a quality problem's existence.

Ideally, quality screens must identify all cases with quality of care problems (sensitivity) while rejecting those with no quality problems (specificity). Missing cases with problems precludes their resolution and hampers quality measurement and sometimes may carry high opportunity costs. Falsely labelling cases as having quality problems when they do not makes extra work for and discourages the expert clinicians who must review them. There may be, and often is, an inherent trade-off between sensitivity and specificity. If so, for practical reasons it may be more important to reduce false positives substantially at the expense of missing a few true positives, if such a strategy is possible.

While screening is far cheaper per case than unaided medical record review, it can still represent a substantial cost if a hospital abstracts (screens) all of its discharges. Moreover, expert reviewers must examine cases failing screens, adding to the cost. Thus efficient screening systems must have high sensitivity and specificity (goals which often conflict), and achieve these goals with the least amount of abstracted medical record information, abstracted as efficiently as possible.

285.43 SCREENS' SENSITIVITY AND SPECIFICITY

The terms sensitivity and specificity refer to classification systems' ability to correctly classify cases according to a critical condition, for example exhibiting a quality problem or not. (See Technical Appendix 'A' of Chapter 3 in this part on page 179.) One can measure a screen's sensitivity and specificity (accuracy) and that of a quality assessment system, for example structured quality review with respect to the identification of quality problems. Generally the term applies to quality assessment (case-based) screens, but applies also to population-based screens.

Case-based screens' utility depends on the extent to which they can accurately classify cases as containing an important quality problem or not. The ideal screen would be both sensitive—identify all cases with such a problem; and specific—not identify cases that have no quality of care problems. Sensitivity is a measure of how well a screen identifies cases with quality problems (or, for a population-based screen, providers whose cases exhibit a high rate of quality problems). Specificity is a measure of how well a screen rejects cases as having no quality problems, that is, does not falsely identify cases as having—when in fact they do not have—a quality problem (or, for a population-based screen, does not falsely identify providers as exhibiting a high rate of quality problems). A screen's accuracy is defined by the proportion of cases (or, for population-based screens providers) it classifies correctly as exhibiting a quality problem or not (or, for population-based screen, as exhibiting a high rate of quality problems or not).

Until recently most quality assessment (case-based) screens had low sensitivity and specificity. Coupled with inherently unreliable traditional peer review (unstructured review of medical records by colleagues) quality assessment was somewhat of a hit-or-miss affair. Recently, systems like QSM (see above) have emerged that provide the means to screen cases cost-effectively to identify genuine quality problems. Their use gives structured quality review a higher sensitivity and specificity than unaided, unstructured medical record review, because outcome/process assessment focuses subsequent review on cases with potential quality problems and specifies their nature. Structured medical record review improves review reliability and accuracy (and hence the entire quality assessment system's accuracy) by reducing the chances that different reviewers would come to different conclusions about whether or not a quality problem truly exists and, if so, its nature. Medical record reviews' accuracy can be increased further by using multiple independent reviewers but this adds to the system's expense.

285.44 GENERIC SCREENS

The earliest case-based screens to be used widely were so-called generic screens. They are individual items for classifying cases into presumed acceptable or those requiring further review. They apply to all of the hospital's cases, hence the term generic. For example: Did the patient die during this admission? A 'no' response means that care would be presumed acceptable; a 'yes' that it requires further review. For quality assessment purposes, hospitals or external review organisations often apply a series of such screens to each discharge. They review further cases that failed any one of the screens in the series. A series of generic screens is often referred to as a generic screen set, or simply as a generic screen (giving rise to confusion with a single item). In this manual, the term screen refers to a set of related items for a particular purpose. Generic screens are simple enough to be paper-and-pencil checklists.

Joyce Craddick of Medical Management Analysis (which is no longer an independent business) developed one of the best-known generic screens, often referred to simply as MMA. In the United States hospitals and external monitoring agencies have used the original and modified versions to screen cases for quality of care problems. Available evidence suggests that such screens are neither sensitive nor specific enough to warrant their use in practice. The major problem with such screens is that they are applied, but inherently cannot be applicable unconditionally, to all cases.

Screens for subsets of cases eliminate items that never apply to the kinds of cases that they intend to screen. For example, the following screen item applies only to patients who underwent a surgical operation: Did the patient suffer a surgical complication? However, simple case-specific screens still suffer from lack of conditionality. In other words, the screen consists of items that are used for all cases of a given type; sometimes an item does not apply to a particular case. For example: Was the specimen sent for histo-pathology? This question is only relevant to certain surgical operations. Thus, either screens must be divided further into those for very specific types of cases (to which all of the items apply) or they must consist of conditional items that apply only to certain cases within the type covered by the screen. Screens with conditional items, for example if . . . , then . . . (sometimes referred to as smart screens), are the most useful but are also more difficult to operationalise.

285.45 SMART SCREENS

Outcome/process assessment screens are smart screens. They match what was done and achieved (processes and outcomes) to what should have been done and achieved for the types of patients whose quality of care they are designed to assess. The most accurate such screens are diagnosis-specific or procedure-specific and review criteria stem directly from explicit practice policies (or practice criteria) that take into account patient characteristics. The items that comprise outcome/process screens are often referred to as screening criteria, see below.

Smart screens are potentially of acceptable accuracy, although formal studies of their sensitivity and specificity have not yet been published. They can incorporate mathematical models to further enhance their performance. For example, death in the hospital is often a quality assessment screen item that invokes further review. However, some deaths may be more expected than others. Screens that could differentiate expected from unexpected deaths would likely reduce the number of cases sent for further review (unless deaths were always associated with other potential quality of care problems that also trigger further review), thereby improving their specificity. Essentially, using the information abstracted from a patient's medical record, the model incorporated in the screen would either use rules to categorise deaths as expected or unexpected or generate an 'unexpected death score'; death in cases exceeding a threshold score would be marked for further review. This threshold would be selected to minimise false positives (deaths occurring in the absence of quality problems) while identifying all (or nearly all) deaths resulting from or occurring in the presence of a quality problem.

285.46 BASIS OF OUTCOME/PROCESS ASSESSMENT SCREENS

For quality improvement purposes, a quality problem exists when:

- care processes and/or outcomes do not conform to specifications (practice policies or criteria), or to providers' or patients' expectations;
- practice policies (or criteria) are invalid or inappropriate, that is, do not produce maximum attainable (within existing technological limits) patient health status

improvement, at least cost and with greatest patient satisfaction (within patients' preferences and society's resources).

Practice policies or, in their absence, practice criteria (sometimes referred to as medical review criteria or review criteria) are the basis of all outcome/process assessment screens. Chapter 7 in this part describes them in detail. To be useful, practice criteria must model the complexities of medical practice. This degree of detail, with its implied complexity of conditionality, requires their operationalisation in automated (sometimes referred to as computerised) screens, for reasons of reliability, validity and economy.

Comparison of performance to specifications assumes that practice policies (criteria) are valid and appropriate. This idea does not mean that practice policies are correct in any absolute sense but rather that there is a consensus of expert opinion (or at least the hospital's medical staff), supported by whatever valid scientific information exists, that the specified practice policies produce desired or expected outcomes (i.e. they are valid) and that, if the practice policies involve social choices, they are socially acceptable (i.e. they are appropriate). Clearly, specifications may change as more or better evidence or technology becomes available, or as different social choices become desirable. Nevertheless, at any point in time some set of specifications is necessary if quality is to be measured and hence improved. Quality is an evaluative concept and all evaluations depend on comparisons, either to a standard (what can and should exist) or to a norm (what does exist, e.g. the best or the average).

Formulating practice policies (or criteria), that is, specifying appropriate processes, is mostly about outcomes: What processes will produce desired outcomes with greatest surety and least cost? Ideally, these specifications would be specific to the patient and encompass all aspects of patient management and the patient's wishes. Conformance to specifications is mostly about processes: Were all necessary (and no unnecessary) processes applied and implemented properly, given the patient's condition and wishes? Was what was done (and was not done but might have been expected to be done) documented properly? In quality assessment, patient and process outcomes serve to alert one to unindicated or unnecessary processes and to those that were botched, that is, implemented improperly. The presence of a maloutcome signifies a potential quality problem that the screen evaluates (e.g. using decision rules or mathematical models) or flags for further review.

In cases failing quality screens, there is no implication that care was inadequate; only that a potential quality problem exists and that further review is required to determine whether or not a quality problem does, in fact, exist. Cases may fail screens because their circumstances are beyond those that the screen was designed to evaluate. Even the most sophisticated screens have limits because of designers' limited knowledge or cost-effectiveness consideration, and some cases' circumstances may exceed them.

285.47 OUTCOME/PROCESS ASSESSMENT SCREENS IN PRACTICE

The earliest outcome/process assessment screens were simple enough to use manually. Today's sophisticated screens require automation for their operationalisation. Structured quality review refers specifically to use of automated outcome/process assessment screens to identify cases that require further review. The Civilian External Peer Review Program (CEPRP), performed under contract for the US Department of Defense, in 1986 developed the first automated outcome/process assessment screens to be used routinely to identify cases requiring further review as part of a quality assessment system. An earlier chapter in this part describes the CEPRP program.

The only outcome/process assessment system available commercially is QSM (Quality Standards in Medicine); see above. This system contains diagnosis-specific and procedure-specific, and specialty, screens, for example those pertaining to obstetrics cases. Hospitals, therefore, can use it to screen all of their discharges. It also supports subsequent further review of cases failing screens. Tools like QSM are both cheap enough to screen all cases (essential for comparing providers who may treat only a small number of cases of any one type during a year) and accurate enough to be useful. Presently, to screen cases for quality of care problems, data must be abstracted from medical records, which tends to be expensive but not prohibitively so. Smart abstracting systems, like QSM, minimise this cost by calling only for that information necessary to operationalise screens or to review further cases failing screens. They can also collect other vital information, for example to construct a disease index or to meet such regulatory requirements as JCAHO or ACHS clinical indicators. The resultant abstracting cost is a small fraction of that for an episode of inpatient care, which may cost many thousands of dollars. With computerised medical records, smart screens can assess automatically the quality of care at virtually no additional cost.

Hospitals would be well advised to purchase existing systems rather than attempting to develop their own. Development of a valid, practical outcome/process assessment system could be expected to cost many millions of dollars and take several years to accomplish.

285.5 | Structured medical record review

285.51 ABOUT STRUCTURED MEDICAL RECORD REVIEW

Structured medical record review (SMR) is a systematic way to:

- confirm quality problems identified by outcome/process assessment screens;
- identify quality problems if the hospital uses unaided review (i.e. does not employ such screens).

Structuring these reviews intends to overcome all of the disadvantages of traditional peer review (as practised in North America). Structured medical record review consists of the following steps (see Figure II-8-9 on page 390):

- initial review (involving one or more reviewers) to confirm (or deny) a quality problem, if outcome/process assessment screening is employed, or to identify probable quality problems, if not;
- if reviewers confirm (or identify) one or more probable quality problems, inviting the doctor who rendered the care (or other person responsible for the care process at issue) to comment on reviewers' determination, in a structured manner;
- final review (involving the same or different reviewers) to confirm (determine a genuine) quality problem exists in light of providers' comments on reviewers' initial determination;
- communication of final review results to responsible providers;
- the possibility of providers' appeal of reviewers' final determination, and ultimate adjudication of whether or not care exhibited a quality problem.

The term potential quality problem refers to the result of outcome/process assessment screening. The term probable quality problem refers to reviewers' initial and (confirmed) quality problem to their final determination (or that of the appeals mechanism).

Structured quality review improves the effectiveness and efficiency of medical record review in two ways. It:

- permits expert reviewers to focus on those cases that exhibit potential quality problems and displays those problems to reviewers;
- structures the subsequent review of cases failing screens.

Outcome/process assessment screens produce a list of problems that expert clinicians can use as the starting point for their quality of care assessment (a distinct advantage over population-based screens). The strength of this advantage depends on screens' sensitivity.

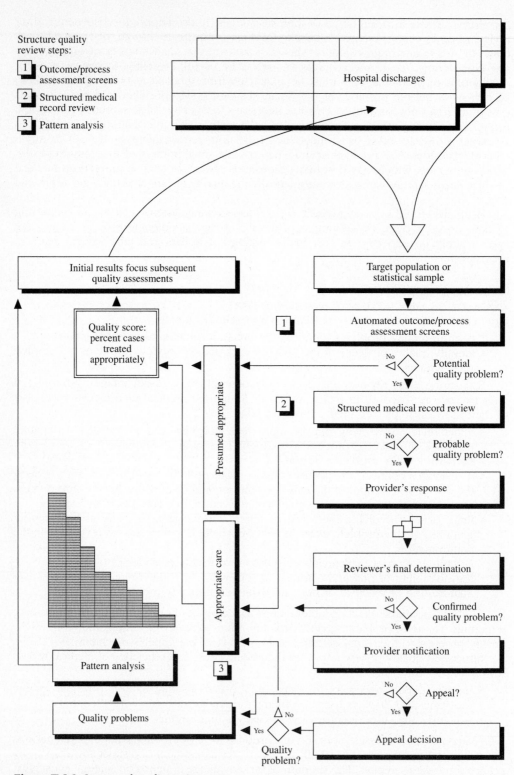

Structure quality review steps:

1 Outcome/process assessment screens

2 Structured medical record review

3 Pattern analysis

Hospital discharges

Initial results focus subsequent quality assessments

Target population or statistical sample

Quality score: percent cases treated appropriately

1 Automated outcome/process assessment screens

No ◁◇ Potential quality problem?
Yes ▼

Presumed appropriate

2 Structured medical record review

No ◁◇ Probable quality problem?
Yes ▼

Provider's response

Reviewer's final determination

Appropriate care

No ◁◇ Confirmed quality problem?
Yes ▼

Provider notification

3

No ◁◇ Appeal?
Yes ▼

Pattern analysis

Quality problems

△ No

Yes ◇ Appeal decision

Quality problem?

Figure II-8-9 *Structured quality review steps*

If they miss important problems, reviewers may be lulled into a false sense of certainty and may not look for quality problems that screens fail to identify. Focusing expert reviewers' attention on potential quality problems should markedly improve the reliability of quality of care assessments. Unaided medical record review is tedious for quality of care reviewers if most cases reviewed exhibit no or only minor care or documentation problems. Structuring subsequent review of cases failing screens to assess the quality of care, and of unaided medical record review, should improve further the reliability of reviewers' assessments.

Specially trained doctors conduct structured medical record reviews. They review only those types of cases that they are competent to judge, for example involving the same specialty or subspecialty in which they were trained and practise currently. They review *all* aspects of the quality of an episode or continuum of care; they do not limit their review to a certain aspect of care, for example a surgical operation, or medical care defined narrowly as what doctors do or for what they are responsible. Expert reviewers:

• focus on cases with potential quality problems, if outcome/process assessment screens are employed;
• are trained in and use a structured approach to conducting such reviews;
• look for all quality problems, not just those associated with doctors;
• record findings in a systematic coherent fashion;
• are subjected to rational argument (rebuttal) by the providers of the care they criticise, so that quality problems must be substantiated and capable of being substantiated.

Usually, structured medical record review focuses on quality problems that pertain to patients' health status. Additionally, reviewers can identify process problems that increase cost or diminish patient satisfaction (whether or not they affect health status). The principles are the same.

285.52 Need for structured medical record review

Careful determination of the quality of care of each individual case is necessary for two principal reasons. Firstly, one must identify only genuine quality problems, that is, criticise processes that are, or providers whose care is, truly deficient, to avoid chasing quality ghosts and wasting valuable quality management resources. Hospitals must not allow reviewers to take pot shots at colleagues' care merely because it is not the way they would do it, if the way it was done was within the bounds of acceptable practice (preferably reflected in hospitals' practice policies). Secondly, the quality of subsequent pattern analyses is inherently limited by the data on which they are based, including reviewers' quality assessments.

285.53 Selection, training and assessment of reviewers

Thinking that all clinicians are endowed with the ability to review medical records to assess the quality of care is far from the truth. Clinicians interested in becoming expert reviewers must understand what is expected of them and be trained in the proper way to conduct reviews and record findings. Such training must also familiarise clinicians with the steps to be followed to conduct the review and the forms to be used to record findings. Hospitals must adopt appropriate review procedures, including recording forms, or, if automated, use an appropriate expert system to support review. No amount of training can be expected to overcome lack of structure. Hospitals must structure review procedures, as well as train reviewers, to produce reliable quality of care assessments.

Given the present state-of-the-art, reviewers' performance is likely to remain an important variable. Thus structured medical review systems must analyse reviewers' performance and, if necessary, hospitals must adjust review processes, including the selection and training of reviewers. Improving the quality of review, like any process, depends on reducing variability.

285.54 STRUCTURING THE REVIEW

Medical record review should follow predetermined steps, with the findings of each step recorded on forms which can be keyed into computer software (or recorded directly into a computerised system) for tabulation and analysis. In principle, expert systems can be designed easily to assist reviewers and record their judgments. In practice, clinicians who are unfamiliar with structured medical record review cannot usually cope with the added unfamiliarity of computer-aided review and are best asked initially to record their judgments using pencil and paper. Subsequently, hospitals can switch to computer-aided, paperless review systems.

Hospitals can devise their own review steps, recording forms, and computer software or they can purchase ready-made systems. Fortunately, the investment in developing a simple system to structure, record and tabulate reviews is relatively modest, unlike that needed to develop outcome/process assessment and pattern analysis or profiling systems. Nevertheless, these costs are not insignificant and hospitals would be well advised to purchase an existing system or obtain expert assistance in developing one of their own. QSM, for example, not only provides automated outcome/process assessment screens but also supports the review of cases failing screens.

To date, there are few systems available commercially that offer much, in part because every hospital, and even individual departments within hospitals, want to conduct reviews in their own way and usually end up doing them less effectively and less efficiently than they could using well-tested, standardised procedures. Hospitals should develop and/or adopt a standardised structured medical record review system.

The review should encompass all aspects of clinical care, by all providers, and its documentation. These aspects include, for example:

- diagnostic workup, including inferences based on test results and other diagnostic information, for example consultations;
- treatment selection, including informed consent;
- treatment implementation, including management of complications;
- patient instructions and follow-up;
- preventive interventions to reduce the risk of, or the severity of disease if, recurrence of the health problem.

Reviewers' task is to identify all deviations from appropriate practices, including care documentation, whether or not they led to maloutcomes. Reviewers must also decide who was responsible for the deviation, lack of an action or an inappropriate action. These deviations or process problems can be subjected to pattern analysis and prioritised for investigation of their root causes, if not obvious. Reviewers must also decide if any maloutcome that the patient may have suffered was the plausible result of malprocess or not. Sometimes reasons for maloutcomes are unclear. Reviewers should only attribute them to malprocess if a plausible, preferably scientifically substantiated, connection exists between it and the maloutcome. Maloutcomes attributable to supposed malprocesses will decline if hospitals rectify such malprocesses and eliminate their root causes.

Usually a single clinician reviews medical records. Clearly, the independent review of each record by multiple clinicians with pooling of or census judgments would likely yield superior assessments, but is prohibitively expensive for routine use. If a reviewer identifies a serious probable quality problem, the hospital may ask a second qualified reviewer to conduct an independent assessment to confirm (or deny) it, to avoid the simple possibility that the initial reviewer overlooked or misread something in the medical record, and to avoid asking providers whose care might have been criticised erroneously from having to respond accordingly. If the two reviewers disagree, a third independent reviewer can break the tie.

285.55 PROVIDER RESPONSE TO REVIEWERS' DETERMINATIONS

Providers whose care (or those responsible for care processes that) reviewers criticise should be given the chance to respond to such criticisms. For example, reviewers may determine that a surgeon performed an unindicated operation, or that he or she did not carry it out properly, for example, failed to do an intraoperative cholangiogram if one was necessary. The surgeon should be given the opportunity to explain why he or she carried out the operation or why he or she did not do the intraoperative cholangiogram. The surgeon's response may reveal that reviewers overlooked or misread something in the medical record, which may be a documentation deficiency or lack of diligence on the reviewers' part. The surgeon may offer a reasoned and reasonable explanation, or may admit that the case was not managed appropriately, with or without explanation. Doctors ought to be encouraged to cite literature or research reports in their responses, since reviewers rarely know everything, rather than to state adamantly that the care was appropriate because that is the way they care for patients.

The same or different reviewers can decide whether or not the provider's response is reasonable and hence the care provided was appropriate (of acceptable quality). If individual clinical departments undertake structured medical record review, which is usually the case, the head of the department may assess the provider's response. If the provider cites studies in support of his or her care, reviewers must assess their relevance and validity, preferably using structured protocols designed for this purpose. Such assessment might necessitate obtaining the opinion of an expert in research methods. Providers can sometimes misunderstand results or rely mistakenly on conclusions from inadequate studies. If the response reviewer finds the quality of care exhibits a quality problem despite or in light of the provider's response, he or she must give a reasoned explanation for this determination. In this instance, the provider should have the right to appeal the response reviewer's determination. Such appeal may be heard by a hospital-wide appeals committee or an expert outside of the hospital.

285.56 QUALITY ASSESSMENT (REVIEW) RESULTS

At each stage in the review process, reviewers must follow structured procedures and record findings in a structured way to ensure their comparability. These findings must be entered into a computer database for tabulation and analysis. They are the results of the quality assessment (review) process that form the basis of subsequent quality improvement efforts.

Structured medical record review (and hence structured quality review) for a specific case should result in:
- a judgment about the appropriateness of care that encompasses all aspects (by all providers) of clinical care (including its support services) and its documentation;
- a list of process problems, deviations from practice policies or criteria, that if resolved would improve the quality of care, and who is responsible for them, for example individual doctor, nursing service, pharmacy, the system of care;
- a list of maloutcomes, with a judgment as to whether or not each one resulted more likely than not from malprocess (for subsequent analysis), and their putative antecedent malprocesses.

285.57 USE OF QUALITY ASSESSMENT RESULTS IN PRACTICE

Through pattern analysis (below), hospitals can use structured medical record review results to identify patterns of care that constitute quality problems. Rarely, review results will identify an imminent danger to patients. For this reason, hospitals must have in place a mechanism to investigate potential imminent dangers immediately after reviewers have identified them and, if warranted, to eliminate confirmed dangers.

Structured medical record review results are also useful in the revision of practice criteria (used for outcome/process assessment screening) and, if existent, practice policies. Structured quality review, because it involves outcome/process assessment screens based on explicit practice criteria, provides a first step toward the establishment of practice policies. Institutionalisation of structured medical record review without case-based screening provides a possible point of entry for the subsequent development of practice policies. They arise from review results, to communicate to everyone in the hospital how each type of patient should be managed.

285.6 Pattern analysis

285.61 ABOUT PATTERN ANALYSIS

Pattern analysis refers to the statistical analysis of data derived from quality assessments (case-by-case reviews). The term is sometimes used synonymously with provider profiling, a broader term that encompasses the statistical analysis of any provider-related data for purposes of describing or assessing their performance. Pattern analysis is an essential supplement or adjunct to case-by-case quality assessment. It intends to describe quality problems' distribution, may identify additional potential or actual quality problems to be investigated consequently, and may guide such investigations. Key analysis variables may relate to person, time, and place, among other factors.

285.62 TYPE OF PATTERN ANALYSIS

There are many types of statistical analyses that can be used to identify patterns of care. The following examples serve to illustrate their use. Detailed discussion of how to search for or analyse patterns is beyond this manual's scope. Often the doctor represents one of the key variables in pattern analysis. For example, a hospital may compare its surgeons' nosocomial infection rates. Clearly, patients' risk for contracting a nosocomial infection may depend, for example, on the procedure involved, disease, comorbidities or age. Structured quality review (or risk adjustment or stratification) can take these factors into account producing more useful information. At some level of specificity and sophistication, the results of the analysis move from being suggestive of a quality problem to confirming one. One should always be mindful that poorly specified analyses may produce misleading results, that is, leading one to conclude a quality problem exists when in fact it does not exist. Obviously, the accuracy of pattern analyses in identifying problems depends on the validity of its specification and the integrity of the data used.

Pattern analyses are often trend (time series) analyses. For example, surgeons' (adjusted) nosocomial infection (improvement opportunity) rates may be displayed for each of the last twelve months. Trends in a deleterious direction (increasing infection rates) may point to a quality problem, especially for a specific surgeon, if the average rate remains constant. Statistical process control methods are valuable in this context, because boundaries must be set, which if crossed likely indicate a quality problem. Natural variation in rates, including apparent trends, must be distinguished from processes that are or are tending out of control (produce results that are beyond statistically significant limits). Failure to account for such statistical considerations can result in wasted effort from chasing quality ghosts, investigating problems that are inferred erroneously and are apparitions and not real.

Hospitals can compare themselves with all, or with similar, others on one or more variables. The validity and utility of such comparisons depend upon the variables used and the sophistication of the analysis. For example, in comparing hospitals' performance based on death rates from CABG (coronary artery bypass graft) one would be concerned with the integrity of each hospital's data and how the analysis handled patient and other outcome-influencing factors that can detract from its validity. The variance between hospitals can be compared to that exhibited by surgeons within a hospital to see if outcomes depend more on the hospital or on the surgeon.

285.63 TYPES OF DATA THAT CAN BE PATTERN ANALYSED

Virtually any process or outcome variable is grist for pattern analysis. As with any analysis, careful thought must be given to its purpose, the appropriateness of the analytic model, the quality (integrity) of data, and the intended use of results. The following types of data derived from structured problem identification mechanisms may be subjected to pattern analysis:

Structured quality review
- Outcome or process data collected for outcome/process assessment screening;
- Structured medical record review results, for example confirmed quality problems (improvement opportunities).

Other quality problem identification mechanisms
- Incident reports, including the results of investigating individual cases;
- Patient complaints/compliments, including the results of investigating individual complaints;
- Utilisation and/or cost data.

285.64 USE OF PATTERN ANALYSIS RESULTS

To some extent, the use of results is predicated on the purpose of the analysis and its specifications. Essentially, hospitals may analyse patterns of review results, among other things, to:
- monitor trends in quality problems;
- identify potential system-wide quality problems that may be masked or too subtle to be revealed by case-by-case review (supplement to structured quality review);
- assess the adequacy of structured quality review (or structured medical record review) and, if necessary, re-review cases in light of particular findings;
- pinpoint problems for further investigation;
- screen populations of cases to identify doctors whose care warrants further review, that is, as a population-based screening tool (see below).

Hospitals wanting to undertake pattern analyses would be well advised to retain qualified biostatisticians, epidemiologists and health systems researchers who are experienced in analysing quality of care data to assist in specifying the analyses and interpreting the results.

285.7 *Quality scores*

Hospitals can construct a simple but meaningful quality score from quality assessment (review) results: percentage of cases managed appropriately (i.e. not exhibiting a quality problem). For example, if a hospital treated all of its cases to quality standards, its score would be 100%. If the hospital deviated from its quality standards in five cases out of 100, its score would be 95%. Hospitals can construct such scores for each type of case they treat and use them to monitor the effectiveness of their quality improvement efforts.

They can also construct quality scores for individual doctors. However, they are less useful than valid hospital-wide quality scores (based on adequate and appropriate samples, etc.) because individual doctors can be criticised only if reviewers said they (rather than the nursing service, for example) were responsible for a quality problem, and most problems stem from poor care systems.

Simple quality scores do not accommodate reviewers' judgments about the seriousness of process deviation or quality problems. Differentiating inadequate care documentation as a quality problem (which it is) from an omission that killed the patient produces additional information for judging and improving hospitals' quality of care. For purposes of constructing quality scores, judgments about the quality of care can be limited to clinical problems, ignoring documentation problems, or even to 'serious' clinical problems. Reviewers may vary in what they consider to be a 'serious' quality problem, although consensus judgments are possible. This approach tends to minimise the importance of documentation problems and provides little incentive to improve. A more complex, but more complete, solution is to rate each process deviation (quality problem) according to its certainty of effect on health status and extent of health status loss. Its consideration, however, is beyond this manual's scope.

285.8 | Population-based screening

285.81 ABOUT POPULATION-BASED SCREENING

Population-based screening depends on the statistical analysis of case process or outcome variables. It intends to identify providers—hospitals, departments or individual doctors—whose cases should be reviewed further to determine if they exhibit exceptional rates of quality problems and to elucidate their nature. The analysis may involve all or specific types of cases, for example those involving hysterectomies. Screening parameters, process or outcome variables, may be taken singly or combined in some fashion to yield decision indicators. The decision indicator represents a threshold or cut-off value that triggers action, that is, review of a provider's cases because results show that he or she is an outlier on a statistical distribution. The term threshold often refers to an absolute value, for example a complication rate exceeding 5%; cut-off (sometimes referred to as a critical value), to a relative value, for example cost per case exceeding two standard deviations (of the distribution of costs for that type of case). As defined here, the threshold may trigger review of 0–100% of providers. By definition, a two standard deviation cut-off value will trigger review of approximately 2.5% of providers (assuming that only high-outliers are to be reviewed further). This latter type of statistical cut-off value assumes that the screening variable is normally distributed. It may not be; the shape of the distribution should be checked, of course.

Population-based screening variables may pertain either to all cases (e.g. length of stay) or to specific cases (e.g. primary caesarean section rate, which pertains only to pregnant women who have not had a prior caesarean section). Population-based screening systems can, but usually do not, employ outcome risk adjustment. Population-based screening systems that do not employ risk adjustment are not quality measures and they cannot identify quality problems. Rather, they identify providers whose cases may contain exceptionally high rates of quality problems. Providers whose cases do not exceed screening thresholds or cut-offs may contain the same or different quality problems than those that the screen identifies, albeit as a lower aggregate rate. A hospital can determine its own thresholds or cut-offs, or, if available, use those derived from larger data sets, for example JCAHO or ACHS indicators (see below).

The validity of such systems depends on the extent to which they can accurately classify providers (not cases). Classification of providers depends on establishing a quality score, for example a threshold rate for acceptable care—for example 95% of cases treated.

In this example, the screening system should identify all and only those surgeons whose care is considered unacceptable in more than 6% of cases. In this way, one can assess the system's accuracy (its sensitivity and specificity) in identifying providers whose cases exhibit high rates of quality problems. The sensitivity and specificity of population-based screens is rarely assessed and therefore largely unknown. Setting up valid population-based screening systems is a complex undertaking.

Population-based systems that risk adjust validly identify quality problems. By definition, a high rate of risk-adjusted operative mortality, for example, is a quality problem, because this technique accounts for patient factors (and other factors that coproduce outcomes) and hence case-mix (whereas surgeons whose patients die at a higher than average rate may not represent quality problems because of the types of patients on which they operate). Risk adjustment is not necessary or is not possible if all patients have essentially the same risk for (are homogeneous with respect to) the outcome or there are no known risk factors. In either circumstance, one still needs to review further providers' cases that exhibit quality problems to elucidate their nature and to investigate their root causes.

Some readers may question the need to identify providers with high rates of quality problems or to risk adjust patient outcomes when the quality ideal is zero defects. For some patient outcomes, such as nosocomial infections for example, one could claim with some legitimacy that the quality goal is zero nosocomial infections. However, pursuing this goal to its logical conclusion, the prevention of all nosocomial infections may not be obtainable practically and, even if practical, may not be the best use of scarce quality management resources. At some point, resolution of other quality problems may yield greater patient health status improvement, greater cost savings, or greater patient satisfaction. If a hospital has a high rate of nosocomial infections or an unusually large variation in its providers' rates, it may decide to determine whether or not the high rate is a quality problem and, if so, to investigate its root causes. Thus, at a minimum, thresholds and cut-offs are essential to determine which cases to review further.

Screening results only represent quality scores if they are based on relevant, completely risk-adjusted patient outcomes. No such validated systems exist presently. Thus, screening results are not quality scores that hospitals can use to judge providers' performance without the need to resort to case-by-case review. Even were such screens to exist, for low scoring providers, whose cases exhibit a high rate of quality problems, case-by-case review remains necessary to elucidate the nature of these quality problems, which relate inevitably to malprocess.

285.82 OUTCOME RISK ADJUSTMENT SCREENS

Outcome risk adjustment (ORA) screens focus on patient or process outcomes, for example mortality, nosocomial infection, and caesarean section rates, as a means of identifying providers exceeding thresholds or lying at the extreme of a statistical distribution, so-called 'outliers'. Risk adjustment is needed to account for case-mix variation. The reality is that providers may treat patients who differ in their risk of suffering a maloutcome independent of provider performance. Apparent variation in outcomes among providers might disappear or shrink to statistically insignificant levels when data are risk adjusted. Conversely, statistically significant differences may appear in apparently uniform results when data are risk adjusted. While risk adjustment does not usually produce such spectacular results, it likely does improve screens' accuracy to identify providers whose care should be reviewed further.

To date, few hospitals use outcome risk adjustment screening systems to identify problems, and few such systems exist. Severity of illness measurement systems, described elsewhere, are unsound theoretically and have yet to be shown to be cost-effective. One practical problem is that a substantial amount of information must be abstracted from medical records. Hospitals willing to invest the equivalent effort in an outcome/process assessment system can identify specific quality of care problems that need to be resolved.

Systems are now emerging that use a limited amount of routinely collected information to screen cases. These systems, such as PRAGmatic (Corporate Cost Management, Rockville, Maryland), must be 'calibrated' using a sufficiently large, acceptable set of cases to yield the norms (expected values) to which individual providers (observed values) are compared for screening purposes. Such calibration is essential because performance norms may vary from place to place or change over time. The need for calibration is a distinct disadvantage of this type of ORA screening system. To date, PRAGmatic (PRAG stands for Patient Risk Adjustment Groupings) has been validated neither as a measure of the quality of a hospital's care nor as a screening tool. It focuses on mortality, nosocomial infections, and long and short lengths of stay. Its major use is by third party payers to choose among hospitals.[2] At best, hospitals could use systems such as PRAGmatic to focus structured quality review on 'outlier' diseases, if they were willing to pay for the analyses.

285.83 CLINICAL INDICATORS

The term clinical indicators is associated mostly with an initiative of the Joint Commission on the Accreditation of Health Care Organisations (JCAHO) in the United States. In Australia, the ACHS has embarked on a similar, but somewhat simpler, exercise. Clinical indicators are population-based screens. They are not quality scores and do not measure hospitals' quality of care; they are not quality indicators.

285.84 ABOUT JCAHO CLINICAL INDICATORS

In 1986, the JCAHO launched its 'Agenda for change (the Agenda), to create a more modern and sophisticated accreditation process'.[3] The Agenda consisted of three initiatives: 'the complete reformulation of Joint Commission standards, the major redesign of the survey process, and the development initially of performance measures, or indicators, and later of interactive indicator database.' These initiatives 'will be fully in place by the end of the decade. This time frame is substantially longer than originally contemplated'.[4] The attempt to collect and report 'performance' data is a centrepiece of the JCAHO's new direction.

The JCAHO's Indicator Measurement System (IMS) intends to assist health care organisations measure and improve their performance. Its goals are ambitious:

- (To) serve as a current national resource of objective data regarding the performance of accredited health care organisations;
- (To) provide comparative performance data to accredited health care organisations for use in their internal quality improvement efforts;
- (To) identify trends and patterns in the performance of individual accredited health care organisations that may call for their focused attention;
- (To) provide a national performance database that can serve as a resource for health services research.[7]

The JCAHO's original plan called for the development of 27 sets of indicators and their full implementation in the early 1990s.[5,6] By 1994, two sets had been developed and tested: obstetrics and anaesthesia (renamed perioperative). Many indicators were tested but only a few survived; some were eliminated because of variability of data. In 1995 the JCAHO added three other indicator sets to IMS: trauma, oncology and cardiovascular diseases. Beginning in 1994, hospitals could volunteer to use the five reportable obstetrics and five reportable anaesthesia indicators. The JCAHO plans to mandate indicators' use for hospitals seeking accreditation, but 'probably not before 1997 . . . they will also be subject to public disclosure.'[7] Deadlines have slipped consistently. Indicator data reporting requirements apply only to hospitals that JCAHO accredits. Hospitals are increasingly restless over JCAHO's accreditation requirements, and are casting about for alternatives.

Hospitals accredited by JCAHO are required to have a computer system capable of collecting and manipulating indicator data. They must submit data on their discharges electronically to JCAHO headquarters, in Chicago, within 60 days after the end of a calendar quarter. JCAHO will tabulate submitted data and then send comparative reports to originating hospitals. These reports will show a hospital's 'performance' in relation to others. By the time hospitals receive their comparative reports about nine to twelve months may have passed since they discharged reported patients.

The JCAHO's clinical indicators approach raises a number of concerns, not the least of which is the practicality of collecting data on every hospital discharge, transmitting them to Chicago, and distributing reports to hospitals. Little attention has been paid to how the JCAHO can use these data in the accreditation process nor to how hospitals can use them to improve the quality of their care. The ACHS' initiative raises the same kinds of concerns; in particular, about how it will fit into the accreditation process and its relationship to the quality of care.

The JCAHO's IMS is likely to prove costly, especially with respect to its utility in identifying and correcting quality problems in hospitals. Structured quality review is likely to prove far more cost-effective and more manageable. Requirements to collect indicator data may invoke high opportunity costs, by diverting efforts away from more productive methods for improving quality of care.

285.85 NATURE OF JCAHO (AND ACHS) INDICATORS

Essentially, the JCAHO's clinical indicators represent specialty specific population-based screens. Each indicator, for example in the obstetrics set, is used independently; the various indicators are not combined, for example, to produce a composite decision indicator. The data can be arrayed by hospital or by doctor, although it is not clear if the JCAHO intends to analyse these data by doctor. A hospital's performance, with respect to primary caesarean section rate for example, can be compared to others generally or of a certain class, for example small, rural hospitals. The inference may be drawn that if a hospital's rate is beyond an absolute or relative standard, for example two standard deviations beyond the mean, the hospital's performance should be examined.

More sophisticated analyses could be performed, of course, but there is no indication that any are planned. How the indicator data are intended to be used is unknown. One way, for example, would be to review the care being given by the hospital's obstetrics department if it exceeded two standard deviations on any indicator in the obstetrics set. The JCAHO also suggests that for rate-based indicators a review be triggered by a noticeable trend over time, presumably in a deleterious direction. Natural rates vary inherently, and statistical guidelines are necessary to define a trend worthy of triggering review of the department's care, which JCAHO acknowledges.

285.86 DATA INTEGRITY, AND SCREENS' VALIDITY AND DISCRIMINATABILITY

The validity of the JCAHO's indicators in discovering quality problems or discriminating among hospitals based on quality of care is unknown; it is not anticipated that they can actually measure quality of care (JCAHO's use of the term 'performance measures' notwithstanding). It would appear likely that the JCAHO's indicators will not be accurate or useful. The clinical indicator project currently under development in Australia by the ACHS also suffers from these same potential weaknesses. They relate to data integrity and screen's validity and discriminatability. We use the term data integrity to encompass all of the problems encountered in eliciting, recording, coding, storing, transmitting and using data for a specified purpose.

Data integrity is always a problem, especially in comparing institutions, because of variability in these respects. There are numerous ways in which comparability may be reduced. They include: adequacy of medical recordkeeping; accuracy of coding and medical record abstraction; differing interpretation of definitions and other operational aspects; and lack of data quality control. Many indicators rely on coding accuracy, which is known to vary substantially (which is one reason that only five indicators remain in the obstetrics and anaesthesia indicator sets of the many that the JCAHO contemplated originally). What plans JCAHO has to assure the integrity of data is unknown, although it does expect hospitals to evaluate data accuracy and completeness, review internal analysis reports, and resolve data edit discrepancies and complete data entry. If the variability in data is greater than that in what is being measured, the static swamps the signal, and the system produces no useful information.

There is little evidence that any of the indicators individually or collectively validly measure quality of care, which is not defined explicitly. Nor is there any evidence that indicators are accurate screening tools, that is, they identify hospitals with quality problems, in obstetrics for example, and do not identify those that have no (or much lower rates of) such problems.

Originally, JCAHO did not contemplate adjusting data for patient characteristics, an inherent flaw when comparing institutions whose case mixes can be expected to vary. For example, a hospital that treats a greater proportion of 'high-risk' cases with respect to a given parameter might exceed the standard or norm, but not represent a quality problem. Conversely, a hospital that treats a greater proportion of 'low-risk' cases might meet the statistical standard, but have a quality problem that is masked by its position in the statistical distribution, that is, its rate is not high enough to exceed the standard, but it is unacceptably high for its case mix. In about 1994, JCAHO decided to risk adjust indicator data. It plans to perform statistical risk adjustment (logistic regression) on each quarter's patient data (so that risk adjustment factors may vary from quarter to quarter). The validity, and hence utility, of any risk adjustment JCAHO might perform is an open question. We discuss problems inherent in risk adjustment earlier in this chapter and elsewhere in this part.

Statistically significant deleterious trends in indicator data may alert a hospital that something is likely amiss. However, a deleterious trend may only trigger review many months after something started to go wrong. Moreover, such data do not depend on comparing institutions, and may be extremely inefficient screens when compared to outcome/process assessment systems.

Indicators, even if valid, must discriminate, if they are to be useful in comparing the quality of care being delivered by hospitals. There is little evidence to suggest that the JCAHO's indicators have sufficient discriminating power to differentiate hospitals based on the quality of their care.

285.9 | Surveys of patient and staff perceptions and suggestions

285.91 THE ROLE OF PERCEPTIONS AND SUGGESTIONS

Systematic surveillance of staff and patient perceptions and improvement suggestions are a valuable adjunct to—but cannot be a substitute for—systematic quality assessment as a source of quality problems and improvement suggestions. This section provides an overview of the methods for collecting staff and patient perceptions and suggestions as part of a hospital's quality management program. Detailed consideration of methods for eliciting staff perceptions and suggestions is beyond this manual's scope. Part IV describes the practicalities of conducting patient satisfaction surveys. A later section in this chapter describes mechanisms for identifying quality problems' root causes, evaluating alternative improvement actions and suggestions, and prioritising them for implementation.

285.92 Staff perceptions and suggestions

Managers design, or at least are responsible for, production and quality management systems, including their improvement. They can accept what they inherit or they can change production processes and quality improvement mechanisms in the expectation that they will improve performance. Rank-and-file employees can be valuable allies in the quest for quality, even though employee participation in surveys or suggestion programs is insufficient to assure and improve patient health outcomes. Some quality gurus suggest that quality can be improved only through employee participation, while others believe employee participation is an essential attribute of the quality of worklife but not essential for quality maturity. Clearly, employee participation is an important factor in managing knowledge-based production, such as health care, but its consideration in this context is beyond this manual's scope.

Various techniques exist for gathering employee suggestions, including the well-accepted if not overly-stuffed suggestion box, employee surveys and focus groups. In addition, employees may suggest improvements to their supervisors during the course of their employment, or form formal or informal groups for this purpose (such as quality circles which we discuss later in the context of group problem-solving techniques). This section deals only with formal mechanisms that systematically canvass employees' views about and suggestions for improving patient care and hospital management.

Periodic surveys of staff perceptions and suggestions may address staff satisfaction and reveal morale and other problems that affect the quality of care, and may be a useful source of suggestions for improving the hospital and its management, particularly personnel management and operational efficiency. While staff satisfaction is properly a means toward high quality care rather than an end in itself, there is every reason to maximise staff satisfaction provided that it does not diminish quality of care, as would, for example, putting staff schedules ahead of patient needs. Satisfied employees stay, easing recruitment and training burdens, provide better care, and care about the care they provide.

Staff surveys may be hospital-wide or focus on a particular area, for example nursing, allowing more in-depth consideration of issues. Personnel departments may conduct hospital-wide surveys and individual departments may conduct their own surveys. The quality management department and/or its consultants should be a valuable resource for advice on the design and analysis of employee surveys, and to the department that conducts them. Low staff satisfaction ratings can pinpoint problems that would bear investigation. The quality management department should analyse survey results for such patterns and if systemic problems emerge, should investigate and remedy their root causes.

The effective elicitation and use of employee suggestions requires top management's support to create the necessary systems, the right climate and the proper incentives. Suggestions are more likely to flow if top management:

- institutionalises systems that facilitate suggestions' collection, evaluation and implementation;
- rewards initiative both tangibly (with promotions, bonuses and so on) and intangibly (with celebration, publicity).

Hospital management must fairly and speedily evaluate employees' improvement suggestions to encourage employees to keep making them. Nothing will kill a suggestion program as quickly as ignoring the suggestions it produces or their half-hearted evaluation. Employees are entitled to know, and should be told, what became of their suggestions. The quality management department may find it useful to institute an automated suggestion tracking system for this purpose.

Improvement suggestions represent staff members' perceptions of implicit problems and their appropriate solution. Prior to implementing suggestions, the quality management department must verify, preferably with objective data, the existence, magnitude and root causes of the implicit problems that they are intended to solve, evaluate the benefits and costs of implementing suggestions, and prioritise cost-beneficial suggestions for implementation. Suggestions' careful evaluation is essential lest their implementation result in unintended untoward effects or cost more than they are worth. For example the introduction of an untested or unevaluated change in the way that laboratory specimens are handled may reduce the costs of tests but adversely affect their timeliness. With comprehensive systematic quality assessment, a hospital would likely pick up such effects if they were a significant quality problem, as well as be able to track improvements in the quality of care. Nevertheless, if possible, prevention of untoward effects is better than their eventual cure. Later sections in this chapter describe these considerations in the context of structured problem resolution.

285.93 Patient perceptions and suggestions

Patient perceptions and suggestions are the only source of information on the interpersonal aspects of the quality of care, and on the acceptability of any trade-offs among quality's various attributes. Further, patients' experiences can help identify technical quality and cost problems, and their suggestions may also lead to quality improvement in these areas. Patient satisfaction surveys are likely to be the principal instrument for collecting patients' perceptions, including satisfaction ratings, and their suggestions. Other instruments that the hospital may use in specific circumstances include questionnaires administered in waiting areas, clinics and wards, and focus groups, in which an independent facilitator invites small groups of patients to talk about such matters as their experiences in obtaining, and how the hospital might improve, care (e.g. at the chronic pain clinic). Patients' satisfaction ratings, for example, can pinpoint areas that the hospital needs to improve. The quality management department should analyse patient survey results for patterns and if systemic problems emerge, should investigate and remedy their root causes.

286 | Incident reports, patient complaints and compliments

286.1 | About incidents

For risk management purposes, all hospitals must have in place mechanisms that:
- permit staff to report and the hospital to analyse incidents;
- record and analyse patient complaints (including threats of or actual malpractice suits) and compliments.

The quality management department should be responsible for these mechanisms (rather than splitting responsibility for them among different departments in the hospital). Further, for quality management purposes hospitals should view these mechanisms as an integral part of a complete problem identification system. They cannot substitute for systematic surveillance but represent a valuable adjunct to a hospital's systematic search for quality problems. This section defines an incident and describes how hospitals should handle them for quality management purposes. Specification of appropriate hospital policies regarding, and mechanisms for reporting, investigating, and analysing, incidents are subjects beyond this manual's scope.

286.2 | Incident defined

For quality management purposes, an incident is something that happened as a result of or in connection with patient care. Incidents can be classified by who reports them:

- staff-reported incidents;
- patient-reported incidents, including those reported by patients' agents, for example family member, lawyer.

Incidents can also be classified by their relationship to care:

- care incidents consequent to patient care which involve either malprocess or maloutcome believed to stem from malprocess—they always involve providers acting on patients;
- environmental (circumstantial) incidents, which may involve:
  —staff–staff interaction (e.g. doctor abuses nurse);
  —patient–staff interaction (e.g. patient murders doctor or doctor strikes patient);
  —patient–visitor, patient–patient or visitor–visitor interaction (e.g. patient rapes visitor or visitor kills patient, or patients or visitors are involved in an altercation);
  —visitor–staff interaction (e.g. visitor rapes staff member or staff member abuses visitor).

286.3 │ Care incident

The term care process incident encompasses maloutcome and malprocess (a deviation from specified process or accepted practice whether or not a maloutcome was evident subsequently). There is no implication that an incident resulted from 'malpractice', a legal judgment that what was (or was not) done did not conform to legally accepted practice standards and resulted in harm to the patient.

The term complications refers to maloutcomes of a disease's natural history or its treatment that diminish patients' health status, whether or not they result from inappropriate care. Complications may be the natural result of a patient's disease or inherent in its treatment, that is, in some cases maloutcomes occur even if all relevant processes were implemented properly (inherent complications), or they may result from unindicated or improper care (potentially avoidable complications). A given type of complication could occur both as a consequence of a disease or its treatment and from inappropriate or improper care. Knowledge may not be sufficient to always distinguish one cause from the other, and treatment of the complication may be the same whether or not it was expected. However, expected complications are likely to be better managed than those that arise unexpectedly, if for no other reason than providers are more alert to the possibility of their occurrence.

The term maloutcome is broader than complication since it encompasses such adverse outcomes as falls from beds, patients struck by providers, fires on wards that injure patients, as well as those that result from specific medical diagnostic or therapeutic interventions. Use of the broad term maloutcome is preferable to use of such terms as 'adverse patient outcome', 'adverse event', 'adverse occurrence' and 'incident' (when used to mean a maloutcome).

286.4 │ Incident reporting

When a staff member or patient perceives—and reports—something extraordinary or untoward occurred in connection with patient care, he or she has reported an incident. In contrast, systematic surveillance examines care or cases to search for and identify things amiss. Incident reporting, therefore, is serendipitous and is less reliable than systematic surveillance as a source of quality problems because it depends on someone's perception of an extraordinary occurrence and willingness to report. Staff reporting of incidents may be very low if it is equated with telling tales about colleagues or if there is fear of retribution. Patients may fear that if they complain they will not receive the care that they need.

Hospital managers can encourage proper reporting of incidents by creating the right climate, making it easy to report them, following up to investigate serious incidents individually and all incidents statistically. Clear hospital policies about what incidents to report, how to report them, and proper follow-up are essential if incident reports are to be a useful source of quality assurance and risk management information.

286.5 | Staff-reported incidents

For staff there are two key questions: What is an incident? When should it be reported? These questions must be answered clearly in hospital policies. Clearly, staff must also know how to report incidents, and forms for this purpose should be simple to complete (or, if the hospital has instituted computerised incident reporting, there should be open and user-friendly access to the system).

Patient care process incidents usually involve only obvious or gross malprocess or maloutcome, and even so are usually under-reported. Consequently, incident reporting is no substitute for systematic surveillance. Nevertheless, in the absence of systematic surveillance incident reporting can still provide useful information about medication errors, swabs left in abdomens, and other such incidents.

Incidents involving interactions between staff, patients and visitors are usually, but not always, better reported, especially if serious and external authorities become involved. A nurse, for example, may be reluctant to report an abusive doctor and a ward orderly may not want to report a fight between patients for fear of being blamed. Staff should be encouraged to report both major and minor interaction incidents because their analysis may reveal patterns and lead to steps to reduce their occurrence. In this regard, hospital policy must balance individual responsibility and creation of a non-punitive atmosphere that encourages incident reporting so that the hospital can improve its systems of care.

286.6 | Patient-reported incidents

Patients may complain about their medical care or allege malpractice, report an abusive doctor, or complain about amenities. Hospital policy should specify clearly how the quality management department should handle such complaints. It must acknowledge promptly all patient complaints and compliments. If a complaint is serious enough to warrant investigation, the quality manager should schedule, and inform the patient when he or she can expect to receive the result of, an investigation. When the quality management department has completed its investigation, the quality manager should report results to the complainant in terms of what was found and what was done consequentially.

286.7 | Investigation of serious incidents

The quality management department should investigate individually all serious incidents and issue a formal report. Hospital policies should specify what constitutes a serious incident that merits such investigation, who is to investigate such incidents and how they are to be investigated, and what is to happen consequentially. In investigating incidents, QMD staff must follow hospital policy to ensure proper attention to natural justice and provide a report to the QM committee through the quality manager (and eventually to complainants).

286.8 | Statistical analysis of incident reports

The quality management department should track all incident reports, including patient complaints, and the results of investigations, that is, enter them into a computerised database. The system should be capable of marrying reports of the same incident by different people. At least annually the quality manager should analyse incidents and investigation reports and prepare a report of this analysis for the quality management committee. If analyses reveal patterns of frequent or serious problems (e.g. among certain types of patient, providers, places), the quality management department should investigate their root causes, if not obvious, and take steps to eliminate them, to prevent problems' recurrence or to reduce their incidence. Later sections in this chapter describe mechanisms to prioritise quality problems identified from this and other sources for investigation and resolution.

The quality management department should also track, analyse and report patients' compliments so that the hospital can reward appropriately individuals' and departments' outstanding performance.

287 | Identifying quality problems' apparent and root causes

287.1 | About identifying causes

Identifying a quality problem is only the first of several steps toward its resolution. (See Figure II-8-10 below.) A hospital's quality management program may identify many problems, necessitating their prioritisation for purposes of investigating their root causes, if not obvious. Hospitals should investigate carefully each apparent quality problem. This investigation should result in a brief report that summarises why it was undertaken, how it was done, what was found and, if appropriate, what options exist for remedying the apparent problem and preferably eliminating its root causes.

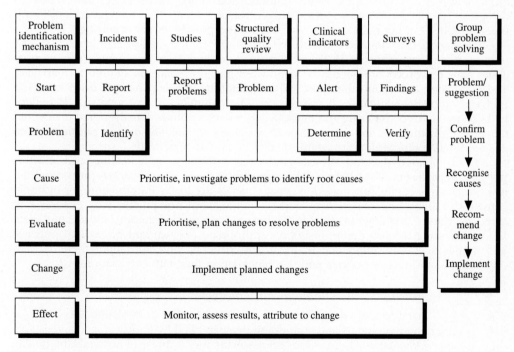

Figure II-8-10 *Structured problem resolution mechanisms*
In group problem solving (GPS) techniques, the same group members both identify and resolve (or recommend changes to resolve) problems. In other structured problem identification mechanisms, different people or groups identify problems from those who investigate their root causes, evaluate alternative improvement action, implement improvement actions and monitor their results. Such mechanisms may identify a problem, or suggest a problem whose existence must be determined, confirmed, or verified.

Sometimes quality problems' causes are obvious; sometimes not. If a surgeon is discovered to be doing operations without documented indications, it may be that his or her medical record documentation is inadequate or that he or she is performing unindicated procedures. In this instance, the quality problem stems from the surgeon's actions (or his or her inaction). But are the surgeon's actions the problem's root cause? Could the hospital's system of care or its organisation be somehow at fault? The next section points out the need to look beyond the obvious to establish quality problems' root causes. Sometimes quality problems' causes are not in the least obvious, and initial conclusions about causes are wrong. An epidemic of nosocomial infections among surgical patients, for example, may require considerable investigation to discover its root causes.

287.2 | Root causes

To fix problems and ensure they remain fixed, one must establish problems' root causes, those that if eliminated would prevent the problem's recurrence; not only their apparent causes, which are merely the problem's antecedent manifestations. The following vignette illustrates the need to, and the difficulty of, identifying quality problems' root causes.

Beneficial hospital's surgical practice quality committee noticed that patient outcomes for a new surgical procedure were highly variable, far more variable than was expected— and many patients suffered maloutcomes. With the quality management department's help, the committee delved into the reasons for the variation. They discovered that surgeons and nursing staff were not adhering to good practices: they sometimes did not implement needed processes, often implemented others improperly, and failed to recognise complications early and to manage them properly. The committee had found the symptoms, but not their cause. Why were these process errors occurring?

Pressing on, the committee discovered that surgeons and nursing staff lacked specific training in and experience with the new procedure, and there was a lack of consensus about how the procedure should be conducted and how patients should be managed. The committee had found the cause of the symptoms but had not yet discovered the problem's fundamental cause. It pressed on. The committee then found that Beneficial had no system for considering and introducing new procedures. Finally, it had uncovered the problem's fundamental cause: lack of a system to prevent quality problems from arising! What could be done to assure quality of care at Beneficial?

The committee decided to strengthen the hospital's credentialling and practice policies mechanisms. Now, before the hospital introduces a new surgical procedure, the new procedures committee: considers what is necessary for its introduction, for example surgeons' training and experience, nurses' training and equipment, etc.; ensures that surgeons, nurses, and other hospital staff have received needed training and are proficient in implementing the procedure; insists on appropriate practice and procedural policies; and monitors closely adherence to them and patients' outcomes until there is high conformance to practice policies and outcomes are in line with expectations.

287.3 | Organising to investigate quality problems

The quality management department is responsible for formulating policies for investigating quality problems and confirming those implied by improvement suggestions (and the appropriateness of suggestions for resolving them). In small hospitals the quality management department may also prioritise problems for investigation and conduct the investigations. In larger hospitals the quality management department may focus only on hospital-wide quality problems, leaving others to individual departments to investigate with the QMD's assistance. This section assumes that the quality management department is responsible for investigating all quality problems. The same principles apply to prioritising and investigating quality problems when individual departments are responsible for these activities (and for reviewing improvement suggestions). They would report results to the hospital-wide quality management committee through the QMD.

The investigation of quality problems may require access to professionals trained in clinical epidemiology, biostatistics, health services research, social science, organisation management, industrial engineering and other relevant disciplines. If the hospital is large enough, it can employ such experts for this purpose; otherwise, it must contract with consultants. Whatever its size, a hospital would be well advised to identify and build working relationships with qualified experts to augment when necessary its own quality management, clinical and administrative staffs.

287.4   *Prioritising quality problems for investigation*

Quality-focused organisations search continually for improvement opportunities. Fully-functioning hospital quality management programs may identify many quality problems of varying importance and complexity. Usually, it makes sense to resolve all quality problems. However, if the number of problems, or the effort required to investigate them all, is large, priorities may have to be established about which problems merit immediate investigation and which can be held for later. Initially, little information may be available about the benefits and costs of resolving problems. The quality management committee, aided by the quality manager and his or her staff, must use its members' collective experience to set priorities. The quality management committee may assign this responsibility to a subcommittee. Priority setting criteria may include the following, for example:

- seriousness of the problem, for example number of cases exhibiting the problem, magnitude of patient health status loss or maloutcomes;
- likelihood that root causes can be identified;
- likelihood that presumed causes can be eliminated or reduced significantly;
- expected effectiveness and cost of potential solutions;
- expected duration and cost of the investigation.

The quality management department should assemble all readily available information that would help the committee set priorities. If little relevant information is available, as a first step the quality management committee may ask the quality management department to conduct a preliminary investigation or gather relevant facts (for example, other hospitals' experience) to assess the quality problem's importance and complexity, and thus assist it to set priorities.

287.5   *Investigating quality problems*

For priority quality problems the quality manager should, depending on their apparent nature and scope, either assign a staff member or constitute a team of appropriately qualified experts (investigators) to develop a protocol, then investigate and report on the problem's root causes. Generally, investigations require only a brief, informal (one to two page) protocol that describes the investigation's purpose and proposed methods, including sources of data and modes of analysis. However, a formal protocol with review by outside experts would be warranted for a large or complex investigation. Even a simple protocol can sharpen an investigation, because it requires the investigator to think through the inquiry in a structured way and permits the quality manager or other expert to review the appropriateness of assumptions and methods.

The appropriate investigative method depends on the type of quality problem. The analysis of existing data is usually the best first step and may confirm or identify causes or suggest useful lines of further inquiry. Such quality problems as poor patient outcomes, for example excess or large variability in mortality from a surgical operation, may warrant formation of a process redesign group to re-engineer the pertinent care system. The next section describes such groups.

Investigators should develop a brief report that describes the purpose and methods of their investigation and its findings. Once investigators have established a quality problem's root causes, the next step is to formulate and evaluate alternative strategies for their elimination and the problem's resolution. Often the same expert or group that investigated the problem can complete this step. But in some cases investigators may lack the expertise to evaluate appropriate solutions to the root causes that they discover. It may be one thing to find out why a process is not working correctly and quite another to know what changes are needed to fix it and how to implement them, especially if they involve human factors (as opposed to technical) changes. In these cases the quality manager should ask another expert or establish another ad hoc working group to explore alternative solutions, starting with the investigators' report of the quality problem's root causes. Conceptually, problem resolution is a distinct step; a subsequent section of this chapter describes it in detail.

The quality manager should track all investigations' progress and the quality management committee should insist on regular progress reports, especially if investigations are protracted. The quality manager should establish a structured quality improvement (SQI) tracking and reporting system, a computerised database to track quality problems, their investigation, investigations' results and recommendations, actions taken to resolve problems, and the cost of investigations, and of planning and implementing improvement actions. This information is valuable to determine improvement actions' effectiveness and the quality management program's cost-effectiveness.

The quality manager should also report and track problems with obvious apparent and root causes, which therefore do not merit investigation, to permit evaluation of strategies to resolve them. This structured report, usually no more than a single page, describes the quality problem and its assumed causes.

287.6 | Process redesign groups

At the production level, quality management's goal is to identify and rectify problem processes, those that if resolved would result in improved product and/or production quality. Production systems are coherent entities or wholes whose constituent processes produce (good, poor, or highly variable) patient outcomes. Examining individual production elements or variables cannot account for their interactions. Consequently, the most important effects may elude analysis. Process redesign groups (sometimes referred to as process action teams) examine entire production systems as integral wholes. The more complex production processes, the greater the opportunity to achieve elegant simplicity, to ensure robustness and competitive advantage. The process redesign group's goal is to re-engineer the offending production system toward achieving this ideal and improving patient outcomes.

The quality manager may establish a process redesign group to investigate a quality problem's root causes and subsequently authorise it to re-engineer the pertinent production system to eliminate them. He or she may also form such groups to benchmark processes, either to describe or re-engineer them. Previous chapters and earlier sections in this chapter discuss benchmarking. Ideally, such groups should consist of people who:

- are responsible for and involved in the processes being examined;
- provide inputs to and are affected by the outputs of these processes;
- can authorise changes to improve processes, if the group suggests such changes;
- are experts who can help analyse processes and suggest changes to improve them.

287.7   *The case of the nosocomial infections' epidemic*

Data showed that an epidemic of nosocomial infections was confined mostly to only three surgeons. Was their technique somehow deficient? Further, analysis showed that they conducted their operations in theatre 'A' (and few other surgeons used it). A review of records revealed that theatre 'A' had been renovated shortly before the epidemic. Inspection showed that the ventilation system had been reinstalled incorrectly and was drawing air from a contaminated area into the operating theatre.

The investigators had discovered the epidemic's root cause. But had they discovered the quality problem's root causes? Why had the reverse air flow not been discovered? Why had the theatres not been checked appropriately before they re-entered operation? Why had the maintenance been faulty to begin with? Clearly, additional investigation is needed to determine the problem's root causes in order to prevent recurrence of this and related problems. Thus an initial investigation may not only provide results useful for resolving an immediate problem but also suggest the need for further investigation to reveal its root causes. This further investigation should proceed immediately, unless it would involve substantial resources in which case it would be referred to the quality management committee for prioritisation.

287.8   *Verifying improvement suggestions' implicit problems*

Improvement suggestions address implicit quality problems—those that the suggestion intends to resolve. If the hospital has an active employee suggestion program, of whatever type, several employees may make the same suggestion or the same quality problem may underlie various improvement suggestions. To identify unique suggestions and underlying quality problems, the quality management department must first collate and classify suggestions. The quality management committee can then periodically prioritise the resultant list of unique suggestions and quality problems. If appropriate, the quality management committee may then ask the quality management department to verify an implicit problem and validate the appropriateness of the suggestion(s) for its resolution. Problem verification involves establishing the implicit problem's root causes. For example, the quality management department may find that the problem is real and important but that the suggested action addresses a symptom and not the root cause of the problem. In this case the quality management department may formulate alternative actions that would eliminate the problem's root causes. The hospital should nevertheless reward the person(s) who suggested the original improvement because he or she did alert the hospital to the problem. The reward may be less than if the person's suggestion would have eliminated the problem's root causes.

The quality management department should evaluate promptly all improvement suggestions and provide written feedback to their originators. If a suggestion warrants investigating, the originator should be so informed and told when to expect to hear about the investigation's results. Investigations prompted by improvement suggestions compete for resources with those for quality problems identified by systematic surveillance of cases or care. The quality management committee should consider simultaneously both types when setting priorities.

288   Structured problem resolution

288.1   *About structured problem resolution*

Structured problem resolution is the second half of the structured quality improvement cycle. It intends to resolve quality problems and eliminate their root causes. Structured problem resolution involves the following steps, depicted in Figures II-8-4 and II-8-10 on pages 370 and 405:

- Selecting among potential quality improvement actions (solutions to problems):
  —formulating alternative solutions;
  —evaluating these alternatives;
  —selecting the most appropriate alternative, or mix of quality improvement actions.
- Implementing chosen solutions:
  —setting priorities among problems to be resolved;
  —planning solutions' implementation;
  —implementing priority solutions for priority problems.
- Measuring quality to ascertain if it has improved:
  —checking that quality improved after solutions' implementation;
  —attributing any observed quality improvement to implemented solutions;
  —tracking and evaluating solutions.

The hospital will need to follow these steps to plan and implement improvement actions stimulated by, for example:

- quality problems to be resolved that it identifies, for example from systematic surveillance, incident reports, patient complaints;
- improvement suggestions, for example from staff surveys;
- structured performance benchmarking;
- structured outcome measurement.

Planned changes may be small, affecting specific practices for example, or sweeping, affecting everyone in the hospital. Their targets may be care processes (practice and procedural policies and their implementation), patient flows, or the organisation itself. (See Figure II-8-11 on page 411.) This section focuses primarily on resolving quality problems and includes improvement suggestions from staff and patient surveys. However, the same principles apply to planning and making changes as a result of structured performance benchmarking and structured outcome measurement, although the latter are more likely to involve process re-engineering and other more substantial changes to specifications, production systems, and hospitals' organisation and management.

288.2 | Organising to resolve quality problems

Hospitals must put in place a system for fixing quality problems and checking that they stay fixed. To date, hospitals have focused their limited quality assurance efforts on identifying problems and have neglected to build the systems necessary to resolve them routinely and systematically. Consequently they have effected little quality improvement. The quality management committee should delegate to the quality manager the responsibility for designing suitable organisational mechanisms to resolve problems. Hospital management, with the full support of the hospital's board of directors, should authorise the organisational changes necessary to institutionalise this system.

Hospitals' structured problem resolution mechanisms should involve actively all relevant organisational levels in the process and devolve decisions to operational units to the greatest extent possible. Usually, existing organisational units can implement quality improvement actions. The quality management department assists organisational units resolve quality problems for processes for which they are responsible, reserving for itself only those quality problems that transcend organisational lines or whose solution involves hospital-wide changes.

The quality management department may co-ordinate process redesign or other ad hoc groups to investigate quality problems' root causes, to evaluate alternative solutions to apparent problems and to eliminate their root causes, and to plan and implement changes. The same or separate ad hoc groups may be charged with carrying out one or more of these structured problem resolution activities. The quality manager is responsible for tracking and reporting progress in resolving quality problems and implementing

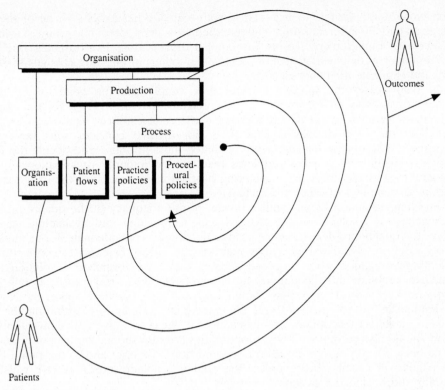

Figure II-8-11 *Structural problem resolutions: A hierarchy of inter-related targets of improvement opportunities*

planned changes—no matter to whom the quality management committee has delegated responsibility for conducting these activities. Further, hospitals would be well advised to train managers (including clinicians) in organisational development and planned change, and to seek expert consultant help when contemplating major changes.

288.3 Selecting among alternative solutions to quality problems

The investigation of quality problems' root causes (see previous section) may include formulation and evaluation of alternative solutions, or this conceptually distinct step may also be undertaken by a different person or group. If the investigation does include the evaluation of alternative solutions, structured problem resolution begins with selection of the best alternative, continues with the planning and implementation of change, and concludes with evaluation of implemented changes.

Quality problems may have both apparent and root causes, and there may or may not be obvious solutions for both. In the case of the epidemic of nosocomial infections (see previous section), repairing the ventilation system is a simple solution to the apparent quality problem (the epidemic). Eliminating its root causes may require changes to maintenance procedures. These changes will likely not only reduce the probability of subsequent epidemics but also the occurrence of other similar quality problems that stem from this epidemic's root causes (faulty routine maintenance procedures). But what should be done about the surgeon performing unindicated operations?

The quality manager may ask the same staff member, consultant, or ad hoc group that investigated the quality problem to formulate and evaluate actions to resolve the apparent problem and to eliminate its root causes (resolvers). Sometimes the quality manager must supplement their expertise with that of other experts, or he or she must engage an entirely different staff member, expert consultant, or ad hoc group to formulate and evaluate improvement actions. In complex organisations like hospitals, one group may be better at elucidating quality problems; another, at effecting changes to resolve them and eliminate their root causes.

In many cases the quality manager may simply ask the head of an existing organisational entity, for example the maintenance department, to fix the apparent problem, to formulate and evaluate alternative actions to eliminate its root causes, and to implement the best alternative if it does not involve considerations beyond the department. The quality management committee must prioritise and decide the fate of proposed solutions to quality problems that involve multiple organisational entities, restructuring a single entity, re-engineering hospital-wide processes, the expenditure of substantial resources, or other major changes.

Problem resolution begins with a review of the adequacy of the quality problem's investigation. If resolvers—those charged with formulating and evaluating actions to resolve the quality problem—believe its investigation was not adequate, for example root causes were not elucidated fully, they may ask the quality manager to conduct a more in-depth investigation prior to proceeding or they may formulate a solution to the immediate problem and recommend further investigation of root causes as one of the actions to be taken. Their report should describe each practical option for resolving the immediate quality problem and eliminating its root causes, including the steps necessary to effect the option, and its chances of success, costs, and implications. The report should also recommend which option the hospital should implement, if any, and the rationale for the choice. Resolvers' reports should be brief and to the point; one or two pages will usually suffice unless the quality problem and/or its root causes are complex and/or demand sweeping changes.

For problems with obvious causes, the way to resolve the problem may be equally obvious, and there is no need to grasp for or contrive 'options' merely to evaluate them on paper (or by email if the hospital employs paperless systems). All cases involve the implicit (if not explicit) option of doing nothing, and the report's recommendation should at least support taking the proposed actions. For each option, resolvers should provide the following evaluative information pertaining to resolution and implementation issues, and document its basis (e.g. studies in the medical, management, or quality improvement literature, studies at or information in the hospital's SQI tracking and reporting system, expert opinion):

Resolution considerations
- Probability of success, for example extent to which the proposed improvement actions (or mix of actions) will resolve the apparent quality problem and eliminate its root causes;
- Aggregate expected health improvement to patients (a function of the maximum possible improvement, the extent to which it can be realised, and the number of patients involved);
- Operational savings or costs (beyond those required to implement the strategy);
- Net savings or costs (a function of initial and recurring implementation costs and operational costs or savings);
- Other benefits expected to result from problem resolution;
- New problems that resolution of the problem or elimination of root causes or the proposed solutions toward these ends might create and how they might be ameliorated;
- Affect on the hospital's ability to make other quality improvements (opportunity costs).

Implementation considerations
- Initial and recurring cost of implementing the strategy, for example training, equipment purchases, additional staff;
- Effect of making the change on the organisation—morale, public relations, etc.;
- Implications of strategy, for example congruence with or need to change existing policies and practices;
- Obstacles to change and how they might be overcome;
- Problems that change might create and how they might be ameliorated;
- Availability of personnel and other resources needed to implement the solution and manage change.

288.4 | *Implementing improvement actions*

288.41 PRIORITISING PROBLEM RESOLUTION EFFORTS

Early on, the quality management committee would necessarily have had to prioritise problems for investigation and subsequent resolution based on information available at that time (see previous section). After the committee reviews the resolvers' report they may reassess the quality problem's importance and priority for resolution. Usually it makes sense to resolve all quality problems. However, if their number is large or their resolution demands many changes and their simultaneous implementation would be disruptive, the quality management committee may have to decide which problems should be resolved first. Resource and other constraints likely mean that not all problems can be resolved at the same time; priorities must be set. Further, while problem resolution may be possible, the cost of improvement may not be commensurate with its benefits.

In some instances the quality management committee might decide that the cost of solving a quality problem outweighs that of its continuance, and recommend the problem be reduced rather than eliminated because beyond a certain point marginal costs exceed marginal benefits; or the committee may implement a solution to an apparent problem while planning changes to eliminate its root causes. The committee may suggest that a solution be pilot tested before its widespread introduction. This strategy is especially useful if the possibility of implementing the solution or its cost-effectiveness is in doubt, or concern exists that it might generate other, even worse, quality problems.

The information for these decisions includes results of investigations that reveal quality problems' apparent and root causes, and resolvers' reports that evaluate alternative solutions, that is, known or best estimates of the extent that the problem can be resolved, and the complexities and costs of implementing the solution.

288.42 PLANNING SOLUTIONS' IMPLEMENTATION

Solutions to resolve priority problems must be implemented successfully. The difficulty of their implementation may vary substantially. For example, if the quality management committee decides that the best strategy to resolve the problem of the surgeon who operates without proper indications is to reduce his privileges, it can simply ask the credentials committee to effect this change. On the other hand, if resolution of a quality problem requires a change in the hospital's admissions policy, for example, considerable planning might be necessary to inform visiting medical staff, referring practitioners and other hospitals of the change and when it would be effective.

Planning is usually required to effect operational changes in the hospital. The quality management committee should routinely delegate the planning of such changes to the executive unit in the hospital responsible for that area of operations, for example nursing department, medical records service. Most investigations are likely to reveal that quality problems' apparent and root causes can be resolved easily within existing organisational units and mechanisms, for example changing a doctor's privileges (by the credentials committee), changing pharmacy hours (by the pharmacy director), changing surgical practice policies (by the chief of the surgical department). For solutions to problems that involve hospital-wide or complex changes the quality management committee may establish an ad hoc working group to plan needed change. Resolvers may also be planners. Process redesign groups may investigate a quality problem's root causes, recommend solutions, and plan and co-ordinate their implementation. However, the quality management committee might want to review the group's progress after each step before authorising it to proceed to the next one.

All planning should result in an implementation plan, which should be a simple but formal document that describes what is to be done, how it is to be done, who is responsible for doing it according to what timetable, with what resources and, if relevant, under what policy or other constraints. Most importantly, the plan must specify expected results, according to a time line if relevant, and expected implementation costs and operational costs or savings. The plan must also specify the means to measure results and costs (or savings) and to attribute them to the chosen improvement actions (or other factors). Measuring the extent of problem resolution, attributing quality improvement to implemented actions, and evaluating their cost-effectiveness provides vital information for assessing progress and improving future quality improvement efforts.

If solutions are to be pilot tested—as they should be if they are risky or their implementability or cost-effectiveness is in doubt—the quality manager should develop a simple protocol stating the test's purpose, the solution to be tested, and end points to be measured and how they will be measured, to determine if the solution resolves the quality problem sufficiently to warrant its adoption, and/or how it should be modified to improve its implementability and/or cost-effectiveness. If a proposed pilot test is extensive or expensive, the quality manager should ask outside experts to review the protocol and, if necessary, he or she should revise it prior to implementation to ensure the best possible test.

288.43 IMPLEMENTING IMPROVEMENT ACTIONS

Hospitals will usually be able to implement planned changes within the context of existing organisational lines and functions. Exceptions include changes in organisation and redesign of hospital-wide care systems or processes or those that transcend organisational units. Improvement actions that affect the entire hospital or process redesigns may require a considerable amount of careful planning, communications and co-ordination for their successful implementation. Quality-focused hospitals must have in place a mechanism, usually the quality management committee, to co-ordinate such planned changes. Solutions to quality problems or the redesign of care processes may suggest competing or even contradictory changes. An organisation can absorb only so much change at one time and continue to function smoothly, which is in itself a prerequisite for assuring the quality of care. Frequent changes to operations can lead to confusion and quality degradation rather than its improvement. Thus the introduction of changes (e.g. too many, too rapidly, too poorly planned) may be a root cause of quality problems—one to be avoided if at all possible.

288.5 Measuring quality and evaluating implemented strategies

Implementing a quality improvement plan should reduce or resolve the quality problems that it was designed to solve and/or eliminate their root causes. In the case of the nosocomial infections' epidemic (see above), repair of the ventilation system should have abated the epidemic (and thus resolved the apparent quality problem). Changes to maintenance schedules should prevent the problem's recurrence. The hospital's infection control program (an integral part of its systematic quality assessment system), which detected the problem initially, can track its resolution.

In accordance with the implementation plan, the quality management department should monitor solutions' implementation and their effects and report progress to the quality management committee according to the specified timetable. If implemented improvement actions reduce the quality problem to the prespecified, expected level and it remains at that level for the specified monitoring period, the quality management department can close the file. If the quality problem diminishes but is not eliminated, or if the problem remains at the end of the specified monitoring period, the quality management committee must decide if additional effort is warranted to resolve the problem or if quality management resources would be better allocated elsewhere. This decision would depend on the lingering quality problem's seriousness, the possibility of discovering its root causes, chances for implementing successfully alternative improvement actions, and so on. In this regard the lingering problem would compete with newly-identified, pending or other lingering problems for attention.

Subsequent attention should focus on checking if the problem's root causes had been identified correctly, determining if the chosen solution is effective, or deciding if the problem's persistence stems from different causes and different solutions are needed now. For example, it could well be that whatever was done about the problem reduced its prevalence by half (whereas the objective was to reduce it by at least 90%). The quality problem lingers but the expected benefits of solving other problems are greater and/or involve less cost. Thus the quality management committee may defer further action on this problem, and/or request the quality manager to continue to track and report progress on its resolution while attending to other quality problems that are now more pressing.

At the conclusion of the planned reporting period—whether or not implemented improvement actions resolved the quality problem—the quality manager should prepare a brief, structured quality problem completion report that documents the extent to which the quality problem diminished after planned changes and evaluates changes' costs and effects. This evaluation should include improvement actions' implementation and recurring costs (or savings) and the extent to which any observed diminution of the quality problem can be attributed to these changes. The report should document the source of information—for example controlled trial, study, data analysis or opinion—to permit conclusions about the certainty of validity of facts and relationships; specifically that between improvement action and problem resolution. This information should become part of the SQI tracking and reporting system.

288.6 | Tracking quality problems and evaluating solutions

As part of their quality management programs, hospitals must set up a structure quality improvement (SQI) tracking and reporting system. Such a system is essential to track progress in resolving problems and to evaluate the results of improvement actions, and to assess the program's cost-effectiveness. Initially this system is likely to be quite simple, because the hospital will undertake only a limited number of quality improvement efforts, and may be no more than an indexed collection of quality problem investigation and completion reports. As the hospital's quality management program matures, the quality management department may need to develop a computerised system to track quality problems and their resolution. Hospitals that use electronic medical records or employ a hospital-wide information network may wish to start with an essentially paperless SQI tracking and reporting system.

Solutions to quality problems may have unexpected or unintended negative consequences, that is, create new problems. A well-functioning systematic surveillance system can usually detect them and subsequent investigation will find the solution to be a, if not the, root cause. If necessary the quality manager may devise additional measures to track particular improvement actions and quality problems that they are designed to solve. If the hospital tracks actions' costs and consequences problem-by-problem (rather than as part of a complete structured quality improvement system), these tracking mechanisms must be capable of detecting problems that quality improvement planners expect or suspect that planned changes might produce. A distinct disadvantage of problem-by-problem tracking mechanisms is their inability to detect unintended costs and consequences, either deleterious or beneficial.

Periodically the quality manager, if necessary with consultants' assistance, should analyse data in the SQI tracking and reporting system (completion reports, evaluations) to compare expected with observed results and to learn from experience. Over time, this experience will be useful in improving the cost-effectiveness of the hospital's quality management program. If documented properly the information may be suitable for publication in journals, to share it with others, thereby advancing the state-of-the-art.

288.7 Evaluating improvement suggestions

Hospitals that conduct patient and staff surveys or employ other mechanisms that result in quality improvement suggestions must establish a mechanism to evaluate promptly the costs and consequences of implementing suggestions and to notify staff, for example, what became of their suggestions and to reward them appropriately. The quality manager should be responsible for developing this mechanism and reporting results to the quality management committee. Obviously, not all suggestions merit the work implied by their formal evaluation. The quality manager can screen suggestions and decide which to evaluate formally, which to refer to operational units and which to discard entirely. The responsibility for evaluating suggestions that involve changes confined to a particular unit can rest with that unit. The quality management department can evaluate changes that transcend organisational units.

Some improvement suggestions will doubtless refer to quality problems identified through structured quality review or by other problem identification mechanisms. These suggestions should be handled as part of resolving the problem to which they relate. Other suggestions may relate to the same implicit problem. The quality manager can group these suggestions for their formal evaluation. Suggestions that merit formal evaluation may compete with quality problems identified through systematic surveillance and by other problem identification mechanisms. Consequently, if resources are limited the quality management committee should prioritise simultaneously both the evaluation of quality problems and of improvement suggestions, and the subsequent implementation of improvement actions.

As a result of formal evaluation, for each unique improvement suggestion, quality management department staff should prepare a brief, structured report that documents the evaluative information specified above for alternative solutions to quality problems. This one to two page report follows that on the investigation of the implicit problem that the suggestion intends to resolve (see previous section) that confirmed its existence, assessed its seriousness, and established that the suggestion would resolve the problem and/or eliminate its root causes. On this basis of the completed suggestion improvement report, the quality management committee should decide whether or not to plan for and implement the changes suggested (and determine what would be an appropriate reward for the suggestion's originator).

For the purpose of prioritising planned changes, the quality management committee should consider simultaneously improvement suggestions and actions recommended to solve quality problems. The same considerations apply to improvement suggestions and actions recommended to solve quality problems. For example, following suggestions' and actions' implementation, the quality manager would prepare a quality problem completion report that would become part of the SQI tracking and reporting system.

289 | Group problem solving

289.1 | About group problem-solving techniques

The problem and its solution is the focus of group problem solving (GPS). The primary difference between systematic surveillance and group problem solving is that with GPS techniques the same group both identifies and solves problems. Some GPS techniques empower the group to implement solutions; others merely to recommend them. Quality-focused organisations may use group problem solving as an adjunct to—but never as a substitute for—structure quality improvement, even if they institute these techniques organisation-wide. Quality management requires the measurement of product (outcomes) and production (processes). Hospitals need mechanisms to identify technical quality of care problems, for example structured quality review, and subjective quality of care problems, for example patient satisfaction surveys. They cannot rely solely on employees' perceptions and experience. Results of systematic surveillance can inform group problem-solving. Group problem-solving techniques tend to concentrate on the cost-efficiency, worker satisfaction and service improvement aspects of quality.

Quality management does not require the use of group problem-solving techniques to improve quality. This section describes the following three GPS techniques:

- Quality circle—developed originally in Japan in 1962 and adapted for use in the West (broadening its focus beyond quality control), this technique has been adopted widely.
- Quality team—developed in the United States in the 1980s as a mandatory, organisation-wide quality improvement mechanism, this technique has not been adopted widely.
- Health accounting—developed by an American health care quality assurance professional co-incident with quality control circles in Japan.

Since GPS techniques involve participatory management, they are useful only to those organisations committed to permitting rank-and-file employees a say in how work is accomplished. Many of these organisations believe quality and participation are inextricably linked. The time needed to participate in groups may impede employees' principal duties unless meetings are infrequent or held outside of normal working hours. The quality circle is the best known worker involvement group problem-solving technique; others include work simplification, quality of lifework and scanlon plans. Emphasis on work group problem solving differentiates these techniques from such other worker involvement programs as zero defects and employee suggestions. Available evidence from industry, with respect to quality circles for example, suggests that group problem-solving techniques provide important but marginal quality improvements.

289.2 | Quality circles

The origin of quality circles is somewhat obscure, even though it is well known that they were developed in Japan in the early 1960s where they are referred to as quality control (QC) circles. They appear to have played an early role in the Japanese quality control movement, being organised primarily to train workers in quality control concepts and techniques, using the magazine *Gemba To QC* (*Quality Control for Foremen*), which began publication in 1962.[8] Today most quality circles are formed to generate ideas and solve problems, often at the lowest levels of an organisation. Lawler and Mohrman characterise present-day quality circles in the United States and other Western countries as follows:

> A quality circle is a group of employees that meets regularly to solve problems affecting its work area. Generally, six to twelve volunteers from the same work area make up the circle. The members receive training in problem solving, statistical quality control, and group process. Quality circles generally recommend solutions for quality and productivity problems which management then may implement. A facilitator, usually a specially trained member of management, helps train circle members and ensures that things run smoothly. Typical objectives of QC programs include quality improvement, productivity enhancement, and employee involvement. Circles generally meet four hours a month on company time. Members may get recognition but rarely receive financial rewards.[9]

The popularity of quality circles has been fuelled by the illusion that they are useful because they started in Japan and are associated with high quality. In addition, Lawler and Mohrman cite the following four features of quality circles as having contributed to their popularity:

- accessibility (managers can buy a turnkey program);
- management can control the number of workers involved, hence program size and cost;
- no decision-making power; easy elimination if they become troublesome;
- fadism; a symbol of modern participative management.

To be successful quality circles must overcome a series of hurdles; many never make it past go; few reach the finish. Lack of agreement on what problems to work on sinks some quality circles at the start. Managers to whom workers present their solutions to problems may not listen, often rejecting solutions outright or taking a long time to respond to them and as a result the program dies. 'Unless some of the ideas are implemented and produce large savings, . . . a significant percentage of QC programs end at this point.'[9] Implementation barriers include: lack of leadership; resistance to change by groups who must implement ideas; insufficient time to fulfil one's duties and make changes; and lack of resources or care.

For programs that surpass the implementation stage, their early success has sown the seeds of their decline, for a variety of reasons. Foremost is that expected savings did not materialise or were less than expected. Other reasons include: creation of a parallel organisation structure, and insider–outsider (participant–non-participant) culture; dissonance between the way participants are treated in groups and at other times; demands to share in savings; and a shortage of ideas that can be tackled by the quality circles after the easiest problems have been solved. Finally, the marginal value of the program may decline as it expands, caused by increased overhead, and time to co-ordinate, facilitate and meet.

Specifically, Lawler and Mohrman identify the following destructive forces that operate at various phases of quality circles' life:

- Startup:
  —low volunteer rate;
  —inadequate funding;
  —inability to learn group-process and problem-solving skills;
- Initial problem solving:
  —disagreement on problems;
  —lack of knowledge of operations.
- Approval of initial suggestions:
  —poor presentations by groups to management;
  —resistance by middle management and staff groups.

- Implementation:
  - —prohibitive costs;
  - —resistance by groups that must implement.
- Expansion of problem solving:
  - —group member–non-member conflict;
  - —raised aspirations;
  - —lack of problems;
  - —expense of parallel organisation;
  - —savings not realised;
  - —rewards wanted.
- Decline:
  - —cynicism about program;
  - —burnout.[11]

In the United States quality circles increased in popularity during the early 1980s. By mid 1985, however, 'one analyst (estimated) that 50% of the quality circle programs that had been started in white-collar environments had subsequently been cancelled'.[10] According to a 1981 survey, only twenty of 238 Japanese-owned factories operating in the United States had quality circle programs.[10]

In Japan, 'most (Japanese) companies had enviable reputations for high-quality products before they adopted quality circles'.[11] Moreover, not all Japanese companies are enamoured by quality circles, citing their lack of effectiveness. The quality guru Juran, for example, believes that 'There is no possibility for the workforce to make a major contribution to solving a company's quality problems'.[12] He believes their main benefit is motivational and morale enhancing. Their utility in hospitals is largely unknown.

Lawler and Morhman suggest using quality circles as a group suggestion program for special projects, for example the integration of a new technology into the workplace, and as a transition vehicle toward a more participative management system, which will replace the quality circles (although they are neither particularly effective nor efficient vehicles to achieve this end).[9]

289.3 Quality teams

The quality team approach was developed at The Paul Revere Companies, whose primary business is insurance.[10] Although successful and the object of considerable praise from some prominent quality gurus, it has yet to be replicated, according to its initiator [personal communication, 1990]. Unlike quality circles, quality team participation is mandatory for all employees. In fact, quality teams represent a complete 'shadow' organisation. Employees are organised into teams along existing organisational lines. The team leader is a member of the next higher team in the hierarchy, all the way up to and including the company president. At The Paul Revere Companies the entire workforce was organised into 128 teams. Originally, team leaders were workplace bosses but subsequently some were replaced by other team members.

Each team leader was trained in conducting meetings and solving problems. The entire effort was supported by management commitment and quality team central, which had a full-time 'chief mechanic' and trained staff. Each team entered its improvement suggestions into a computerised information system and periodically updated the status of each suggestion. With the quality team approach, changes were implemented by the team who identified and solved the problem. There were no presentations to 'management' (who would decide whether or not to implement a quality circle's suggestion). If a change was beyond the scope of the team's work, the suggestion was passed to the next higher team until it could be acted upon. The linking pin system in which the leader of one team was a member of the next highest one facilitated this step.

The Paul Revere Companies made a major financial and organisational commitment to the idea in 1984. This commitment involved a change in its culture to one focused on 'quality'. A key aspect of this change was to train all employees in preparation for the process and in order to sustain it. Top management promised no one would be laid off as a result of a quality team idea that might have reduced staffing as a consequence. Teams, that is employees, who improved operations received recognition and rewards even if the improvement in quality cost the company more money than it saved; about 60% of ideas did save money.[10]

Paul Revere's loss of its leading market share was the impetus for its quality team program. Within two years the company had regained its number one position. After three years the company had improved its correspondence response from 90% in ten days to 100% in five days.[10] In the first year employees logged 7135 suggestions into the computerised tracking system, of which 56% were certified. Recognition costs were US$80 000, but annualised savings amounted to US$3.25 million. The following year the number of suggestions rose to 9259 (of which 62% were certified) and savings increased to US$7.46 million. Ideas had to do with production efficiencies, like moving a file cabinet closer to the desk, as well as those that might affect the quality of the company's product.

Implementing the quality team approach required a commitment of substantial resources. Members of the group planning the initiative spent two hours per week each for six months; core staff consisted of the equivalent of 4.5 employees; 10% of the company's employees received thirty hours of training; groups met extensively on company time; rewards had to be given for certified ideas, and time spent celebrating teams' successes. Nevertheless, Townsend estimates Paul Revere received a 10:1 return on its investment. He cites two key factors for success: top management's commitment and rewards to employees. If he had to do it again, he would place greater emphasis on measuring quality as well as costs and benefits [personal communication, 1990].

289.4 *Health accounting teams*

289.41 HEALTH ACCOUNTING IN PERSPECTIVE

Health accounting is an innovative approach to quality improvement that predates health care's fascination with TQM/CQI. John Williamson, a medical practitioner who specialises in medical education and quality assurance, developed and elaborated health accounting between 1963 and 1979. Although it was tested in a variety of settings, 'health accounting' was never adopted as a permanent quality assurance program and the term died. However, health accounting's underlying principles are now widely accepted and are being implemented in many parts of the world in a variety of guises. Health accounting was probably the first demonstration of a complete cyclic approach to improve the quality of health care using traditional clinical problem-solving methods.

Health accounting focuses on the outcomes of care; not operational efficiencies. It relies on structured group judgment to identify and prioritise quality problems, with the precautionary step of their empirical verification (because at the time of its introduction systematic quality assessment was not practical). The emergence of structured quality review has largely solved the problem of identifying genuine quality problems and it has the added advantage of measuring quality and identifying deficient care processes. Nevertheless, hospitals embarking on a quality management program may wish to adopt the health accounting approach until they can institute structured quality improvement. While useful for initial quality assurance studies, health accounting cannot substitute for or achieve the benefits of structured quality improvement based on systematic surveillance.

289.42 HEALTH ACCOUNTING DEFINED

> Health accounting is a problem-oriented approach to quality assurance with the goal of assessing and improving both the effectiveness and efficiency (utilisation) of health care. This combined emphasis on both quality and utilisation review is essential to a co-ordinated accountability program.[13]

Health accounting is a philosophy, not a set of rules. When implemented, it is an organisation-wide program. At the institutional level it requires creation of a quality assurance executive board (policy group), a multidisciplinary priority setting team, and expert study teams, all of which are supported by trained staff. This structure may be replicated at the department level for intradepartment (as opposed to interdepartmental, institution-wide) projects. Health accounting involves five stages: (1) priority setting; (2) initial outcome assessment; (3) definitive assessment and improvement planning; (4) improvement action; and (5) outcome reassessment.

289.43 STAGE 1, PRIORITY SETTING

To start, priority teams 'meet only once to establish a ranked list of topic priorities for quality assurance projects'.[13] Problems are scored in terms of achievable benefits not being achieved and projects rank-ordered based on their cost-effectiveness.

> The team should consist of 5 to 13 members of the facility's staff and should represent the whole facility as well as an area of primary focus such as paediatrics, nursing, or occupational therapy. The teams should include health care professionals, administrative personnel and a consumer.[13]

289.44 STAGE 2, INITIAL OUTCOME ASSESSMENT

A study team is constituted for each project that the executive board selects for study. 'The purpose of stage 2 (initial outcome assessment) is to verify the priority problem identified by group consensus in stage 1.'[13] The study is terminated if the team's analysis does not verify the priority team's judgments about the achievable benefits of the topic or if any study does not appear to be feasible.

289.45 STAGE 3, DEFINITIVE ASSESSMENT

Stage 3, definitive assessment and improvement planning, begins if the executive board agrees that deficient outcomes identified in stage 2 warrant further action. First, the study team determines what needs to be corrected (known as definitive assessment). Next it plans improvement actions.

> Frequently, both tasks are conducted simultaneously with new improvement action ideas suggesting the need for additional assessment of the need for or feasibility of certain approaches. Consequently, definitive assessment does not usually end until improvement planning has been completed.[13]

289.46 STAGE 4, IMPROVEMENT ACTION

'The objective of stage 4 (improvement action) is to carry out and evaluate the improvement actions developed in stage 3.'[13] This evaluation focuses on the extent to which planned change is effected; the changes' impact on patient outcomes is considered in stage 5. The study leaders implement the improvement plan after it has been approved by the executive board.

289.47 STAGE 5, OUTCOME REASSESSMENT

The purpose of outcome reassessment (stage 5) is '(1) to determine if the stage 4 improvement efforts have resulted in improved outcomes, the final goal of the entire five-stage health accounting system and (2) to establish evidence that measured changes can be reasonably attributed to the implemented improvement actions.'[15] Further:

> Stages 3, 4, and 5 are repeated one or more times until acceptable improvement is achieved or until it becomes evident that the effort is outweighing the potential benefit. Stage 5 can be repeated at intervals in the future to monitor maintenance of improvements.[13]

289.48 SOME COMMENTS ON HEALTH ACCOUNTING

The one-shot prioritisation of quality problems was an obvious drawback, although logically there is no reason why the exercise cannot be repeated periodically and priorities revised. Indeed, in subsequent health accounting demonstrations, 'priority teams' met initially to start the process and annually thereafter to select new topics and, if advisable, substitute them for those of lesser priority selected previously.

Health accounting teams identify and examine problems, identify their causes and implement solutions. In this regard, they may operate in a manner similar to process redesign groups or TQM/CQI process action teams. Health accounting teams may encounter two problems. Firstly, the expertise needed to identify and solve problems, that is, recommend solutions, may differ from that required to implement solutions. Secondly, and more important, vesting implementation powers in ad hoc teams can blur lines of authority and responsibility, and undercut an organisation's functioning, especially if problems (and their resolution) cross existing organisational boundaries. Like many programs intended to improve quality, health accounting was instituted within the existing organisational architecture, including, for example, departmental structures and lines of authority.

Effective quality management often requires redesigning an organisation's architecture to facilitate continuous change to production processes toward improving product quality. Organisations should not be considered immutable and should change, or be changed, if other forms would be more functional. Structural problem resolution (described earlier in this chapter) recognises these considerations explicitly. Teams of affected decision makers working together, such as occurs with health accounting, may be an effective device for gaining commitment to change (in contrast to half-hearted compliance with orders from on high). But changes that cross organisational boundaries may be beyong the team's reach, or, if they have the authority to make them, may result in other problems because they are not fully conversant with changes' effects on processes beyond their purview.

Keeping responsibility for improvement actions within existing (or appropriately restructured) organisational channels has much to recommend it, assuming that one can devise effective mechanisms to combat inertia, foot-dragging, and other barriers to appropriate change. Creating an adaptable organisational architecture—one that has the ability to continuously realign itself to facilitate process improvement—is perhaps one of the greatest quality management challenges, which if not met will, at best, produce only initial and incremental (rather than sustained and substantial) quality improvement.

In health accounting, plans have to be made to track progress on each problem separately. Careful monitoring of progress to know if further actions would be worthwhile is a plus, but does not permit the benefit of additional work on an existing problem to be compared to that expected from working on a newly-identified problem. Further, the need to monitor maintenance of improvements separately for each problem was an obvious drawback and drain on resources. No single mechanism can identify all types of quality problems, nor can it always track their resolution with sufficient granularity. However, comprehensive systematic surveillance, involving structured quality review and other mechanisms described earlier in this chapter, diminishes, if not eliminates, the need for systems geared to individuals' problems.

Ultimately, all quality improvement actions must result either in improved specifications or process changes that facilitate their attainment, including reduction of production (and hence product quality) variance. Thus successful and meaningful quality improvement actions will manifest themselves in better conformance to (improved) process specifications and greater attainment of expected patient outcomes, both of which structured quality review can measure. Process cost accounting can track the cost of care; patient satisfaction surveys, patients' satisfaction with care; survey of enrollees or the entire community can facilitate decisions regarding value trade-offs.

289.5 *The case of the nosocomial infections' epidemic*

Differences and distinctions between structured quality review and group problem-solving approaches to quality assurance may seem very abstract. How would systematic surveillance by a hospital quality management department (QMD), a quality circle of ward nurses, and health accounting teams identify and resolve an epidemic (unusually high incidence) of nosocomial infections?

The QMD's systematic surveillance system, for example structured quality review, would pick up the epidemic of nosocomial infections. Reliance on quality circles or health accounting could well result in the problem never surfacing, especially if the excess rate of infections was not obvious, that is, noticeable only by systematic surveillance. Once the epidemic had been identified the QMD would decide what priority it should be accorded relative to other problems, and investigate its root causes, essentially work for clinical epidemiologists. If a quality circle, for example of ward nurses, thought there was an excess of nosocomial infections, it may not have the expertise or organisational ability to confirm or deny the epidemic's existence, let alone solve the problem. If the epidemic had been recognised by the health accounting priority setting team, a problem-based team would be set up to confirm its existence, investigate its causes, select and implement remedies and monitor progress and take whatever further action was appropriate. Certainly, the team could include epidemiologists and others who would be capable of elucidating the epidemic's causes. However, the team may or may not include people who have the authority to eliminate a particular root cause because that would require knowing a problem's root cause when constituting the team. Certainly, the team could communicate what needs to be done to those who could effect needed changes, but giving it the authority and resources to effect them is another matter. The epidemic's cause turned out to be faulty maintenance. It would be unlikely that the original health accounting team included anyone from maintenance.

In contrast, after finding out that the epidemic was caused by facility maintenance—inhaling rather than exhaling operating theatre air—the QMD would ascertain what it would take to fix the problem and to prevent its recurrence. The quality management committee would evaluate alternative quality improvement actions and decide which ones to implement. Clearly, fixing the theatre ventilation system would be very cost-effective and it would be done immediately, but it illustrates the need to balance one improvement against another. The quality management committee, through the hospital manager, would direct the head of maintenance to effect the repairs immediately and to revise maintenance routines, checklists and so on to prevent the problem's recurrence. The directive to change would be made through existing organisational management channels after careful consideration of implications and impacts, which admittedly, in the case of this example, are trivial, but need not always be so. The QMD's systematic surveillance system, which tracks nosocomial infections among other quality problems, would demonstrate the epidemic's abatement.

References

1 QSM. Boston: Quality Standards in Medicine, 1991.
2 Patient risk adjusted grouping methodology: what is PRAG? Rockville, Maryland: Corporate Cost Containment, 1994.
3 O'Leary D. Agenda for change initiatives: setting the record straight. Joint Commission Perspectives 1991; Mar/Apr: 2–3, 16.
4 News Release. Chicago: Joint Commission on Health Care Accreditation, 15 Aug 1990.
5 Provost J. Structural measures. In working paper 87–4, proceedings of a quality of care symposium. Baltimore: US Department of Health and Human Services, Health Care Financing Administration, 1987.
6 The Joint Commission's 'Agenda for Change'. Chicago: Joint Commission of the Accreditation of Healthcare Organizations, 1986.
7 Joint Commission on the Accreditation of Healthcare Organizations. Data collection software functional specifications manual: IMSYSTEM. Chicago, 1994.
8 Kusaba I. Quality control in Japan. In: Reports of QC circle activities. Tokyo: Union of Japanese Scientists and Engineers. Cited in Schonberger RJ. Japanese manufacturing techniques. New York: The Free Press, 1982.
9 Lawler EE, Mohrman SA. Quality circles after the fad. Harvard Business Review 1985; Jan/Feb: 65–71.
10 Townsend PL. Commit to quality. New York: John Wiley & Sons, 1990.
11 Hayes RH. Why Japanese factories work. Harvard Business Review 1981; Jul/Aug: 57–66.
12 Juran JM. Product quality—A prescription for the West. Management Review 1981; 70(7): 55–61.
13 Williamson JW, Ostrow PC, Braswell HR. Health accounting for quality assurance: a manual for assessing & improving outcomes. Rockville, Maryland: American Occupational Therapy Assoication, 1981.

Chapter 9

MANAGEMENT OF QUALITY MANAGEMENT

---

290 | Contents

For many hospital professionals, the idea of managing quality in a hospital is a new one. The idea of managing quality management is even more novel. This chapter details the concept of managing quality management under the following headings:

- **291.** Purpose of this chapter
- **292.** Key concepts
- **293.** Industrial analogies
- **294.** Quality as a management function
- **295.** Quality management in hospitals
- **296.** Planning quality management
- **297.** Evaluating quality management
- **298.** Evaluating the quality management department
- **299.** Cost and value of quality and its management

291 | Purpose of this chapter

Quality really matters. Quality is not an aspect of a product or service, it defines it. By managing quality one can improve products and services and give customers greater satisfaction and better value for money. Managing quality costs money; but the lack of quality (quality-cost) can be, and almost invariably is, even more costly, even though an organisation may be oblivious to these costs right up until the end when it goes out of business.

Quality management is required for, and is synonymous with, good management. While management has many aspects, such as financial and personnel management, its central function is achieving the organisation's purpose, viewed from the customer's perspective. Quality management intends to improve this aspect of management, an organisation's production function: what it produces that attracts, pleases and retains customers. It is an integral part of production or service delivery, not something separate. The management of quality management can, and should, be subjected to the same scrutiny as that to which quality management subjects an organisation's production function. The management of quality management refers to the process of implementing and improving quality management. Hospitals should strive to improve their processes for managing quality, as well as those for producing health status improvement.

Providers, doctors especially, are often sceptical about the value of 'peer review', quality assurance and similar programs. They are quite right to be sceptical. Moreover, because they are trained to be so, one should not be surprised that they are sceptical. Doctors' scepticism about the value of quality management might be a self-defeating prophecy. Given they feel it has dubious value, they may not participate or, at best, engage only half-heartedly, virtually ensuring little of value results and fulfilling their prejudice that it has little value. To allay scepticism, hospitals must periodically evaluate their quality management program to document its value and to improve its cost-effectiveness.

This manual describes the authors' best thinking about how to begin to manage quality in hospitals. Obviously the approaches suggested here are not perfect; they cannot fit every hospital's exact circumstances nor are they necessarily the only or best approach for every circumstance. Through experience, hospitals will be able to improve on the authors' suggestions. Quality management is about continuous improvement in products and production processes, including quality management. This chapter examines the management of quality management, encompassing a set of critical, but often overlooked, issues:

- quality as a management function;
- managing quality in hospitals;
- planning quality management;
- evaluating quality management;
- cost and value of quality and its management;
- the bottom line: quality management will improve quality and may save money.

---

292 | Key concepts

This chapter elaborates on the following key concepts essential to understanding the management of quality management.

- Worldwide, industry has realised that it is quality or else. As the years pass, the gap between the best and the rest grows exponentially. Companies are devoting considerable time, attention and resources to quality management; not for competitive advantage, but for their survival. Hospitals should view quality management in this same light.
- In many companies the quality revolution is on paper rather than on the shop floor. Lip-service to quality management, the installation of amorphous, isolated, or window-dressing programs, cannot and will not improve quality. In other companies, quality management programs have simply ground to a halt because they have failed to produce expected results. Often they focused on the structure of quality management processes rather than their outcome or effectiveness, and failed to focus on what matters most to customers: the quality of goods and services.
- Health care has yet to come to grips with the quality revolution. Medicine poses a far greater quality management challenge than does manufacturing, even though the same basic principles apply. In this decade, and beyond, quality management—rational decisions about health care's products and how best to produce them—will be one of the hospital's most significant challenges.
- Quality management is, or should be, an essential component of hospital management. It provides the information to reassure patients about the

hospital's quality of care and to improve continuously the quality of that care. Today, in most hospitals quality management is conspicuous by its absence.

- Quality management offers a different, more useful perspective on the organisation and delivery of health care for purposes of improving its quality. This paradigm requires managers, doctors, nurses and others to view the hospital as a production system designed to improve patients' health status; commit to quality; and measure performance.

- The hospital is a health-producing facility; its purpose is to improve patients' health status. Everything that the hospital and everyone in it does must be geared to accomplishing this purpose. Managers, doctors, nurses and others are all necessary, and no one and no group alone is sufficient to achieve the hospital's purpose.

- There are no quick fix solutions. Managers must stay the course and avoid sounding the retreat at the first sight of resistance. Managers must back demands with deeds. They must recognise excellence and reward success. Managers' failure to change can doom quality management efforts every bit as much as their lack of commitment or the absence of supporting structures and processes.

- Quality management means meaningful measurement. Health care has been devoid of meaningful feedback to improve its quality. Experience can be misleading; perceptions can be wrong; and so-called solutions may not yield much improvement. Actions may be hit or miss, and without feedback no one will know that anything has really improved. Managers must provide the will, the means and the incentives to measure care processes and outcomes, and to use the resultant information to improve quality.

- Quality management must include all of the hospital's activities, especially clinical care, the core of its production function. Improving the hospital laundry, while a laudable, useful and achievable goal, will make very little difference if the quality of clinical care remains unaltered.

- Today there are virtually no incentives for hospitals to implement meaningful quality management programs. There are powerful disincentives, including the need to fund quality management from existing budgets without any way of increasing revenues by offering higher quality care or better value for money. Effective quality management requires bringing rewards in line with value added. Positive incentives (carrots) are far more powerful and important than negative ones (sticks); presently, managers lack both.

- Ultimately, the hospital's board of directors is responsible for the quality of its care. Operationally, this responsibility rests with the manager. His or her instrument for policy guidance is the hospital-wide quality management committee (QMC). The manager's principal resource is a qualified quality manager, who sits on, and may chair, the quality management committee, and heads the hospital's quality management department (QMD). Without a qualified quality manager and supporting professional staff, the hospital's chances of implementing an effective quality management program are slim to none.

- Quality assurance and improvement activities should be based as close to the point of production as possible. Quality is produced by front-line health professionals who treat patients; not by quality managers. The quality manager's function is to provide front-line workers with the circumstances and systems that they need to do their jobs well, to measure performance, to reward excellence, and, if necessary, to change circumstances, systems and people to bring out the best in those willing and able to deliver the highest possible quality of care.

• A hospital's quality management plan focuses its quality management efforts. Its most useful aspect is the process for developing the plan. The strategic plan embodies the hospital's quality management policy, a written statement of its commitment to quality. It must aim to make quality a routine part of hospital operations, not the isolated concern of the quality management department. The annual implementation plan specifies what will be accomplished in the coming year. At year's end, the hospital must evaluate its progress in relation to its plans.

• Planning is not dreaming. Quality management plans must specify potentially achievable objectives and describe plausible means for their achievement, including budgets that represent financial commitments. Problems in the hospital, including an inability to provide services within budgets, may occasion an increase—not decrease—in quality management activities and the QMD's budget.

• A hospital's quality management program can, and should, be subjected to the same scrutiny and continuous improvement to which the program subjects clinical care and hospital operations. Changes must be justified by their effect on improving the quality of care and the cost of attaining such improvement.

• Program evaluation, gauging a program's worth, is an essential element of managing quality management. Every year the hospital should compare what the program achieved and spent with what it planned to achieve and to spend. The quality manager should explain variances from plans or previous performance as part of preparing next year's plan. This annual evaluation and planning cycle, repeated endlessly, permits the hospital to progress toward quality maturity.

• A proper external audit of a hospital's QA/QI mechanisms and accomplishments is the most useful evaluation because it provides an objective assessment of the hospital's quality of care and a direct means of evaluating its quality management program. Whenever possible, hospitals should compare their performance to learn where they stand and what level of performance is possible.

• Whether or not to have a quality management program is not a relevant question. The only relevant question is: Which quality management program best suits the hospital's circumstances? To improve the management of quality management, the hospital must measure what its quality management program is achieving and how much it is costing to achieve it.

• Initially, quality management may increase costs because the hospital must pay for the quality management program and, in some cases, doctors may be undertreating cases now (in comparison to best practices).

• In principle, a quality-mature hospital can expect lower costs from: reduced liability insurance premiums, malpractice claims and monetary damages; reduced iatrogenesis, specifically preventable errors and clinical complications; reduced unnecessary tests and treatments; improved clinical efficiency resulting from quicker diagnosis, better treatment selection, etc; improved operational efficiency, with resultant better use of resources; and improved productivity through enhanced employee job satisfaction and morale.

- Reduced costs may only result in savings if wards are closed, staff are laid off, or other similar measures are taken to cut expenditures because the same or more health status improvement can be achieved with fewer resources. Keeping the same resources in place would mean that some services are idle some of the time, or that the hospital is providing services to additional patients. In either case, no savings would result. Savings can only accrue to the hospital if government alters present perverse incentives. If quality management is to be truly successful, payment for care must be based on its quality and the efficiency of its production.
- The bottom line: We do not know how much money quality management can, let alone will, save. Its main benefit is improving the quality of care and reducing variability, giving patients more health status improvement with greater certainty. If quality-focused care costs the same as or less than present care, that is an added benefit. Certainly it provides better value for money.

293 | Industrial analogies

293.1 | Quality or else

Industy has become enamoured with 'quality'. Quality management focuses an organisation's attention on what value its products add to customers' quality of life, expressed usually in terms of meeting their latent or overt needs or wants. While production management is only one aspect of management, quality management puts the spotlight on what an organisation produces and how well it produces it. In business, the customer is always right, and the best and most lasting way to make a profit is to produce what the customer wants at or below the price that he or she is willing to pay. Competition drives manufacturers' quest for quality and productivity. This philosophy is best, and most simply, illustrated in the manufacture of goods, such as automobiles and customer electronics. Virtually all existing quality management concepts and techniques stem from manufacturing. For the most part, they are elegantly simple. Success depends on applying these concepts systematically and constantly and consistently.

Worldwide industry has realised that it is quality or else risk the loss of one's business.[1] Quality does not always cost more; production system can produce better quality and lower costs. Companies are devoting considerable time, attention and resources to quality managment. There is no other choice if they want to survive. A company's survival depends on how well it anticipates and meets customer needs. In a global economy, companies in far-flung countries compete in the production of almost all goods and services. Economic dominance, competitiveness and people's standard of living rest on quality. Quality is a management philosophy manifest in an organisation's production system; an organisation's products are its raison d'etre. The products' quality determines whether or not the organisation survives or dies.

293.2 | Successful strategies

In his foreword to the book *Health care quality management for the 21st century*, the American Joseph Juran, a giant of industrial quality management, writes:

> During the past few decades many of our manufacturing companies encountered crises arising from intensified competition in quality. These companies tested various new strategies for making themselves more competitive. Some of them achieved stunningly successful results—much higher quality at much lower costs. The companies that achieved such results did so mainly through some combination of the following strategies:

—Their upper managers personally directed a new approach toward quality management by creating and serving on a guiding quality council. In effect, the upper managers took charge of quality management.

—They adopted the concept of 'Big Q', which applies quality management to business processes as well as to traditional operating processes and to the needs of internal customers as well as external customers.

—They adopted the concept of mandated, annual quality improvement at a revolutionary pace. To this end, they created an infrastructure to identify the needed quality improvements and to assign clear responsibility for making those improvements.

—They adopted the concept that planning for quality should involve participation by those who will be affected by the plan. They also adopted a modern quality-focused methodology to replace empiricism in quality planning.

—They undertook to train all members of the managerial hierarchy in the modern processes of managing for quality: quality planning, quality control and quality improvement.

—They provided the workforce with opportunities to receive training and to participate actively in the processes of managing for quality.

—They enlarged strategic business plans to include quality goals, as well as the means for meeting those goals.[2]

293.3 Lessons for health care

Health care has yet to come to grips with the quality revolution. Improving the hospital catering service, while a laudable, useful and achievable goal, will make very little difference if the quality of clinical care remains unaltered. Medicine poses a far greater quality management challenge than does manufacturing. However, the same principles apply, even if the methodologies must be necessarily more complicated and sophisticated. The basic technologies necessary to improve medical practice exist now and more sophisticated versions are on the way. Their use will stimulate still further improvements. The longer one waits to get started, the further behind one will be. As the years pass linearly, the gap between the best and the rest grows exponentially. Manufacturing industry has already seen it happen. Any industry that falls behind has to try that much harder to catch up, let alone move and stay ahead.

Sitting in a hospital in Australia, it may be hard to envision how the Japanese or anyone else could compete with you in improving health care. True, hospitals may be full of foreign-made equipment and drugs may be products of multinational pharmaceutical companies, and Japanese computers might be seen in clinics, if they have any at all—but Australian doctors are still providing the care. How could this change? Biomedical technology and medical practice, like manufacturing, services, and virtually all aspects of business, are becoming global. The cost of pharmaceutical research and development is now so high that it can be recouped only if its products are sold worldwide as fast as possible after their discovery. Only truly global companies can expect to survive as world-class players.

Advances in medical informatics (management of health science knowledge, and clinical and patient information), fuelled by advances in artificial intelligence, computer technology and telecommunications, will revolutionise the practice of medicine within the next thirty years. Uncontrollable increases in the cost of care and patients' desire for the best possible care, will all but make their use inevitable. Artificial intelligence will manifest itself in all areas of medical practice from robodocs (robots assisting surgeons) to compudocs (desktop computers assisting doctors diagnose, treat and manage patients' care). Digitised images taken in remote clinics can be interpreted by expert clinicians in Sydney or London or Boston—and will be if they provide better service at less cost than is available locally.

In the near future, hospitals are unlikely to be filled with DSTs (decision support technology) labelled 'Made in Japan', but that day may come. The knowledge base they incorporate may come initially from the United States, adapted to Australian preferences and practices. When that day arrives Australian hospitals will be delivering care based on American knowledge whose quality is assured by Japanese technology. The public will demand its use because outcomes will be demonstrably better and the cost of care measurably less; millions of dollars will be added to the trade imbalance.

Even if that day never comes, Australian health care will be under pressure from other countries that may offer better care at lower prices, tempting people abroad for treatment. The cost of everything depends on input costs, including that of health care. Certainly, the United States' vast health care spending (over 14% of GNP and rising) is not helping its international economic competitiveness and is depressing its workers' wages. Employers must divert a large share of productivity gains to health care, money that otherwise would be available for wage increases. Industries that lag in productivity gains—like health care—experience cost inflation unless they cut workers' wages.

Perhaps the Dutch or someone else will master the technology of health care quality management and set up competing hospitals that offer guaranteed outcomes at fixed prices. Certainly they can be kept out, but only until people realise that they could be getting better value for money. Perhaps those other hospitals might even be in a different Australian state. Even without direct foreign competition, the winds of change are likely to blow with sufficient force to make business as usual a remote possibility. Health care has a preference for the status quo; for the semblance of change for any real change; and for token initiatives over fundamental reforms. Quality management demands no less than total commitment to continuous change.

In every industry there is a complacent giant and a thousand start-ups. The giant believes it can safely ignore the start-ups; most of them will die. But those few that survive can wipe out a once mighty and seemingly impregnable giant or force it to make painful adjustments to a new reality. There is no reason not to make a good thing better. By being proactive one can stave off unpleasant changes dictated by others. Manufacturers have found this out, often at the cost of their business.

293.4 What it takes

The appearance of concern with quality, form over substance, is doomed to failure from the outset: hospitals must institute genuine quality management. Even with the best possible intentions, success is not guaranteed and hospitals must manage quality management. In many Western companies quality management programs have simply ground to a halt because they have failed to produce expected results. Often they focused on the structure of quality management processes rather than their outcome or effectiveness, and failed to focus on what matters most to customers: the quality of goods and services.

The organisation's chief executive officer must also be its chief quality officer. He or she must enlist the assistance of a quality manager who reports to him or her directly, and who heads a team of quality management professionals. Quality management cannot be the concern of a lowly individual or of an isolated group. Successful quality management programs pervade the entire organisation and everyone is engaged in quality improvement efforts. To succeed in the quest for quality, organisations must institutionalise quality management as their way of doing business, focus on end results, and subject quality management programs to the same rigorous scrutiny to which they subject their production function. Quality management is the business of improving product quality. Quality management of QM is the business of improving quality management.

294 | Quality as a management function

294.1 | Quality management is good management

Experienced managers know that attention to quality is simply 'good management'. Highly successful companies have long been mindful of their products' quality. Health-producing facilities have long been one of the worst managed sectors of the economy. Only recently has health care even been thought of as an important part of the economy. Indeed it is. In many developed, postindustrial countries the health sector is, or will soon be, one of, if not the, largest economic sectors. Despite the size of our largest hospitals, health care is still predominantly a cottage industry, at least in terms of its management. Virtually no attention has been paid to health care's product nor to the production of health. Before reading this manual how many readers would have conceived of health improvement as a product, let alone the nature of its production? With the ever increasing cost of health care, the dawn of the era of quality, and the advent of technologies to assess and measure the quality of health care, this situation is about to change. In this decade and beyond, quality management—rational decisions about health care's products and how best to produce them—will be one of hospitals' most significant challenges.

294.2 | Quality management: time for a new view

Quality management offers a different, more useful perspective on the organisation and delivery of health care for purposes of improving its quality. As with any paradigm shift it involves viewing, and then doing, things differently. All change is painful to those who must change. With continuous change the pain can become unbearable unless organisations manage it appropriately. Change can be challenging, even fun, if one participates meaningfully in the process rather than being a victim of others' decisions. Participation can be threatening to managers, especially those who believe or fear that they are inadequate for the task. Quality management should threaten no one and help everyone do his or her job better. It substitutes confidence for fear and replaces deficiency and demise with the common goals of satisfying customers and survival. This new quality management paradigm requires managers and doctors and ultimately all of the hospital's staff members to view the hospital as a production system designed to improve patients' health status, commit to quality, and measure performance.

294.3 | Hospital as a production system

The hospital is a health-producing facility; its purpose is to improve patients' health status. Everything that the hospital and everyone in it does must be geared to accomplishing this purpose. Managers, doctors, nurses and others are all necessary, and no one and no group alone is sufficient to achieve the hospital's purpose.

Hospitals have often been seen to be or been run as doctors' workshops. Historically, hospital managers minded the laundry, food preparation and so on, while doctors got on with the important job of healing the patient. Just as the doctor's job has become more complex, so has the task of running a hospital, in part because of the increased complexity of medical technology. This new complexity requires a new breed of manager, as it has required better educated doctors. Most importantly, it requires the realisation that only by viewing patient care as a total production function can it be improved. Better trained surgeons will not necessarily lead to better patient outcomes if the hospital's nursing care and other services are substandard.

Managers must realise that they are the leaders of the quality team, not the hospital's custodian. Hospital directors must emphasise and delegate this responsibility to the manager, and give him or her the authority to carry it out. Doctors must realise that their efforts alone are not solely responsible for patients' outcomes; rather, it is the hospital that produces outcomes. The quality of the hospital's management, organisation, staffing and so on is an important determinant of patient outcomes. Thus no matter how dedicated they might be, neither doctors and nurses nor any other group can assure the quality of patient care. But nor can managers improve the quality of care, which depends on the totality of care and services provided by doctors, nurses and other caregivers. They can, and should, sustain and support a management climate that permits and encourages providers to participate effectively in improving the quality of their care. A quality management program is the key manifestation of such support. Quality management provides the framework and means for managers, doctors, nurses and others to collaborate effectively toward common ends: improving patients' health status, reducing the cost of care and increasing patient satisfaction with care.

294.4 | Commit to quality

In many companies the quality revolution is on paper rather than on the shop floor. Managers have failed to progress beyond the belief stage and to commit to quality. At best, they practise management by mirrors, form over substance. Lip-service to quality management, the installation of amorphous, isolated, or window-dressing programs, cannot, and will not, improve quality. Similarly, quality management programs in hospitals must have substance as well as form. They must be adequately resourced, employ competent people and operate in a climate conducive to success. And, above all, they must be integrated fully in the way that the hospital delivers care. Quality management must include all of the hospital's activities, especially clinical care—the core of its production function. Managers must avoid focusing on minor activities. Focusing on the laundry or kitchens because it is simple or easy might yield some benefits but they will be minor compared to what can and should be achieved.

Quality management requires sustained effort. There are no quick fix solutions. The early stages of a quality management program may yield no tangible benefits. Managers must avoid sounding the retreat at the first sign of resistance, especially by doctors. They must stay the course. Sustained, unwavering effort, often in the face of considerable resistance, is required to yield tangible benefits. This effort must be continued if one wants to maintain the flow of benefits. Managers must back their demands with deeds that reinforce their words. They must recognise excellence and reward success.

Quality management is never being satisfied with products' quality, production costs, how products are produced, how production is organised, or any other aspect of how the organisation achieves its purpose. Managers, doctors, nurses and others must strive for excellence and they must never tire of asking, and answering, the question: What could be done differently and better?

294.5 | Quality management means measurement

Quality management involves measuring care processes, immediate outcomes and end results of care. For the most part, health care provision has been devoid of meaningful feedback. Today hospitals have little, if any, meaningful information to improve quality. Quality management requires that the hospital measure its performance in meaningful ways and to use this feedback to improve the quality of care. Without being able to describe accurately what one is doing and with what results, systematic improvement is simply not possible. At best, actions may be hit or miss, and no one will know that anything has really improved. People need to measure their progress to maintain their commitment to quality. They cannot be expected to improve unless they know how well they are performing. Surgeons, for example, cannot improve their care unless they know its end results. Their noble motives must be reinforced by appropriate incentives to improve and the reward of knowing that they are improving.

Quantification is quality management's most essential tool. Firstly, measuring the quality of their care allows hospitals to quantify performance and to identify deficiencies and improvement opportunities. Secondly, it permits effort to be focused on what is important. Thirdly, it provides the only means of knowing if one is truly improving. Only through careful measurement can one know how well one is doing and the extent to which intentions result in improvement. Certainly one can attempt to identify and resolve problems by committee; but without measurement one cannot anchor judgments in reality. Perceptions can be wrong and so-called solutions may not yield much improvement.

In one doctor's experience, patients returning to the clinic after discharge seemed to be doing remarkably well. He was surprised to learn that only 50% of similar patients treated at a centre of excellence survived, according to a journal report. How could it be that his patients did so much better than those of the best centre? He forgot that the dead don't return to the clinic. After careful study of records the doctor found his patients' survival was identical to that of the best centre. His clinical impressions were entirely misleading. This same story can be repeated countless times: data, properly collected, analysed and interpreted, are essential for quality management. Hospitals must specify practice policies and measure the extent of conformance to them. They must also measure immediate and long-term patient outcomes and relate them to care processes. Quality management means meaningful measurement.

294.6 Measurement must be meaningful

The hospital must know and not assume what is done (care processes), what is achieved (outcomes), the cost of producing outcomes, and the extent of patients' satisfaction. To date, if they have measured anything, hospitals have focused on service activities, such as numbers of separations, operations and so on, and have simply assumed or been unconcerned about their utility or the cost of their production. Today the tools exist to measure quality in meaningful ways. Managers must provide the will, the means and the incentives to measure care processes and outcomes and to use the resultant information to improve continuously the quality of the hospital's product: more health status improvement at less cost with greater patient satisfaction.

Surgeons, for example, may draw immense satisfaction from completing operations successfully, especially difficult ones. The trouble is that for centuries they, and providers generally, have focused too often on inadequate measures of success—the number of items of service provided—rather than what matters most to patients—end results, health status improvement. Surgeons, for example, simply assume that if they perform operations successfully (i.e. to their satisfaction), and if they perform the right operation and perform it correctly, that benefits would flow to the patient. Quality management cannot tolerate such assumptions. Emerging techniques and tools mean that they no longer have to be tolerated.

While surgeons may have had the will to measure outcomes, they often lacked the means to do so successfully. Certainly they had (and still have) no incentive to inquire about end results (beyond the noble motive), as Codman pointed out almost a century ago.[3] They were not paid to collect data, nor were they paid based on performance. In fact, such measurement would be an added expense and outcomes might prove to be worse than imagined.

294.7 Quality management environment

The environment in which hospitals operate shapes their management and operations, including the hospital's interest in and the nature of their quality management programs. In turn, the environment that hospital managers create in which quality management programs must operate determines their effectiveness. Incentives, including when necessary sanctions, are a powerful, and often determinant, part of the environment.

Today there are virtually no incentives for hospitals to implement meaningful quality management programs. In fact there are powerful disincentives. What incentives do exist for quality management are largely regulatory sanctions, including hospital accreditation, or the threat of litigation, including professional liability insurance. Unfortunately, in Australia hospitals barely recognise the link between litigation and effective quality management, if they recognise it at all. The disincentives include the need to fund quality management from existing budgets without any way of increasing revenues by offering higher quality care or better value for money, and managers' lack of incentives to engage (and lack of carrots and sticks to encourage doctors and other hospital staff to get involved) in quality management. Managers need the means to overcome people's reluctance to quality management and to change.

Enlightened providers and the general public, through government or industry associations, must insist on quality and provide the incentives and sanctions for effective quality management. Essentially, effective quality management requires bringing rewards in line with value added. A simple solution to this complex problem might be for hospitals to publish their quality scores and prices and for patients to decide where to seek care; payment would follow the patients. The cost of lack of quality would be going out of business. In Australia, where there is no market in hospital care, all prices being effectively controlled by government, at the present time, it is unlikely to occur. For a truly free market to operate, to exercise effective choice, consumers must be able to discern the quality of the goods and services that they intend to buy.

If managers' and everyone else's salary depended on meeting quality goals it would not be long before quality improved or managers found another line of work. If a hospital guaranteed its, or produced better, outcomes, patients might be inclined to prefer one hospital over another, spurring real competition if patients controlled funds. While education and incentives that reinforce enlightened self-interest are clearly the best approach, ultimately sanctions must include mechanisms either to allow substandard hospitals to go out of business (which may be unlikely) or to change their management (which may be difficult, but possible to effect). Further discussion of health care financing reforms to promote quality management and hence improve the quality and productivity of health care, is beyond this manual's scope. Short of informed consumers empowered to choose, bureaucratic oversight coupled preferably with incentives and sanctions related to quality and to cost may be the only alternative.

294.8 | Carrots and sticks

Quality management is a special aspect of management—one that focuses on an organisation's product—but it is first and foremost about getting things done through other people, who must be informed, educated and motivated. Theories about managing people apply to medicine as much as they do to other types of enterprise. Medicine is the quintessential knowledge industry where positive incentives (carrots) are far more powerful and important than negative ones (sticks). Realistically, however, both must be used, even if the balance is tipped heavily in favour of the positive.

The North American criticism, often repeated in Australia although in reality occurring rarely, is that classic quality assurance activities are inspectorial in nature: rooting out bad apples. This rather simplistic connection is often made: errors occur; doctors are responsible for these errors; we must identify and remove bad doctors; quality will improve. The hospital certainly has a fiduciary responsibility to protect patients from aberrant medical practitioners and doing so can only improve the quality of care. However, this limited perspective has many disadvantages. Chief among them are the following. Firstly, the inspectorial approach creates a defensive climate: doctors become fearful of possible sanctions, refuse to co-operate in quality assurance activities, try to cover themselves against all possible criticism by practising defensive medicine, and get criticised for overservicing patients and practising bad medicine, reinforcing a vicious cycle of distrust. Secondly, it perpetuates the myth that when something goes wrong, someone—not the system in which he or she works—is solely to blame. Thirdly, rooting out all aberrant practitioners will only improve quality to a very limited degree.

Effective quality improvement depends on everyone in the organisation working toward that end. Almost everyone wants to do a good job. The extent to which he or she can do so depends not only on his or her abilities but also on the environment in which he or she works. An organisation's management creates that environment. Management must be committed to quality improvement, provide the means to improve quality and, above all, be an integral part of the process, accept criticism, and change. Management's failure to change can doom quality improvement efforts every bit as much as its lack of commitment to supporting structures and processes. If jobs are to be done well, management must provide the training, resources and so on for optimal performance. Only when every other factor has been eliminated can management blame workers for failure to perform. Managers and doctors must recognise that they are responsible and accountable for the quality of care. Managers must be concerned with the practice of medicine, what doctors do in the hospital. Doctors must recognise that their performance depends on the hospital and hence that they are part of an organisation and must take an active role in its management.

295 | Quality management in hospitals

295.1 | *Quality management is an essential production element*

The hospital's central purpose is to improve its patients' health status beyond that which would have occurred without its intervention. Clinical care is the hospital's core activity; doctors and nurses are the minds and hearts of this core. In addition, the hospital provides or contracts for a variety of other services that support this clinical core. They include: laboratory, imaging and other clinical support services that furnish information essential to clinical decision making; food services that sustain patients and staff; housekeeping, groundskeeping and other ancillary services that maintain hospital operations. All of these services must be managed, and the hospital's staff includes a complement of managers, bookkeepers and others who provide the information, co-ordination and direction that allow the hospital to accomplish its mission. Today, in most hospitals quality management is conspicuous by its absence.

Quality management is, or should be, an essential component of a hospital's management. It provides the information to know how well the hospital is accomplishing its mission and how well constituent departments and services are contributing to the whole. In this respect, constituent departments can be viewed as having 'customers' in the hospital. For example, doctors who order laboratory tests can be viewed as the laboratory's customers. If the laboratory does not produce timely reports or produces invalid results, clinicians' work will be affected adversely. Similarly, if the laundry has problems in doing its job, there may be spot shortages of clean linen or costs may be higher than necessary and the quality of patient care will be diminished.

Quality management must be concerned with all of the hospital's activities that affect the quality of care, encompassing health status improvement, cost, patient satisfaction and any trade-offs that there may be among these aspects of quality. This manual focuses almost exclusively on improving patient health status improvement, primarily because it is the hospital's defining purpose and because it is the most unique, the most difficult and, to date, the least well-explored aspect of quality improvement. The same principles apply to improving clinical care and all of the services and functions that support it, including the laundry. However, focusing on the laundry while ignoring clinical care, which has characterised many quality improvement efforts, is akin to rearranging the deckchairs on the *Titanic*.

295.2 *Scope of quality management*

Quality management's principal functions are to determine what is the right product and to produce it right. In the hospital's context its principal function is to operationalise the quality improvement spiral and, particularly, conformance improvement (quality assurance). (See Chapters 6 and 8.) Quality assurance involves identifying and resolving quality problems through the quality assurance cycle:

- specifying products (practice policies that specify how the hospital intends to diagnose and treat patients);
- measuring the extent to which processes conform to policies and achieve intended outcomes (to identify quality problems);
- identifying root causes of deviations from processes and intended outcomes;
- evaluating alternative improvement actions;
- implementing chosen actions to remedy problems and eliminate their root causes; and
- checking to see that quality problems have been and remain fixed.

Most hospitals are struggling with quality assurance, an essential prerequisite for other, more sophisticated quality management strategies. In medicine, because of the difficulties of measuring end results and attributing them to preceding interventions, conformance to practice policies (and achievement of intended outcomes with low variance) virtually defines practical quality management. Moreover, for the most part information to formulate practice policies comes from outside of hospitals, from professional colleges or societies for example. With the institutionalisation of quality management programs in hospitals, they will begin to generate the information needed to revise practice polices. Eventually hospitals must measure long-term patient outcomes, the end results of care (to validate practice policies), assess medical technologies (to improve health care interventions, the technology of medicine embodied in practice policies), and conduct health services research (to improve care delivery and processes). Presently hospitals rarely fund research, even though research funded by government may be conducted within their walls. Research on patient care processes is rarely done anywhere.

295.3 *Responsibility for quality management*

Ultimately the hospital's board of directors is responsible for the quality of its care. The board delegates this responsibility to the hospital manager. Operationally, responsibility for the quality of care rests fairly and squarely on the hospital manager's shoulders. He or she cannot, and should not, pass it off to others, for example by pretending it is the responsibility of medical staff. Doctors alone do not and cannot improve patients' health status.

As with any management responsibility, the hospital manager must seek the counsel of others and get things done through other people in the hospital. The hospital manager's instrument for policy guidance is the hospital-wide quality management committee (QMC). His or her principal resource for quality management, including the design and implementation of the hospital's quality management program, must be a qualified quality manager, who sits on, and may chair, the quality management committee, and who heads the hospital's quality management department (QMD).

Medical and other hospital staff are an integral part of an effective quality management program. When all is said and done, quality depends on the actions and attitudes of the front-line health professionals who treat patients. The manager's function is to provide them with the circumstances and systems that they need to do their jobs well, to measure performance, to reward excellence, and, if necessary, to change circumstances, systems and people to bring out the best in those willing and able to deliver the highest possible quality of care.

295.4 | *A quality management department and the quality manager*

A quality management department (QMD), headed by the quality manager, is the hospital's resource for assessing, assuring and improving the quality of its care. Today this vital resource is absent from most hospitals in Australia and other countries or, if it does exist, does not have the broad and necessary responsibilities described here.

The quality manager is an essential member of the hospital's management team and second only to the hospital manager in responsibility for its product. Without a qualified quality manager and supporting professional staff the hospital's chances of implementing an effective quality management program are slim to none. Part III discusses the practical aspects of establishing a quality management department, including a job description and personnel qualifications for a quality manager.

Worldwide there is a shortage of trained, experienced quality management professionals. This shortage is perhaps the greatest barrier to improving the quality of health care. Urgent attention must be given to resolving this problem. Hospitals can help alleviate this shortage by pressing for and allowing staff to participate in training programs, and by offering on-the-job training and, most importantly, providing opportunities for quality management. Quality management is a demanding and difficult job and, like clinical practice, applies knowledge and skills for practical purposes and, ultimately, can be perfected only through experience.

295.5 | *Quality management at the workface*

Quality assurance and improvement activities should be based as close to the point of production as possible. Quality is produced by clinicians, nurses and many others, not by quality managers. The quality manager's job is to insist on, and to facilitate the achievement of, quality. Achieving quality requires first defining it, second measuring it, and finally using this feedback to adjust processes to assure conformance with specifications. This manual focuses primarily on clinical care including, for example, use of structured quality review to assess its quality. This section looks at a critical input to clinical care—the clinical laboratory—to illustrate three points: the need to:

- manage the quality of all facets of a hospital's operations;
- devolve authority and responsibility as close to the operational level as possible; and
- co-ordinate quality management activities.

295.6 | *The clinical laboratory as example*

The product of a clinical laboratory is accurate, precise, timely tests. Responsibility for designing and implementing proper quality assurance systems rests with the head of the laboratory, whether or not the laboratory is owned by or located physically in the hospital. Systems external to the laboratory (e.g. those for which the quality management department is responsible) monitor the internal system's effectiveness in producing accurate, precise, timely tests. If the laboratory has an exemplary record for test accuracy and so on, the hospital's management may and should reward the director and give him or her discretion to reward the staff for their good work. Conversely, if the laboratory's performance is inadequate the hospital manager can warn the director, give him or her the means and incentives to improve (including access to quality management expertise) and, ultimately, if he or she fails to correct the situation, replace him or her. Whether or not this replacement would produce more accurate tests depends on the reasons for poor performance. If they rest in the resources the hospital made available, for example inadequate equipment or other constraints, replacing the laboratory's director is unlikely to improve its performance. Hospital management must realistically assess performance, including quality problems' root causes, and respond appropriately.

Laboratory tests account for a substantial fraction of health care costs. Beyond test accuracy, precision and timeliness, for what should the laboratory director be held accountable? For example, should his or her quality assurance responsibilities encompass test use, as is sometimes suggested?[4] Clinicians order tests. They should be responsible for what they order, since they understand why they ordered the test. Giving the laboratory director responsibility for test use implies putting on him or her the onerous and impossible task of policing, or at least monitoring, the appropriateness of clinicians' test ordering. The laboratory director's responsibilities in these regards should be limited to participating in activities to establish practice policies about test use and interpretation, specimen collection, and other matters that go on outside of the laboratory but about which he or she has expertise.

The laboratory director is responsible directly for deciding how to do tests and report results, for example selecting the equipment, determining laboratory practices etc. minimising the costs of testing, in-process utilisation control and reporting test use. The hospital's practice policies, for example, may dictate that certain tests must be ordered or concurred in by the clinical laboratory director. If so, he or she must set up an appropriate preprocess verification system. He or she should report test use so that the hospital's quality manager, with the director's assistance, can analyse patterns of use as a means of identifying potential quality problems, for example inappropriate test use, in lieu of or preferably as a supplement to the hospital's structured quality review or other quality problem identification systems. Quality improvement requires a hospital-wide, systematic approach. The laboratory director, for example, is directly responsible for some things (exactly which things depends on how the hospital divides functions and responsibilities), and participates in others. The quality manager is responsible for co-ordinating all quality management activities.

295.7 *Quality management in clinical departments*

The quality management department (QMD) is responsible for co-ordinating quality management activity throughout the hospital. The essence of quality management in hospitals involves facilitating the formulation of practice policies (or equivalent specifications), assuring conformance to specified care processes and immediate outcomes, for example using structured quality improvement (described elsewhere) and, to the extent practical, improving practice policies based on feedback from within and outside of the hospital.

With appropriate input from clinical departments, the quality management committee establishes the policy framework needed to formulate practice policies. The quality management department assists clinical departments to adopt and adapt existing practice policies to the department's circumstances and, when necessary, to elaborate and/or revise them. While individual departments formulate practice policies within their domain, mechanisms must exist for involving other departments or units when appropriate. For example, development of clinical practice policies would benefit from interdepartmental co-operation—for example between medicine and surgery, because for some health problems both medical and surgical interventions are acceptable; and between neurology and psychiatry, because for behaviour disorders symptoms may be organic or psychological in origin.

With the advice or consent of the quality management committee, the quality management department decides which types of cases to review and how to review them for quality management purposes. The quality management department or individual departments may screen medical records or delegate this activity and the review of patient medical records to clinical departments. The quality management department analyses or assists departments to analyse review results for patterns of care and integrates these data with those from other quality information systems. The quality management committee prioritises quality of care problems and the QMD is responsible for identifying or assists others to identify their root causes. If a quality problem involves clinical care, the QMD engages the appropriate clinical departments in discussions about how best to resolve them, and determines the costs and other consequences of their resolution. Ultimately the relevant clinical department is responsible for planning and implementing improvement actions (sanctioned by the quality management committee, if they transcend departmental responsibilities or have hospital-wide implications); the QMD, for following-up on their implementation, and measuring and documenting quality improvement, including its attribution to improvement actions.

Clinical departments must engage meaningfully in quality management if hospitals' quality of care is to improve. Individual departments may also initiate quality improvement activities in accordance with their quality management plan (discussed later). The quality management department's role is to co-ordinate the hospital's quality management activities, to communicate its quality management policy to clinical departments, and to assist them improve the quality and productivity of care. Through communication channels that the quality management department establishes and maintains, one department can pass on improvement suggestions that only another department can implement, or those that require the quality management committee's consideration because their implementation requires interdepartmental collaboration or they have hospital-wide effects.

295.8 | Deciding among improvement opportunities and actions

Usually a plethora of opportunities exist to improve quality. Quality managers are often confronted with the question: Which opportunities should we address first? Clearly there is no simple answer. The best approach is to consider explicitly the amount of health status improvement that can be expected to result directly or indirectly from each improvement opportunity and the cost of its realisation. This same calculus can be applied to deciding among alternative ways of solving a given problem and deciding among competing improvement opportunities (actions to resolve different quality problems). Aggregate health status improvement is a function of expected average improvement per case and the expected number of cases in an appropriate predetermined period. Costs include the cost of making and, if applicable, sustaining the change, and any additional costs (or savings) that result from changed practices or processes.

This cost-effectiveness approach requires a substantial amount of information, or judgment in lieu of measurement. Decisions about which changes to pursue can be made either by establishing a maximum amount per unit of effect (cost-effectiveness ratio) and making all changes that exceed it (the ratio can be changed if opportunities exceed the money to realise them all), or by periodically rank ordering all potential improvements and funding changes until the available amount of money has been allocated. In Australia, in public hospitals especially, precise measurements of cost-effectiveness will be difficult, if not impossible, until quality management becomes entrenched. Thus, initially at least, such decisions will be made inevitably on the basis of best judgment.

Use of a predetermined ratio permits decentralisation of decision making because it becomes a decision criterion, whereas periodic evaluation of opportunities centralises decision making but may result in more consistent evaluations. Funding constraints can obviously affect how many and which opportunities to implement beyond cost-effectiveness considerations. For example, if the hospital insists on budget neutrality, one can only fund improvement actions that increase costs from the resources liberated by those that save money (or from off-budget spend-to-save funds). This constraint will obviously affect the selection of improvement opportunities and actions.

295.9 | *Information needs*

Quality management requires information. Information requires data. Collecting and ensuring the integrity of data is often expensive. Any such expense, however, pales in comparison to the money spent on poor or ineffective health care, especially if one also adds the cost of lost economic productivity, human suffering and other such factors. Effective quality management requires both science information management and patient information management. Science information management involves generating, evaluating, disseminating, and using information about health care interventions' development, delivery, cost-effectiveness, and impacts (see Chapter 3 of this part). Patient information management involves these same processes applied to patient care (see below).

Assessing, delivering and assuring patient care requires increasingly prodigious amounts of data. To date, we have paid scant attention to satisfying this fundamental need for efficient recordkeeping by clinicians and effective use of recorded data. The spectre of additional, burdensome, useless paperwork always seems to be raised in doctors' minds whenever mention is made of the need to improve medical records. Can the extra work pay off? Firstly, there need not be any extra work if only useful information is recorded in efficient ways. Secondly, recordkeeping, like any other resource consuming activity, must be seen as producing commensurate benefits. The minimum amount of data must be collected and maximum use must be made of collected data for quality management purposes.

The greatest determinant of medical records' utility is what data are collected and how they are used. High quality care requires not only appropriate care but also its proper documentation. The medical record's primary purpose is to manage a patient's care effectively. Carefully recording what was done not only improves the management of the patient's current care but also improves the patient's subsequent care. The patient's record represents a core resource for improving the quality of care and health care practices.

Medical records, considered broadly, represent a complex subject encompassing not only technical issues (such as computerisation, coding and continuity) but also ethical, legal and social issues (such as truth, privacy and access by patients). For quality management purposes, data collection must be clearly relevant to patient care, quality assurance, measuring outcomes, or assessing medical technology or its delivery. To the extent practical, the collection of irrelevant data should be avoided, as it is expensive to collect and may obfuscate more useful data. The totally computerised medical record may prove to be a boon to quality management; however, in the meantime hospitals can improve their information for quality management in the following ways:

- Providers should develop practice policies for what must be in the medical record of all cases, for certain types of cases (e.g. surgical patients), and for given diagnoses. Where appropriate, guidelines can be developed for what need *not* be recorded (especially if record reviews find that such irrelevant material is often recorded).

- Medical record specialists should devise check lists, forms, charts and so on to aid and speed recording.
- Doctors should delegate recordkeeping whenever appropriate, checking and assuring its completeness and accuracy.
- Medical records should be abstracted routinely to provide the information necessary for quality management. Abstraction is facilitated by use of standardised records (e.g. with specified filing order within the medical record for forms or types of data), structured data entry formats and discharge summaries coded for analysis.
- Abstracted data must be used for quality management to justify the cost of their abstraction. Some simple computerised database management system is essential for this purpose. Someone, if not everyone, should be trained to interpret these data correctly.
- The results of structured quality review, and any special quality assurance studies, should be integrated with routinely abstracted data to maximise their utility for quality management purposes.
- Samples of patients should be followed-up to ascertain their outcomes and these data should be integrated with other data. Outcome data must be analysed to determine interventions' cost-effectiveness. Such analyses and their correct interpretation are essential for improving practice policies and patient care processes.
- Results of all analysis should be used to improve practices and to revise what data are relevant to collect.

The development and use of computerised systems, depending on their sophistication (the amount of incorporated intelligence), can be expected to aid medical recordkeeping in a number of ways, including the following:

- avoid multiple entry of identifying and other data;
- structure the medical record and promote its completeness;
- allow patients to enter data about themselves, including their preferences, for example for different health states;
- prompt providers to enter certain information, follow-up on answers, and even ask the right questions;
- offer suggestions for diagnostic tests and the therapeutic interventions, question the doctor's diagnosis or therapeutic plan if it appears at odds with the facts, and eventually suggest the correct diagnosis or therapeutic interventions for the patient's circumstances, based on the most current medical knowledge, the patient's preferences, the hospital's facilities and capabilities, and such other factors as payment policies;
- monitor progress and suggest remedial actions, for example to prevent physiological parameters drifting out of control or managing complications;
- provide the means for routinely assessing the quality of care;
- obviate the need to abstract records (because all of the needed data will have already been collected);
- permit real-time analysis of data and use of the resultant information for patient care, to promote quality and facilitate improvement in practice patterns;
- with standardisation of data and coding schemes (and appropriate data integrity assurance), permit valid comparisons among providers and facilitate appropriate development or revision of practice policies.

296 | Planning quality management

For industry, quality management is no longer a matter of competitive advantage, it is a matter of survival. Hospitals should view quality management in this same light. Isolated quality improvement efforts, CQI training without supporting structures and processes, and amorphous TQM programs are unlikely to achieve anything useful. Quality management programs must focus on the most important aspects of the hospital's work, for example care of its most common high-risk, high-cost cases, and on the most decisive interventions, for example simplifying care processes to resolve quality problems. A hospital's quality management plan focuses its quality management efforts, and must encompass both strategy and implementation.

Strategic and annual implementation plans are the cornerstone of every quality management program. The hospital's strategic quality management plan stems from and embodies the hospital's quality management policy, a written statement of its commitment to quality. The strategic quality management plan describes how the hospital intends to manage the quality of its products and its quality management program. The quality management plan must aim to make quality a routine part of hospital operations; not the isolated concern of the quality management department.

Typically, a strategic plan has a five- to ten-year horizon, and describes the intended situation at the end of the planning period and the steps necessary to produce this desired outcome, given the hospital's present situation. The annual implementation plan specifies what will be accomplished in the coming year. At year's end, the hospital must evaluate its progress in relation to plans. Based on this information, the hospital can extend its strategic plan and, if necessary, revise it, and formulate its implementation plan for the coming year. This planning and evaluation cycle is repeated endlessly. To begin the cycle, the hospital must assess its current quality management activities. Detailed exposition of how to assess hospitals' quality management activities and develop quality management plans is beyond this manual's scope. This section intends to give the reader an appreciation of the essentials. Part III provides additional practical advice.

Hospitals must design their quality management programs to achieve objectives using the best available technology for their circumstances. Hospitals must define exactly what they want the quality management program to achieve; clarity of purpose is essential for success. Vague statements about high quality and doing better cannot suffice because measures of effectiveness flow from statements of objectives; without measurement improvement cannot be documented, if it is possible at all.

In setting objectives, decision makers must assess the external and internal environments. The climate for quality management will obviously affect what can be accomplished realistically. Further, if the internal environment is not conducive to quality management, the plan's objectives may include changing the environment as well as launching or continuing specific quality management activities. Objectives have four essential attributes. They must:

- state exactly what is to be achieved by when (in this context, the planning period);
- be potentially achievable within technical, personnel, financial, organisational, cultural and any other relevant constraints;
- be measurable and preferably suggest measures of effectiveness (for evaluation purposes);
- contribute to achievement of higher-order objectives.

Planning is not dreaming. Plans should be realistic and based on what should and can be accomplished. Quality management plans must specify potentially achievable objectives and describe plausible means for their achievement, including budgets that represent financial commitments. Budgets (expenditure plans) should be based on activities and not vice versa. Each year the budget should be based on what needs to be done (sometimes referred to as zero-based budgeting), and not be merely an extension of last year's budget. Because of quality management's centrality to the hospital's functioning, quality management budgets cannot be subject to across the board reduction. Clearly, if the hospital reduces its operations substantially, some reduction in quality management activities will likely be in order. However, problems in the hospital, including an inability to provide services within budgets, may occasion an increase—not decrease—in quality management activities and budget.

The quality management plan can be a very useful document. It represents the cumulation and integration of individual departments' quality management plans. The most useful aspect of quality management planning is the process for the plan's development and its subsequent evaluation. Quality management planning should involve everyone in the hospital whom the plan affects. Quality management plans produced in isolation are unlikely to be effective. Quality management is not done unto others; it is a process in which providers, the people who produce the hospital's product, must participate. The quality management plan must address the management of the hospital's quality management program with this same incisive logic. Every change to the quality management program must be justified in terms of its effect on improving the quality of care and the cost of attaining such improvement.

297 | Evaluating quality management

297.1 | Perspective

A hospital's quality management program can, and should, be subjected to the same scrutiny and continuous improvement to which it subjects clinical care and hospital operations. A quality management program that does not result in high quality care, conformance with practice policies and intended outcomes, is itself of poor quality and of little value. Program evaluation, gauging a program's worth, is an essential element of managing quality management. The principles underlying the evaluation of a quality management program parallel those elaborated in this manual for assessing, assuring and improving clinical practice. This section describes the basic elements of evaluating a quality management program. Detailed exposition of how to conduct such an evaluation is beyond the manual's scope.

297.2 | Evaluation reference frames: standards versus performance

All evaluations are comparative. 'How's your wife?' the comic asked. 'Compared to what?', the stooge replied. Two dimensions define four possible points of reference for comparing a program's value. The first dimension relates to criteria—absolute (standards) versus relative (performance); the second, to perspective—internal (the program's) versus external (e.g. the program's sponsor). Absolute and relative criteria are described further below, from both internal and external perspectives.

A standard describes what should be done and achieved; performance, what is done and achieved generally. Standards can be expressed in the form of ideals—what should be done or achieved ideally; or of objectives—what the program or others have decided should be done or achieved, which may approach, but are usually less than, the ideal. Clearly, objectives may be set by the hospital's quality manager or its board of directors, or, as occurs most often, result from negotiations based principally on practicalities. The quality manager may be concerned about the technicalities of the board's quest for the ideal; conversely, the board with the cost of the quality manager's quest for the ideal.

While objectives may vary from hospital to hospital, ideals, by definition, encompass all hospitals, although their manifestation in a particular hospital may vary according to its circumstances. As used here, ideal refers to a set of expectations to which the most dedicated and able can aspire, even if they cannot satisfy it completely, rather than absolute perfection, something beyond everyone's reach in most or all respects. By comparing its objectives to a set of idealised objectives, a hospital can establish a sense of what it intends to achieve compared with what it might strive to achieve. This comparison is akin to comparing one's performance to that of the best performer (see the next section). This manual's content suggests a set of idealised objectives for quality management in hospitals.

Performance can be expressed in terms of norms—what most people do or achieve; and excellence—what the best achieve. A hospital's present performance can also be related to its past performance to gauge the extent of its progress. Performance measures are clearly most suitable for ratio (rather than categorical or scalar) data. For example, a hospital may monitor the proportion of obstetrical cases it treats within commonly accepted practice standards. This proportion will lie somewhere on a distribution of such scores for all hospitals. The hospital may be satisfied with lying at the centre of the distribution—average performance—or it may aspire to achieve the performance of the best hospital—that lying at the extreme right-hand of the distribution. In the near term, hospitals may only have access to their own data for comparison purposes. They can tell whether or not their performance is improving. External comparison (often referred to as benchmarking) is essential to know where one is relative to others' performance and what it is possible to achieve.

297.3 Levels of program evaluation

To evaluate a hospital's quality management program one can examine the program's structures, processes, outcomes and impacts. Structures refer to the program's operational elements, their organisation and inter-relationships, for example the quality management and quality management department, which shape processes. Processes refer to the program's activities, for example identifying and resolving problems to improve outcomes. Outcomes refer to the end results of activities, for example improvement in the quality of care. Impacts refer to the value of outcomes.

Impact assessment involves equating outcomes to the cost of their production and making value judgments, principally about alternative use of resources to achieve outcomes or higher-order objectives. Operationally, outcomes are the most important indicators of a program's success or failure. Assessments of structures and processes are more immediate and simpler levels of evaluation. However, they are more suitable for identifying failure than success. For example, a program that fails to identify problems that exist cannot expect to improve care. Similarly, a quality management program that cannot seem to find time to look for problems is unlikely to find any, no matter how good the tools at its disposal. On the other hand, identifying all of a hospital's quality problems will only improve the quality of its care if the hospital resolves them and eliminates their root causes. Only by measuring actual improvement in quality can one know that it has improved. Even if a hospital's quality of care does improve, it still must attribute the improvement to specific actions rather than to other factors. Often hospitals must assume plausibly that if they fix quality problems and they stay fixed, their actions produced the observed improvement.

297.4 Information for program evaluation

To improve the management of quality management, one must measure what the hospital's quality management program is achieving and how much it is costing to achieve it. Today hospitals are not used to measuring either the quality or the cost of their care, let alone those of actions to improve it. Quality management must begin to provide this information and must collect the same type of information about its own activities. The hospital must build information systems for this purpose and eventually they will have to be computerised. Initially, evaluation efforts are likely to be primitive because of insufficient information. However, their sophistication must evolve rapidly if quality management is to be managed adequately. The quality management department should check the accuracy of information to be used to evaluate the quality management program's cost-effectiveness, since the evaluation's validity is limited by the information's accuracy. When external information is used for comparative purposes, the QMD must assess both the limits of its comparability and its accuracy.

297.5 Setting up the evaluation

The hospital should conduct an annual evaluation of its quality management program. The evaluation plan is an important component of the hospital's quality management plan, specifically its strategic and annual implementation plans. The evaluation must be thought about at the beginning and must be elaborated on as the program develops, not left to the end or to chance. Early on, comparisons with the structures and processes recommended in this manual may be satisfactory. However, once the program becomes operational emphasis must shift to outcomes. The next sections discuss evaluating the program's progress relative to its plans, and its activities and outcomes. Simultaneous conduct of all three levels of evaluation provides the best picture of the program's value and how well it is performing.

297.6 Quality management program plans and progress

Each year the hospital's quality manager should compare what the quality management program achieved and spent with what it planned to achieve and to spend, expressed in the previous year's implementation plan. For carefully prepared plans, analysis of variance between what was planned and what was actually accomplished is most instructive. The quality manager should identify unplanned activities and describe why they were undertaken and planned activities that were not undertaken and describe why not. Using this information in the context of the hospital's quality management policy, the quality manager should recommend any necessary revisions to the hospital's strategic plan and draft next year's implementation plan for the approval of the hospital's policy decision-making body, for example the quality management committee. This annual evaluation and planning cycle permits the orderly evolution and improvement of the hospital's quality management program. It should be the occasion to celebrate success, to renew the hospital's commitment to quality and to improve quality management.

Each year the quality manager should also compare the hospital's quality management program structures, organisation, interrelationships and activities to those suggested in this manual (or other similar set of quality management program specifications). This comparison will yield a sense of where the program is relative to where it could, if not should, be. The quality manager might want to explain why the program has been able to approach or fall short of the ideal, and what it will take to keep it on track or to catch up, as the case may be.

In comparing hospitals' quality management programs to the structures and processes useful for assuring and improving the quality of care that we describe in this manual, quality managers must bear in mind that they cannot be considered absolute standards, for two reasons. Firstly, quality management programs must be tailored to individual hospitals' circumstances. What may be appropriate for a large hospital may not be appropriate for a small one, for example. Secondly, quality management technologies are still emergent; we are just beginning to develop and use them. As knowledge increases and solidifies, new, more cost-effective technologies can be expected to supplant older, less cost-effective ones. Thus a stronger sense of the ideal will emerge as hospitals gain and report their experience in implementing quality management programs.

297.7 Quality management program activities

Essentially, quality management in hospitals is about identifying problems, resolution of which would improve the quality of care. A hospital's quality management program may be evaluated in terms of its ability to identify and resolve quality of care problems. Applying the evaluation framework described previously, one can examine problem identification and resolution mechanisms being used in the hospital, and their outcomes, from both internal and external perspectives.

Each year, as part of its quality management strategic and implementation planning, the hospital can review the adequacy of its structures for and the ways it carries out problem identification and resolution activities. This review should include the documentation of actions intended to resolve problems, their results, and mechanisms to improve subsequent quality management activities. The hospital may want to retain a consultant to assist the quality manager to complete this task. Accrediting bodies, such as the ACHS, may also perform some or all of this function as part of their accreditation surveys. The structures and mechanisms suggested in this manual represent a useful point of departure for such a review.

The hospital should also examine the results of these activities in terms of the number of problems identified and prioritised for investigation of root causes, and those problems for which remedial actions were implemented, followed-up and documented. It should also review the cost of undertaking these activities. Results can be compared to current plans and those for past years. The quality manager should explain variances from plans or previous performance. If actions intended to resolve problems failed to do so or if actions were not taken to resolve important problems, subsequent lessons learned should be used to redesign problem resolution strategies. The quality management department can target costly activities, especially those that seem to have low yield, for investigation to see if it can improve their efficiency or devise more cost-effective alternatives. The scope of such an inquiry would depend on review results and may involve the redesign of the entire quality management function if it is not performing satisfactorily.

The most useful evaluations are external audits of the hospital's quality of care. Firstly, they provide an objective assessment of the hospital's quality of care. Secondly, they provide a means of evaluating its quality management program. Hospitals with good quality management programs can identify and resolve problems. Thus they will have already found a high proportion of the problems the auditors identify. Furthermore, the auditors will report that the hospital's quality of care is high. When such audits are conducted, the quality manager should review results with the auditors to look for ways of improving the hospital's quality management program.

297.8 | Quality management program performance

Fundamentally, quality management activity is only useful if it improves the quality of the hospital's care. Once again, internal and external frames of reference are both useful. The quality manager should keep track of the proportion of cases treated to standards (ascertained through structured quality review, for example). Initially, the hospital may focus on high-risk or high-cost cases, extending its activities to other types of care as the quality management program matures. The proportion of cases managed appropriately should reach and be maintained at a high level. If not at a high level, the proportion should increase steadily. Variance in outcome may be a manifestation of failure to follow policies or their improper implementation (which can be ruled out by structured quality review), or inherent limitations of the adequacy of those policies or the technologies that they embody.

If the proportion of cases meeting standards is low, efforts should be made to investigate and remedy root causes. If the proportion of cases performed to standards remains low, the types of and reasons for variation should be scrutinised. If the same problems keep recurring, actions intended to resolve them were obviously ineffective (assuming that sufficient time has elapsed for them to take effect), perhaps because investigators discovered the problem's apparent, but not its root, causes. If different problems keep arising, the reasons for this state of affairs should be investigated. For example, it may be that practice policies were changed but not communicated to all concerned, or that surgeons introduced a new operation for which neither they nor the hospital were prepared adequately. In such instances, hospital policies and practices should be changed to avoid recurrence of such circumstances.

Whenever possible hospitals should compare (benchmark) their performance, both in terms of the clinical quality and the cost of care. Such comparisons are important not only to avoid the potential for self-delusion that exists without the benefit of objective external assessment but also to learn what level of performance is possible. Clearly, such comparisons should be valid otherwise they will be misleading, which is worse than useless. To ensure comparability, the same standards must be applied uniformly to sufficient numbers of like cases. These conditions would be met, for example, if external auditors were to use structured quality review to assess coronary artery bypass grafts at different hospitals that perform this procedure. The variation in acceptable care rates would be most instructive. The shape of the distribution would reveal the range in performance and the variation around the mean. The mean would indicate how much the average hospital could improve compared with the best one. The range would show what the best hospital is achieving and just how bad is the worst hospital's performance.

Assuming that all hospitals intended to provide the same quality of care, poor performance, beyond statistical chance, would be an indictment of poor management generally or quality management specifically. There is no inherent reason why hospitals' standards should be the same, of course, although they might have to explain to their patients why they should be satisfied with lower standards, or risk patients going elsewhere. Providing slightly lower quality care at half the cost might be a satisfactory answer, especially when or if patients have to pay for care directly. Hospitals wanting to improve their performance might visit the best hospitals to see what they were doing differently, with a view to changing their own care processes.

Presently, we have little idea about attainable levels of practice performance. Based on what limited experience exists, hospitals with rates of cases treated within specified practice standards below 85% should be very concerned about the quality of their care. A rate of 95%–97% might be considered acceptable; 97%–99%, good; and above 99% excellent. Even if a hospital treated 99% of its patients within specified practice standards, it could still improve the care of one in 100 of its patients. While this figure might not sound alarming, with one million hospital discharges per year it would represent 10 000 patient care episodes. Obviously a hospital's rate would depend on the strictness of the standards and the type of care assessed. Regrettably, today, for certain high-risk procedures external auditors may find that the quality of care could have been better than it was in 33% or more of cases.

298 | Evaluating the quality management department

The quality management department, headed by the quality manager, is responsible for developing and implementing the hospital's quality management program. Thus the program's accomplishments are one measure of the quality management department's and quality manager's accomplishments, but not the entire measure. What the quality manager can accomplish depends on the resources at his or her disposal and the hospital's environment. While these factors should have been taken into account in producing the implementation plan, they are often beyond the manager's control. People are always overestimating their chances of success, especially if they desire the outcome: the perpetual triumph of hope over experience. Further, eventualities can vary from expectations. Ultimately, all useful comparisons are situation specific: what was achieved compared to what could reasonably be expected to have been achieved under the circumstances. This comparison is the only useful one, but is difficult to make because determining realistic expectations involves considerable judgment, beyond measurement capabilities.

Evaluation of the quality management department's performance should start by comparing the assumptions in the previous year's implementation plan with what happened, for example regarding resources to be provided, and expected co-operation of doctors in quality management activities. For example, if doctors were more resistant to participation in quality management activities than expected, evaluators must decide to what extent this reality influenced what could be accomplished or represents a fault in program design or implementation. For evaluation purposes, the program's objectives must be tempered by this assessment. For example, if through no fault of his or her own the quality manager was not able to gain doctors' participation in quality management activities, objectives related to these aspects of implementation plans should be excluded from the evaluation of the quality management department's and the quality manager's performance. The evaluation should focus on the achievement of remaining objectives, and any additional ones that the quality management department was able to achieve, and the cost of their achievement. The hospital manager may also want to gauge the quality manager's performance and those of his or her staff on the basis of more traditional personnel review practices, but those considerations are beyond the manual's scope.

299 | Cost and value of quality and its management

299.1 | Types of cost and ways to consider value

Cost and quality are inextricably intertwined. Efforts to control cost are met routinely by chorus chants of 'Quality will be diminished'. Efforts to improve quality are met with cries of 'We don't have the money'. How can one afford not to improve quality? You may well ask. Only by considering cost and quality simultaneously can one make rational decisions about what constitutes an improvement. The highest quality care can provide a lot, cost a little, and satisfy patients.

The relationship between quality and cost is often a source of confusion and this section intends to sort it out. It examines the cost of quality (or more precisely the lack of it), quality management and the management of quality management. The final section answers every manager's bottom line: Will quality management save money?

299.2 | The cost of production quality: Is quality free?

Quality gurus are often fond of saying that quality is free; one even wrote a book with that title.[5] Others, extolling the virtues of health care quality management, say that high quality care costs less than inferior care. But can the highest quality care be the least expensive? We know that the very best is often expensive (and that the most expensive is not always the best). Fundamentally, one must differentiate the desired product from the cost of its production.

Production's goal is to produce a product that conforms to its design specifications. In manufacturing, quality is often defined simply as conformance to specifications, product designs. The cost of manufacturing a product depends on product and process designs, and manufacturing performance. Product designs are often the most important determinant of costs. Obviously, it costs more to manufacture a Rolls Royce than a Ford, based simply on their respective design specifications. Process designs, the way the product is actually manufactured, including worker capabilities, training and incentives, determine the ease of conforming to specifications. Production costs consist of manufacturing, rework and scrap, and quality control costs. Often rework and scrap account for 30% of total costs. In this case, it pays to increase manufacturing and/or quality control costs if they can be offset by reduced rework and scrap. Here quality is free: higher quality production (conformance to specifications with less rework or scrap) costs no more (and conceivably less) than business as usual. The savings (profits) accrue directly to the manufacturer. But how about in medicine?

299.3 | Production quality cost in health care

Quality management can reduce iatrogenic disease that occasions additional care expenditures, and unnecessary tests and treatments (including hospital admissions and days of care), both of which would save money. What scant evidence exists points to the potential for substantial savings. For example, in the United States one estimate suggests that 'the average 250 bed hospital loses $1 million a year because of nosocomial infections. ... On average, a surgical wound infection adds a week to the patient's hospital stay'.[6] Since iatrogenesis and unnecessary care can only diminish health status, their avoidance would improve quality. The situation is not that simple of course.

Presently, medicine lacks the detailed practice policies that are the equivalent of manufacturing product and process specifications. Such policies are the cornerstone of health care quality management. Were they to exist, conformance to practice policies and their proper (competent) implementation would result in high quality care, and would inherently constitute potentially the lowest cost of care within design constraints (i.e. the practice policies and care processes that implemented them). The actual cost of care, however, would depend on adherence to specifications (cutting corners would cut cost and quality), provider performance (lack of skill in implementing designs would also increase cost and reduce quality), and the cost of production (an efficient hospital could do it all for less than an inefficient one). Whether or not this cost would be less than the present cost of doing business is an open question. Part of the problem, of course, is that no one knows what care really costs, nor the cost of the lack of quality.

Depending on the cost of iatrogenesis and unnecessary care, in medicine higher quality care (greater improvement in patients' health status through conformance to practice policies) could actually cost more, not less, for two reasons. Firstly, some patients may not be treated according to appropriate practice policies and improving their care may represent a net increase in costs. Secondly, the cost of quality management may exceed savings from extra and unnecessary care. Even if these latter circumstances prevailed, the quality of care would be higher, with less variability in outcomes. Whether or not such improvements were worth any costs they might entail is a sociopolitical judgment.

299.4 | The cost of product quality: What is product quality?

Quality management or, at a minimum, ensuring conformance to practice policies, is a cost of doing business and may save money rather than increase costs. But what about product quality, manufacturing specifications or the contents of practice polices that specify health care's product?

High quality products delight customers. Chances are that almost everyone can name products whose very name is the epitome of 'quality'. Rolls Royce may come to mind, Swiss chronometers, Cross or Montblanc pens. These products are the very best. They are also the most expensive, not the cheapest, so perhaps quality is not free after all. These expensive products perform better than others, with greater reliability. While competitors may offer comparable products at a lower price, for example Japanese compared to German luxury cars, luxury cars will always cost more than basic models, whose price also varies and depends on competition among manufacturers. Ultimately, quality is in the user's mind. Does a pen costing hundreds of dollars really write better than a disposable one purchased at a small fraction of the price? Both products may write well, be quality products; one certainly costs a lot more. People are willing to pay a premium for prestige; a product's high quality may be inherent in its high price. One way that manufacturers compete is on the quality of their products, especially in relation to their price, that is, perceived value for money.

299.5 The cost of health care's product

Health care quality management can strive to achieve any given level of health status improvement at lowest cost. In this case the problem is reduced to one of production quality, as described above. Some people believe that health care's goal is to achieve maximum possible health status improvement, a goal limited only by existing technology. Others confuse high quality health care with spending the most money possible. Obviously, services provided with neither rhyme nor reason are just as likely to reduce as to improve health. Nevertheless, the highest quality care (that set of practice policies which produces maximum achievable health status improvement) may also be, and often is, the most costly.

The problem, of course, is knowing what set of practice policies (production specifications) produces maximum improvement in patient health status. If there are several sets of alternative specifications, each known or assumed to be essentially equivalent in terms of health outcomes, we could and should choose the lowest cost set. However, reducing the specifications, for example accepting 10% less health status improvement, may reduce costs by 50%. Such care would not be the highest possible technical quality but it certainly would be much better value for money. Thus in medicine, as with goods and services generally, highest quality health care may be the most costly, in the same way as a Rolls Royce costs more than a Ford, and a Swiss chronometer costs more than a Hong Kong watch.

299.6 Quality management: an essential cost of doing business

How much does a proper quality management program cost? This question is often the first one asked, especially by those responsible for budgets. The answer, of course, depends on a variety of factors, including the hospital's size, the complexity of its case mix and services, and the stage of development of its quality management program. There is no doubt that quality management costs money, often a great deal, even if the amount is a small fraction of the hospital's total budget. However, the sheer size of expenditures can never be an excuse for not making them unless one is truly destitute. Hospitals' budgets are very substantial. Quality management programs can be funded simply by not spending so much on other activities, even patient care. After all, iatrogenic care is hardly a boon to patients.

The problem is that hospitals usually have little idea about the quality of their care. That is why they desperately need a quality management program. Essentially, quality management is simply a cost of doing business, in the same way that the manager's salary or financial accounting is a cost of doing business. Doctors may think erroneously that they could get by without either of these types of expenditures. However, their fees are also a cost of doing business. Presumably the patient expects something of value in return for the payment. The same is true for quality management.

Quality management has two essential functions: to reassure patients about the hospital's quality of care, and to improve continuously the quality of that care. The first is a fiduciary responsibility, the second a social obligation—if not a business necessity, because of existing perverse incentives (discussed later). The hospital must carry out these functions as cost-effectively as possibly. Thus whether or not to have a quality management program is not a relevant question. The only relevant question is: Which quality management program best suits the hospital's circumstances? A secondary question is: How much to spend on quality management generally and on each of its constituent activities specifically? Conceptually, marginal utility is a good test, but difficult to apply in practice because of insufficient information. Under this test, the last dollar spent on quality management should have generated at least as much quality improvement as would have the next best use of that dollar.

299.7 Accounting for the cost of quality management

Quality management involves two kinds of cost: cost necessary to assess quality and that needed to improve quality. Initiating quality management may require substantial expenditures, especially if huge problems were the stimulus for action, or simply because little or nothing may have been done. The cost of fixing whatever problems quality management uncovers cannot properly be called a quality management expense. These costs must be assigned to the affected department or service.

After this initial burst of expenditures, quality management may bear financial fruit—reduced quality costs from iatrogenic disease, for example—and improvements in production efficiency that offset its cost. For this reason, quality management information systems must track costs incurred in running the quality management program and estimate those avoided as a result. In quality-mature organisations that have built quality into processes to the greatest feasible extent, quality assessment can be quite sophisticated and resource sparse. The cost of quality assessment continues indefinitely, of course. The cost of simply assuming quality exists can be devastating.

As the hospital's quality management program develops further, expenditures for outcomes measurement may become substantial. They can be properly counted as quality management costs in that they assess the end results of care and provide information necessary to improve practice policies, and thus to improve care further. Without clear, mandated responsibility for outcomes measurement hospitals might be reluctant to incur these expenses and incentives must be created to bring about this desirable state of affairs. The cost of research to assess existing and to develop new medical technology would generally not be considered a quality management cost and would, therefore, be assigned to a separate cost centre, in the same way as manufacturing goods or providing services represent separate cost centres.

There is a cost even to managing quality management. Information is required to manage quality management; information has both a value and a cost. Developing strategic and annual implementation plans, conducting annual evaluations and other procedures all bear a cost. But they also have great value and are essential to progress toward quality maturity. Nevertheless, their cost must bear some reasonable relationship to their expected utility. In the long run, money spent on managing quality management must result in better use of remaining quality management funds. The quality manager's job is to generate and use the information necessary to assure cost-effective quality management, recognising that a great deal of uncertainty will always remain, calling for judgment at every step.

299.8 The bottom line

299.81 QUALITY, QUALITY COST AND THE COST OF QUALITY MANAGEMENT

Will quality management save money? Will it even improve quality? Little empirical information exists to answer either question because no one has tried consistently and continuously to improve the quality of health care using the comprehensive, integrated approach described in this manual.

299.82 QUALITY AND QUALITY MANAGEMENT

With respect to quality of care, the logic supporting quality management is compelling: agreeing how best to treat patients and making sure they are treated that way must at least reassure people that they are receiving 'best' care. Whether or not 'best' practices lead to maximal health status improvement is an empirical question, one that quality management intends to answer. For the foreseeable future, practice policies will be based mostly on the consensual judgments of clinicians or experts, supported with what little empirical information exists. Moreover, eventually they will reflect social choices about what should be done and, in this eventuality, the achievement of maximal health status improvement is rarely determinant.

Some people would argue that since we do not know what are best practices we should let doctors decide individually. Firstly, or course, doctors formulate, or at least influence heavily, practice policies. Secondly, certainly if everyone agrees that any treatment is as good as any other, practice policies should be appropriately permissive. In such a circumstance, research would seem urgently indicated to determine if any treatment is worthwhile and if so which one. This situation is encountered rarely. Even if competing schools of thought emerge, and lacking further information each is acceptable, some practices can usually be ruled out or questioned. At the same time, hospitals can gather outcomes data to shed light on practice policies' validity, as a result of which, if appropriate in light of this new information, they can change them. Certainly explicit practice policies are necessary to provide a point of reference from which to improve the quality of care.

299.83 COSTS, SAVINGS AND RED TAPE

Whether or not quality management can save money is an entirely different question. Again, empirical evidence is lacking presently. Logic would suggest that: some costs would increase and some could be expected to decrease; some real savings might result; but, likely as not, few savings will accrue to the hospital unless government alters present perverse incentives.

299.84 INCREASED COSTS

Hospital costs will increase initially because the hospital must pay for the quality management program that will lead eventually to cost savings. These initial costs should be viewed as spend-to-save funds. In some cases the cost of patient care may increase if doctors are undertreating cases now (in comparison to best practices). Certainly better recordkeeping may require more attention to detail, if not more time, and may also be a source of increased cost in the short run even if automation, for example, can produce savings in the long run. Hospital managers and doctors are notorious for their focus on costs rather than value resulting from expenditure; perhaps because of the perverse incentives under which they must operate.

299.85 REDUCED COSTS

In principle, a quality-mature hospital can expect lower costs from:

- reduced liability insurance premiums, malpractice claims and monetary damages;
- reduced iatrogenesis, specifically preventable errors and clinical complications;
- reduced unnecessary tests and treatments;
- improved clinical efficiency resulting from quicker diagnosis, better treatment selection etc.;
- improved operational efficiency with resultant better use of resources;
- improved productivity through enhanced employee job satisfaction and morale.

299.86 SAVINGS

Reduced costs may only result in savings if wards are closed, staff are laid off, or other similar measures are taken to cut expenditures, because the same or more health status improvement can be achieved with fewer resources. Keeping the same resources in place would mean that some of them would be idle some of the time and no savings would result. These 'fixed' costs would be spread over fewer days of care or fewer cases and the cost per case could well increase. Alternatively, some of the freed-up resources could be used to:

- offset the cost of the quality management program that made possible improved quality and productivity;
- reduce workloads or the pace of care, if that would improve its quality;
- improve documentation, if that were necessary;
- treat more patients, if there are any going untreated now.

However, the hospital's annual budget would remain the same even though cost per health status improvement unit or per case might, and likely would, have decreased if more health benefits were gained or more patients were treated with the same resources.

299.87 TO WHOM SAVINGS ACCRUE

A hospital's revenues and providers' incomes bear little if any relationship to product quality. In fact, doing it right may increase rather than decrease cost, if the costs of quality management and remedying any deficiencies that it discovers exceed the cost to the hospital of lack of quality. In these circumstances, instituting quality management will be seen as an additional, net cost to the hospital, because of its inability to increase revenues based on improved quality.

The people to whom savings accrue may be different from those who have to pay any additional costs. If quality management results in quicker, more accurate diagnosis, more appropriate treatment selection, quicker, better treatment implementation and so on, as it should, these improvements may also result in fewer days lost from work, improved economic productivity and reduced disability payments etc. However, none of these savings will accrue to the hospital even though it bears the cost of their realisation unless payment mechanisms are changed to provide hospitals with tangible incentives to achieve such benefits. Under present health care financing mechanisms, if quality increases the patient (and society) will benefit, not the hospital. Further, if quality management decreases cost, the hospital's only tangible reward may be a decrease in its budget, because it would ostensibly require less money to operate. If quality management is to be truly successful, payment for care must be based on its quality and the efficiency of its production. Hospitals, managers and doctors must not only be educated about the need for and provided the means to achieve quality maturity but must also be given performance-based incentives to promote quality of care. Discussion of health care payment reform is beyond this manual's scope.

299.9 | The real bottom line

The real bottom line rests on the question of alternative use of resources. Could money devoted to quality management be used elsewhere to effect more health status improvement or reduce the cost of care? Doctors and other providers often want to purchase new equipment; politicians, to extend coverage or services to those who do not have them. Certainly both represent valid demands. However, the resultant health improvement is likely to pale in comparison to spending the equivalent amount of money on quality management. Certainly additional expenditures for more services harbour no potential to reduce the direct cost of care, and thereby liberate money to fund doctors' and politicians' agendas. Quality management can document and improve quality—twin benefits not achievable by any other means—and may decrease costs, freeing resources for additional care and other desired uses.

A much more difficult issue is the balance between quality management, specifically quality assurance and improvement—delivering the best care we know how; and research—improving know-how. Quality assurance fulfils an important fiduciary responsibility and offers immediate improvements in care. While quality assurance activities can provide information about conformance to specifications, they generate relatively little information to solve problems with production processes or to design better products. Medical technology assessment and other types of health systems research are needed to improve practice policies and such research costs money. Research can save money only if it finds cheaper, not more costly, ways to achieve present or higher levels of health status improvement. While research promises to improve care (and quality management), the probability, magnitude and timing of its benefits are all uncertain. A recent review of outcomes for surgical care of colorectal cancer is illuminating:

> At present considerable effort and resources are being poured into large multicenter studies of adjuvant chemotherapy and radiotherapy in an effort to provide marginal improvement in survival of patients with colorectal cancer. If by more meticulous attention to detail the results of surgery could be improved, and our results suggest that this would not be difficult, the impact on survival might be greater than that of any of the adjuvant therapies currently under study.[7]

If the major health care problem is finding sufficient resources to treat patients exhibiting florid pathology with proven, cost-effective interventions, it might be hard to justify extensive quality management programs or even maintaining adequate medical records. In industrialised countries people are concerned about an oversupply of doctors (rather than a shortage), overservicing of patients (rather than underservicing), unnecessary operations (rather than masses of people denied their benefits), the introduction and use of unproven technology with its attendant costs (rather than the inability to apply proven interventions), and the quality of care they will receive from a medical practitioner (rather than ability to find one when needed). Under those circumstances, an incremental increase in effort applied to recordkeeping, data analysis and use of information will likely improve the cost-effectiveness of health care. Nevertheless, the principle of assessing an activity's cost-effectiveness applies to quality management as much as it does to medical technology.

Whether or not quality management programs will generate more savings than they cost is an empirical question. The bottom line on quality management is that we do not know how much money it can, let alone will, save. Its main benefit is improving the quality of care and reducing variability, giving patients more health status improvement with greater certainty. We know that it can accomplish these desirable goals. If quality-focused care costs the same as or less than present care, that is an added benefit. Another additional benefit of quality management is its positive impact on the development of sound, socially acceptable practice policies, the information and knowledge with which to formulate them, and the quality and productivity of health systems research.

On balance, in the long run cost savings will equal if not exceed any cost increases, especially if one considers improved medical knowledge and indirect social benefits that are among the important by-products of quality management programs. These expectations can, and should, be compared eventually to experience. The cost-effectiveness of quality management programs can, and should, be assessed and improved. The principles described in this manual for clinical care pertain also to the management of quality management programs, as this chapter explains.

References

1 Dobyns L, Crawford-Mason C. Quality or else: The revolution in world business. Boston: Houghton Mifflin Company, 1991.
2 Juran JM. Foreword to Crouch JB. Health care quality management for the 21st century. Tampa, Florida: American College of Physician Executives, 1991.
3 Codman EA. A study in hospital efficiency as demonstrated by the case report of the first five years of a private hospital. Boston: Th Todd & Co, 1918.
4 Dorsey DB. Evolving concepts of quality in laboratory practice. Arch Pathol Lab Med 1989; 113(12): 1329–34.
5 Crosby PB. Quality is free. New York: New American Library, 1979.
6 Evans G. Infection control staffing: is one ICP for 250 beds enough? Hospital Infection Control 1991; 18(16); 17–79.
7 McArdle CS, Hole D. Impact of variability among surgeons on postoperative morbidity and mortality and ultimate survival. BMJ 1991; 302(6791); 1501–5.

PART III

BUILDING AN EFFECTIVE QUALITY MANAGEMENT PROGRAM

SUMMARY

This part describes the essential administrative and organisational elements of an effective quality management program. Unless a hospital puts these essential elements in place all of its efforts, and those of its staff, to introduce such programs will fail. The principles expounded here apply generally to hospitals and other health care facilities throughout the world. Necessarily, the situations we describe and the steps toward effective quality management that we prescribe apply specifically to hospitals in Australia. Hospitals elsewhere will need to recognise their particular situation and, guided by prescribed principles, adjust specific steps to suit their context.

This part of the manual defines and describes the several elements that are intrinsic to a program of quality management and their interrelationships. None of the elements mentioned in this part, with the possible exception of a quality management department, are unfamiliar to anyone associated with hospitals. Nevertheless, hospitals often fail to recognise the critical importance of these various elements to an effective quality management program. In a high percentage of hospitals these critical elements' performance is either less than satisfactory or the interrelationships between them have received little or no attention; and in many instances some of these important elements are absent altogether. Accordingly, here we place considerable emphasis on both elements and their interrelationships. Hospitals can only achieve effective quality management if all of the elements exist and function properly, including their interrelationships.

To implement quality management effectively, it is necessary to set objectives and to provide resources, just as is the case for any other hospital activity. In addition, achieving objectives requires a range of techniques and an organisational structure to deliver them. To date, all too frequently objectives have been blurred, resources have been minimal, techniques have been less than sophisticated, and the lack of organisational structure has meant that very little has been delivered.

Chapter 1

INTRODUCTION TO AND PURPOSE OF PART III

---

310 **Contents**

This chapter deals with the need for a coherent program and an organisational framework for quality management. It covers the following topics:

311. Purpose of this part
312. Contents of this part
313. Purpose of this chapter
314. The missing link
315. Quality management: the clinical/management interface
316. Requirements for quality management
317. Hospital size and quality management
318. Attitudes towards committees
319. Education for quality management

311 **Purpose of this part**

An effective quality management program will not simply happen. It requires an extensive organisational structure to drive, manage and support the many and varied elements that comprise such a program. This part describes the components of the organisational structure necessary for a quality management program to be successful and, indeed, in the absence of which a quality management program cannot possibly exist. Most of the elements of this organisational structure are often ignored or taken for granted in hospitals—particularly by health professionals—and hence the devotion of this part to them.

However, even when all these crucial elements are present and functioning, most hospitals still have some difficulty deciding how and where to get started on the difficult road to effective quality management. Included in this part, therefore, is material aimed at assisting hospitals with the task of getting started. Many hospitals will already have some quality management activities, so that readers must use this material as a guide, adapting the suggestions to the specific requirements of their own individual hospital.

312 | Contents of this part

This part contains six chapters. Each chapter deals with one of the essential elements necessary to implement an effective quality management program. The organisational elements described here represent the structure that is necessary for a successful quality management program. Hospitals must possess each of these elements and operate them efficiently. The contents of this part consist of:

* Introduction to and context for an organisational structure.
* Governing body, management and by-laws—the vital role these elements play in successful quality management.
* Quality management committee and an effective committee structure. Quality management cannot succeed without a well-functioning committee structure. Appendix A of this chapter provides model terms of reference for a quality management committee.
* The quality management department and the quality manager. We detail the functions and role of the quality management department and provide a job description and qualifications statement for a quality manager.
* Medical records are critical. Quality management is about measurement. Assessing or measuring the quality of clinical care depends on the documentation in the medical record. We describe the background, current status and directions for the future.
* Getting started is often a hospital's greatest difficulty. This chapter provides a framework to assist a hospital to map its direction and some signposts to help it to find its way.

313 | Purpose of this chapter

For most people in hospitals engaged in quality management or any of its subsets, the concept of a program or even an organisational structure is still foreign. This chapter provides the rationale for the remaining chapters of Part III and serves as an introduction to what we regard as the most important element of quality management: the organisational framework for its accomplishment. In the hospital's context this includes an appropriate committee structure, including interrelationships among committees.

314 | The missing link

For almost twenty years a great deal of effort has been expended in trying to introduce quality management activities into Australian hospitals. In spite of these efforts very little real progress has been made. While it has been easy to blame the reluctance of medical staff in particular to involve themselves in quality assurance activity for this lack of success, the problem is a much more fundamental one. Effective quality management depends heavily on management commitment and its manifestation in an appropriate administrative structure. For reasons which we explore below, this administrative framework is the weak link in the chain. Indeed in many hospitals it is missing altogether.

315 | Quality management: the clinical/management interface

Quality management (QM) pertains to all of a hospital's activities that intend to assure and improve quality of care; in short all of them. In contrast, hospitals have usually applied the term quality assurance to performing some limited aspects of clinical care to standards. Quality management (QM) includes, at a minimum, quality assurance (QA), quality improvement (QI), utilisation review (UR) and risk management (RM). (See Figure III-1-1 below.)

Quality management presents a problem for some medical staff who have a conceptual difficulty drawing the distinction between assuring the quality of care for an individual patient, and a program or system which ensures quality of care and services for patients admitted to the hospital. The former is not possible without the latter. Clinical care is all about individuals; quality management and quality assurance are about systems for assuring that individuals receive quality care.

Quality management is in reality a subset of hospital management and is concerned primarily with the hospital's production function: improvement of patients' health status. The important difference is that this aspect of hospital management cannot be conducted by managers alone, but must have clinical and especially medical staff input. Traditionally, however, both managers and medical staff have tended to view each other's role as quite separate. Hospital management has shown a reluctance to intrude into what was perceived as purely clinical activity, and doctors have both disparaged and diminished the importance of the management function. A quality management program not only demands joint involvement by management and doctors, but perhaps is the means whereby both these groups could achieve a better understanding about the importance of each other's role in assuring and improving patient health care. We still hear of managers of hospitals of all sizes who claim that 'quality assurance' is something for doctors and nurses. It is still possible to meet with directors of hospital boards who quite clearly have no idea what quality assurance or quality management mean, nor any perception that they have a role in the initiation and implementation of such programs.

Quality assurance, for its part, implies action to implement changes in systems, patterns of service or care processes. In the complex environment of even a small hospital, such action is impossible unless the organisational and management structure

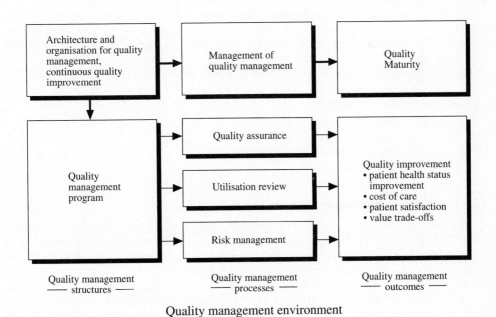

Quality management environment

Figure III-1-1 *The dynamic of quality management and quality improvement*

is present to translate decisions into action. The absence of an effective organisational and management structure for quality management has been the main reason for the failure of most initiatives in this area around Australia.

316 | Requirements for quality management

This part of the manual looks at the structural and organisational arrangements that are essential for successful quality management. In our experience, medical staff have little patience for what they see as unnecessary formality in, and for what we describe as the essential 'structure' of, committee activity and decision formulation. Only this formality and a structured process of committee activity will provide medical staff with the legal protection they seek, and will ensure that their efforts and the time that they spend on committees is not wasted; in short, that the energy they direct toward quality management or quality assurance will produce results.

A successful quality management program requires:

- the will to carry it out;
- the data and information to make decisions about quality of care;
- the structure to implement improvements;
- the knowledge about what to implement and how to implement it;
- the means and resources to implement it;
- measurement of results and use of this information to improve the program.

317 | Hospital size and quality management

In Australia a very high percentage of hospitals consist of 150 beds or less, although the majority of hospital beds are in hospitals of 150 beds or more. The comments and suggestions made in this part dealing with the organisational and administrative structure for quality management refer generally to hospitals of 150 beds or more.

Smaller hospitals present special difficulties. Due to their size small hospitals cannot support the structure necessary for all the elements of an effective quality management program. Small hospitals can manage quality provided they can draw on the resources of a larger program elsewhere. We recommend that small hospitals base their quality management program on a regional arrangement which can provide a centralised organisation. In this way a small hospital becomes part of a larger group for the purpose of quality management. Examples of such regionalised arrangements might be:

- geographic, such as country regions;
- ownership, such as private hospital chains;
- loose associations for QM purposes only;
- linkages with larger hospitals.

318 | Attitudes towards committees

One has only to sit in at a number of hospital committees to see another reason why efforts to implement quality management have not succeeded. An understanding of committee function, the importance of well-prepared agendas and minutes, and the ability to adequately chair a committee meeting, are not usually included in the training of either doctors or nurses or any other health professionals. In most hospitals very little attention is paid to the sort of detail necessary to ensure proper functioning of a committee. Partly, we believe this deficiency is a cultural attitude, where behaviour and performance is passed from one generation to another. Partly, however, it exists because management has not provided the training and support necessary for committees to function adequately. While a large number of hospitals can and do function almost in spite of their inadequate committee structure and performance, such an environment is not one in which a quality management program can succeed.

319 | Education for quality management

Throughout the manual readers will notice references to attitudes of either hospital boards, managers or medical and nursing staff to a variety of aspects of quality management and to quality management itself. To implement a quality management program successfully means that, in many instances, key players' current attitudes and understanding will need to change. For those working in a complex facility such as a modern hospital, changing attitudes means sustained, widespread education. One of the features of present 'QA' efforts in most hospitals is the limited attempt to educate any staff about QA, let alone quality management.

While such organisations as ACHS make available extensive programs of seminars and workshops, at an individual hospital level this educational effort is seriously diluted. In practice, this dilution often translates into a situation where there may be, at best, only one or two individuals in the hospital who have any real comprehension about what is being attempted. Hospital boards and managers are left to their own devices and yet their understanding of QM is quite critical to its successful implementation. Medical and nursing staff receive little, if any, education about QM or its subsets and are left to work through their anxieties and concerns. Their reaction is often one of indifference if not hostility—attitudes hardly consistent with success.

Successful quality management requires a considerable educational effort for all hospital personnel. Hospitals must also direct information to non-clinical staff about what is being attempted and what is expected of them, and provide them with proper instruction when necessary. This educational effort must be planned, professional in its execution and ongoing. A rough estimate suggests that hospital personnel will require, on average, at least one day (eight hours) per person per annum of education, although of course the actual amount per person will vary substantially and will depend on the person's role. Managers will require three to four days of leadership training per year and, ideally, to reach quality maturity each employee should receive five days of training in the first year and about three days in each subsequent year, to learn about and reinforce quality concepts and such special topics as clinical quality assessment. The quality management department is responsible for this education effort, which may involve arranging participation in hospital courses provided by QMD staff and consultants or contractors or sending staff to workshops and other educational experiences provided by associations, universities, or other organisations.

Chapter 2

GOVERNING BODY, MANAGEMENT AND HOSPITAL BY-LAWS

---

320 | Contents

This chapter describes the critical role of the governing body and management in the establishment of a quality management program and emphasises the commitment which must be present. It covers the following topics:

321. Purpose of this chapter
322. Role and function of hospital boards
323. Management's role
324. Hospital by-laws

---

321 | Purpose of this chapter

The successful implementation of a quality management program must start with the hospital's board of directors and its management. This chapter describes in some detail the role of directors and managers in a quality management program and the responsibility which they must shoulder to meet the demands of such an initiative.

322 | Role and function of hospital boards

322.1 | Boards are ultimately responsible for quality

The role of the hospital board or the governing body and consequently of its management is quite crucial if any quality management initiative is to succeed. In the final analysis, the board is responsible for the quality of care that pertains in the hospital. Board members need not become experts in QM nor should they become involved in the day-to-day functioning of a quality management program. However, if they are to fulfil their responsibilities as directors, board members have an obligation to take all practical steps to prevent unnecessary and, certainly, avoidable risk to the facility, its staff and patients. This obligation includes receiving regular reports about the quality of care and possessing sufficient knowledge of the process of quality management to be able to understand and act upon such reports, and to judge the adequacy of the hospital's QM systems and activities.

322.2 Board education for quality management

Board members should take whatever steps are required to properly inform themselves about the problem of medical and hospital quality of care and its manifestation, for example malpractice. It is management's responsibility to see that the board clearly understands what is meant by quality management and quality assurance, and what the broad thrust of such a program should be. If management itself does not have this knowledge, it must take steps to obtain it.

The board should understand, for example, some of the complexity involved in the implementation of a quality management program and the likely reaction of medical staff in particular, and the extent of attitudinal change that such a program of quality management demands throughout the hospital. For a board of directors to achieve an adequate understanding of quality management and its ramifications requires more than a five-minute mention by the hospital manager during the course of a busy board meeting. In a quality-mature hospital one might expect the majority of the board's time to be spent on quality management matters. One approach to achieve such understanding is to hold a one-day seminar for directors with presentations about the various aspects of quality management and its essential constituent elements. Hospitals will need to hold additional seminars periodically as the hospital's quality management program develops and the sophistication of its activities and hence the information they provide increases.

322.3 Board responsibilities

In order to fulfil its responsibilities for the quality of care, the board should:

- insist on being kept current about developments in health care quality management;
- develop a policy on quality management;
- insist on a plan to implement the policy, which would include establishing a QM program to implement the plan;
- allocate the resources needed to implement the plan successfully;
- require periodic reports on quality management activities and the hospital's quality of care;
- hold management responsible for implementing the quality management program, and assessing and improving the quality of care.

322.4 Keep current

Consistent with our comments regarding the need for education in the area of quality management, it is important that board members are constantly brought up to date by the manager on the rapid development of quality management issues. If health professionals have difficulty understanding these matters, it is so much more difficult for a board member who has to make important decisions in relation to them.

322.5 Develop policy

The hospital board is responsible for developing a policy about the quality of care, including quality management. The policy should encompass a vision of what is needed and why it is needed. However, the board's responsibilities do not begin and end with what might be described as a policy statement of high-minded words. As described later, the board's responsibility is also to see that its policy is implemented. Policy decisions relating to quality of patient care and quality management may well sit in a document which sets out the 'Charter, Objectives and Strategies' for all functions of the institution. Whether or not such a document exists, the board needs to state in writing its objectives and policies and to approve and endorse a quality management plan.

322.6 | Adopt a plan

Having developed policies relating to quality of care and quality management, the board now has to approve a plan to achieve its policy objectives. The plan should state the hospital's quality management program's objectives, and the strategies and steps necessary to reach the objectives. The essence of such a successful plan includes:

- being realistic in terms of the resources available and the obstacles which are likely to be faced;
- setting clear goals and objectives, which in turn demands a vision of what is to be accomplished;
- selecting a strategy for and specifing the steps needed to achieve objectives;
- programming the resources needed to carry out the steps, including organisational arrangements, personnel assignments, timetables and budgets;
- establishing a management information system to monitor progress, guide implementation and facilitate revision of plans.

Objectives need to be set and management must explain to the board its strategy to achieve these objectives. For example, the objective may be to improve continuously the quality of patient care. However, these words mean little to anyone, including board members, without the addition of a strategy necessary to reach that objective and the steps to be taken. The statement of strategies for use by a hospital board should be, of necessity, briefer than that adopted by the quality management committee and to be used by hospital staff. The plan should include immediately some and eventually all of the following elements:

- if not accredited, seek, as soon as practicable, and maintain accreditation by the Australian Council on Healthcare Standards;
- in accordance with the quality management plan, institute a quality management program embracing quality assurance, quality assessment, quality improvement, credentialling of medical staff, utilisation review, risk management etc.;
- establish a variety of monitoring and surveillance mechanisms and processes, including those to investigate, track and analyse, for example:
  —consumer (patient) complaints/compliments;
  —patient, staff and visitor incidents;
  —patient satisfaction;
  —patient processes/outcomes;
- develop mechanisms to implement and co-ordinate changes to improve care, to monitor their effects and costs and to use the resultant information to improve quality management.

This list of quality management activities will vary from hospital to hospital depending on the need to spell out such detail in the strategy. The matters listed above are intended as examples and are by no means a complete list of QM activity. This chapter spells them out to ensure that the governing body understands the range of activity to which it is committing itself, and to assist the board to assess the degree to which such policy is being implemented.

322.7 | Allocate resources

Many people are concerned about the cost of quality management. However, they should be more concerned about the cost of quality or its lack—such as needless deaths, iatrogenic illness, extra days in hospital, defending and paying malpractice claims, low staff morale, and disillusionment with medical care. Often these consequences can be prevented at very little if any cost, provided an effective quality management program is put in place. Surprisingly, an effective quality management program including quality assurance in its early stages can amount to less than 1% of a hospital's operating expenditure—an amount which might be far less than the cost of one malpractice suit. Very often the quality management program's early costs are in more appropriate resource allocations (including staff reassignments).

Unlike most other hospital activity, which at the present time is not (but should be) subject to cost-benefit measurement, we believe that the costs and benefits of a quality management program should be measured to enable a board to appreciate the cost-benefit trade-offs incurred. All hospital activity, including the care delivered, must eventually be judged in terms of effects and costs. The quality management program should become the vehicle for making this transition. Setting up the quality management program in this vein provides the necessary example.

To document the value of a hospital's quality management program, it is necessary to track its costs and benefits. To be complete, such tracking must include the cost of errors that are occurring. It is easy to measure the cost of the program; quite another to measure the value of improvement, and the cost of existing or residual lack of quality. The costs/effects of various quality management activities must be measured to ensure that the program is effective and that the desired effect is achieved at the lowest cost; that is, to choose rationally among the range of QM activities and the intensity with which they should be applied. It is not a question of whether or not a quality management program should exist, but rather a question of how much to spend and of allocating resources among competing activities. Before voting any allocation of funds for a quality management program, hospital management must reassure the board about the quality of the proposed program and how these resources are to be spent. This reassurance is embedded in a comprehensive quality management plan, the essence of which is described above.

'All that glitters is not gold' applies as much to quality management and quality assurance as anything else. We are aware of two major hospitals in Australia that committed significant expenditures to 'quality assurance' activities; however, after some twelve or eighteen months they were unable to demonstrate one problem solved or one positive change in patient care. The reason, we believe, was that both hospitals focused their attention on the QA methodologies necessary for quality assessment but ignored the organisational framework necessary to resolve problems. Having identified a range of problems, there was no satisfactory mechanism available to resolve them. The need to demonstrate success reinforces the need, as part of the quality management program, to collect data on problems solved or improvements made and the costs and savings made by the hospital quality management program.

The board must be advised what is and what is not realistic, particularly in regard to resources, and it must also be properly advised about the likely difficulties which will be faced in the implementation of such a program. Few boards we have encountered have any understanding of these issues. A successful quality management program demands that the full spectrum of essential elements (detailed later in this chapter) functions effectively. Implementing parts of the whole cannot produce the effects of the whole.

322.8 | Assess results

To this point, the board's responsibilities have only just commenced. In the course of developing the quality management plan, key measures of success and progress should have been identified. Adequate management information systems are required to enable a board to receive appropriate reports concerning progress and success. The board must insist that management provides such regular reporting. The board must ensure that its policy is translated into effective action and above all must follow-up to see that the policy is being adhered to and is working. Regular review of reports is crucial to fulfilling this responsibility.

322.9 Hold management accountable

The board must see that management does not devolve responsibility for the quality management program to health professionals or anyone else. The board must insist that management accepts and understands this responsibility and is accountable to the board for all aspects of the quality management program and ultimately the quality, cost, and acceptability of care delivered in the hospital.

323 Management's role

The successful implementation of policies relating to a quality management program will rest heavily on the management's shoulders. Management cannot stand by assuming, as has been frequently the case up until now, that medical and nursing staff can carry this responsibility unaided. However, managers, as is the case with other health professionals, are not born with an instinctive understanding of quality management programs and quality assurance concepts. One of the reasons managers have tended to pass the responsibility for 'quality assurance' to health professionals is their own lack of understanding and expertise in the areas of both clinical matters generally and quality management specifically. Nothing will test the skills and capacity of managers more rigorously than the implementation of a quality management program. However, product quality is, or should be, the raison d'etre of management. Quality is not something to be regarded as an extraneous burden to be passed lightly to others or to be seen as a task to fill in one's spare moments. It is management's main mission.

Many hospitals may already be engaged, to a greater or lesser extent, in some 'quality assurance' activity. However, neither boards nor managements can assume that implementing a coherent quality management program will be anything but a complex and at times difficult undertaking that requires sustained and continued effort and commitment. The hospital's quality management program must be structured and organised; it will not simply happen. The manager is responsible for structuring this activity in the way best suited to his or her hospital. Each hospital is unique, and management all too commonly has to face the hurdles of a highly individualistic medical staff and power plays between individuals and groups. The approach and strategy to be adopted will therefore vary from hospital to hospital.

Medical staff must also have the 'will to implement', if quality management is to be successful. In our view, the necessary response will be forthcoming from most medical staff if the program is presented and implemented as a co-operative endeavour intended to improve patient care and not primarily as a means of controlling doctors nor focused exclusively on weeding out 'bad apples'. Regardless, we would emphasise that the final responsibility for the successful implementation of a quality management program in any hospital must be that of management, whose motto must be 'Quality is the job'.

324 Hospital by-laws

324.1 Aspects of hospital by-laws

Hospital and medical staff by-laws play an important role in the entire quality management initiative. By-laws are discussed under the following headings:

- definition;
- current situation in Australia;
- by-laws and quality management.

324.2   Definition

By-laws constitute the internal legislation of a hospital. They provide the legal and administrative framework by which a hospital can achieve its objectives. By-laws therefore can have a major impact on the operation of a modern hospital. Not only do they govern the relationship between a hospital board and management, and the direct providers of care and services, but they also provide the hospital medical staff with a stable and predictable environment in which they are able to make decisions commensurate with the hospital's objectives and policies.

324.3   Current situation in Australia

There is considerable variation between public and private hospitals in Australia as to the manner in which by-laws are structured. Public hospitals' by-laws are usually incorporated in the one document that describes matters relating to the hospital in general and to medical staff in particular. Private hospitals, while mostly incorporated organisations, do not include in their Articles of Incorporation material which is found in hospital by-laws. Some private hospitals separate hospital and medical staff by-laws, while others combine them in a way similar to public hospitals. However, in general private hospital by-laws tend to give greater weight to the activities relating to medical staff activity than to matters relating to the hospital itself.

324.4   By-laws and quality management

Hospital by-laws should include a section that stipulates that involvement by all staff, clinical and non-clinical, in quality management activity is mandatory. In many public hospitals the increasing use of 'terms and conditions of appointment' provides an additional avenue for emphasising to medical staff their obligations in relation to quality management, such as serving on committees and attention to quality of documentation. Private hospitals in general do not subject medical staff to a formal contract that includes written 'terms and conditions of appointment'. In our view such a contract is long overdue, to protect the hospital, the doctor and patients.

The inclusion of provisions for mandatory involvement in quality management in the hospital by-laws serves to reinforce the authority of the board and management and to underscore their commitment to a quality management program and to assuring the hospital's quality of care. The by-laws should provide enough detail to make it unequivocal for medical staff to understand what is expected of them in relation to quality management. In particular, they should make clear that while all medical practitioners will not necessarily be actively involved in quality management or quality assurance activity all of the time, they must, if and when requested, be prepared to participate in such commitments as committee activity.

The by-laws should also spell out the responsibility of medical staff to maintain adequate medical records. The poor standard of documentation in medical records in many hospitals frequently represents a greater legal risk to the hospital and its medical staff than any clinical negligence or inadequacy on the part of members of the medical staff.

By-laws should also define sanctions that might apply to medical staff who continually flout the sort of requirements referred to above, or whose care is persistently or irremediably substandard. Limitation on clinical privileges or even termination of hospital appointment should be recorded as possible sanctions. If sanctions are described for particular infractions of the by-laws, fact-finding and adjudicatory mechanisms must be described clearly, so that procedures are clear and documented and so that every practitioner is treated fairly and uniformly and has the right to question findings and appeal decisions.

<h1>Chapter 3</h1>

<h1>THE QUALITY MANAGEMENT COMMITTEE AND AN EFFECTIVE COMMITTEE SYSTEM</h1>

<h2>330 | Contents</h2>

An integrated committee system is crucial to any quality management program. This chapter explores the system of quality management committees and looks at the interrelationships of the various committees under the following headings:

331. Purpose of this chapter
332. Why committees?
333. Quality management and committees
334. The quality management committee
335. Interrelationships of committees
336. Characteristics of quality management committees
337. Functioning of committees
338. Well-functioning committees
339. Education for committee skills

<h2>331 | Purpose of this chapter</h2>

Quality management and quality assurance simply cannot succeed in any hospital without an effective system of committees. This chapter emphasises this view and discusses in some detail the most important aspects of a quality management committee system.

<h2>332 | Why committees?</h2>

Most hospital doctors hate committees, for reasons mentioned elsewhere. However, committees and the committee system in a hospital of which they are part represent the institution's nervous system. Committees are a necessary forum for discussion and decision making. They form a critical element in democratic or participatory management.

Committees permit the orderly generation and transfer of information, the bringing together of diverse expertise and perspectives, and the orderly taking and implementation of decisions. One of the factors which makes hospitals so complex is their number of highly skilled and independent health professionals, all of whom have differing perspectives on the many issues that arise. Communicating with and accessing the skills and views of this range of professionals would be difficult, if not impossible, without committees.

As well as being a mechanism for communication, committees also have the responsibility for problem solving and decision making. For reasons which are multiple and at times not always clear, committees in Australian hospitals seem to have great difficulty with the decision-making role. Decision making requires empowerment and entails a commitment to action—a commitment which all too often is missing.

Many modern management movements, including total quality management, emphasise permanent or temporary 'teams', people working together toward common goals, principally in this context to produce goods and services or improve their quality. One can regard teams as committees, stripped of their formality and the need for members to report to 'constituencies', since in theory teams are purely functional entities. In this chapter we eschew the word 'team', but readers should recognise that what we say about committees also applies in principle to teams, even though they may be consituted less formally. For example, a committee should have written terms of reference, whereas a team's 'terms of reference' may be no more than a manager's verbal communication to a subordinate to get the right people involved to solve a problem. Teams' functioning and success—or failure—depends on the types of committee 'dynamics' that this chapter details. Ad hoc formation of teams—and committees—may create more problems than it solves, a point that this chapter emphasises.

333 | Quality management and committees

333.1 | Successful quality management depends on committees

The success of any quality management program depends not only on the existence of a committee system, but, more importantly, on the capacity of hospital medical and nursing staff to understand how the system works and how they fit into it. If hospital committees are to function effectively, medical and nursing staff have to have some grasp of committees' 'greater purpose'. Such a perspective should be acquired through the development of a quality management plan, terms of reference for the various committees, and training aids and materials for staff.

The quality manager, in concert with the chairperson of the quality management committee, is responsible for explaining the larger picture of committee activity to committee members and to the wider hospital staff. An important element in this education of hospital staff is a brief document describing the hospital's commitment to quality management and how it assures quality, including committee activity. This document should be distributed to each staff member. Similarly, in hospital by-laws and in terms and conditions of appointment for medical staff, reference should be made to this commitment to quality management.

333.2 | Current situation

It is difficult to generalise about the current situation of committees in hospitals in Australia. Public hospitals, for reasons that are uncertain, tend to have a myriad of committees. Indeed, our experience suggests that in many hospitals there are too many committees. This situation often results from an ineffective committee system, so that failure to achieve results often leads to the establishment of yet another committee to carry out the task. Whatever the reason, many larger public hospitals have 'committee mania' and management (or lack of it) by committee prevails, leading to an extraordinarily cumbersome process of decision making.

Private hospitals, on the other hand, tend to have a less than optimal number of committees, and in many a medical advisory committee is frequently all that exists. It is only relatively recently that most private hospitals, the majority of which are small (less than 100 beds), have developed any semblance of medical staff organisation or committee structure. There has been a tendency on the part of private hospital managements to be satisfied with a medical advisory committee that, in many private hospitals, plays only a token role.

In hospitals where there is a committee system, the problem is often how the committees function and their interrelationships. Experience suggests that there are very few hospitals where the chairpersons and members of committees have a clear understanding of the overall purpose of their committee and what its function is in the overall management of the hospital. Certainly the concept of committees being an integral part of quality management is absent.

333.3 | What is needed

There can be no fixed rule about precisely what committees any one particular hospital should have, of course. Most hospitals will need the following committees, whose interrelationships are depicted in Figure III-3-1 on page 474.

333.4 | Hospital-wide committees

- Quality management committee—responsible for quality management in the hospital and can co-ordinate such activities for the entire facility.
- Credentials committee—responsible for the annual assessment of privileges of every member of the medical staff and for the review of any individual member when and if appropriate.
- Medical appointments advisory committee—responsible for advising the board of directors concerning the suitability for appointment of each new and existing member of the medical staff on a triennial basis or at such other interval as the board decides.
- Quality of care committee—responsible to the quality management committee for the quality of clinical care; may have a number of committees relating directly to it including the following:
  —Quality assessment/measurement committee—responsible for a range of activities relating to quality measurement, such as structured quality review, patient satisfaction surveys, incident and complaints reporting and tracking etc. (See Parts II and IV.)
  —Practice policies committee—responsible for developing practice policies. (See Part II.)
  —Medical record (clinical information) committee—responsible for all aspects of clinical information recording, storage and retrieval, and whose responsibility extends to ensuring the availability of data for patient care, administrative and quality management and quality assurance purposes.
  —Special studies committee—responsible for special quality of care studies including nosocomial infection (infection control), and tissue audits.
  —Infection control committee—responsible for supervision of all procedures relating to maintaining an infection free hospital environment, including sterilisation procedures, for both clinical and non-clinical areas.
- Services, technology and research committee—develops policies, procedures and protocols for the acquisition of technologies which exceed certain unit or aggregate

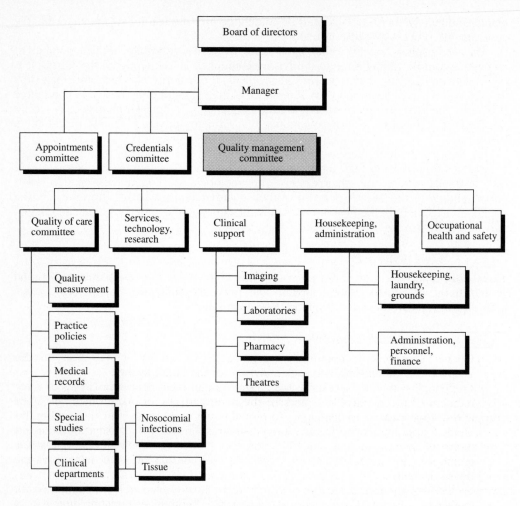

Figure III-3-1 *Quality management committee structure*

acquisition or use costs. This committee guides and assists the assessment of technologies for decision by the board, and makes recommendations to the board concerning services to be provided having regard to technology available or required. In large hospitals it may also be responsible for the overview of all research projects (or a separate committee may be established for this purpose).

• Clinical support committee—responsible for quality of services relating to imaging, laboratories, pharmacy:

—Pharmacy (drug) committee—responsible for decisions relating to storage, distribution, control and usage of all medication in the hospital, and policies and procedures relating thereto.

—Operating theatre committee—responsible for all aspects of the operating theatre environment and functioning.

• Housekeeping/administration committee—responsible for quality of services in these areas including:

—Housekeeping, laundry and grounds committee.

—Administration, personnel and finance.

- Occupational health and safety committee—responsible for the health, safety and welfare of all employees and staff. (See Part V.)

333.5 | *Departmental or divisional committees*

Matters which need to be considered at departmental level might be described as 'production' effectiveness. To what extent each department or division will need committees relating to quality of care activities will depend largely on the hospital size and the sophistication of its services. Where obstetrics is conducted, for example, a delivery suite committee responsible for all aspects of the delivery suite function may be required or it may be considered adequate to combine such activity with the operating theatre committee. The decision to establish departmental committees, and their terms of reference, are matters for decision by the hospital's quality management committee.

Each clinical department or division will have its own quality of care committee that is responsible for practice policies and the review of practice criteria and standards, operational efficiency, for example such matters as waiting times, and various aspects of patient satisfaction.

Many small hospitals, because of their low volume of activity and the high workload placed on only a small number of medical staff, will find it more satisfactory either to participate in a regional arrangement and/or to combine one or more committees in order to use their available human resources to best advantage.

333.6 | *Changing the committee structure*

Changing a committee structure, either by introducing new committees or changing the terms of reference of existing committees, including terminating them, is a good deal easier to do in theory than in practice. Chairpersons and committee members who have been accustomed to a particular committee structure, perhaps for many years, will often strongly resist any attempt to change it. Territorial issues and power structures within the hospital are bound up in the arrangement of committees and change will quite often threaten the status quo. Accordingly, any change to the committee structure needs to be carefully thought through and planned, and the change itself should be a staged process. Members of the existing committees should be involved in the preliminary discussions and the planning. Perhaps the worst of all situations is where the resistance to changing committees is so great that a decision is finally made to leave the existing structure in place while superimposing a new committee structure on the old. We have witnessed the results of such a decision, which could only be described as producing chaos.

334 | **The quality management committee**

Each hospital should have a committee that is responsible for quality management throughout the entire hospital. Such a committee might have a number of subcommittees dealing with such areas as medical practice standards, the process of structured quality review, and so on and such non-clinical quality assurance activities as occupational health and safety. (See Figure III-3-1 on page 474.)

The quality management committee is the most important committee in the hospital, making recommendations to the manager and, through the manager, to the board of directors. Doctors and nurses, generally speaking, may have little understanding about management but they certainly understand quality of patient care. Most of the committees reporting to and relating with the quality management committee should have as their major if not exclusive focus the quality of patient care. For this reason we have designated the hospital quality management committee as the most important of these committees. While it may be considered an issue of semantics, the terms 'patient care review committee' and 'clinical services committee' do not provide a sufficiently clear focus for most clinical staff of this key committee's prime purpose.

The quality management committee chairperson should usually be a senior respected medical practitioner and the committee will comprise members who come from most if not all the major clinical and non-clinical departments or divisions in the hospital. Like all committees, with the exception of the credentials committee and the medical appointments advisory committee, it will be multidisciplinary. It will have the power to co-opt additional personnel when additional expertise is required. A useful approach to develop skills among committee members and to assist with the difficult task of co-ordinating committee activities is to select the best person to chair its various functional subcommittees and appoint them to be committee members (somewhat the reverse of the usual situation in which committee members are appointed first and then picked to head subcommittees).

The hospital quality management committee will have the following functions. They are elaborated in terms of reference provided in the Appendix to this chapter. These terms of reference have been provided because the current activities of similar committees in most hospitals are far too limited and they are not sufficiently detailed in most instances. The quality management committee is responsible for:

- managing all quality management activities, hospital-wide, including quality assurance, utilisation review, risk management, and plans and policies relating to quality assurance to be conducted in departments or divisions;
- making recommendations to the manager and to the board, which has an overriding responsibility in relation to quality management policy matters;
- recommending actions to administrators and other line officials;
- monitoring the work of the quality manager and quality management department;
- receiving and acting upon reports about quality management activity and the quality of patient care, which will come from departments, divisions, or subcommittees to the quality manager, and providing reports to management, including the board of directors;
- providing guidance, recommendations and support to heads of departments or divisions about quality management and quality assurance;
- providing and facilitating communications and problem resolution across departments and divisions and across various services;
- monitoring all clinical quality assurance activity;
- ensuring that all quality management and quality assurance issues referred from other committees are properly tracked and accounted for;
- evaluating the cost-effectiveness of all aspects of quality management.

335 | Interrelationships of committees

In essence, committees and the data which flow between them represent the hospital's nervous system. They provide the sensors to tell what is going on, the means to make sense of it all, and finally the instrument for taking action to assure and improve quality of patient care.

The quality management committee is the overall co-ordinator of all quality management activity. This does not mean that the members of the quality management committee have the sole responsibility for all such quality management functions. Rather, it has to delegate effectively much activity to a number of other hospital committees, many of which already exist in most hospitals, and, most importantly, to division heads and their staff who deliver or support services to patients.

Figure III-3-1 on page 474 depicts the range of hospital committees that is required and that commonly exists in hospitals. All these committees individually must function effectively and must relate meaningfully to the others. One of the quality management committee's principal roles is to see that this happens. The quality manager and the quality management department provide the resources and support necessary to ensure that it does happen.

Figure III-3-1 also provides some indication of how the various committees connected with some aspect of quality management relate to the quality management committee. These relationships are, of course, much more complex than can be demonstrated by such a simple chart. As anyone who has sat on hospital committees knows only too well, the biggest difficulty is keeping track of issues as they flow from one committee to the next, and deciding which committee is responsible for what action. All too frequently issues become lost and it is not uncommon for members in a committee, their memory triggered by the current discussion, to ask: 'I wonder what happened about such-and-such a matter that we were discussing some months ago?'

The quality management department and its manager, working through the quality management committee, must track and follow-up on issues and see that issues do not become lost. The quality management department should also ensure that the committees involved in the quality management system are liaising appropriately with each other and that they are reporting regularly in an approved manner to the quality management committee. The pivotal position and role of the quality management committee is not simply a question of 'control' but of integration of functions. This important committee is designed to avoid confusion, contradictory changes and policies, and the needless upsetting of existing operations.

From time to time an issue will arise that will require the authority of the hospital manager rather than falling into the realm of quality management. In these circumstances the matter will be referred to a committee other than the hospital QM committee, or directly to the manager. It is our view, however, that if the committees referred to earlier in this chapter are fulfilling their correct role, most of their business will have implications for the quality of care in the hospital.

336 | Characteristics of quality management committees

The most important feature of a quality management committee system is its capacity to move away from the inadequate current practice of 'quality assurance' for doctors, 'quality assurance' for nurses, 'quality assurance' for physiotherapists, and so on. Patient outcomes are produced by the hospital, not by individuals working in isolation within its walls. To achieve this goal of hospital-wide quality management, most of the committees need to be multidisciplinary—by which we mean medical and other health professionals, together with management, sitting on the same committee. For a committee system to support a quality management program effectively, mechanisms must be found to provide for:

- appropriate input by those involved in patient care or service delivery;
- the collection, analysis and evaluation of information;
- problem identification;
- problem resolution;
- appropriate follow-up.

The system must be able to deal with the wide range of issues which arise when quality of care is under review and accordingly will have the following characteristics:

- It will consist of a number of committees, the precise number of which will vary from hospital to hospital depending on:

—size of the hospital;
—complexity of services
—management structure of the hospital.

* All the (sub)committees must relate to one main central co-ordinating committee, which we call the quality management committee, responsible for all aspects of quality of care and services.
* In large hospitals there may be a number of departmental or divisional quality assurance committees reporting to and relating with the central quality management committee, either directly or through a functional subcommittee, such as a quality of care or a clinical support subcommittee.
* All committees, except the medical appointments advisory committee and the credentials committee, which should comprise medical practitioners only, must comprise medical and other health professionals, managers and other relevant types of hospital staff.

337 | Functioning of committees

337.1 | Committees have various, distinct functions

All committees involved in the quality management process will find themselves faced with a variety of functions. Many of the issues that have to be dealt with are complex and to reduce this complexity to a minimum, various functions should be identified and dealt with separately. In addition, factors such as time and expertise will necessitate that separate committees will handle different functions more effectively.

When considering committee functions it is important to distinguish between the functions of:

* data collection and data analysis;
* recommendations or decisions concerning actions that might be initiated;
* the actual implementation of actions decided upon.

All these functions may well take place in the same committee, but not necessarily so. It may well be that recommendations from a committee may only be implemented by a decision of management or even the board of directors.

By way of example, let us assume that as a result of data provided, the quality management committee reaches the conclusion that there is a problem relating to medication errors. Having identified the problem, the QM committee authorises the QM department (QMD) to investigate the cause or causes of the medication errors. This step may involve establishing a working party or a subcommittee. At the completion of this task the QM department finds the causes of the problem are: firstly, legibility of handwriting of one or two medical officers; and secondly, the inadequacy of the system by which nurses distribute medication to patients in the hospital. The action taken to solve each of these causative issues is obviously different and each is referred by the QM committee to the appropriate committee or individual for solution. The solutions reached and actions taken are eventually reported back to the QM committee. A QM committee has neither the time nor expertise to conduct all the functions required in our example and it must delegate some of these steps to others.

In the final instance, however, it is the QM committee which must choose between competing solutions and differing approaches to solving a problem especially when they overlap organisational responsibilities. The quality management committee is the point in the hospital where 'the buck finally stops'. It may be, of course, that resolution of a problem ultimately may require management or board decision. The recommendation relating to the problem, however, must be that of the QM committee.

337.2   *Lines of reporting*

To whom or to what other committee any committee reports is an important aspect of quality management. Remaining mindful of this reporting responsibility will assist committee members to focus their decisions more effectively and at the same time ensure that those decisions are more relevant. Reporting relationships is a matter for inclusion in a committee's terms of reference, and it is the responsibility of the chairperson to remind his or her committee of these relationships when appropriate. All the committees, which we have enumerated as part of a quality management program, are ultimately responsible through the manager to the board of directors. Committees' terms of reference need to state clearly the degree of autonomy with which decisions in these individual committees may be made.

337.3   *Size and composition of committees*

We suggest that rather than creating a large and cumbersome committee which often becomes difficult to manage, in many instances a smaller core group should be appointed as members of the committee. When an issue arises which requires otherwise non-existent expertise, the committee will have the power to co-opt additional personnel on an ad hoc basis.

Who should sit on committees is an issue which will vary from hospital to hospital and will depend on the committee's function. The individual personalities of committee members is just as important as to which disciplinary group they belong. The selection of chairpersons is even more critical, and the credibility and standing of the chairperson with colleagues is also important. Medical staff are not the only professional group in the hospital, but the reality of patient care is such that if quality management is to succeed, the medical staff must feel comfortable with the composition of the committees and the chairpersons must have credibility in the eyes of the medical staff.

337.4   *Attendance at committees*

If quality management is to be effective, attendance and participation in these committee activities is essential. It is also important to ensure that the burden of participating in quality management and its many aspects is shared by as wide a group as possible. A preparedness to participate in quality management activity should be mandatory for all staff, and for medical staff should be a condition of appointment.

Continual failure to attend meetings should be a matter for discussion between the chairperson and member, and ultimately the hospital manager. At the very least, continual failure to attend meetings should result in termination of the individual's position on the committee. The rules governing attendance at committees must be stipulated by the hospital and clearly understood by all concerned.

Before accepting appointment to committees, medical staff must be prepared to arrange their activities such as theatre lists and clinic times so as to ensure that these do not conflict with attendance at meetings. Unfortunately, on occasions important committee responsibilities, essential to the effective functioning of the hospital, are given second priority to the demands of a busy private practice. The nature of medical practice is such that such conflicts will inevitably occur. Good planning and foresight should reduce this problem to a minimum.

337.5   *Authorisation of committees*

While it is the board's responsibility to determine and authorise the hospital's major committees, establishing other working committees is management's responsibility. Management is responsible for ensuring that the committee system functions as an integrated whole and that individual committees function adequately.

337.6 Confidentiality

Members of any committee should consider the committee's business confidential to its members. However, when considering committees involved in a hospital quality management program, the need for confidentiality becomes even more important. Legal action against members of such committees may be precipitated by members' lax attitude to confidentiality. Some committees, such as a credentials committee, have such a need for absolute confidentiality that even a minute secretary is dispensed with, the minutes being kept by one of its members.

338 Well-functioning committees

338.1 Requirements for effective committees

Nothing is more crucial to quality management than an effective committee system. An 'effective committee' refers to a committee that functions well and fulfils its objectives to members' satisfaction. We are constantly amazed at the poor standard of committee activity which we see regularly in hospitals of all sizes, public and private. This ineffective committee activity is an important cause of the poor success rate for quality management implementation in Australia and, ironically, doctors' dissatisfaction with committees.

It is a common misconception that if a number of well-meaning individuals sit together in a discussion, all else will automatically follow and an effective committee will result. If those responsible pay attention to certain basic elements of committee activity, there will be a corresponding improvement in the attitude of the medical staff, many members of which currently see such activity as a timewasting exercise (which it often is the way many committees are run now).

While some committees are a forum for the exchange of knowledge and information, others must serve the purpose of formulating and implementing decisions. However, nothing is so deadening to enthusiasm as for members of a committee to believe that whatever they do or whatever decisions they may make or recommend, nothing will result. The output of a committee must be taken seriously and be seen to be taken seriously. If members of a committee believe that what they do is valuable and valued they will make the necessary effort.

There are a number of critical elements that are essential if the time spent by busy hospital professionals is not to be wasted in many hours of fruitless effort. These elements consist of:

- properly constructed terms of reference;
- membership appropriate to role and function;
- skilled chairmanship;
- deliberate formality;
- who can and cannot attend;
- well-prepared agenda;
- concise but meaningful minutes;
- adequate accommodation.

338.2 Terms of reference

It is important that every committee should have prepared terms of reference which delineate the committee's purpose and role. Essential matters when preparing terms of reference include:

- authorisation for the committee, for example hospital board;
- purpose of the committee;
- membership of committee:

—number of members
—qualifications of members
—method of selection of members
—length of service for the committee members
—initial membership conditions, if any
—how chairperson is appointed;
* whether the committee is a 'standing' (in perpetuity) committee or an 'ad hoc' (time limited) committee;
* functional relationships to other committees;
* reporting relationships;
* mechanics of the committee:
—agenda
—minutes
—notice of meetings
—frequency of meetings;
* quorum;
* voting procedures, for example simple majority;
* guidelines for committee functions;
* general statement about the relationship with hospital by-laws and conformity with hospital policy;
* mechanism to change terms of reference;
* other relevant considerations.

At the inception of the committee such terms of reference must be approved and adopted by the committee to ensure that they have been formally accepted and, in the process, that every member of the committee has had an opportunity to discuss them. At this time or subsequently, members may recommend amendments to the terms of reference to the authorising body for its consideration. The chairperson is responsible for ensuring that the committee does not stray outside its terms of reference. A chairperson's failure to guide the committee in this way is a common cause of rambling discussions which have very little relevance to the committee's business and which leave everyone feeling dissatisfied. Model terms of reference for quality management committees are set out in the Appendix to this chapter.

338.3 Membership of committees

Committees can be classified as functional or representational in character, and in many hospital situations these two types of committees are often confused. Most hospital committees belong to the functional type and as such membership should be small with a maximum number of nine and with a minimum number of five persons. However, committees established to review medical records using the process of structured quality review, which is referred to in Part IV, may only consist of three members and it may be appropriate for a hospital's QM committee to have as many as fifteen members.

Each member on the committee should be an expert, or at least be able to make a meaningful contribution, and should be seen as an equal contributor. Representation, of course, usually does play a part in selecting committee members in most hospitals, and the aim should be to see that those selected can represent relevant points of view as well as structural groupings in the hospital.

The chairperson may be appointed or may be elected from among committee members. If appointed, he or she may participate in the process of selecting the members of the committee. Where the chairperson is selected by the members of the committee, it is often a worthwhile practice for the position of chairperson to rotate among the committee.

338.4 | Chairmanship

The quality of committee chairmanship determines its effectiveness. Few people, whether they be senior medical personnel or other hospital staff, are born with the skills to chair a committee. Such skills do not come naturally; they have to be acquired. The chairperson must be familiar with meeting procedure, and anyone faced with the responsibility of chairing a committee should purchase any one of a number of simple texts on meeting procedure. In general, meeting procedure is based on British parliamentary practice, which, while not essential to apply strictly, requires some experience to handle adeptly.

A good chairperson must accept the responsibility of guiding, steering and facilitating the discussion. This responsibility is fulfilled by identifying the task or issues at hand and seeing to it that all members of the committee understand what is required. It is also necessary to ensure that all members have the opportunity to speak and play a part in reaching a decision. The chairperson must also be able to terminate the discussion in a manner which, while not pleasing everyone, nevertheless is able to leave the committee with the feeling that the best was achieved under the circumstances and that it is adequate. The chairperson is also responsible for ensuring that the agenda is properly prepared and that the minutes are adequate prior to their distribution. This view does not imply that the chairperson actually writes and distributes the agenda or is a minute secretary.

During the meeting, the chairperson is also responsible for ensuring that the wording of all motions is clearly understood by all present, and in particular by the minute secretary. Failure to fulfil this rather obvious responsibility often results in continual arguments at subsequent meetings about what was actually said and what was really decided. The chairperson's responsibility does not end with a structured procedure for the committee. He or she also has to be the driving force for the committee. This means continually keeping an overview to ensure that the committee is functioning adequately in the total hospital and, in this instance, quality management framework.

338.5 | A structured procedure

Hospital committees and in particular those that form part of the quality management framework, will not be effective unless they are conducted with a significant degree of formality. The degree to which meeting procedure is structured will depend largely on the size of the committee, but in general should embrace the following points:

- the quorum to be strictly observed;
- formal opening and closing of meeting;
- corrections, if any, to the minutes of the previous meeting and their formal acceptance as an accurate record;
- discussion only permitted after a formal motion is proposed and seconded, or at least no protracted discussion to proceed until a motion has been formally proposed to the meeting;
- no discussion to proceed until members understand clearly the wording of the proposal;
- all motions to be put to the vote;
- business not on the distributed agenda not to be discussed except with the committee's approval;
- meeting times to be strictly observed. Meetings should start on time and finish on time. Meetings which continue to extend over the prescribed time suggest greater care is required in agenda preparation or that the meeting is not being adequately controlled. If the allotted time has elapsed before business has been completed, uncompleted business should be deferred to another meeting. In general, meetings should only last for one hour, or less. Occasionally, committees may have to

consider matters that require an exception to this rule. However, hospital staff members are busy people, and like all busy people, they find it difficult to attend lengthy meetings, and, more importantly, they can only concentrate effectively—in a way necessary for a productive meeting—for relatively short periods.
- before closing the meeting, the chairperson should review briefly the actions and decisions determined during the course of the meeting, both as a reminder and to ensure concurrence by those present.

We lay great stress on these issues because lack of a structured meeting procedure inevitably leads to timewasting, and more importantly may inadvertently expose many committees and the hospital itself to unnecessary and avoidable legal risk.

338.6 Who can and cannot attend

From time to time guests, observers or presenters of reports, experts who may be resources for decisions, or other such people have a legitimate place at a committee meeting, although they will not be members of the committee. Such attendees should be present only with the specific invitation of the chairperson, who in turn should have his or her actions approved or endorsed by the committee.

Persons other than properly appointed members of a committee have no right to participate in the business of the meeting, including moving or seconding motions, speaking or voting. Their right to speak is dependent on an invitation by the chairperson. Presenters of a report, having presented the report and answered questions related to the report, may be requested to leave the meeting. In all these circumstances and whatever the limitations placed on attendees other than members, the utmost courtesy needs to be extended, as would be done to a guest in one's home.

338.7 Agenda preparation

Preparation of an agenda is a key factor in the success or otherwise of a committee. This task should not be left to a clerk; it must have the oversight of the chairperson. It is simply not good enough to merely transfer a list of items for discussion from one month's agenda to the next. This not uncommon approach merely results in the committee continually discussing the same matters over and over again. The responsibility for avoiding this situation lies with the chairperson and not the minute secretary.

The agenda, together with the minutes of the previous meeting, should be in the hands of committee members at least seven days prior to the meeting to enable them to prepare for it. We have witnessed occasions when the agenda was handed out to members of the committee on their arrival for a regularly scheduled meeting. The key to effective participation in committees is preparation. Unless the agenda and accompanying documentation are available in ample time prior to a meeting, adequate preparation is not possible. Committee members have a corresponding duty to prepare for meetings so that meaningful discussion of agenda items can ensue.

338.8 Minutes and their preparation

The minutes of a meeting form a legal record of that meeting and as such deserve special care and attention. Ideally, the hospital should make available a minute secretary, who is not a member of the committee, for the sole purpose of taking the minutes. Pressure on resources at times may make this difficult or even impossible. Moreover, if concise, accurate and useful records of important meetings are to be achieved, the person designated to record and prepare the minutes, whether a minute secretary or a member of the committee, must be given instruction on what is required to complete this task correctly.

Minutes should record only decisions and actions to be taken. With few exceptions, minutes should not record names of individuals. The chairperson is responsible for indicating what additional information relating to the decision or action should be recorded. Some system should also be adopted to clearly indicate who is responsible for implementing decisions or taking actions decided at the meeting, and for reporting the outcome back to the committee.

The minutes should be checked by the chairperson or the hospital manager (or designee) before distribution in order to ensure that no obviously defamatory material has been inadvertently included in the minutes. In any case, the chairperson should always check the minutes for accuracy prior to distribution. For reasons similar to those made in the case of the agenda, the minutes must accompany the agenda and be available to members at least seven days prior to the meeting if adequate preparation is to be achieved. This reading and acceptance should be the first item of business of each meeting.

338.9 | *Accommodation*

Adequate facilities should be provided for committee meetings, in terms of space and comfort, and ideally each person attending should be given writing materials. We have participated in meetings held in a corridor, with people walking through committee members. Papers were balanced on knees and the atmosphere was hardly conducive to serious deliberation and decision making.

339 | **Education for committee skills**

Hospital management has a responsibility to ensure that those hospital staff appointed to committees understand sufficient of the principles we have outlined to enable the quality management committee system to work effectively and with minimal legal risk.

A routine orientation program for all new appointees to committees is a positive step that management can take to ensure members have at least a rudimentary insight into committee skills. Where a particular problem is apparent, management may need to organise a special training workshop. This type of orientation is especially important for committee chairpersons. Hospital management is responsible for ensuring that hospital staff understand how to organise committees, how to conduct themselves effectively in a committee and the rudiments of committee chairmanship.

Without such training, committees will not function effectively and, in multidisciplinary meetings, medical staff will tend to dominate the proceedings without necessarily being effective. Even in those meetings comprised solely of medical staff, the vocal and those with strongly held views will take over the meeting unless a competent chairperson guides the proceedings.

Appendix A

MODEL TERMS OF REFERENCE FOR QUALITY MANAGEMENT COMMITTEES

33A0 │ Contents

33A1. Purpose of this appendix
33A2. Terms of reference
33A3. Authorisation
33A4. Purpose of the committee
33A5. Committee membership
33A6. Meetings
33A7. Process considerations of the committee
33A8. Committee recommendations and reporting

33A1 │ Purpose of this appendix

Terms of reference for a hospital quality management committee (or its equivalent) are often insufficiently detailed and generally do not acknowledge the breadth of activity that this committee should encompass. This appendix provides a detailed description of the terms of reference for a quality management committee, the key committee in a quality management program.

33A2 │ Terms of reference

Terms of reference need to address the following matters at a minimum:

- authorisation—what is the source of the committee's authority, the board or the manager;
- purpose or role of the committee;
- membership—such matters as the number of members, their qualifications, method of selection, length of service, and how the chairperson is appointed;

- process considerations;
- whether a standing or ad hoc committee;
- functional relationships to other committees;
- reporting requirements;
- mechanics of the committee—meetings, agenda, minutes, notice of meetings and frequency of meetings;
- quorum;
- voting procedures;
- guidelines for committee functions;
- mechanisms to change terms of reference;
- other relevant considerations.

33A3 │ Authorisation

The board of directors of Beneficial Hospital has authorised the hospital manager to establish a quality management committee for purposes of monitoring and improving quality of care and requires reports to the board about these matters.

33A4 │ Purpose of the committee

The quality management committee has the following roles:

1. making recommendations to the board, which has overriding responsibility for quality management policy;
2. taking responsibility for assuring the quality of care and services throughout the entire hospital, including plans and projects relating to quality management to be conducted in departments or divisions. Such activity will include, for example:
   - establishing service and quality control, including utilisation review and risk management, including occupational health and safety;
   - conducting quality of care assessment and improvement;
   - credentialling and appointing medical staff;
   - planning and evaluating QM projects.
3. receiving reports about quality management activity through the quality manager;
4. taking responsibility for and monitoring of all clinical and non-clinical QM activity;
5. monitoring the QM program;
6. monitoring the work of the quality manager and the quality management department;
7. providing guidance and support and recommendations to heads of departments or divisions about quality management and its various aspects;
8. taking responsibility for the integration and co-ordination of all QM issues referred from other committees, and the tracking and accounting of such issues;
9. providing and facilitating communications and problem resolution across departments and divisions and across various services;
10. recommending actions to administration and other line officials.

33A5 │ Committee Membership

1. The committee will consist of a minimum of five (5) and a maximum of fifteen (15) members. The chairpersons, or their designees, of the functional committees relating to quality management will be members of this committee.* Three committee members will be individuals in their own right who by virtue of their knowledge, expertise and commitment to quality management, would be an asset to the committee.† The remaining members will be persons or occupants of

positions critical to hospital functions. The committee has the power to co-opt other members from appropriate departments or professional groups.

2. Members are appointed by the hospital board from the list of names recommended by the hospital manager, on the advice of the quality manager. Depending on the size of the hospital, two or three members of the committee should be elected by hospital staff to the committee. In addition, where appropriate the board may appoint an individual from within the hospital who, after advice, it considers can bring needed skills and expertise to the committee.

3. Members of the committee will serve for two years and will be eligible for reappointment or re-election.

4. A member of the committee can be removed from membership of the committee if they fail to regularly attend meetings of the committee without good reason, or in matters relating to conflict of interest,‡ or when the board of directors has reason to believe that a member's behaviour and conduct in the hospital is inconsistent with his or her role on the committee. Such a decision will be that of the board of directors on the advice of the committee on the vote of two-thirds (2/3) of the membership of the committee.

5. In the case of a vacancy on the committee due to death, resignation, or removal the manager, on the advice of the quality manager and after consultation with the chairperson of the committee, may nominate a candidate for approval by the committee. The nomination will go to the board for appointment. The nominee when appointed would serve the remainder of the two-year term.

6. The chairperson of the committee may be appointed by the board from the members of the committee on the advice of the manager, or elected by the members of the committee. If elected by the committee such election should be approved by the board.

7. The quality manager and the hospital manager are ex-officio members of the committee.

* See Figure III-3-1 on page 474.
† Within this formula, it is important to ensure that the committee is multidisciplinary and that medical and nursing staff are adequately represented. The possibility of including outside experts on this committee should be considered.
‡ See paragraph 33A.6, point 2, following.

33A6 | Meetings

1. A quorum for the committee to begin and to continue to transact business is a majority of members or five (5) members, whichever is less.

2. Where a member of the committee is the subject of a submission to the committee, or where for any reason there may be a conflict of interest, real or apparent, he or she must absent himself or herself from the deliberations of the committee for that subject or submission. If a member does not voluntarily absent himself or herself, the committee will be the sole judge as to whether such a conflict of interest exists. In the event that a member has, but does not reveal, an apparent conflict of interest, discovery of such conflict shall be grounds for removal from the committee.

3. The business of the committee shall be formally conducted and all decisions properly recorded.

4. An agenda shall accompany a notice of regularly scheduled meetings, and it shall be distributed not less than ten (10) days prior to the meeting.

5. Minutes will be distributed with the agenda.
6. The committee shall meet monthly or at such other frequency as will be decided by the committee. However, the chairperson, or in his or her absence any two members, may call for an emergency meeting of the committee without notice or agenda being distributed prior to the meeting. The hospital manager or the quality manager may also request a meeting.
7. Matters coming before the committee shall be decided by a simple majority vote of those members present and voting in favour of the motion. The chairperson has a casting vote in the case of a tied vote. Proxy voting is not permitted. Co-opted members will be in attendance for special business relating to their particular expertise only and will not have the right to vote.

33A7 | Process considerations of the committee

1. The quality management committee is a 'standing' committee.
2. The committee will, when appropriate, in the process of its deliberations make use of subcommittees and ad hoc committees or working parties. Both standing subcommittees and ad hoc committees or working parties (formed to conduct special studies or working parties) will be provided with terms of reference, and the membership of such committees will be expressly stated and approved by the QM committee. Where feasible, at least one member of the QM committee will sit on each subcommittee and ad hoc committee or working party.
3. The committee has the authority to refer matters to any other committee as is deemed appropriate. Such referral may be for a decision and action or merely for information.
4. The decisions and actions of the committee will at all times be in accordance with the hospital by-laws and policies, and relevant statutes and regulations.
5. Confidentiality of the business of the committee shall at all times be paramount. Members will only discuss the committee's business with other members and such other persons who are authorised to provide or receive such information.

33A8 | Committee recommendations and reporting

1. The committee will report on a regular basis through the manager to the hospital board. The frequency of such reports will be determined by the size of the hospital but will be no less than three-monthly.
2. Decisions made by the committee will be those which the board, and the manager acting for the board, has delegated to it. Recommendations of the committee will be transmitted to the manager for action, and where recommendations relate to policy, at the manager's discretion they will be referred to the board.
3. The committee may recommend modifications to these terms of reference from time to time, such modifications to be endorsed subsequently by the board before taking effect.

Chapter 4

THE QUALITY MANAGEMENT DEPARTMENT

---

340 | Contents

This chapter examines and details the role and function of a department of quality management under the following six major headings:

- **341.** Purpose of this chapter
- **342.** Context necessitating a quality management department
- **343.** Functions of the quality management department
- **344.** Managing the quality management program
- **345.** Support and resources for quality management
- **346.** The quality manager

341 | Purpose of this chapter

This chapter introduces the concept of a quality management department as a technical and administrative resource unit for quality management in a hospital. It also describes the range of functions of and the staffing and resources for such a department.

342 | Context necessitating a quality management department

342.1 | Quality demands attention

Imagine you are an assembly line worker in a motor car factory. What would be your reaction to being told that you and your fellow workers, who have never been involved in, nor have any knowledge of, quality control, are solely responsible for the quality control program for the cars that you assemble? Moreover, management is not willing to let you take time out for quality control activities nor to support this effort. We believe that the end result for most factories adopting this approach would be considerable turmoil, no effective quality control program, and bankruptcy because the car-buying public can judge the resultant product. But that is precisely what has happened in hospitals around Australia, the nation's principal health-improving 'factories' (whose individual demise is precluded by lack of information about how much or how little they improve patients' health).

The common attitude encountered among hospital managers, and even within some areas of government, is that quality management and clinical quality assurance is a side issue to the main business of caring for patients and that it is primarily a task for health professionals. A small minority of managers understand that quality management should be an integral part of hospital activity. Unfortunately, at the present time there are very few hospital managers or those in government who fully comprehend the resources required to properly manage quality; nor the benefits from an effective quality management program. In addition, in relation to quality managers some argue that we have too many managers now or too many types of health professionals. They argue that to create another type is merely to compound many of our current problems in hospitals, in terms of fragmentation of care and increased costs. But these arguments are incorrect. If we have too many managers they are of the wrong type or they focus their efforts on the wrong activities. Quality managers and quality management are essential to integrate hospital activities, to improve quality and to contain costs.

The argument concerning the lack of need for specialist quality managers needs to be refuted. Creating further categories of health professionals merely for industrial or political reasons is clearly undesirable. However, our experience in Australia is of most hospital 'quality assurance co-ordinators' struggling to introduce 'quality assurance' projects in the hospital with inadequate knowledge and almost no authority. Because, in general, they lack the necessary knowledge and because they are often part of the nursing establishment, for the most part they are ignored by medical staff. The type of program described in this manual demands a senior health professional (who may well be a nurse) with a wide knowledge base and placed in a position of authority in the hospital, if a program is ever to be successfully implemented.

Quality of care is an integral part of clinical activity and of hospital management but it has to be properly managed. Quality managers are essentially specialists in a particular area of management. They assist the manager in a special area of activity in the same way as a financial manager or a marketing manager, or more to the point a quality manager, would assist the manager of a business enterprise.

Like it or not, quality management and its subset, quality assurance, has now developed a wide and discrete body of knowledge and should be seen as a subspecialty of management, with a special focus on the quality of clinical and other services. Such activity requires the input of special professional skills. This chapter explores the nature of such a professional person and his or her role and skills.

342.2 | *Need for a quality management department*

The functions of the quality management department (QMD) form an integral part of hospital management. Some few Australian hospitals, mainly teaching hospitals, already boast such a department. However, they are still a very small minority and, in the past at least, have been perceived by the rest of the industry as participating in an unnecessary indulgence. None of these 'departments' conforms fully to the concepts we describe in this manual.

All hospitals should have a quality management department, but in the case of small hospitals some regionalisation will be necessary. This arrangement is not only necessary because of their small size relative to staff and other costs associated with this initiative, but also because of the desirability of minimising the problem of variability of standards and policies. Units in a common group of whatever variety would not be autonomous but would be subject to QM policy determination by a common co-ordinating committee. This committee would set quality management policy and lay down such matters as performance standards, practice policies and review criteria; how the programs are to be assessed; and uniformity of information systems. Such an arrangement will ensure not only that scarce expert resource personnel are used most effectively, but it will also play a major part in achieving that hospital- or system-wide integrated characteristic which is so important.

342.3 │ Attitude of medical staff

Not uncommonly, when the idea is mentioned medical staff react almost spontaneously by concluding that a quality management department is merely an instrument of management to control them, and by implication interfere with their clinical activities. A quality management department is certainly a management tool, but one which is designed to support medical, nursing and other hospital staff do the best possible job for patients. More importantly, it is an instrument which they themselves should have the task of shaping, implementing and monitoring through the hospital QM committee. Resistance by the medical and other health professionals to sensible solutions may ultimately result in changes far less palatable to them as it perpetuates the public perception of problems. In the case of the medical profession, such changes may further erode its autonomy.

The wariness of medical staff to the concept of a quality management department will inevitably be shared by others in institutions where power plays and structural politics have such important roles. Some of this concern may be allayed by emphasising that such a department reports to and is monitored by the hospital QM committee, and as a department it is accountable to the hospital manager.

343 │ Functions of the quality management department

343.1 │ Quality improvement resources

The quality management department is the principal resource for implementing the hospital's quality management program and hence assuring the quality of structures (inputs, including staff and working conditions) and processes that impact on care outcomes. The quality management department's functions are listed and contrasted with those of the quality management committee in Figure III-4-1 and Figure III-4-2 (on pages 492 and 493) and must include the following:

- credentialling/appointment of medical staff;
- measurement of the technical quality of care;
- monitoring/surveillance of quality;
- structured quality review;
- abstracting/case screening;
- incident reporting;
- patient complaints/compliments;
- utilisation review/control;
- patient satisfaction surveys;
- risk management, including OH&S;
- management of QM implementation.

At the present time some of these activities, at least, are conducted in a number of administrative areas in most hospitals. The lines of authority of the personnel involved are to a variety of departmental or divisional heads within the administrative structure of the hospital. We believe that there is an inherent advantage in having them in one administrative unit.

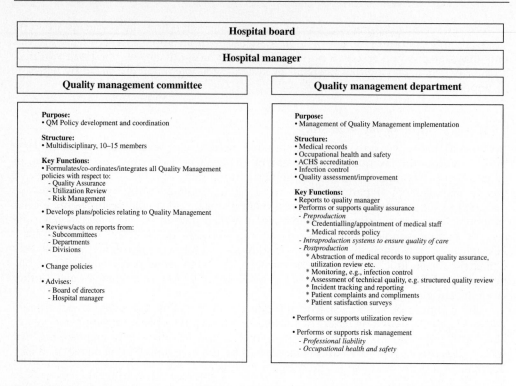

Figure III-4-1 *Comparison of role and function of quality management committee and quality management department*

343.2 *Credentialling/appointment of medical staff*

Any hospital which purports to be serious about the quality of care provided to its patients must have a system in place which enables its governing body, through its medical staff, to ensure that those doctors working in the hospital are only undertaking the care of patients within the limits of their training, experience and competence. In general, in Australia the absence of effective credentialling systems for medical staff has exposed hospitals, both public and private, and medical staff themselves to unnecessary risks of medical and hospital negligence actions.

In many Australian hospitals, the hospital administration or, in larger institutions, the medical administration already conduct the appointment and credentialling process. However, because the process is vital to the entire quality management program, it should be within the responsibility of the quality management department. In addition, just as credentialling is part of quality management, quality assurance activities and processes that assess the quality of clinical services are themselves essential for an effective and objective credentialling process. If clinical privileges are to be withdrawn or modified, the objective evidence to support such action can only be obtained from processes which measure and evaluate the care of the provider in question. To the present time, the absence of an effective quality management program to produce such evidence has rendered the appropriate restriction of clinical activity of doctors not only administratively difficult, but legally hazardous.

The following activities fall into the general category of 'credentialling', and their conduct should be the task of the quality management department:

• checking qualifications of medical staff;

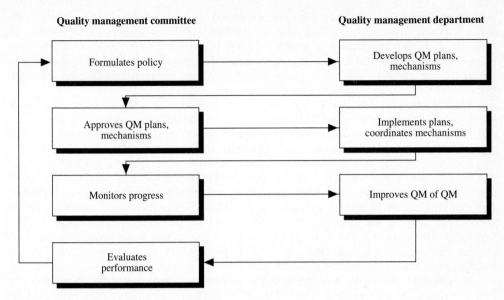

Figure III-4-2 *Functional relationships between quality management committee and quality management department*

- checking the insurance status of medical staff. This should occur annually and no doctor should be appointed or permitted to continue to work in a hospital unless he or she carries and provides proof of current medical indemnity insurance against professional negligence;
- checking the registration of medical staff annually. The number of doctors who simply forget to register themselves is quite surprising. Non-registered medical practitioners, if involved in an episode of negligence, place themselves and the hospital in a particularly invidious position;
- providing the organisational arrangements for the reappointment process, which in most Australian hospitals occurs every three years;
- providing the organisational support for the credentialling process. Credentialling should occur annually; Part IV details the credentialling process;
- maintaining profiles on medical staff. The quality management department should keep confidential accounts of awards for excellence and examples of good quality care as well as any malpractice awards or other evidence of deviations from accepted practice by members of the hospital medical staff. Such sensitive information must not only be confidential, but strict protocols must be developed concerning right of access to such information;
- keeping track of current problems as revealed by the quality assurance activity of clinical services. This information is important for the board of directors and members of the hospital's credentials committee. Doctors do not wake up one morning with the idea that: 'Today I am going to be negligent'. Most episodes of negligence by medical staff reveal a long trail of episodes sometimes stretching back for several years.

343.3 Measuring quality

343.31 MEASUREMENT OF THE TECHNICAL QUALITY OF CARE

Quality measurement or assessment is one of the most important and key functions of a quality management department. The attention of most Australian health professionals, doctors in particular, has been directed mostly to this aspect of quality management. When medical or nursing staff ask how to conduct 'quality assurance', it is usually the function of quality assessment to which they are actually referring. In spite of this focus however, and despite the existence of appropriate technology, the routine assessment of the quality of clinical care is rarely conducted in Australian hospitals despite the often grandiose claims to be a 'centre of excellence'.

Surgeons in particular have been attracted to a variety of software programs which would enable them to conduct a surgical audit. As valuable as these programs are in obtaining and collating data relating to surgical activity including complications, they represent only one small part of a comprehensive quality management program.

While medical and other hospital staff should have some general understanding of the appropriate methodologies, detailed day-to-day involvement by medical and other health professionals in the methodologies for quality assessment is not the key to effective quality management or quality assurance in hospitals. The participation and involvement of medical staff in the process of structured quality review is an exception to this statement. However, for the most part the staff of the quality management department should be capable of advising on and implementing all the necessary quality measurement and assessment methodologies.

As a general principle, it is not possible to improve quality of care unless you can first define and then measure it. The failure of most 'quality assurance' initiatives is in the failure to define quality adequately. Moreover, if care is found to be deficient, repeated measurements are needed to see if changes actually improved the quality of care and, if possible, to establish that the measured improvement can be attributed confidently to the implemented changes.

There are several aspects of quality which demand a variety of approaches and methodologies. They are:

- technical quality expressed as performance of providers, infection rates etc.;
- some aspects of the use of resources and costs of care, such as unnecessary investigations and lengths of stay. While utilisation review addresses the number of services used, the actual measurement of costs of hospital care is outside the scope of this manual;
- patient satisfaction. This is an important aspect of quality, reflecting the interpersonal quality of care provided. It can be measured by patient satisfaction surveys and the tracking of complaints or compliments (which may also reveal problems in the technical aspects of care).

343.32 Monitoring/surveillance of quality

Monitoring or surveillance of quality related variables is a key function in any quality assurance program and is a component of measuring the technical quality of care. There are many forms of monitoring and all require the time and skills that should be available within a department of quality management. Infection control, and review of all unexpected deaths or other sentinel events are examples of surveillance techniques to identify possible areas of poor quality care. A vital function of the quality management department is not only to run these data collection and surveillance systems, but also to integrate their results and to paint a coherent and complete picture, and to highlight any inconsistencies that might exist.

343.33 Structured quality review

The term peer review was first introduced into the Australian health scene in 1977. Initially it was poorly understood by the medical profession and in retrospect probably should not have been used. It is still used synonymously, by some people, with quality management and quality assurance. The term literally refers to the process whereby the work of medical staff under certain circumstances is reviewed by their colleagues. Essentially, in North America where the term originated, it refers to reviewing colleagues' medical records as a means of assessing the quality of care. In Australia such a review of medical records by colleagues has never been a routine activity and is performed rarely. For this reason, and to avoid even further confusion, in this manual the term structured medical record review is used to describe the process whereby peers (medical, nursing or other) assess the quality of clinical care by reviewing the medical records of colleagues. Where structured medical record review is preceded by the use of outcome/process assessment screens and followed by pattern analysis, the process has been named structured quality review (SQR). In general, the authors have tried to avoid the use of the term peer review altogether.

Many Australian hospital medical staff have come to use the term 'peer review' to apply to almost any meeting of medical staff where cases are presented and discussed. The usual meetings commonly held in hospitals by medical staff do not represent effective review of quality of care by peers. The open nature of these meetings makes frank examination of the performance of a colleague not only almost impossible, but also legally hazardous should such an examination be attempted. Such clinical meetings should not be called peer review meetings but 'clinical case conferences'.

Without becoming involved in a semantic argument, it is necessary to merely state that peer review's purpose is to assess the quality of care provided to an individual patient for an episode or a continuum of care. It is essentially a means of identifying practices which are beyond acceptable boundaries. Peer review or what from here on will be referred to as structured medical record (SMR) review is the first step toward effecting improvement in the technical quality of care. The premise of such a process is that doctors can judge other doctors' work.

The reviewer depends on the medical record for information and this, in turn, emphasises the crucial importance of adequate medical records. Similar to the situation in a court of law, when considering quality of patient care the principle must be that 'if it isn't in the medical record, it didn't happen'. This principle applies particularly to the recording of 'negative' findings. Obviously the doctor has an obligation to record everything relevant that was done to the patient, including what was not done that might reasonably have been expected to have been done and why it was appropriate not to do it.

While case-by-case review via the medical record does occasionally identify significant problems, the real advantage to be gained is when such medical record review is part of structured quality review. In the absence in Australia of more sophisticated technology, we believe that the process of structured quality review, correctly implemented, is likely to be the mainstay of quality of care measurement for some years. Such review should be seen as a technology in its own right. Such review must be properly structured and adopt a procedural and reporting formality if it is to play the important role it should in clinical quality assurance. The structure is necessary to maximise the validity and utility of the information derived.

Structured medical record review and structured quality review are labour intensive and hence some selectivity is needed to focus efforts. Cases may be selected on the following bases, for example:

- those where problems of quality of care are suspected (such suspicion can be enhanced by use of screening systems);
- those where medical intervention represents a high risk;
- those diagnoses or interventions where the volume of cases is significant;
- those where costs are particularly high.

While only health professionals can participate in the process of structured medical record review (SMR) and structured quality review (SQR), the organisation and administration of this system will need to be the responsibility of an administrative unit if it is to function effectively. The quality management department is the obvious instrument for this purpose.

For a review process to be effective and legally safe, the following conditions must apply:

- the review should be a routine ongoing exercise and a continuing part of quality assurance activities;
- it must be in camera and not in a public forum;
- it must be fair, objective, and motivated solely by the desire to improve patient care and protect patients' welfare;
- there must be strict confidentiality;
- doctors must be convinced that the process is undertaken fairly by their peers, or by qualified experts;
- the process must be free from local bias and potential accusations of malice;
- where freedom from bias or malice cannot be guaranteed in a hospital, those conducting the review must be recruited for the task from another hospital, another area health service, or even another state;
- the entire process must be documented and structured, a system which is replicated on each occasion. In so doing, all practitioners understand exactly what is to take place, and those conducting the review are protected from accusations of malice and denial of natural justice;
- whenever a medical practitioner is to be subjected to the process of SMR or SQR he or she must be informed of the fact. In addition, terms and conditions of appointment should describe the hospital's quality assurance mechanisms including the mechanism of structured quality review;
- in the case of an adverse finding by peers about a colleague there must be the right of appeal.

For committees engaged in structured quality review or in credentialling of medical staff, to be effective and provide adequate safeguards against the possibility of subsequent legal action, the following principles must apply:

- the committee must be properly constituted;
- the committee must have appropriate terms of reference which are strictly adhered to;
- the minutes must be carefully prepared and checked;
- the affairs of the committee must be kept confidential;
- strict adherence to the rules of natural justice is essential;
- the committee should adopt a carefully designed formality about its procedures;
- all medical staff must be subjected to the same form of review process.

The process of structured quality review by peers, if all or valid samples of cases are reviewed, holds out the possibility of enormous progress into areas previously thought impossible. Such possibilities include:

- a meaningful measure of quality of care;
- an examination of the patterns of care including the relationships between the processes and outcomes of care, and leading to the improvement of quality;
- the gaining of insight into the effectiveness of medical interventions.

The idea of manually reviewing every record is too daunting to contemplate. However, as is described elsewhere, the advent of computer technology has now rendered even this daunting exercise a relatively simple, effective possibility.

Structured quality review, as outlined above and as described in detail in Part IV, does not exist to our knowledge in any hospital in Australia. Further, most hospital committees function in such a way that it would be difficult for most of them to meet the previously listed requirements.

343.34 ABSTRACTING/CASE SCREENING

Case abstracting is the process of extracting data, usually from the medical record but sometimes from other sources, relating to some aspect of either the process or the outcome of care, and placing them in a single file for storage and analysis.

Case screening is the process of reviewing all or a sample of case abstracts (or medical records) to separate them according to certain explicit criteria into two or more categories. The purpose of separating records into two or more categories is to focus subsequent effort differentially. For example, cases may be separated into those presumed to be acceptable and those requiring further review. This process of screening thus ensures that effort is focused on cases where something is more likely to be amiss. Effective case screening can improve both the effectiveness and efficiency of quality assurance. This activity can be time consuming and requires skills which should be found in the staff of the quality management department. Case screening is an integral element of the process of structured quality review.

The decision to abstract or screen medical records for a particular issue, and the conclusions to be eventually reached about the results, will require input from the health professionals themselves. However, practising doctors and nurses should not and cannot be expected to carry out the actual process of abstract/screening of medical records.

The medical record is the usual source of information but other supplemental sources may be used also. Abstracting information from the medical record will continue to be necessary until all clinical information is in an electronic form. Once such electronic information exists, the relevant data for quality assurance can be extracted from the wealth of other data stored in automated records.

While much is and can be done manually, in recent years considerable progress has been made in the abstracting and screening of medical records by use of computer technology. The use of artificial intelligence in screening systems permits more sophisticated screening at a level closer to clinical reality than is possible with manual systems (see Part II).

343.35 INCIDENT REPORTING

In many Australian hospitals, still, 'incidents' are seen merely as mishaps which occur to either patients or staff as a result of physical accidents. Incidents are really much wider than this traditional perspective. The purpose of recording incidents is to identify patterns of care or circumstances which expose the hospital or its staff to unnecessary risk or which represent opportunities for improving the quality of care.

Incidents can be grouped into the following categories:

- staff/patient/visitor accidents (patient slips in shower);
- staff–patient mishaps (staff hits patient);
- staff mistakes (swab left in abdomen; nurse drops patient);
- patient–patient incidents (patient hits patient);
- patient–staff mishaps (patient rapes staff member);
- visitor–staff, visitor–patient incidents (visitor kills patient).

While incident reporting does occur in Australian hospitals, in most hospitals incidents are directed to either nursing administration, medical administration or the hospital manager. In some hospitals that is about as far as they go. In addition, we frequently find that many incidents are not reported for a variety of reasons.

Nurses fail to report medication errors for fear of retribution; doctors react very strongly when requested to report medical incidents, seeing it as unwarranted criticism; and one head of a service department admitted that his sole understanding of a hospital incident was an episode of angry confrontation that had occurred between himself and a patient. In a quality-mature hospital self-reporting of incidents would be the rule rather than the exception. However, the main problem is that incident reports frequently are not collated and tracked in a way that enables the detection of patterns of behaviour, events or circumstances that could lead to effective preventative action and hence improved quality of care. It is important to know that a surgeon left a swab in an abdomen. It is much more important to know how many times this particular surgeon or this particular theatre team have left swabs in an abdomen. In other words, one must determine if swabs left in the abdomen represent the failure of a person or the hospital's operating room procedures.

While it is important to collate incident reports, it is the responsibility of the quality management department to analyse and present the results of such an analysis in a form that is meaningful to clinicians and administrators. It is also the department's role to work with the clinicians and administrators to track down causes of apparent problems, find ways of remedying them, and thereby improving the quality of care, including staff and patient satisfaction, and reducing risk.

343.36 PATIENT COMPLAINTS/COMPLIMENTS

Patient complaints may often represent the tip of an iceberg of hospital problems. All too commonly, monitoring of patient complaints is poorly co-ordinated and feedback to clinical staff is frequently absent. The quality management department should monitor and track all patient complaints to ensure that patterns of complaints that could disclose problems of patient care are identified and addressed adequately. As inadequate as such feedback obviously may be, its systematic organisation is a step toward quality improvement.

The prompt handling of complaints by someone trained to do so is a potent preventative measure in malpractice litigation. The angry patient who has his or her anger turned around by an attentive and receptive senior representative of the hospital is far less likely to vent his or her frustration via the legal process. One way of turning away this anger is to take the complaint seriously, investigate it and tell the complainant what was found and done.

In many cases patient compliments provide the only positive feedback that hospital staff receive concerning the services they are providing. Patterns of compliments too should be analysed, and staff or departments performing outstandingly should be recognised and rewarded.

343.4 | Utilisation review/control

An ongoing analysis of the hospital's services and their resource use is a very important function of the quality management department. Utilisation review is that aspect of quality management that relates to the appropriate use of services. This function enables the hospital and its medical and nursing staffs to know how and in what way the hospital utilises its resources. Whether it be a review of lengths of hospital stay, or the use of investigations, or the number of certain types of procedures, the review should be undertaken as an ongoing monitoring process and, in addition, whenever there is good reason to believe that a problem exists, or specific information is required for a specific purpose. Reviewing one problem area may lead to information about another. Such a situation occurred at one hospital when a physician who conducted a review of the delay in admitting patients to the coronary care unit from accident and emergency found that the number of ECGs carried out on these patients in the course of their transfer from one area of the hospital to another was grossly excessive and unjustifiable.

The interest and enthusiasm of medical and nursing staff in this activity will only be sustained when a clear decision has been made concerning precisely what information is to be collected, how such information is to be used, and if it assists the hospital staff to solve a problem. The time and methodological skills necessary to undertake reviews of this nature make it essential that staff other than medical and nursing personnel are available. There is no way that busy medical practitioners can be expected to conduct this type of activity themselves, even if they possess the required knowledge and skills to do it. The input of medical and other health professional staff should be obtained in the interpretation of data and in the decisions relating to the implementation of subsequent action.

343.5 | Patient satisfaction surveys

Doctors in general tend to disparage patient satisfaction surveys as far too simplistic a method to be of any value in the evaluation of the quality of patient care. This attitude is again a reflection of the tendency by medical staff to concentrate solely on the technical aspects of the care and services provided by doctors. Hospitals and doctors should never forget that satisfied patients rarely become litigants, regardless of the type of misadventure that may befall them.

While the construction of good questionnaires is never an easy task, patient satisfaction surveys are important to evaluate the subjective aspects of care. Moreover, they can play a very important role in identifying areas of real concern even to medical staff, as the following examples demonstrate:

- A survey which reveals widespread dissatisfaction with meals and food preparation may well lead to a realisation that important special diets for patients such as diabetics are not being prepared adequately.
- A survey which reveals dissatisfaction with an X-ray department might result in the discovery that patients were being left half-naked on hard and uncomfortable stretchers for hours on end.
- A survey which reveals patients were inadequately instructed in the use of appliances or medication, or demonstrated a failure on the part of health professionals to communicate with patients, provides valuable information on patient compliance—an important aspect of patient care.

If the patient is regarded as a consumer instead of simply an occupier of a hospital bed, such surveys reveal important community attitudes about the hospital and become an important tool in evaluating consumer/patient satisfaction. The development of patient satisfaction surveys and the organisation of such a project is properly part of the role of the quality management department. Part IV details the technical aspects of patient satisfaction surveys.

343.6 | Risk management

343.61 MINIMISING RISK OF FINANCIAL LOSS

To date in Australia risk management has not been seen as a discrete element of hospital activity. Risk management is an integral part of quality management, and one of the greatest risks faced by hospitals and their medical staff is the possibility of malpractice litigation. In Australia the term 'risk management' has been used usually in reference to general insurance risk, workers compensation and, perhaps, occupational health and safety. The term is used in this manual to refer to the processes of minimising the risk of financial loss to the hospital. The objective of risk management is to reduce such risk to the lowest level commensurate with achieving the organisation's purpose. Occupational health and safety of employees is a significant part of risk management and should be part of the responsibility and function of the department of quality management.

There are three aspects of risk management:

- risk avoidance;
- damage control; and
- risk transfer (insurance).

343.62 RISK AVOIDANCE

The reduction of malpractice litigation is an important goal of risk avoidance in hospitals. The employment of properly trained and experienced medical and nursing staff, the effective credentialling of medical staff and the maintenance of adequate medical records, are all aspects of risk avoidance in hospitals. Similarly, the maintenance of registries of devices used in the hospital, especially implantable devices, and awareness of product recalls are additional aspects of risk management. Part V deals exclusively with risk management, including occupational health and safety.

343.63 DAMAGE CONTROL

Any hospital, particularly in today's environment, can assume that at some time an incident will occur which will have public consequences and attract considerable public and media reaction. An unexpected death under circumstances where the competence of the hospital or its staff is suspect, can often propel the hospital into a frightening arena of media and public controversy. Part of the responsibility of the quality management department is to see that the hospital has a properly prepared plan of action to meet such situations. Who is to be the hospital spokesperson? Where is he or she to obtain guidance and advice? Who notifies the insurer about potential adverse events? Other aspects of damage control include: ensuring that detailed notes are kept about such events at the time; and paying attention to such matters as relations with a patient's family and relatives.

Whether or not the quality manager is the appropriate hospital spokesperson in such a situation, the quality management department should be responsible for planning the steps to be taken in such circumstances, both inside and outside the hospital. Certainly, the QMD must be able to demonstrate convincingly that the 'incident' was a rare, and not a frequent, occurrence.

343.64 RISK TRANSFER (INSURANCE)

While general risk transfer (insurance) may well be the responsibility of the quality management department, a discussion of insurance is certainly beyond the scope of this manual. Most hospitals need and indeed probably have outside expertise to advise them on their insurance requirements.

344 | Managing the quality management program

344.1 | Management of quality management

In the complex service environment of any hospital, it is clearly simply insufficient to initiate quality management activity and assume it will automatically be carried through successfully and without difficulties. This conclusion is no reflection on the health professionals, but rather a realistic position to adopt for activities which are new and, because of the very complexity of hospital services, are subject to a variety of obstacles and difficulties.

Due to the very nature of quality management, it is very easy for a hospital and its staff to assume that effective quality management is in place when in reality there is merely a facade of activity with little or no results to show after the outlay of much time and money. To ensure that this does not occur requires skilled staff who are responsible for implementing the quality management plan which has been approved by the QM committee. The range of QM activities which is involved requires expert guidance and control throughout the hospital and this is the task of the quality manager and the QM department. Monitoring the QM program is the only effective method of ensuring that activities are really worthwhile, that the program is meeting its predetermined objectives, and that time and resources are not being wasted. In other words, the QM program itself must be assessed in ways similar to those suggested for clinical services.

The quality management department must set up an information system to measure what improvements have been achieved and how much it cost to achieve them and what savings may have resulted. There are a number of obvious costs such as committee meetings (staff time and perhaps opportunity costs for visiting medical officers (VMOs)); employees of the QMD; consultants; surveys and so on. Ultimately it should be possible to convert improvements to dollars so as to be able to equate them with the costs of realising the improvements. We realise that at the present time some of these suggestions are easier to make than to implement. However, we believe that the QM program should be as accountable as possible, and its costs and benefits must be subjected to assessment.

The following situations represent examples of program monitoring:

- Incident report analysis. The analysis of incident reports is a very important element in quality management and an example of monitoring. Keeping track of incidents, and knowing which incidents to follow-up and how they should be followed-up, is by no means as simple as it may seem.
- Quality assessment. Measuring the quality of a particular modality of care is of little value without analysing this activity's effectiveness and its implications. A good example of this idea is the management of infection control. Having determined the standard acceptable, once an agreed deviation from that standard has been detected it is important to determine the cause of the deviation. Why is the infection rate in this hospital higher than the acceptable level? Not only does the cause of the problem need to be determined, but also there needs to be action initiated to correct the problem and subsequent checks to ensure that the correction has taken place. It is the role of the QM department to see to it that these various elements have been put in place.
- Quality improvement actions analysis. Having recommended corrective actions, have they been implemented? For example, having determined that medication errors were in large part due to doctors' handwriting legibility, has the recommended corrective action been taken and has it resolved the problem of medication errors?

The management of the implementation of a quality management program is a good example of the sort of function that must be conducted by the quality management department. Busy doctors and nurses will not have the time to conduct this type of activity, even if they have the necessary expertise.

344.2 | *Hospital accreditation*

The process of hospital accreditation as conducted by the ACHS is a complementary activity to quality management within the hospital. Most hospitals in Australia already have one of their staff members, usually a nurse, who is responsible for leading the hospital through the preparatory process for hospital accreditation. This staff member should be part of the staff complement of the quality management department, responsible to the quality manager.

344.3 | Planning and evaluation

Planning and evaluation is one of the most important areas that requires the support of the quality management department. In the first instance the quality management committee approves a quality management plan prepared by the quality manager. The quality management department's role is to supervise and control the implementation of that plan and to evaluate progress against the plan. The quality management committee's task is to hold the quality manager responsible for developing the QM plan, implementing it and evaluating progress against the plan.

We often find ourselves talking to doctors and other health professionals keen to embark on some 'quality assurance' activity. The question asked so frequently is: 'Where do we begin?' This is such a frequently encountered difficulty that we have dedicated an entire chapter to this topic. (See Chapter 6 in this part.)

Every hospital needs an expert group of quality management professionals who are available to answer this and a whole range of similar questions. How to start? How to develop a QM plan that is realistic for the circumstances? What should be the role and function of the quality management committee? Such plans and activities have to be supervised and monitored to ensure that they are implemented and revised appropriately in light of experience.

Other planning and development functions of a quality management department include:

- development and evaluation of new quality assurance technologies and policies for their introduction;
- evaluation of new therapeutic and diagnostic technologies, known as technology assessment. This activity is carried out by the technology assessment committee;
- evaluation and supervision of research initiatives as they affect quality of patient care;
- co-ordination of continuing medical education with quality measurement and credentialling.

344.4 | Outside liaison/keeping up-to-date

An important role for the quality management department is ensuring that the hospital is made aware of current trends and attitudes elsewhere in quality management. The introduction or discussion of new methodologies is of particular importance, as is the capacity to interpret new ideas and to assist medical staff to develop the right questions to ask about them.

Legal issues are becoming increasingly important to the whole area of hospital quality management and its various facets. The quality management department is responsible for keeping track of legislative changes—such as recent federal legislation and that in various Australian states to introduce some form of legal 'privilege' to provide protection for medical and other hospital staff engaged in certain aspects of quality management activity—and communicating their relevance to hospital operations.

345 | Support and resources for quality management

345.1 | Where there is a will there must also be resources

While clinical staff, particularly medical staff, must be involved in a quality management program and must see it as their program, they cannot run such a program without proper support. A quality management program requires resources; one of the most important— and presently scarce—resources is skilled personnel. It also requires an organisational structure and consequentially an allocation of funds. The responsibility for such support and resources rests with management, it does not rest with medical or nursing staff.

Provision of a quality management program has its own costs, just as other hospital functions such as accounting or administration have their own costs. It is certainly true, for example, that the establishment of effective support systems for a quality management program, such as an efficient clinical information system, where none exists, will occasion costs. However, it is difficult, for example, to imagine a hospital (or more to the point funders of care) denying the need for an accounting function because it carries a cost. The critical issue is that the value of the resultant information exceeds the cost of generating it.

345.2 │ Staffing the quality management department

As most Australian hospitals do not have quality management departments, any build-up of staff should be slow and gradual to meet the demand for service and activity. Certainly, in the case of hospitals of 200 beds or more, there will need to be one person with quality management skills; one assistant to the quality manager, for ACHS accreditation for example; one infection control officer; and secretarial support. For hospitals of 350 beds additional staff members with quality management skills will be required. If all the staff of a hospital who are engaged currently in QM activities were to be brought together under the QMD umbrella—such as the infection control staff, the nursing 'QA' officer, the OH&S staff (fire and safety officer), the officer responsible for the hospital's accreditation efforts, and a pro rata amount of secretarial resource staff—the quality management department would immediately have significant human resources. Recently, while in the United States we had the opportunity to visit one 1100 bed hospital whose QM department had a staff of twenty-one persons. Quality management departments in US hospitals may employ twenty or more professionals. Here current QM resource issues revolve principally around their productive use rather than their quantity. Specific issues include the value of externally-mandated QA activities and the effectiveness of internally-oriented QI efforts. Utilising levels of quality management resources currently found in US hospitals in ways advocated in this manual would immediately improve their productivity and lead to substantially more quality improvement. To increase the value of their quality management activities, US hospitals would have to create a culture conducive to QA/QI, employ properly qualified quality managers as part of the senior management team, enhance quality management employees' knowledge and skills, and work to eliminate counter-productive external mandates and perverse incentives.

345.3 │ Clinical information

Historically, the medical record department in most hospitals has been seen and treated as the poor relation of all hospital departments. The role of this department is quite critical to the successful implementation of any aspect of quality management. Accordingly, we believe that the true value of the medical record department will be best appreciated if it is part of the quality management department. In such circumstances the medical record administrator would report to the hospital manager through the quality manager. In those hospitals that have a separate medical record and clinical information departments, both should become united within the quality management department.

345.4 │ Skilled personnel

Even small hospitals will need to identify one person as the quality manager even though the position may be part time or occupied by a consultant. However, one of the current difficulties in Australia is the small pool of people with any experience or skills in the broad field of quality management. There is, however, an increasing number of hospital professionals with the requisite background, educational requirements, and the potential to develop the requisite knowledge and necessary management skills to fill the role of quality manager. We note with acclaim the recently established postgraduate diploma course in quality management and quality assurance at La Trobe University's Lincoln School of Health Systems Sciences. Specially designed programs leading to masters degrees are beginning to emerge in the United States.

Until such programs of formal training programs for quality managers become widespread, hospitals must consider the need to provide this training themselves with the use of outside consultants, or to send key personnel overseas for training. Apart from the role of quality manager, positive initiatives are necessary to overcome a deficiency in training programs by establishing courses for all professionals who are engaged in quality management. One- or two-day seminars do not represent an adequate training program for the demands of this activity.

345.5 | Role and standing of quality management personnel

Not least because the implementation of quality management implies considerable attitudinal and organisational change, especially on the part of medical practitioners, it is absolutely essential that the quality manager occupies a position of authority and seniority within the hospital hierarchy, and that he or she reports directly to the hospital manager. Quality management professionals should be seen as an integral part of the hospital's senior management team.

We have encountered quality assurance co-ordinators selected because there was no one else to fill the role. These professionals, usually nurses at middle management level or lower, have very little understanding about quality management or quality assurance and, what is worse, in some cases very little motivation. Those who are motivated suffer considerable frustration due to lack of authority to influence changes in policy or organisation in the hospital, which is often essential to enable an effective quality management program to proceed. Because the co-ordinator is a nurse it is not uncommon to have him or her reporting to the director of nursing. From the point of view of medical staff, such an appointee can have little if any credibility as a change agent unless the line of reporting is to the hospital manager.

The quality manager who is seen as part of a particular professional group (medical or nursing) will certainly experience great difficulties in implementing hospital-wide attitudinal and behavioural change. Equally unsatisfactory is the quality manager who is not a health professional, and who consequently has an insufficient grasp of hospital culture. The chance of such an officer influencing hospital professionals is very small. This picture of the 'QA' co-ordinator, while not universal is not uncommon, particularly in smaller country hospitals, and is a recipe for failure before the program even commences.

345.6 | Outside resources

Even for the most highly qualified and skilled quality manager, circumstances will continually arise where outside consultant or specialist advice and assistance will be required. The quality management department and the quality manager have the responsibility to develop networks of experts whom they can approach when necessary. A good example relates to the provision of legal expertise.

Hospital medical staff have become extremely anxious about their legal exposure to quality management activities including credentialling. New legislation and an accurate picture of the legal position of medical staff needs to be fully explained to them. In Australia much of this concern is misplaced, as Part VI points out. However, the failure of hospitals to provide an authority to explain legal issues has resulted in medical staff, and surgeons in particular, having become unnecessarily concerned. The quality management department should arrange for legal experts to explain these issues to medical staff rather than allowing bush lawyers among hospital staff, spurred on by misleading anecdotes from the United States' media, to paint a totally distorted picture of the situation in Australia.

346 | The quality manager

346.1 | Role and responsibilities

The quality manager is responsible for the overall implementation, integration and co-ordination of the hospital's quality management program. These goals are achieved by:

- implementing an integrated program designed to enhance the quality of patient care and promote the efficient use of hospital services and resources;
- assuring that the program meets the ACHS requirements and is in conformity with hospital policies;
- providing administrative, technical, and educational assistance and support in the development and maintenance of the quality management program to the extent appropriate at both departmental and hospital-wide levels.

346.2 | Relationships

The quality manager reports directly to the hospital manager and works in close association with:

- the medical staff;
- administration;
- nursing service;
- ancillary and allied health professionals;
- other hospital employees;
- patients;
- the wider community.

346.3 | Major duties and responsibilities

Medical staff often assume erroneously that the quality manager is someone whose role is to tell them how to conduct their clinical work. We mention this misconception merely to refute it. The quality manager is a skilled professional whose task is to administer a program. The QM professional plays an important role in helping to shape hospital and practice policies, which form part of the organisational constraints and incentives on clinical care. However, the quality manager should not be involved in moment-to-moment patient care or in telling doctors or any other health professional what to do or how to do it.

Due to the importance we attach to this function we provide a job description of and personal qualifications for the quality manager in the Appendix to this chapter.

Appendix A

MODEL JOB DESCRIPTION AND QUALIFICATIONS FOR A QUALITY MANAGER

| 34A0 | Contents |

34A1. Purpose of this appendix
34A2. Job description
34A3. Qualifications

34A1 | Purpose of this appendix

Most hospitals in Australia in recent years have acquired a staff member whose primary responsibility relates to quality. Usually he or she is designated 'quality assurance co-ordinator'. As Chapter 4 emphasises, the job is not one of co-ordinating but rather one of managing. The task of managing the hospital's quality management program described in this manual demands a great deal more than that expected of today's quality assurance co-ordinator. Similarly, the qualifications needed to meet the demands of this expanded role are correspondingly greater than those usually encountered with today's co-ordinators. This appendix intends to assist hospitals when they are recruiting a quality manager by providing a starting point for an appropriate job description and statement of qualifications.

34A2 | Job description

34A2.1 | *Policy development*

- Monitor pertinent state and federal regulations and Acts and advise medical staff and administration concerning same.
- Manage the development of a QM plan for the hospital.
- Manage clinical information systems.
- Advise and assist management on matters relating to liability insurance and the handling of malpractice claims.

- Liaise with outside organisations concerning quality management.
- Co-ordinate and organise an annual appraisal and review of the quality management program, to update plans and if necessary revise policies.

34A2.2 Data collection and analysis

- Provide support for data collection and analysis, including the identification of data sources and studies to evaluate patient care, and any corrective actions taken.
- Monitor the use of hospital services for the appropriateness of admission, length of stay and discharge planning procedures.
- Develop data collection arrangements and report formats to enhance uniformity and prevent duplication of effort across hospital departments and service functions.
- Identify opportunities to co-ordinate concurrent and retrospective data collection from patient medical records, analysis, and reporting with risk management, incident reporting, infection control and patient safety.
- Develop and administer medical record abstracting.
- Identify, investigate and resolve patient care problems, and monitor patterns of patient care.
- Develop patient and staff satisfaction surveys to identify problems and suggestions for change.
- Analyse and evaluate patient complaints and compliments.
- Investigate, track and report incidents.
- Supervise and co-ordinate matters relating to OH&S.

34A2.3 Communication and reporting

- Prepare and disseminate quality management communications, for example quality assurance, utilisation review, and patient and staff satisfaction reports.
- Attend meetings of medical staff where appropriate, and of quality management and other committees where considered appropriate after consultation with the manager. Oversee the preparation of agendas, reports and minutes.
- Prepare, receive and review all pertinent data, minutes, reports and results, and summarise them for presentation to management, the medical executive committee and the board.

34A2.4 Education and support

- In the area of quality management, assist the hospital and medical staff and the relevant committees to identify important aspects of care and establish indicators and criteria for evaluating patient care and services. Assist the hospital and medical staff to identify and analyse inappropriate utilisation, high costs or inefficiencies.
- Serve on QM committees and assist with the integration of such committees.
- Assist hospital and medical staff to identify and give priority to problems, and to determine action for problem resolution.
- Assist in development and presentation of in-service education programs for medical staff, hospital support staff, management and the board.

34A2.5 Administrative

- Manage staff and professionals.
- Oversee medical records.
- Provide administrative support for the credentialling of medical staff.
- Obtain and access outside resource assistance for medical staff concerning such matters as legal issues relating to quality assurance, and access to greater expertise in quality assurance when or if necessary.

34A3 | Qualifications

34A3.1 | *Knowledge*

The quality manager must have knowledge of:

- state and federal Acts and regulations and ACHS standards in relation to quality management;
- concepts of quality management, quality assurance, medical record management, utilisation review and risk management;
- basic statistical concepts and applications;
- data collection, analysis and display techniques, both manual and computerised;
- group dynamics and organisational change theory.

34A3.2 | *Skills*

The quality manager must be able to:

- work effectively as a member of the senior management team;
- communicate effectively, both orally and in writing;
- plan, establish and achieve objectives;
- function independently and under pressure;
- organise efficiently with attention to detail;
- initiate and guide problem resolution across departments and promote the acceptance of quality management activities.

34A3.3 | *Education and experience*

The quality manager needs the following qualifications and experience:

- a degree or qualification in medicine, nursing, medical record administration or related health care field. Higher qualification in quality management or such related field as change management, education, administration or associated clinical field, helpful but not required;
- three to five years experience as a practising health professional in an acute care facility with two to three years experience in quality management;
- one to two years supervisory experience.

Chapter 5

MEDICAL RECORDS

| 350 | **Contents** |

Clinical data is a key prerequisite for assuring quality of care. This chapter explores the following issues relating to clinical information:

| 351 | **Purpose of this chapter** |

A clinical information system consists of medical records and the capacity to extract, aggregate, and analyse the information from records for clinical and other purposes. Traditionally, while hospital professionals understand the purpose of and need for adequate medical records, they have tended to honour them in the breach. A patient's medical record is the core of the totality of information relevant to patient care, quality management, and health care administration and policy. For quality management purposes, hospitals can link administrative, cost, patient outcome, and other relevant data to the clinical contents of patients' medical records to create patient records.

This chapter stresses the important role that clinical information plays in high quality patient care including a successful quality management program. The chapter also highlights current deficiencies in clinical information, which militate against the effective implementation of a quality management program, and how they can be rectified.

| 352 | **Historical background** |

In the late 1950s a handful of key figures of the New South Wales Branch of the AMA met and decided that something had to be done about the appalling state of medical records in public hospitals in New South Wales. At that time the question of private hospital records did not even rate a mention. The common wisdom of the day was that whatever transpired between patient and doctor and the private hospital was not an issue for the public domain. Moreover, at that time the private hospital sector in New South

Wales, somewhat more so than in other states, was seen as an insignificant part of total hospital activity. This meeting—over thirty years ago—was the stimulus for the beginning of hospital accreditation in Australia and with it, eventually, the Australian Council on Healthcare Standards. Part I details this historical account.

Those early pioneers confidently believed that accreditation would go a long way to provide the incentives and sanctions that would solve the problem of hospital medical records, as well as the problems associated with many other aspects of the organisation and management of hospitals in Australia. The adequacy of medical records has been and continues to be an Australia-wide problem. Results of the hospital accreditation program have subsequently confirmed that medical records are a problem in all Australian hospitals, public and private.

353 | Current status of medical records and recordkeeping

353.1 | Progress to date

What progress has been made in the past thirty years in relation to the quality of hospital medical records and the expectations in general concerning hospital accreditation? Medical records have improved considerably when compared with the situation that existed in the 1950s. However, requirements and expectations have also risen and the resulting gap remains wide. Much of the improvement that has taken place can be attributed reasonably to the program of hospital accreditation conducted by the Australian Council on Healthcare Standards. However, to date hospital accreditation has failed to bring about the level of improvement in medical records anticipated by its founders. A number of factors account for this situation including:

- the lack of effective incentives or sanctions;
- a lack of will on the part of hospital managements in the face of resistance from some sections of the medical profession;
- the extensive use of voluntary surveyors, who inevitably interpret standards in the light of difficulties and achievements in their own hospitals, producing a self-perpetuating cycle of low, substandard expectations.

353.2 | Hospital information needs

In general, hospitals and hospital boards in Australia in the past have failed to adequately appreciate the importance of clinical information in the overall management of their hospital. Turning again to an industrial analogy, one can appreciate and reflect on how important it is for a factory to know precisely how many cars, and of each model, it makes in any one year; how many defects have resulted in the course of the manufacturing process, and what those defects are; and even to know for certain that the factory is meeting predetermined objectives, and that the factory's 'outcomes' are within certain anticipated standards.

Translated to the hospital, the purpose of clinical information is very similar. Many doctors may find such an analogy somewhat distasteful. However, the parallels that exist between assuring quality in industry and in the hospital, while not complete, are quite marked. Readers will find these linkages in Part II. In some instances considerable expenditure and effort will be required to bring clinical information services and medical record departments to an effective functioning level. There is, fortunately, considerable evidence that several states in Australia have at last recognised this need.

353.3 | Facilities and working conditions

In the past, terms of remuneration for medical record administrators, working conditions, and resources in general have been such that it would certainly appear that the hospital industry itself has not attached much importance to medical records and the process of storing and retrieving clinical information. After all, if the governing body and management do not believe that medical records and effective clinical information systems are important why should the medical staff! One has only to ask the average visiting medical officer where his or her priorities of spending in the hospital lie, and it would be surprising indeed if he or she even remembers to mention the medical record function.

353.4 *Demands on clinical information*

The hard truth is that medical records and the related clinical information systems in many, if not most, of our hospitals are generally speaking far from adequate to meet the present-day needs of hospitals. They also fall short of the level of documentation demanded by good clinical practice. Quality management programs must have as one of their principal objectives the assurance of the quality of documentation, which is a vital aspect of clinical care.

Today's hospital environment differs dramatically from the relatively carefree hospital world that existed immediately after World War II. To manage and be accountable in today's world places burdens of sophistication on hospitals which were undreamed of fifty years ago—and much of that sophistication focuses on information. Of all the information that is needed in order to manage a hospital, the most vital is clinical information. Health professionals need to know what they are really doing and how well they are doing it; hospital management needs information to effectively manage scarce and increasingly costly resources. On a macro scale, government needs to know what to fund, how much to fund, where to fund and how to fund.

Suddenly it is being realised that the smarter one becomes in terms of attempting to manage finances, or to better allocate resources within complex organisations such as hospitals, or to look at the quality of care being produced, the more important becomes the basic clinical information on which all rational decisions must ultimately rest. In addition, the provision of high quality care demands good medical records.

353.5 *Medical and hospital litigation*

Information from medical defence organisations and other professional liability insurers all points to the inadequacy of the written record as one of the major contributing factors in the problem of medical and hospital litigation. On many occasions a weak case for negligence against a hospital or doctor is impossible to defend due to the inadequacy of the medical record. Lack of information, illegible records, defamatory statements and errors are as much, if not more, of a problem than actual clinical misdemeanours. Correcting this situation is perhaps one of the most important elements in a hospital's risk management program.

354 Deficiencies in clinical information

Current standards of medical records and the related collection of clinical data in Australia remain significant problems throughout the country, in both private and public hospitals. The situation is a composite problem consisting of the following elements:

- Many individual records in many hospitals are inadequate in terms of diagnosis and progress notes.
- In as many as 60% of cases, records in some hospitals lack a principal diagnosis for encoding purposes, which has been authenticated by the responsible medical officer on discharge. (While there is some lack of uniformity between states in Australia, the definition of the principal diagnosis used in this manual is that used by the New South Wales Department of Health namely: 'the condition accounting

for the majority of hospital days stay'.) In contrast, in the US, principal diagnosis refers to the condition that was determined after investigation to have resulted in the hospitalisation. Note: It is important to include this definition to avoid confusing US readers and those in countries that follow the US model.

- Where the doctor has recorded a principal diagnosis, there is reason to believe that coding accuracy is very poor because the task of determining the principal diagnosis is left to junior medical staff.
- The illegibility of handwriting is important, particularly in the case of treatment sheets.
- Medical record departments are under-resourced in terms of facilities, equipment and staff, so that the real benefit of well-trained information professionals often falls short of what might be considered basic, and the dividend of good hospital information for medical staff and management is often missing.

Most medical practitioners agree about the need to keep accurate and timely medical records; yet experience shows that when one looks at their compliance with this position, there is a large gap between the agreed need and actual practice. Only in recent years have some doctors ceased to argue that while they might have an obligation in relation to medical records in a public hospital, the situation in private hospitals was different. In spite of protestations by hospitals, medical staff insisted that what happened in the private hospital was purely a matter between themselves and the patient.

Today this point of view is probably far less prevalent than previously, largely due to the effect of the accreditation program of the Australian Council on Healthcare Standards. However, in spite of attitudinal changes due to accreditation there is no doubt that the problem of hospital medical records remains a matter for concern, with what appears to be little tangible evidence that anything is being done to correct it. We can only conclude that either:

- accreditation standards are not sufficiently explicit; or
- surveyors are not willing to penalise a hospital for less than adequate medical records (the 'glass house effect'); or
- it is not possible within the time frame allowed for an accreditation survey to adequately review the quality of medical records.

Recently-adopted changes to ACHS standards for medical records—if effectively implemented and if surveyors demand compliance—might reasonably be expected to result eventually in some tangible improvements.

Wide variations exist in the adequacy of medical records between hospitals and even within the same hospital. If quality is conforming to requirements, establishing recordkeeping standards and reducing the variation in the quality of hospital medical records within the same hospital would result in immediate quality improvement.

355 | Some illustrative case studies

355.1 | *Experience points to typical problems*

We describe below some of the medical record situations that we have encountered over a wide range of private and public hospitals. Clearly, scientific surveys of hospital medical records would be more informative. However, such surveys have not been conducted and in the circumstances we can only point to particular, typical problems.

355.2 | *The case of the absent medical notes*

During an unannounced visit to a small private hospital, which is part of a large well-regarded hospital group, we randomly selected a medical record. The patient was about to be discharged following an abdominal hysterectomy from which she had made a good recovery. We were advised by nursing staff that during the procedure the patient had sustained a cardiac arrest. Examination of the medical record revealed not one word had been recorded in the surgeon's operative report or the clinical progress notes to document this fact.

In our view, doctors have an obligation to record everything. Should legal action have followed, the doctor would wish to defend himself on the basis that he did everything possible to resuscitate his patient. The absence of any written record to support this contention might well have resulted in a judgment not in his favour. The situation adopted by the courts is that if it is not recorded, it did not happen. It is quite possible that the doctor in this situation had meant to render it apparent that the maloccurrence did not happen by recording nothing. Had legal action taken place, the number of witnesses, both doctors and nurses (supported by nursing notes) who would have asserted that the event did happen, would have been overwhelming.

355.3 | *The case of the non-recording obstetricians*

We became aware of an attitude by obstetricians at one small private and a large public hospital in relation to making entries into the medical record in relation to normal confinements. At both hospitals, which were in no way related, obstetricians had adopted the practice of not making any entry when the confinement had been normal. The attitude of many doctors is that: 'If we didn't say anything, there was nothing to say'.

At the private hospital a patient had a confinement which ended in caesarean section. The baby was normal. Two years later the same woman was again in labour and on this occasion the obstetrician judged it prudent to allow a vaginal delivery. As the confinement was considered normal, no record was made by the obstetrician. However, some eighteen months later the second child was found to have a mental deficit and the hospital and the obstetrician were sued successfully because the mother had not been given the benefit of a caesarean section and, it was alleged, that during trial labour the child had suffered consequential cerebral damage. With no medical notes relating to the confinement, neither hospital nor obstetrician had any defence whatsoever, and premiums for doctors' indemnity were notched up yet again. This case emphasises the importance of recording negative findings.

355.4 | *The case of the missing principal diagnosis*

In a small public hospital of 100 beds, only 10% of separations on discharge had a principal diagnosis for encoding purposes, which had been authenticated by the responsible medical officer. Medical record staff also pointed out that the accuracy of that principal diagnosis was suspect when compared with the case notes. The principal diagnosis was determined by junior medical staff with no supervision by visiting medical staff. Visiting medical staff should be responsible for recording and validating the principal diagnosis in the patient's medical record.

355.5 | *The case of no clinical data and no principal diagnosis*

At a large public hospital of some 400 beds, only an estimated 20% of separations had a principal diagnosis. Junior trainee medical staff in this hospital often refused to complete the discharge summary sheet, which contains the principal diagnosis. As the principal diagnosis is essential for coding, the capacity to retrieve aggregated data from the medical record department was severely limited. In the same hospital, however, specialist medical staff complained that the medical record department was incapable of meeting their requests for clinical data. As ye sow, so shall ye reap!

355.6 | Some further examples

- In another large hospital a record was picked at random It related to a patient admitted for gastroscopy. Not one word appeared on that part of the medical record reserved for medical information and progress notes.
- A pathologist working in a teaching hospital complained that in the course of post-mortems, clinical information necessary to support a clinical diagnosis was frequently absent from the medical record.
- In another public hospital, the medical record department claimed that they were embarrassed to receive requests from other hospitals because the information requested, while clinically relevant, was simply not present in a high percentage of cases.
- In one large public hospital where the state of medical records was particularly poor, the visiting medical staff, while admitting that the quality of the medical record was part of their responsibility, claimed that a large part of the problem was their inability to effectively discipline junior medical staff. What was really absent was adequate supervision and teaching of junior staff by the complaining visiting medical staff.

356 | Quality not quantity

One major problem with medical records is their overwhelming bulk. In recent years most hospitals in Australia have moved to a unitary record system in which medical and nursing notes follow one another on the same continuation sheet. This produces not only a very bulky medical record, but increasingly medical staff are complaining of the difficulty in isolating medical from nursing notes. Because of these problems we are aware of some hospitals reverting to separate medical and nursing notes. There is also no doubt that the more junior the professional, generally the more voluminous the material.

Better structuring of the record, with 'pro-forma' sheets, boxes and clearly designated spaces which will need to vary according to the medical discipline, will aid the usability of the medical record. The same principles applied to discharge summaries would make them more useful. The very bulk of many medical records reinforces the need for complete, concise discharge summaries. Not nearly enough effort and resources have been applied to the medical record to make it easier to enter and retrieve data. A serious review of the policy of 'unitary' records, in which medical and nursing and all other provider data are written on the same continuation sheets, needs to be undertaken. Pilot studies should be initiated to test better designed medical record and continuation sheets, better use of colour coding and of dividers in bulky records, and other such procedures. Use of computer-based (electronic) medical records will overcome many of the limitations inherent in paper-based medical records. However, their consideration is beyond this manual's scope, and regrettably their wide-spread use in Australian hospitals likely lies many years in the future.

No one seriously questions the importance of the medical record or of the clinical data it contains to patient care, quality management, hospital management and, in the near future, hospital funding. Yet it is difficult not to assume that if industry generally found itself in the same position, enormous resources and effort would be applied to explore better alternatives or at least ways to improve the current situation. If the relationship between the medical record and such matters as quality of patient care and financial management can be emphasised and demonstrated to medical staff, one might reasonably assume that the quality of medical records would improve, especially if sanctions were applied to chronic laggards.

357 | Clinical information for the 1990s

357.1 | The demands of quality management

The medicolegal environment of the 1990s and the increasing complexity of medical technology demands even more accurate and detailed medical records than in past years. Quality management itself makes the following demands on a clinical information service:

- the ability to assess retrospectively processes and outcomes of care depends on the quality of the information in the medical record;
- the capacity to screen records to determine patterns of care depends on coding which in turn depends on timely entry of an accurate principal diagnosis;
- the abstraction or screening of records and the capacity to provide aggregated clinical data rests heavily on the resources of the medical record department.

Quality management is therefore a major reason in itself to improve the state of medical records, and improvement in the adequacy of the medical record often results from the introduction of an effective quality management program. High quality care is not only care that improves the patient's condition clinically, but that which is documented well. Good care must not only be given, but also must be documented to have been given. Further, the adequacy of the documentation of one episode of care may affect the quality of the next episode or the next admission. The demands of clinical outcomes research also place great emphasis on the adequacy of the medical record. Every medical record is a potential research observation, or would be if well-documented.

People often overlook the important role that the medical record plays in areas which are just as if not even more important today than previously. They represent the elements of good medical care, namely the recording of:

- facts about the patient's condition, tests ordered, treatments considered and implemented;
- diagnostic inferences;
- patient progress, response to treatment, instructions;
- patient's desires and satisfaction.

357.2 | Case mix funding

Developments on the horizon relating to hospital funding and the assessment of hospital activity are all related in some way to the capacity to categorise hospital activity by reference to the range of clinical case mix that the hospital is servicing. Without accurate and detailed medical records, hospitals will find themselves seriously disadvantaged and their funding compromised because of their inability to accurately describe their case mix.

357.3 | Screening of records

Problems in the area of patient care generally do not happen as isolated situations; usually they fall into recurring patterns. Such patterns, whether of untoward events by medical practitioners or related to nursing services, or any other of the many service divisions in a hospital, can only be identified if there is a capacity to screen significant numbers of patient records retrospectively. A clinical information system with analytic capabilities is needed in order to display patterns of care. Patterns of care enable the hospital to know when and where to investigate the adequacy of management of individual cases. Such techniques make it possible to distinguish between normal and acceptable variations in clinical management on the one hand, and the truly aberrant practitioner on the other.

The surgical team which has a bout of wound infections can only be identified reliably as having a significant problem if by reviewing and abstracting a series of records in certain categories over the previous six or twelve months an abnormal pattern of wound infection emerges. Only after a problem has been identified as significant should resources be devoted to investigating the cause, lest money be wasted chasing phantom problems. Moreover, vigorous pursuit of artefacts leads clinicians to believe that quality assurance activities are a waste of effort. Computerised analysis and reporting of patients by disease codes is a critical element in the total framework of effective quality management because it permits analysis of patterns of care.

358 | The way forward

358.1 | Technology

To an increasing degree computerisation of medical information is occurring at a rapid rate in hospitals. Initial steps have been in the areas of laboratory reports and radiology. While the traditional medical record is still mainly manual, systems do exist to computerise them in whole or in part, and their use is growing. Even though medical records are created manually, there is growing interest in computerising selective data from them. These automated abstraction systems are currently seen most often in surgery and obstetrics but there is a trend for them to become universal.

While the raw data entered into medical records needs to be complete and accurate, accessing that data in aggregated form and in a way that is meaningful in today's world requires computer technology. The ability to aggregate clinical data by diagnosis, by provider, and by complications is no longer a sophisticated addendum but a fundamental necessity. The ability to aggregate clinical information enables patterns of practice to be identified by diagnosis, by provider, by hospital and so on. Aggregating information is the basis of clinical research and also enables the use of hospital resources, so-called utilisation review, to be effectively conducted. The next few years will see enormous technological progress in the area of computerised analysis of the process and outcome data from medical records. Indeed, some of that technology is already here. Such systems, however, demand a standard of medical recordkeeping which is still unusual in Australia. While information automation can help to improve medical recordkeeping, without the will there is unlikely to be the way.

358.2 | Improving hospital medical records

This chapter draws attention to serious weaknesses in hospitals' medical records and information systems. To assist hospitals to improve, we describe below actions the various actors responsible for hospital care and its recording should consider taking.

358.3 | Board and management

The people who hold statutory responsibility for the hospital's activities should first recognise that many aspects of clinical information are quite unsatisfactory at the present time, and that considerable resources and energy are required to rectify these current deficiencies. A modern hospital is a large commercial enterprise. Hospital directors and managers must quickly accept the fact that managing the hospital, financing the hospital, managing risk and minimising litigation, and assuring the quality of care and services, all depend heavily on the calibre of clinical information.

The financially constrained environment of the 1990s demands that a higher proportion of resources be directed into clinical information and its related functions. The department of clinical information cannot continue to be treated as the poor relation among the hospital departments as it has been treated in the past. Hospitals must be prepared to devote adequate resources to all aspects of recordkeeping, including automated abstraction systems and the coding they require. Managers of hospitals that employ medical record administrators should use these highly qualified staff appropriately as middle managers with responsibilities for clinical information policies and practices.

Once the board is seen to take the medical record and clinical information seriously, others, including medical staff, are more likely to do likewise.

Much more money must be spent on research and development to find better ways to keep records, to record information, to activate records and other such procedures. If industry in general were faced with such an issue that was so critical to its daily operation, large funds would have long ago been directed to the problem.

358.4 *Clinical information and the quality management department*

The role of the clinical information department is to constantly monitor medical records' quality and contents to ensure that they meet all necessary requirements. Using the criteria from the ACHS' accreditation guide, hospitals should undertake regular audits of medical records and report results through the medical records committee to the quality management committee, and to the medical staff and management. Further, the process of structured quality review will also provide objective evidence of the adequacy or otherwise of medical record documentation.

Clinical information is such a vital component of quality management that the clinical information (medical record) function should come under the jurisdiction of the quality management department and the medical record administrator should report through the quality manager to the hospital manager. All too frequently in large hospitals a separate medical record department falls under the jurisdiction of medical administration. Unfortunately, this arrangement merely ensures that traditional attitudes become enhanced and opportunities for change remain marginal. Hospital managers either directly, or most appropriately through the quality manager, must take a personal interest in the area of clinical information if the commitment which we advocate for the hospital board is to be adequately transmitted into effective action.

358.5 *Medical and nursing staff*

The hospital's medical staff must understand from the time of their appointment that the hospital board and management are serious about the need for high quality medical records. Junior staff must be encouraged to achieve high standards of recording and considerable efforts should be made to train junior staff in the skills required. Nothing, however, is more effective with junior staff than that of example. If visiting medical staff and staff specialists do not place much value on the medical record, the junior staff will leave that hospital sharing the same indifference.

Quality management and, in particular, practice policies give a lead on what is important and what is less important in documentation in medical records—a constant problem for junior doctors. Doctors and nurses in training need to be taught what to write in medical records and how to write it. Such education carries a cost, but is essential for quality management and indeed for high quality care. Further, all hospital staff, but doctors in particular, require continual in-service education on the skills needed for and the importance of medical recordkeeping. Visiting medical staff should review trainees' notes so that medical records become a potent teaching tool. Doctors and nurses must make time to complete medical records adequately, and in busy hospital schedules, particularly for junior trainee medical staff, time must be allowed for proper medical recordkeeping. The completion by medical staff of discharge summaries and the principal diagnosis within one week of discharge is as important as other aspects of medical recordkeeping.

Doctors make the vital clinical decisions in hospitals and our comments, therefore, are mainly directed at medical staff. Nursing notes, however, are an important source of information and we do not wish in any way to minimise their importance. Like medical staff, nurses should be taught how to make appropriate nursing notes. At some stage prior to discharge, nursing notes should be summarised for easy reference later, including incorporation in the patient's discharge summary when appropriate.

Continual failure to meet the hospital's recordkeeping policies should result in significant sanctions against offending medical staff. Such sanctions, however, must be set out in hospital by-laws and drawn to the attention of medical staff on appointment. We have not set forth a series of sanctions, which may vary from hospital to hospital, but a withdrawal of all clinical privileges for a three-month period may be appropriate when all attempts to persuade a medical practitioner to modify his or her behaviour have failed. While sanctions must be present, incentives are much to be preferred and are usually much more effective. Clinicians whose medical records are exemplary should be extolled as models and proclaimed publicly. Well-deserved praise depends on the ability to measure performance.

358.6 | *The Australian Council on Healthcare Standards*

The ACHS criteria for medical records are sound, but in too many instances not observed in practice. The time has now come for the ACHS to demonstrate to hospitals in Australia that it is serious about its requirements for medical records. Given the number of surveyed hospitals which fail to meet these criteria, failure by one or two hospitals to achieve accreditation because of their inability to meet the medical record requirements would be a salutary lesson for the industry.

Chapter 6

GETTING STARTED

---

360 | Contents

This chapter details a plan of procedure for a hospital wishing to establish an effective, hospital-wide, multidisciplinary, integrated quality management program. It covers the following topics:

361. Purpose of this chapter
362. At square one
363. Hospital assessment
364. Organisational and attitudinal change
365. Expectations
366. Outside resources
367. Order of implementation
368. Building a firm foundation: more steps toward quality maturity
369. Managing QM implementation and assessing progress

361 | Purpose of this chapter

Our experience with hospitals demonstrates how difficult it is to begin a quality management program from scratch. At the present time in Australia there are few if any models of such a program (since few have been attempted) which can be used to signpost the way. This chapter intends to provide some signposts and to offer benchmarks by which a hospital can map its progress.

362 | At square one

Hospital managers find that knowing where to begin is one of the great difficulties. Not knowing where to begin is sufficient rationale for some to justify inaction. There is no doubt that where to begin is perhaps the most difficult step in the entire process of quality management implementation. For this reason we have devoted this chapter to laying down a coherent series of steps to enable a hospital to see its way through what for many is an endless maze. Not every hospital will wish or need to follow our suggestions precisely, but at least they will have some benchmarks against which they can measure their progress.

We are very conscious of the number of small hospitals in Australia. These comprise not only small rural hospitals but also private hospitals of less than 100 beds. We recognise that such facilities must have a somewhat different approach to the

519

implementation of a quality management program than a large referral hospital with many hundreds of beds and a considerably greater range of resources. We are also aware of the wide range of activity and available resources that exist in hospitals both large and small, so that generalisations of almost any sort are likely to be seen as irrelevant to some, while useful to others.

Establishing the sort of quality management program we advocate is not a simple side issue for any hospital, large or small. For this reason most hospitals will require outside help at some stage to implement such a program effectively and with a minimum of difficulty. In the end, we believe that successful implementation of quality management will be driven by three factors: commitment, resources and planning.

363 | Hospital assessment

Our first encounter with a client hospital usually consists of an account about the 'quality assurance' activities which are already occurring, followed by the request for some help with this current activity or an acknowledgment that in spite of their present efforts they do not seem to be getting very far. While we recognise that the very process which leads a hospital to call for help reveals that considerable progress has been made, most hospitals' perceptions about quality assurance and quality management still remain rather limited. Most calls for help reveal a hospital that has remained focused on individual activities, projects or studies, and where the concept of a program for the entire hospital has not even been considered.

Initially, we accepted a hospital's account of its current 'quality assurance' activity at face value, only to discover, on assessment, that many of the key elements necessary for an effective program were missing; that the current 'quality assurance' was far from effective; and that many of the hospital staff were frustrated and disillusioned by lack of progress and results. As far as 'quality assurance' is concerned there is, on the part of hospital managers in particular, a perception and performance gap which is usually matched throughout all professional areas of the hospital.

Accordingly, it is essential for any hospital to undertake a detailed assessment of all quality management activity in the hospital in order to provide a realistic picture of what is occurring and what needs to be done. This assessment usually consists of a series of one-on-one interviews with a representative sample of staff, but particularly medical staff. It is helpful to make use of structured questionnaires that, when collated, provide a surprisingly full picture of what is actually happening in the hospital. Included in these interviews are management and directors of the board.

The statement, for example, that the obstetric department is engaged in significant 'quality assurance', when tested in a face-to-face interview with a senior obstetrician, may result in a very different picture. More importantly, such interviews permit the examination of attitudes, particularly of medical staff, to such matters as aberrant practitioners, medical records, credentialling, and concerns relating to quality management and the effectiveness of the hospital's committee activity. Attitudinal obstacles to quality management become an important element to be considered in a quality management plan and in the subsequent implementation process. Moreover, in one-on-one interviews, conducted by consultants who are themselves experienced medical practitioners or nurses, medical staff are prepared to discuss many of these contentious issues. The resultant rapport that can result from such encounters enables the interviewer to commence the long process of attitudinal change that is so critical to the implementation of an effective quality management program.

In addition to personal interviews, the assessment needs to include time spent sitting in on a sample of committee meetings to assess their performance in such terms as agendas, minutes and the capacity to function effectively. Interviews and assessments should be followed by a detailed report to the hospital, and this report becomes the key element in developing the subsequent quality management plan.

364 | Organisational and attitudinal change

By now the reader will have realised the implications of the sort of quality management program being advocated. Required activity is far more extensive than that usually seen, as when an individual or a small group of professionals involve themselves in some incidental aspect of quality assurance. The program being advocated involves every aspect of hospital activity on a continuing basis; not a small add-on to the usual daily activity of doctors and nurses. This concept is new in Australia and the perception gap is so great that it is either rejected out of hand or received with a mixture of scepticism and bemusement.

This reluctance is seen not merely on the part of doctors, nurses and other clinical staff, but also particularly with management. One of the greatest difficulties in commencing a quality management program is to persuade management that this activity has anything to do with them. Likewise, members of hospital boards are only just starting to realise that they too must become committed to quality management if it is ever to become a reality.

Throughout the almost twenty-year history of 'QA' in Australia, governments (state and federal) and hospital managements have placed the onus for implementing 'quality assurance' mainly onto medical and other hospital professional staff. However, if a program of quality management, including quality assurance, is to be implemented, the greatest change in attitude is that required of management itself. Management must be deeply involved in the hospital assessment and all subsequent phases of 'getting started' activities. For the broad concept of quality management advocated in this manual to be successful, management will need to change its attitudes every bit as much as it expects other hospital staff to change theirs.

Nursing staff, because of their employed status and in general their better understanding of organisational structure than doctors, have tended to go their own way with 'quality assurance'. Nurses, in some instances, seem even more reluctant to enter into multidisciplinary quality management activity than doctors. This isolation may have more to do with power plays than concern about quality of care.

Implementing an effective quality management program represents a major organisational challenge. Implementing the type of program we advocate entails a considerable switch in the total mind-set of the institution. It sees quality as the main function of the hospital, and all services and activities should be geared to that purpose. The depth and extent of this change in approach must be constantly kept in mind. Proper allowance, in terms of communications, training and incentives, must be made so as to ensure that everyone in the hospital understands the objectives and the philosophy this entails.

There are, of course, other attitudinal hurdles that have to be faced. Once the hospital has made the difficult decision to embark on an effective quality management program, clinical staff, and doctors in particular, just want to get on and do something that can demonstrate their conversion to the faith. We have found it extremely difficult to bring medical staff to the point of understanding how important the planning and initial steps are in ensuring ultimate success. Many hospitals will dismiss as unnecessary some of the basic elements in the program, claiming that they already exist in their hospital. Unfortunately these claims in many cases fall far short of necessary levels of achievement, subsequently resulting in significant difficulties in implementation unless the hospital is prepared to initiate prior corrective action.

365 | Expectations

A hospital-wide, integrated, multidisciplinary program cannot be developed overnight without any outlay of resources. It would be unrealistic to believe otherwise. Given the assumption that the hospital board and management support the program and have the will to see it through to full implementation, and that a core of medical staff have a commensurate level of commitment, we believe that such a program can reach a useful stage within one to two years. However, reaching the state of quality maturity could take from five to ten years, or even longer. Building such a program requires prolonged and sustained effort and resources. Moreover, the process is never fully complete because it evolves as the hospital evolves. While clinical care is for ever, so is assuring the quality of that care for ever.

Having implemented an effective program, it is also unrealistic to believe that there would no longer be episodes of poor quality care, or that the threat of malpractice litigation would entirely disappear. Indeed, if one looks for quality problems one is likely to discover them. However, it is realistic to anticipate that serious malprocess will become rare. Further, one might expect morale in the hospital to rise as all staff realise that the quality of their care and services is constantly improving. From the patients' viewpoint, better quality of life, quicker recovery, and longer and more productive lives are all very important outcomes—something which health professionals, immersed busily in their daily activities, sometimes overlook as the main reason they are in business.

366 | Outside resources

There will be few hospitals that will be able to implement all the aspects of a hospital-wide, integrated quality management program without requiring some outside assistance in the course of this activity. While larger teaching hospitals will, without doubt, have many of the skills and resources necessary, because of their very size and staff sophistication they are nevertheless usually very rigid institutions. Introducing significant change in such organisations presents a special level of difficulty. Initiating such change from within will be particularly difficult. Outside consultants, who are not part of the organisation, can play the role of 'change agents' enhancing chances of success.

The initial challenge to introduce quality management in Australian hospitals in the late 1970s (then referred to as 'peer review') was directed at the medical profession. With the benefit of hindsight, this challenge was probably misdirected. The initiation of such major organisational change must start with management based on policy directives of the board of directors. Increasingly, managers are beginning to see quality management, including quality assurance aspects, as part of their responsibility, but unfortunately the majority still view the undertaking as solely the responsibility of clinical staff. Those who do understand something of the wider implications lack sufficient knowledge and expertise in the area to enable them to know just where to start. The hospital manager is the most important figure in the successful implementation of hospital-wide, integrated quality management. Given the environment and the context in which they work, hospital managers will require considerable assistance to be able to launch such a program.

367 | Order of implementation

367.1 | Steps in establishing a quality management program

We list the steps for getting started in a predetermined order, recognising that some hospitals will not need, or will not be able, to follow this order religiously. It is also possible that in some situations more than one of these steps may be attempted at the same time. However, we caution that in our experience each one of these steps has its own hurdles to be overcome, involving personalities and existing hospital organisation—all of which will prove more difficult in reality than they may appear to be on paper. The worst possible situation is to promise the hospital everything and deliver little or nothing. It is with this in mind that we counsel caution and slow but steady progress.

In summary, suggested implementation steps, depicted in Table III-6-1 below, are as follows:

- obtain the commitment of the board and management;
- establish a QM planning group—the eventual QM committee;
- appoint a QM manager/resource officer;
- conduct a QM assessment;
- develop a QM policy and plan the QM program;
- set implementation strategy—establish the QM program and implement the QM plan;
- initiate communication/education;
- establish the structure/process of the program—including committee restructuring and education;
- hire professional/administrative resources;
- upgrade the medical record/clinical information system;
- formalise risk management including occupational health and safety;
- credential medical staff;
- hire additional QM resource staff;
- form additional committees if/when warranted;
- initiate quality assurance activities, for example studies, quality measurement and monitoring;
- manage QM implementation;
- assess progress and revise plans.

Table III-6-1 *Getting started*

The time frame for completion of these activities will vary greatly from hospital to hospital depending on individual circumstances. The three-year implementation suggested here may be reasonable for some hospitals and overly optimistic for others. Achieving quality maturity may take 10–12 years.

When	What	Who
To start	obtain board commitment	hospital manager
after commitment	establish QM planning group	medical nursing staff/hospital manager, outside consultant
next	appoint quality manager	hospital manager, outside consultant
next, or at same time	assessment of QM activities with report	outside consultant

continues

Table III-6-1 *continued*

When	What	Who
next	develop QM policy, QM plan	quality manager, planning group
next, or at same time	begin hospital-wide education for QM	quality manager, planning group
next	form QMC from planning group; terms of reference	quality manager, chair planning group
next	commence committee restructuring; agenda, minutes, chairmanship	quality manager, consultant
at end of 1st year	review progress and revise plans	QMC, quality manager
next	consolidate 'QA' activities, functions in separate QMD	quality manager, MRA, OH&S officer etc.
with committee restructuring completed	establish mechanisms to effect changes identified by assessment, monitoring activities	QMC, QMD
next	begin to implement QM plan	QMC, quality manager
at same time	plan and initiate patient satisfaction survey	quality manager, outside experts
at same time	review and co-ordinate system for recording & tracking incidents, complaints, compliments	quality manager, DON, OH&S officer
at same time	reinforce education, communication program to hospital staff	quality manager
next	review needs to focus attitudinal behavioural change program	QMC, quality manager
next	commence upgrade of medical record dept. if necessary	quality manager, MRA
next	initiate simple projects e.g. study blood products' usage	relevant clinical, support depts., quality manager, QMC
at same time	review and upgrade infection control	quality manager, infection control sister, clinical & support depts.
at end of 2nd year	review progress and revise plans	quality manager
QMC, QMD functioning well	formalise risk management, including OH&S, programs	quality manager, OH&S officer, chair QMC, HM
12 months before reappointment triennium	commence discussions with medical staff about credentialling	quality manager, HM, medical staff, consultant
next	review need for additional QM staff	quality manager
next	form additional committees if necessary	quality manager
QM program established and a core of supportive medical staff	commence quality assessment using SQR	quality manager, medical staff, MRA, consultant
next	review needs to focus contents of education program	quality manager, QMC
next	begin process of charting progress in improving care	QMD
at same time	expand studies, extend quality assessment, extend monitoring	QMC, quality manager, clinical, other staff

continues

Table III-6-1 *continued*

When	What	Who
at end of 3rd year	review progress and revise plans	quality manager
at end of 5th, 10th, 15th years	evaluate QM program, revise policies, structures, activities etc.	quality manager, QMC, HM, board, medical and other staffs
on continuing basis	assess, improve, and continue hospital-wide education program	quality manager, QMC
on continuing basis	manage QM implementation	quality manager
on continuing basis	monitor QM program's cost-effectiveness	quality manager, QMC, HM, board

List of abbreviations:

DON	director of nursing	QM	quality management
HM	hospital manager	QMC	quality management committee
MRA	medical records administrator	QMD	quality management department
OH&S	occupational health and safety	SQR	structured quality review
QA	quality assurance		

367.2 Obtain commitment

Commitment, commitment, commitment! No three words better sum up the first basic essential for the implementation of quality management. Primarily there must be commitment on the part of the hospital board and the management. Commitment must also be present on the part of medical, nursing and all other hospital staff. However, unless the board and management have a deep commitment to this concept, it will be well nigh impossible to generate the attitudes necessary throughout the remainder of the hospital. One important and tangible manifestation of commitment is adequate resourcing of the quality management program.

While we have listed 'commitment' as the first implementation step, the reality is often that only after the hospital engages a consultant does the board and its manager fully comprehend what is expected of them. Nevertheless, achieving this commitment is the single most crucial part of quality management implementation. Next in order are continuity of leadership and constancy of effort.

367.3 Establish quality management planning group/committee

The hospital must establish early on a quality management planning group. We describe this group as a 'planning group' because initially it will spearhead the hospital's planning for quality management. Eventually, however, this committee will become the quality management committee and as such will be the most important committee of the hospital. Great care needs to be taken with its composition, its chairperson, and its terms of reference, all of which in most hospitals will require some outside advice and assistance. This committee should not be chaired by a board member, but rather by a senior, respected member of the medical staff, at least at the beginning. It is inappropriate to have directors of the hospital board on a quality management committee. Doctors are the most important participants in any quality management activity. If they are to be involved they must be able to identify with the program.

The manager should develop terms of reference for the planning group/QM committee, if need be with outside consultants' assistance. Given current perspectives, without outside help most terms of reference for this committee will be far too limited. For this reason, the Appendix to Chapter 3 of this part provides model terms of reference for a QM committee.

367.4   *Appoint quality manager*

The hospital should appoint the quality manager early in the program's staged implementation, before it has developed the QM plan, to ensure that he or she is involved in the planning process and can take 'ownership' of the plan. One of the most important and at the same time the most difficult tasks is to identify persons with adequate educational skills and background to head the quality management department and, as quality manager, to direct the quality management program. Review of Part III, Chapter 4 (on the quality management department) highlights the difficulties that most hospitals will experience. Moreover, the implementation of subsequent steps will depend heavily on a permanent resource in the hospital. While consultants can play an important role, it is essential that in the developmental phase of the program the hospital can rely on some in-house leadership and expertise to carry the program forward.

Quality managers require two essential skills: the capacity to administer the program, and the knowledge about what to do. In Australia, most of the persons filling this role lack one or both of these requirements. In addition, while there will always be the exception, an understanding of the complexities of hospital culture is a prerequisite for the position. While hospital managers will ultimately decide who they want to employ as quality manager, they would be well advised to pay greater attention to candidates' management skills and understanding of hospital culture than their formal knowledge, of quality management methodologies, for example. Quality managers can more easily acquire the specific knowledge that they need to implement a quality management program, through training or retaining consultants, for example, than they can become competent managers or understand the culture of health care or how hospitals function, including the complex relationships among the professionals who work in them.

367.5   *Conduct QM assessment*

Reference has already been made to the need to have an outside expert assess the hospital on the many aspects and elements that form a quality management program. Experience suggests that it is an unusual hospital that can assess itself in this regard. Such an assessment involves more than a survey of the type conducted currently by the ACHS. Accreditation is no guarantee of an effective quality management program. An assessment of the hospital should result in a detailed report which responds to the following and related issues, for example:

- the level of meaningful quality management and quality assurance being conducted in the hospital, and whether or not there is documented evidence of this activity;
- documented evidence of changed patterns of practice or service as a result of existing quality management activity;
- the extent of multidisciplinary activity, and the integration and co-ordination of current activity;
- the effectiveness of committees in terms of agenda preparation, minutes, decisions, subsequent action, and the capacity of chairpersons and committee members to conduct themselves adequately in a committee;
- the presence or absence of a quality management committee or its equivalent. The role and authority of such a committee and its relationships with other hospital committees;
- the reporting mechanisms for quality management activities, including lines and frequency of reporting;
- mechanisms for dealing with aberrant medical practitioners, and the presence of a formal system of appointment and credentialling;
- mechanisms for documenting practice policies, for both medical and nursing staff;

- an assessment of attitudes towards, and understanding of, quality management by board members, management, medical staff, nursing staff and others;
- the level of sophistication of the clinical information system in the hospital. The adequacy, from the point of view of quality management and quality assurance, of the content of the medical records, and of coding and discharge summaries with a principal diagnosis.

367.6 Develop quality management plan

The assessment report should provide the essential background for developing a QM policy and plan that will set out what the hospital wants to achieve, and how it intends to close the gap between its existing QA activity and what is required for an effective quality management program. The assessment report should also suggest an appropriate implementation strategy.

A proper quality management plan is the cornerstone of an effective QM implementation strategy, both at the early stage of getting started and throughout subsequent continuing quality management activity. The quality manager is responsible for producing the QM plan and it must be approved by the QM committee or the planning group. The plan will indicate who is to be responsible for, and will also attempt to put some time scales on, its implementation. The QM plan should be reviewed and, if necessary, amended annually.

The key elements in a quality management plan are:

- being consistent with the policy and objectives adopted by the hospital board;
- being realistic, in terms of the resources available and the obstacles that are likely to be faced;
- setting clear goals and objectives that can be measured;
- selecting a strategy for and specifying the steps needed to achieve objectives;
- establishing a process of implementation including the proper use of outside consultants, with clear responsibilities and schedules;
- identifying key measures of success and progress.

367.7 Set implementation strategy

The sheer size, complexity and structural politics of larger hospitals may render our preferred holistic or 'hospital-wide' approach, involving a hospital QM committee with divisional or departmental QA committees at a later stage, impractical. Doubtless, the success of a QM program depends on the ability to manage its implementation and operation. The holistic approach, which we emphasise, aims to put in place the entire structure of such a program in a logical sequence to provide the essential management structure that improves chances of success, and has much to commend it. Nevertheless, other factors may militate against such an approach.

The most likely obstacle to the holistic approach in the prevailing climate is the apprehension of medical staff when faced with what some of them see as the introduction of a new, and what they imagine to be a large, meddlesome hospital 'bureaucracy'. The refusal of either the hospital or its medical staff to accept a hospital QM committee means in essence there is no program. However, in a large hospital establishing a QA committee in one of the departments or divisions may be all that is required to enable medical staff to see some early results and overcome their apprehension. Such an initiative will provide them with some idea of the need for a quality management program, the process involved, and likely benefits to them and their patients. The hospital quality management committee, with its hospital-wide coordinating role, may have to follow at a later stage. This piecemeal or 'demonstration' approach can be a non-threatening exposure to quality management. However, its success still depends on management's committment to creating the requisite QA/QI culture. With management's commitment this nucleus of activity can be replicated in other departments and expanded ultimately to become the hospital-wide integrated program that is essential for meaningful quality management. Nevertheless, we recommend this departmental approach only as a last resort when, for whatever reason, a hospital-wide approach is impossible initially. We take this stand for the following reasons:

- The department-by-department approach is not a miniature version of the hospital-wide model, but rather the selective implementation of some aspects of QM.
- Instituting QM in a single department can only implement some aspects of QM that are appropriate to that department.
- The effect of the whole can only be realised by a hospital-wide approach.

While larger hospitals initially may be attracted to an incremental approach, experience suggests that the lead time to achieve an integrated program is considerably lengthened. It leads to considerable fragmentation of effort and patchy results, so that after one or two years the hospital may still be wondering just what it has achieved for its efforts. The variations in attitudes and understanding between departments in large hospitals and structural politics, which are always present, could mean that an integrated quality management program might never be realised.

To take a simple example: A study to examine the management of pneumonia is undertaken by the department of internal medicine, which has decided to embrace a QM program. Review of medical records, however, reveals that the major problem would appear to be with the department of surgery whose members seem to need some further education in this area, but who have refused to participate in a QM program. The end result is that nothing will be achieved to improve the quality of care for patients suffering from pneumonia, and a good deal of frustration and hostility is created along the way. Consistent with our general approach to hospital quality management, we believe that the refusal or inability of hospital staff to implement a hospital-wide QM program is an indictment of that hospital's board of directors and its management.

367.8 *Initiate education/communication*

368.1 READ THIS MANUAL

Nothing will guarantee success more than proper education of and frequent communication with the entire hospital and its staff concerning the purpose and mechanisms of quality management, specific objectives, plans to achieve them, and identified quality problems and their resolution. Such a level of education and communication, even in a small hospital, is far from easy and planning must include this important aspect. Perhaps a start should be made by requiring all of the key players to read this manual, because it was written for just this reason. In this regard, special attention to the following groups of hospital staff is essential.

367.82 THE BOARD AND MANAGEMENT

From the outset, the hospital board and management must fully understand what is to be undertaken and formally adopt a policy of commitment to quality management. We recommend that board members and the management team participate in a short seminar at which there is ample time for questions and discussion. If health professionals have difficulty with quality management concepts, how much more difficult it must be for laypersons, many of whom have only a marginal understanding of hospital activity. However, it is these people who bear the ultimate responsibility for allocating resources and whose support and understanding is essential for success.

367.83 MEDICAL STAFF

Nothing better illustrates the attitudinal difficulties to be faced in quality management implementation than the lack of interest so frequently presented by medical staff. Generally speaking, medical staff's understanding of quality management is marginal, and yet their lack of interest results in enormous difficulty persuading them to sit still long enough to learn something about it. It is often difficult to organise a meeting that requires a significant number of busy doctors to be in the same place at the same time. It will often be quite impractical to run a quality management seminar as an isolated event for medical staff. Opportunities must be sought at existing events, such as medical meetings, hospital reunions, and divisional or departmental meetings at which information about plans and progress can be conveyed. Medical staff's refusal to participate in such activity may well reflect their lack of commitment, or a belief that what is going on is a waste of time. For all these reasons, organising weekend retreats for key members of the medical staff is an approach that offers some hope of overcoming some of these obstacles. The question of how much and when to involve medical staff becomes an important element in planning. At the very least, medical staff must be kept informed about the plan and how it is progressing.

367.84 NURSING STAFF

Members of the nursing staff, other than nursing administration, are often taken somewhat for granted in explaining and conveying information about quality management programs. Nurses are the largest single element in a hospital's workforce and it is imperative that all nurses from the most senior to the most junior should understand what is taking place in the hospital and the implications for the nursing staff. Once again, it is difficult to find an opportunity at which a significant proportion of nursing staff can be brought together at the same time. However, nursing unit managers' meetings and departmental meetings do present opportunities to tell nursing staff about plans and progress.

367.85 QUALITY MANAGEMENT BULLETIN

Most hospitals have some form of hospital bulletin which carries internal information about a range of activity within the hospital. In spite of its existence, a hospital can emphasise quality management by developing a modest but QM-specific newsletter. The objectives of such a newsletter are to:
- communicate what is going on;
- highlight accomplishments;
- celebrate success.

Education and training for quality management commences in the hospital with the original planning group and continues as an ongoing exercise. It will be an unusual hospital that will be able to manage such educational activity initially from its own internal resources. We see this role falling to outside consultants. Some of the educational process can be accomplished by presentations, but the use of videos, workshops, seminars and discussions will all have a useful place.

Some of the important educational elements that require constant reinforcement are:
- the identification, in the early stages, of leaders and those who have an interest in quality management;
- the role, importance and responsibilities of the QM committee, and its relationship with other hospital committees;
- the need for some formality in committee procedures, for members of committees to understand rules of procedure, and the need for chairpersons to have some training in good effective chairmanship.

367.9 | Establish structure/process of the program

There has been a failure in Australian hospitals to draw the distinction between the techniques of assessing and measuring quality of care, and the program or system that must exist for effective quality improvement. In setting up an effective quality management program, two aspects are especially critical: the quality management department and interrelationships of a system of committees. Medical and nursing staff have neither the time nor skills to engage in extensive quality management activity in a way that is effective. Having in place the QMD with the resources, knowledge and skills to manage the QM program becomes the crucial element in its success. Because hospitals historically have given scant attention to committees and their effectiveness, this phase of implementing an effective quality management program will require time and patience.

368 | Building a firm foundation: more steps toward quality maturity

368.1 | Hire professional/administrative resources

Once the board has approved the quality management plan, hospitals should establish the quality management department (properly part of such a plan). The quicker such a department can be established, the more readily will resources be available to provide the essential support necessary to continually improve quality of care.

Initially, the only professional resources available to the quality management initiative may be the recently-appointed quality manager, and perhaps outside consultant help. Periodically, hospital management must review these resources and assess their adequacy for the workload the hospital is likely to face in the next implementation period. At the appropriate time, the hospital must bring together the infection control staff, any independent quality assurance personnel such as nursing 'QA' staff, who exist in many hospitals, and OH&S staff with a pro rata of secretarial support. In small hospitals it may be wiser to proceed more slowly, expanding the role of the quality manager and gradually adding to the support available as the quality management activity in the hospital increases. However, even in a small hospital a basic level of support resources is essential.

How quickly a hospital can develop its quality management department will depend very much on staff attitudes, particularly those of medical staff who, if the purpose and role is not carefully explained to them, may see another administrative unit as somewhat threatening. However, if such a department is seen as the rationalisation of administrative functions, as we have proposed, it should be perceived in a positive light. The role of the quality management department and the role of the quality manager should be clearly and precisely defined. To re-emphasise a key point: the quality manager's role is not to tell doctors or other health professionals what to do nor how to do their job, but rather to help them make possible the continuous improvement in patient care.

368.2 | Upgrade medical record/clinical information system

Most public hospitals already have a medical records committee. Generally the committee spends more time arguing about the details of forms than such important issues as the content of the record, the link between the medical record and quality management and quality assurance, and the importance of written policies governing the record, discharge summaries and the final diagnosis. In addition, the medical records committee should be prepared to play a role, together with the quality management committee, in explaining to medical and nursing staff the vital importance of the medical record and the data that they have the responsibility to record. Given current attitudes, there is a need to constantly reinforce the importance of the medical record for any quality management initiative, and also for the medicolegal security of the doctor and the hospital.

Many small hospitals do not have their own medical record administrator and in some cases the medical record system is fairly primitive. Increasingly, small hospitals are making use of regional arrangements to upgrade these facilities. Every hospital should have a medical records committee to check and report on the following elements of the clinical information system:

- the content of the medical records in the hospital and the conformity of medical records with the criteria set out in the Accreditation Guide of the Australian Council on Healthcare Standards;
- the presence in each record of a final (principal) diagnosis, entered by the medical officer responsible within one week of discharge (legitimate exceptions being those records awaiting results of clinical investigations);
- the presence of a, preferably structured, standard discharge summary, whether it is sent to the patient's outside doctor or not;
- the availability of a disease index with the capacity to statistically manipulate data from the medical record. Computer software for use by small hospitals is now available but the sharing of data manipulation facilities on a regional basis may also be a possibility for small hospitals;
- the development of appropriate policies and procedures, if not already present, and a mechanism for ensuring compliance with these policies and procedures.

Once the quality management department is operational, it should assume responsibility for the hospital's medical record and clinical information system functions.

368.3 Formalise risk management, OH&S

A quality management program is largely about managing risks—the risks of poor quality outcomes for patients, the risks of medical and hospital litigation and the risks of inappropriate use of resources. This perspective is generally unfamiliar to most hospitals and their staff. Explaining this approach becomes a further task for the educational effort and must be communicated to all hospital staff.

Occupational health and safety is an important aspect of risk management and one which receives low priority in most hospitals. (See Part V.) Early on in the development of the quality management program, the QM committee and the quality manager should accept responsibility for the occupational health and safety of hospital staff, as well as patients. Such responsibility will add considerably to the profile of the QM effort and do much for hospital morale. The first step should be a survey of the hospital and its work environment. Since most hospitals have few skilled OH&S resources, they will need to retain an occupational health and safety consultant to conduct this assessment. Subsequent actions will rest heavily on the recommendations contained in the report following such an assessment.

Other risk minimisation actions include: credentialling of medical staff (see Chapter 2 in Part IV); patient complaints tracking, incident reporting, and patient satisfaction surveys (see Chapter 3 in Part IV); and mechanisms to elicit staff suggestions for improving patient care (see Chapter 8 in Part II).

368.4 Credential medical staff

To institute an effective system of credentialling of medical staff, the following steps should be taken:

- enter into detailed discussions with the medical staff to explain why the system is to be introduced, what are the benefits for them, and how the scheme will function;
- involve one or two respected senior members of the medical staff in developing the scheme;
- establish the credentials committee, whose members should select the chairperson;

- train credentials committee members in meeting procedures, provide firm guidance concerning confidentiality, and reassure members concerning their legal position;
- ensure that all documents including minutes and relevant forms are carefully prepared and checked, and the mechanism for appeals is in place.

Part IV provides additional details of credentialling and appointment mechanisms.

368.5 | Hire additional resource staff

The establishment of the credentialling process should be the occasion for reviewing the level of support and resources available to the department of quality management. Credentialling, which should occur annually, requires administrative support, and it may now be opportune to look at a rationalisation of administrative staff and provide the quality manager with additional resources.

368.6 | Form additional committees if/when warranted

The whole purpose of the QM committee structure is to be able to:

- collect and act on data relating to quality of care;
- measure and compare quality of care to standards;
- establish mechanisms to identify problems;
- determine the cause of problems;
- resolve problems and, eventually, check that the problems have been resolved.

Now is the time to establish or, if extant, review the functioning of the other essential committees. See Chapter 3 in this part. Attention must be paid to terms of reference, interrelationships, lines of reporting of the entire committee system, and how the committees are to be serviced and supported. In addition, as we have described for the QM committee, instruction in how to conduct meetings and meeting procedure will need to be extended to a wider hospital group. Large hospitals with divisional or departmental organisation will need to establish committees to deal with QA/QI studies and practice policies, and specify their relationship to the hospital QM committee, their reporting arrangements and their degree of autonomy.

368.7 | Initiate quality assurance activities

Some months may elapse while the hospital establishes, with varying degrees of pain and difficulty, an appropriate committee structure. During this period it is important to initiate some studies to examine quality of care issues. The appropriate time for this examination will vary from one hospital to another. However, some activity should commence as soon as practical. An important principle is not to attempt too much at once, especially initially. Viewing hospitals as systems for improving patient's health status permits viewing quality management and quality assurance as a way of looking for deficiencies in the care system to be resolved, rather than as mechanisms for finding fault with doctors, nurses, or other care providers. The quality manager should guide quality improvement studies regarding such matters as quality management committee authorisation for the activity, the appropriate methodologies to use, the correct implementation approach, and documentation of results.

All the following activities can be done with minimal resources and will help to show progress and some early results in a process that to date may have seemed somewhat tedious for many hospital staff:

- in the early stages, do not attempt more than one issue at a time;
- look initially at suspected problems with strong circumstantial evidence that something is amiss, rather than attempting to review routinely all activity;

- start with special studies or projects, for example, the use of blood and blood products;
- initially explore the use of techniques such as explicit criteria for retrospective audits on relatively uncomplicated but important cases. Only after adequate explanation to medical staff attempt the use of structured quality review (see Part IV);
- survey patient satisfaction, a useful source of information if conducted correctly and non-threateningly;
- establish effective mechanisms for reporting and tracking incidents and complaints/ compliments, if they do not already exist;
- document and disseminate practice policies, some of which may well exist but have never been documented, or if documented, never distributed;
- survey staff for suggestions regarding improvements in patient care.

Monitoring or surveillance is a most useful technology for assessing quality of care. However, monitoring is only useful if mechanisms have been put in place to investigate the causes of identified problems and to rectify them. Some examples of monitoring are:

- monitoring and tracking incidents;
- monitoring and tracking patient complaints and compliments;
- infection control;
- monitoring of sentinel events such as unexpected deaths, readmissions to hospital within a specified time frame, and unplanned admission to the intensive care unit.

369 | Managing QM implementation and assessing progress

369.1 | *Annual review of progress against plan*

Twelve months after commencement and annually thereafter is the time to evaluate progress, to check the results of the early stages of implementation and to determine whether there has been real achievement or merely a lot of talk. The hospital needs to consider the following aspects, and consultant advice may again be advisable.

QM program structure and process
- Compare progress, for example in terms of committee structures and function, with those recommended here and with the plan originally developed. The QM plan will need to be updated each year as a result of such assessment.
- Identify deficiencies in the program.
- Decide how deficiencies should be corrected.
- Prioritise and implement corrections.
- Follow-up subsequently to see if the corrections have been implemented, with the expected effects.

Quality of care
- Review the problems that have been identified and the suggestions for improvements that have been made.
- Review the solutions that have been implemented to address the identified problems.
- Review the changes that have been made in either patterns of care or systems since the program commenced.
- Review and celebrate documented improvements.

369.2 | Evidence of success

How successful the program is likely to be in any particular hospital depends heavily on the degree of continuing commitment and the resources applied. Indicators of success for the first five to twelve years would include:

- improvement in employee morale;
- improvement in patient satisfaction;
- diminution of patient complaints;
- diminution of malpractice litigation;
- reduction in incidents involving patients and staff;
- improvement in medical records;
- presence of practice policies for a wide range of contentious clinical activities;
- documented improvement in the technical quality of care;
- capacity to inform the board in a quantitative form of the quality of patient care.

369.3 | The small hospital

We are well aware that small hospitals may feel quite overwhelmed by the organisational requirements that we have described in this chapter. However, every hospital does not have to do everything at once to move meaningfully towards the goal of an effective quality management program and a quality-mature hospital—a point we have made from the start. Just as a 300-bed metropolitan hospital does not have the resources to conduct coronary bypass surgery, many small hospitals of fifty beds or less will not have the resources in-house to conduct every aspect of quality management. To re-emphasise an obvious point: small hospitals (of 100 beds or less) will need to obtain some of the necessary resources from regional or organisational groupings.

However, even the smallest hospital should have its own QM committee and a quality manager—even if the latter is part time and perhaps one and the same person as the hospital manager himself or herself. In addition, at a bare minimum these small hospitals should have:

- adequate medical record policies;
- effective clinical and QM information systems;
- mechanisms to identify and resolve problems, and improve continuously the quality of care.

369.4 | Time frame

One of the first questions hospital management usually asks is: 'How long will it take?' The real question is: How long does it take to become a 'quality-mature' organisation? Once a quality management program commences it never stops.

Industry, which has embraced the concept of total quality management—a concept very similar to our model of hospital-wide, integrated, multidisciplinary quality management—believes that it may take five, ten or more years of intense, concerted activity to reach the stage of a 'quality-mature' organisation, and this accomplishment is where success begins.

Certainly the introduction of a quality management program that involves the magnitude of organisational change described here cannot be achieved overnight in any hospital. Indeed, the too rapid introduction of such change would be impossible for an organisation of the complexity of a hospital to digest. Starting from the situation existing in most Australian hospitals, benefits from a quality management program would be tangible after the first one to two years, depending on where it starts and how fast it goes. From that point on, the benefits will progressively increase. A fully functioning program which becomes an integral part of hospital activity could not be anticipated in under five years.

The time frame for implementing an effective program will obviously vary from hospital to hospital. Every hospital will have differing needs and will probably be at different stages of knowledge, commitment and implementation of aspects of quality management. However, as a guide we suggest:

- Board education, establishing the quality management committee and the quality management department could take one to two years.
- Getting activities underway to produce meaningful results could take two to five years.
- Refinements to the program could take an additional two to five years.
- Achieving quality maturity will take five to twelve years.

QUALITY MANAGEMENT METHODOLOGIES

SUMMARY

This part describes the methodologies that hospitals can use to assess and improve the quality of care. We have chosen those methodologies that are the most useful for the Australian scene and that, in the main, are not being effectively implemented presently. Hospitals in almost all—especially industrialised—countries could also use these methodologies to improve the quality of their care. Whether or not their implementation is practical presently depends on local circumstances, of course. Credentialling, for example, would require adaptation to local customs, but the principles would remain constant. Hospitals would need to tailor patient satisfaction surveys in accordance with local culture. Implementation of structured quality review depends mostly on hospitals' and doctors' commitment to, and the absence of incentives that militate against, quality improvement. None is superior to any other, and the reality is that over a period of time and on different occasions, hospitals will need to employ them all. Adopting all of the methodologies described in this part is necessary but not sufficient to produce a quality-mature hospital.

This part describes methodologies in some detail—firstly because it is difficult to read such detail anywhere else, and secondly because failure to pay sufficient attention to process details seriously compromises their outcomes. Poor implementation produces poor results in quality management as surely as in clinical practice. Nevertheless, the level of detail that we can provide here falls short of a blueprint for installing the methodologies in hospitals. Hospitals that wish to install them would be well advised to obtain expert, consultant assistance, if it is not already available among the hospital staff.

Chapter 1   *Introduction to and purpose of Part IV*—provides a context for the part and its purpose, discusses the three methodologies described in the part and the framework for their selection.

Chapter 2   *Credentialling and appointment of medical staff*—describes the difference between appointing and credentialling, discusses the importance of credentialling in quality management and details the mechanics of implementation.

Chapter 3   *Patient satisfaction surveys*—describes the purpose of patient satisfaction surveys as a means of assessing the interpersonal elements of quality and details the methodology of conducting such a survey.

Chapter 4   *Structured quality review*—is devoted to the details for the implementation of this methodology for assessing and measuring quality of care.

Chapter 1

INTRODUCTION TO AND PURPOSE OF PART IV

---

410 | Contents

This chapter introduces readers to three key methodologies for quality management and describes a variety of such methodologies while recommending only a few. It describes:

411. Purpose of this part
412. Contents of this part
413. Purpose of this chapter
414. Rationale for methodologies described in this part
415. Preproduction quality management
416. Intraproduction quality management
417. Postproduction quality management
418. Implementation of quality management methodologies

411 | Purpose of this part

This part describes selected methods that are useful for managing the quality of care and should be an integral part of a quality management program. They were selected for their relevance to the current Australian scene. There is no implication that all methods must be used from the start—even though all can be—nor that one method can substitute for another. A quality-mature hospital will employ all three methodologies in some form and many others besides. The appropriate mix of quality management methods depends on a hospital's particular circumstances.

The informed reader may be surprised by the small number of methodologies we have chosen to describe in this part. There are many other methodologies that a hospital may already have in place or may want to consider using. Activities such as infection control and incidents and complaints monitoring are examples of common enough techniques in most hospitals and are referred to without detailed description elsewhere. However, implementing all of the methodologies described here will provide the hospital with the tools it needs to get started and achieve substantial improvement in its quality of care within the resource constraints under which most Australian hospitals must operate.

412 | Contents of this part

This part provides the framework and subsequently the detail of three methodologies selected for their ease of application (encompassing mechanics, interpretability of results and use of results to improve practice) given the present state of quality management in Australian hospitals. The absence of a particular methodology from this part does not imply that it should not be used; rather that it may already be applied in hospitals, it may not be appropriate for the average Australian hospital, or its use may be appropriate only under certain circumstances that are beyond the manual's scope. Methodologies described in detail are:

- credentialling and appointing visiting medical staff, including:
  —model terms of reference for medical appointments advisory committees
  —model terms of reference for credentials committees
  —domains and other matters for credentialling;
- structured quality review (SQR);
- patient satisfaction surveys.

413 | Purpose of this chapter

The remainder of this chapter provides a rationale for the various methodologies that are included in this part, using the framework developed in Part II. It also summarises some key points about the implementation of quality management methodologies. It sets the context in which these methodologies are used and re-introduces readers to the terms preproduction, intraproduction and postproduction quality management—industrial analogies that are used to broaden an understanding of quality concepts.

414 | Rationale for methodologies described in this part

Part II of this manual provides a framework for understanding the production of health and quality improvement. Here we use the framework exemplified in Figure IV-1-1 on page 540, to comment on the different types of quality management methodologies and provide a rationale for selecting those included in this part. Chapter 6 in Part II describes this framework in the context of a health production system.

This part is a guide for particular elements of a quality management program, not as an encyclopaedic reference. These elements are concerned primarily with the technical and interpersonal aspects of the quality of care. The methodologies included here focus on quality improvement through quality assurance, rather than improved product specifications (i.e. practice policies). This part does not describe methodologies for generating new knowledge or developing new technologies; nor for setting or revising product specifications (practice policies); nor for undertaking industrial engineering or other efficiency improvement programs; nor for conducting employee suggestions or other participatory management programs; nor for exploring the ethical or value dimension of quality; nor for trading-off health status improvement, cost and patient satisfaction.

Even though we describe selected methodologies in some detail, necessarily the level of detail that we can provide here is insufficient to represent a step-by-step blueprint for implementation. Each hospital's objectives, policies and circumstances will vary, necessitating some adjustments to or elaboration on the general descriptions we offer. Any hospital that is considering implementing a quality management program or specific

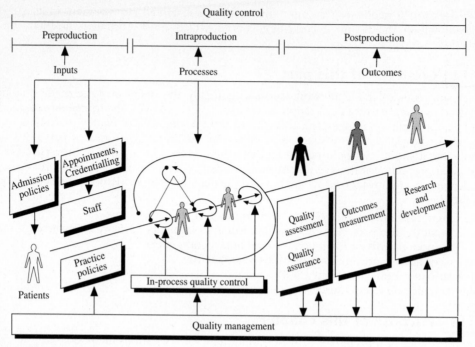

Figure IV-1-1 *Health care quality management system*

methodologies as part of such a program would be well advised to obtain expert, consultant assistance, if it does not have the necessary expertise among its staff.

We cannot overemphasise a key point that we have emphasised repeatedly: the management commitment and organisational structure necessary to implement quality management must be in place if the program is to succeed. Isolated implementation of methodologies, no matter how adequate and appropriate, cannot produce quality improvement. To be fruitful their implementation must take place on fertile program ground cultivated by management commitment.

415 | Preproduction quality management

415.1 | Credentialling

Deciding who to allow to do what in the hospital is a fundamental quality management mechanism. It is also relatively easy to implement. For these reasons we devote a chapter in this part to describing a process of credentialling and appointing medical staff. Credentialling is inherently based initially on qualifications and experience, not measured performance. Incident reporting systems and patient complaints/compliments can be important sources of information for credentialling decisions. Structured quality review and patient satisfaction surveys (which are both described in this part) can generate performance information that ultimately can and should be used in credentialling decisions.

415.2 | Services and admissions policies

The quality of care depends in part on what services the hospital chooses to deliver to whom. This obvious fact is often overlooked when a hospital is pressed to add a service that it is ill-equipped to deliver or to treat definitively everyone who turns up at its doors.

An effective quality management program may reveal that the hospital is not delivering certain services or failing to care for some types of patients to standards. If the hospital cannot obtain or upgrade the resources necessary to improve such services, it is probably better to discontinue them and to refer patients to other hospitals that can deliver these services to standards. In some circumstances there may be no other hospital to which patients can be referred. This problem is not the sole concern of the providing hospital. In Australia it is often dealt with by the public hospital authority, and indeed in some states the so-called role delineation of hospitals attempts to deal with the issue. Ultimately consumers, who may become patients, must decide if they are willing to accept substandard local care or acceptable care at a distant location. Alternatively, they might be willing to pay an extraordinary premium to upgrade resources, where this is a practical option.

The hospital's quality management committee is responsible for recommending which new services and technologies should be added, that is, are within the hospital's ability to provide to standards; and those that should be discontinued, that is, those being provided now that are not within the hospital's ability to provide to standards. This committee is also responsible for determining appropriate admission policies—which patients to treat and which to refer. Information for making these decisions will come from various sources, including, for example, the availability of doctors with necessary training and experience (determined by credentialling) and performance (determined by structured quality review).

415.3 | *Practice policies*

Few hospitals have established practice policies. In those that have, they are generally limited to special units, for example the intensive care unit, and then cover only quite limited aspects of practice. Beyond such policies, hospitals rely on doctors to treat patients as they consider best, without knowing the exact nature of the doctor's implicit policies nor how faithfully he or she follows them, except by manifest outcomes (which the hospital rarely if ever monitors). Hospitals would do well to insist that clinical departments develop or adopt practice policies, at least for the most common problems that the hospital admits.

Developing useful practice policies de novo is a difficult and resource consuming task, one likely beyond most, if not all, hospitals' present expertise and means. In any case, practice policies are unlikely to be the best place to start when embarking on a quality management program. Nevertheless, where practice policies have been developed anywhere in the world they can be evaluated, and if judged valid adopted, and if need be adapted to local circumstances. Practice policies can be developed from structured quality review results (which will highlight where they are most needed), or, if in place initially, modified as a result of such review.

Once adopted, hospitals should make practice policies known to the medical staff and insist that a grant of privileges (and, in the case of new staff, appointment) is conditional on their acceptance. Hospitals should withdraw privileges from practitioners who deviate from policies without reasons acceptable to peers. This idea should not be taken to mean that innovation must cease. Quite the contrary. A system of explicit policies coupled with process and outcome monitoring will likely reveal inadequate practices— those that need to be rethought or those requiring innovation. Innovations should be introduced formally, either as experiments or subject to other means of formal evaluation, rather than surreptitiously without the benefit of learning about their cost-effectiveness.

Practice policies define the hospital's production processes (and hence its products) for quality management purposes. They must never be immutable. The hospital must establish mechanisms to review and revise practice policies both periodically and when needed by a new regulation or medical breakthrough, or simply as the result of experience gained through quality management mechanisms. Practice policies define acceptable medical practice. They also define expected (hence acceptable) outcomes, because they are based on such explicit considerations as desired patient outcomes and available resources. Without defining acceptable practices hospitals cannot assure the quality of care; at best, they can merely assess it using criteria developed by others.

415.4 Preadmission review

At first blush, preadmission review looks very attractive, especially to payers. The idea of preventing unnecessary operative procedures and admissions setting length of stay expectations, and ensuring that the patient's discharge is planned before admission, is very appealing to payers and to patients. For the hospital and payers, however, such reviews can be very costly. The issues addressed by preadmission review can be addressed more efficiently by (retrospective) structured quality review (SQR). Certainly, SQR cannot prevent an unnecessary operation that has already been performed, but it can help avoid them among a surgeon's subsequent patients. Further, SQR can examine what was actually done and achieved and generate substantial additional quality improvement information. Eventually hospitals will be able to use decision support technologies for intraproduction quality control that includes the very best features of preadmission review and structured quality review.

416 Intraproduction quality management

416.1 Decision support technology

A variety of decision support technologies is beginning to emerge that would permit intraproduction quality management. However, their routine use for this purpose is likely many years away. In general, Australian hospitals are quite unprepared for their use, which should be limited to properly evaluated pilot studies for the foreseeable future.

416.2 So-called concurrent review

Support for so-called 'concurrent review' as a quality assurance tool stems from the idea that it can prevent delays in treatment and maloutcomes. As explained in Part II, concurrent review is an expediting system—for example reminding doctors to discharge the patient; or immediate retrospective review of care that may harbour the potential to improve or avoid further loss of health status if prompt action is taken—for example in the case of an accidental overdose. Certainly hospitals should have in place procedures for efficient and effective care, including, for example, spotting complications and managing them promptly. However, concurrent review is an inefficient method for these purposes. The considerable resources necessary to operate such systems could be used better elsewhere.

417 Postproduction quality management

417.1 Assessing the quality of care

Assessing the quality of care given to hospital patients has been and for the foreseeable future is likely to remain the mainstay of quality management. In this part we describe two methodologies for this purpose. They are:
- structured quality review, which focuses primarily on the technical quality of care; and
- patient satisfaction surveys, which focus primarily on the interpersonal aspects of care, amenities, availability of services and the hospital's standing in the community.

The information that these two methodologies produce can be used in all aspects of quality management, particularly, in this part's context, credentialling of medical staff (further strengthening this methodology's utility of assuring quality of care) and improving provider performance.

417.2 | Structured quality review

The resources and systems necessary to implement structured quality review are relatively modest and within the means of almost all hospitals, especially with the support of expert consultants. The major barriers to the implementation of such methodologies to date have been: lack of management commitment and therefore the necessary structure; the complacency of the medical staff; and a lack of a clear understanding of what is involved. For structured quality review to succeed, the hospital must upgrade its medical records and clinical information systems. The introduction of structured quality review provides both the impetus for and the means to focus such improvement.

417.3 | Patient satisfaction surveys

Patient satisfaction surveys are well within the means of the average hospital. If designed properly they can provide useful quality improvement information that complements that obtained from structured quality review.

417.4 | Clinical indicators

Conceptually, clinical indicators—population-based monitoring of the quality of care—are very appealing especially to payers and regulators. For hospitals, especially those starting quality management programs, they can often require considerable effort without generating much quality improvement information. Their best use is to identify processes that are out of control, or providers or types of cases whose care may be deficient. However, the confirmation and investigation of problems requires case-based review. Case-based surveillance systems, such as structured quality review (SQR), are likely to prove a far more effective and efficient way for hospitals to start to identify problems and improve the quality of their care.

417.5 | Structured outcome measurement and research

Eventually Australian hospitals will need and want to progress to structured outcome measurement and focused health systems research to improve product specifications—that is, practice policies—and to resolve important issues about interventions' effectiveness and efficiency. For the foreseeable future, however, hospitals will need to focus on structured quality review. Only the largest hospitals with established quality management programs should implement structured outcome measurement, and then only on a pilot basis. Similarly, few hospitals in Australia can justify establishing health services research units to conduct studies to improve the effectiveness and efficiency of their care. Where they exist, such units can help implement quality management methodologies.

418 | Implementation of quality management methodologies

None of the quality management methodologies described in this part of the manual is a panacea; none will work if implemented in isolation. Improving the quality of care requires a total commitment—the education and participation of all employees from the hospital's board of directors and manager to part-time staff.

The hospital's management must announce, commit to, and be active in quality management. The structure to improve quality (described in Part III) must be in place. Then the methodologies described here will help improve quality. But they will not produce miracles, and the process never ends nor does their use end. These methodologies, in some form or other, must be implemented for ever; they represent the essence of the hospital's purpose and its activities.

One methodology is not a substitute for another; all must be used sooner or later. While it may be wise to phase in these methodologies (see Part III, Chapter 6), eventually they will all be in use simultaneously. To summarise implementation:

- Quality is the job, not an afterthought.
- Quality improvement is an approach to management: it never ends.
- To work effectively, the hospital must be organised for quality improvement; the structure must correspond to the objective.
- Management must support quality improvement from the outset and reinforce it continuously.
- Everyone, from hospital manager to part-time staff, must be oriented to and educated for quality improvement; this education must be planned and funded.
- Resources must be provided to operate QM activities.
- One cannot expect miracles; to realise the full effect of quality improvement activities will take up to ten years of continuous sustained effort, even though some results will materialise immediately.
- Quality is everyone's job; it cannot depend on voluntarism.
- Quality is doing the right thing; doing it right the first and every time.
- Select the key items to measure and control; health care's primary goal is to improve patient health status consistent with the patient's values and society's resources.
- QM professionals require support and resources; their efforts alone cannot improve quality.
- Quality pays; people must be rewarded for improvements. Financial and other incentives and rewards are keys for success; no one's job should be threatened merely by improvement in effectiveness or efficiency.
- Everyone must have a shared notion of quality; the concepts in this manual serve this purpose.

Chapter 2

CREDENTIALLING AND APPOINTMENT OF MEDICAL STAFF

| 420 | **Contents** |

This chapter deals with the credentialling (also known as the delineation of clinical privileges) and the appointment process of medical staff. The chapter looks at:

421. Purpose of this chapter
422. Prerequisites for successful credentialling of medical staff
423. Managing credentialling and appointments
424. Credentialling: delineating clinical privileges
425. Credentialling procedures
426. Appointments
427. Appointment procedures
428. Evaluating credentialling and appointment efforts

| 421 | **Purpose of this chapter** |

This chapter details the organisational, conceptual and administrative steps necessary to introduce a meaningful system of credentialling and appointment for medical staff. Toward this end, it includes the following three appendices:

- Appendix A—model terms of reference for medical appointment advisory committees to assist hospitals in the functioning of these committees.
- Appendix B—model terms of reference for credentials committees to assist in the functioning of these committees and to explain their role.
- Appendix C—domains and other matters for credentialling. The concept of domains when identifying procedures and details regarding anaesthetic credentialling are described.

545

422 | Prerequisites for successful credentialling of medical staff

422.1 | Relationship between credentialling and appointing

The interface between the appointment process and the activity of credentialling is usually not well understood in Australia. Credentialling is the formal matching of what the doctor wishes to do in the hospital at any one time and his or her competence to do it. While certain aspects of a practitioner's suitability for appointment may remain unchanged from the time of his or her first appointment, his or her competence to undertake certain clinical activity may not. Good-for-life qualifications are no longer an adequate measure of competence.

The decision process relating to credentialling and that bearing on an appointment should be seen as separate functions. The credentialling process comes first, followed by the appointment process, and for this reason we discuss credentialling before appointment. Nevertheless, they should be a functional whole. (See Figure IV-2-1 on page 547.)

A formal credentialling/appointments system is one of the mainstays of a quality management program. Credentialling, in particular, if correctly applied is one of the most important elements of a hospital risk management program, protecting the hospital and its medical staff from a significant proportion of malpractice claims. Quality management and credentialling have a back-to-back relationship: QM cannot be effective without credentialling, and credentialling cannot be appropriately applied without an effective QM program.

422.2 | Need for a complete system, systematic processes

Figure IV-2-1 on page 547 illustrates the process of credentialling and appointments.

The credentialling and appointment processes must be formal and carefully structured. Legal protection for all concerned depends on a routine process which is formalised and carefully documented. Such a process for appointments already exists in most large hospitals, but in many small public hospitals and many private hospitals it does not. Given the traditional open nature of private hospitals where medical staff establishments generally do not apply, it becomes of even greater importance to ensure that the appointment process is successful in fulfilling its proper function of carefully screening those practitioners permitted to work in the hospital.

Credentialling of medical staff depends heavily on other key elements of a quality management program if it is to be effective, successful and, above all, credible. The administrative process to ensure a smooth and efficient operation must be in place before any effort is made to commence credentialling. This administrative process is part of the organisational structure so essential for a quality management program (see Part III). Further, the capacity to reduce or limit a provider's privileges depends, in turn, on the capacity to measure a provider's performance.

Assessing the quality of a provider's care and being able to measure the provider's performance is an essential prerequisite to effective credentialling. To be able to reduce a doctor's privileges fairly—and in a way that can withstand legal challenge—demands an objective measure of his or her performance. The process of structured quality review (see Chapter 4 in this part) provides the necessary information. Failure to have these other elements of a quality management program in place will mean that the credentialling process, often established only after considerable negotiation and discussion with medical staff, becomes discredited before it even commences.

422.3 | Need for policies

Every hospital will have attitudes and rules that have developed over time in relation to appointments and which impinge on the question of delineation of clinical privileges.

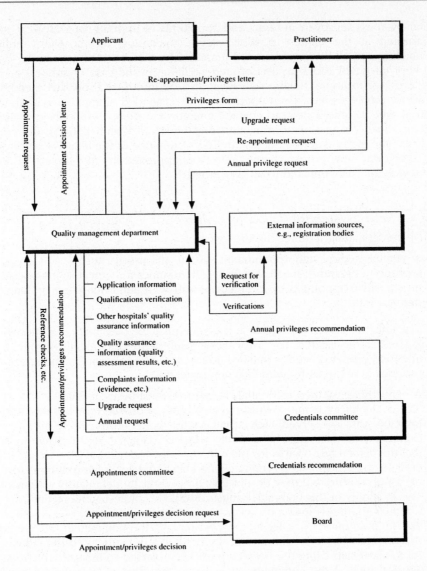

Figure IV-2-1 *A flow chart showing interrelationships of credentialling and appointment of medical staff*

Such matters should not be passed on by word of mouth but should be carefully developed and agreed upon in documented policies. Examples of such policies include the frequency of credentialling and appointments, those pertaining to an appeal mechanism, and the appointment of medical practitioners who have reached the age of sixty-five years. Further, hospitals need to develop policies regarding both upgrading and downgrading clinical privileges; the situation regarding locums; and the question of emergencies. During the course of operating a credentialling program, hospitals may encounter other situations that merit establishing an explicit policy.

Whatever policies the hospital develops, they should be clearly documented and disseminated so that all concerned understand what the rules are under a range of circumstances. Policies should not be communicated by word of mouth. Policies regarding the credentialling and appointment of medical staff should be included in the hospital by-laws, and even in terms and conditions of appointment. Medical staff must be informed at the earliest possible stage concerning the hospital's policies on credentialling and all the issues related thereto. The medical staff are not the only ones to be kept informed about aspects of credentialling; in the case of surgical or obstetric procedures, for example, theatre staff must also be informed about any member of the staff whose privileges have been upgraded or downgraded, granted or withdrawn.

From time to time a need to change, amend or develop new policies will become necessary. Such changes may originate from the medical staff council, the credentials committee, the medical appointments advisory committee or the board of directors. In all cases, however, any policy change must be approved by the board of directors, documented and disseminated to all concerned.

422.4 | Need to establish, follow procedures

Effective credentialling requires the existence of:

- a parallel medical staff appointment system (discussed later);
- a properly organised medical staff, which assumes a medical staff association, and an executive appointed by the medical staff with authority to act on behalf of the medical staff.

To be effective and to prevent or at least minimise the possibility of a successful legal action against medical staff or the hospital as a result of the credentialling program, certain basic rules and proper processes must be adhered to. The following summarises the rules and processes of a successful credentialling program:

- A properly constituted credentials committee must be established.
- The credentials committee must have carefully prepared terms of reference which must be strictly observed. (See Appendix for model terms of reference.)
- Committee minutes must be carefully prepared. Hospital management must ensure that the person responsible for the minutes fully understands how to undertake this task. In some hospitals the minutes are checked prior to distribution by a second person to ensure that they do not contain potentially defamatory statements.
- The members of this committee must observe absolute confidentiality.
- Committee process must observe the rules of 'natural justice'.
- The application for privileges, the decisions of the committee and the advice to doctors must be done with a carefully designed and structured formality.
- All medical staff using the hospital must be subjected to the same process.
- All decisions of the committee must be in the form of recommendations to the board of the hospital or to the appropriate appointments committee, which would need to see any recommendations regarding privileges, before a conclusion is reached in relation to the committee's recommendations concerning an appointment.

422.5 | Quality management plan

Prior to introducing credentialling for medical staff, the hospital must develop a plan for its introduction. This plan is normally part of the hospital's quality management plan. It includes:

- developing policies and procedures for how credentialling is to be conducted;
- ensuring that the linkages between credentialling and the appointment process are in place;

- ensuring that the process of structured quality review for assessing and measuring quality and performance is in place; and
- informing the medical staff, in particular, about the process of credentialling and what their participation will be in the process.

422.6 *Quality management department*

Before a hospital commences credentialling it should have established a functioning quality management department, with a quality manager. Credentialling demands the department's resources. Effective annual credentialling can create a substantial administrative workload. This workload raises the question of cost-benefit. While annual credentialling creates a cost, it also provides assurance of a practitioner's competence and hence is a potent mechanism for avoiding preventable maloutcomes that can prove costly to both the patient and the hospital. As a significant risk management tool, hospitals can expect credentialling to diminish the incidence and cost of litigation in the long run.

422.7 *Education/communication*

For many if not most Australian hospitals credentialling as described here will be a new experience. It is important that before introducing a credentialling program the hospital explains to members of the hospital board, management, senior nursing staff and, in particular, all medical staff what is envisaged and how it will work on a day-to-day basis.

423 Managing credentialling and appointments

Significant management support is required for credentialling and appointing. A structured turnkey process will not only minimise this workload but will also add to the protection for both hospital and medical staff against legal actions by aggrieved practitioners. Such support includes:

- checking qualifications of medical staff;
- checking insurance status of medical staff;
- checking registration of medical staff;
- keeping profiles on medical staff;
- tracking any malpractice claims history;
- supporting the credentials committee.

The quality manager is responsible for administering the credential and appointment system. The quality management department (QMD) provides the required administrative support. In a moderate to large size hospital, credentialling may impose a substantial annual workload. The QMD must develop a systemised approach to the task, and preferably automate as much of it as possible.

Many Australian hospitals do check the qualifications of medical staff prior to appointments, and some may even check practitioner's registration (medical licences). Hospitals should check annually the registration and the insurance status of each member of its medical staff. In the case of registration, the hospital should check with the Medical Board in each State to ensure that the registration is valid and current. At the very least, the hospital should require each applicant to produce a valid current receipt for registration and legal indemnity insurance.

424 Credentialling: delineating clinical privileges

424.1 *Context*

All too commonly in Australian hospitals—particularly, but by no means exclusively, in the private sector—the hospital or its medical staff attempt to curtail a member of the visiting medical staff from conducting a specific clinical activity. This action comes out of the blue, usually in response to a situation of incompetence, mishap or illness. More often than not, no precise method of delineating clinical privileges exists. The practitioner in question immediately defends himself or herself by making a charge of bias. 'You haven't dealt with any of my colleagues like this, why all of a sudden pick on me?' It is then very easy for the practitioner to justify in his or her own mind that bias exists by a competitor in a powerful position and the next step is the threat if not the actuality of legal action against the hospital and some of its medical staff or both.

Often in such cases, while members of the medical staff have been talking about the situation informally, sometimes among a wide circle of people, perhaps for weeks or months, the first time that the affected practitioner learns about the concern is when he or she is suddenly, without warning, prohibited. Inadvertently, therefore, not only may the doctor have been defamed but also natural justice has been denied. In the end, because a proper process was not followed, the practitioner wins the ensuing legal battle even though a curtailment of some of his or her clinical activities would have been in the best interests of patient care. The hospital is, as a result, left with a worse situation than the one in which it started. A properly conducted credentialling process can avoid such problems.

While most doctors determine their own capacity to conduct procedures and other clinical activity with great responsibility, a small number, like any other members of the community, may become psychotic, alcoholic or suffer any number of disabling diseases. The doctor under such circumstances who was perfectly competent some months previously may suddenly become quite dangerous without in any way recognising this fact. A very much smaller percentage of medical staff, it seems, have an inborn inability to recognise their own limitations or lack of competence. In the absence of an effective credentialling program, dealing with this group in any hospital, public or private, is probably a hospital administration's greatest problem.

Under Australian law the termination of a medical practitioner's appointment is very difficult. The withdrawal or limitation of privileges as a result of a deliberate and formal process by one's peers is another matter.

424.2 | Purpose of credentialling

In the late 1960s two episodes involving doctors in hospitals in New South Wales triggered the demand for a system to determine who should do what in hospitals at any particular time. The first episode involved the death of a young woman during a thryoidectomy in a well known Sydney private hospital. The surgeon was a fully qualified anaesthetist and the anaesthetic was administered by a series of three general practitioners. The second episode involved a small country hospital where a solo general practitioner conducted a total hindquarter amputation on a patient with the Director of Nursing administering an open ether anaesthetic. These two episodes became important catalysts in the development of quality management in Australia. Unfortunately, Australia still has not succeeded in introducing effective mechanisms for credentialling, despite the pioneering efforts of the New South Wales Branch of the AMA, and despite the fact that such systems have been in place in North America for more than fifty years.

Credentialling of medical staff is a critical element in a quality management program. It assures that practitioners are qualified and competent to conduct procedures and that the hospital can thereby adequately reduce the risk of preventable maloccurrences. Any hospital interested in assuring the quality of patient care and concerned about protecting itself from malpractice litigation must be prepared to institute a program of credentialling or delineation of clinical privileges for its medical staff.

424.3 | The nature of credentialling

In Australia there is a common misunderstanding that credentialling merely refers to the sighting of a doctor's qualifications during the process of appointment. This means in practice that the possession of a higher qualification, together with a doctor's claim to be proficient in a specialty or subspecialty, will result in privileges being granted automatically for whatever the doctor wishes to do within that specialty.

Credentialling or the delineation of clinical privileges is the process whereby the medical staff itself, on behalf of the board, determines precisely what any individual medical practitioner can or cannot do in the hospital. The credentialling concept is an extremely flexible tool by which a hospital, through its medical staff, is able to match medical staff's clinical competence with the hospital's mission and resources. Credentialling may also be appropriate for other professionals such as independent nurse midwives and nurses working in intensive care units. Any mechanism for credentialling or delineating of privileges for medical staff must also include mechanisms to ensure that adherence to privileges granted is assured prospectively, if possible, and that appropriate sanctions are brought to bear in cases where practitioners deliberately undertake practices for which they have not been granted privileges.

Credentialling may be categorised into three types based on the stage of its implementation as follows:

* in association with the initial or new appointment;
* annual (routine), including the circumstances of a reappointment;
* non-routine, which in turn can be described as:
  —locums (including 'emergencies')
  —upgrading (when new training has been completed during the yearly cycle)
  —downgrading, for example as a result of a complaint or problem involving patient care.

Contrary to the usual practice in Australia, credentialling is a process which should be distinct from the appointment process and should occur annually as a routine for all medical staff. The process should allow for 'emergency' credentialling, for example when an unannounced locum appears and requires authority to work in the hospital.

424.4 | Timing of credentialling

Credentialling aims to ensure that all activity in the hospital is carried out within the limits of the doctor's training, experience and competence. For most medical practitioners an annual credentialling process is purely perfunctory in that most doctors limit their practices instinctively. However, for legal and other reasons it is essential that all staff are routinely submitted to the same formal process annually. Where complaints arise, evidence of incompetence appears, unsuitable procedures are carried out or documented, or objective evidence of a less than acceptable standard of care can be demonstrated, a special review of privileges may be considered necessary.

All medical practitioners wishing to practise at the hospital shall make application to the manager setting out their qualifications, training and experience. In addition they must define the details of the clinical activity that they wish to perform. This application for granting of clinical privileges will be made annually, and will as described above be combined, initially, with an application for appointment and every three years with the application for reappointment.

Three months prior to the end of the triennium the hospital should send each medical practitioner both an 'Application for Reappointment' and an 'Application for Privileges'. This latter form (or a cover letter) should list privileges granted previously and request advice regarding any changes sought. In his or her reappointment request, the medical practitioner must include a request for privileges, one that may include changes to those in effect.

424.5 | Emergencies

In cases of life-threatening emergencies and when no other medical assistance is available, regardless of privileges granted any medical practitioner is expected to do whatever he or she considers to be necessary to save life or limb. In such a situation, however, if not fully qualified, the practitioner involved must be able to demonstrate subsequently that no other more qualified medical practitioner could have been called upon under the circumstances.

424.6 | The credentials committee's role and function

The credentials committee is the instrument for determining the privileges of members of the medical staff. Its role is to ascertain and certify that the medical practitioner is, at any one time, competent to carry out requested services in the hospital and to evaluate any matter relating to the privileges of a medical practitioner referred to it by the manager or the medical staff association. The credentials committee is responsible to the hospital manager and through the manager to the board.

424.7 | The credentials committee's structure and organisation

The credentials committee consists solely of medical practitioners. Its membership should comprise a core group of five respected medical practitioners. The medical staff should nominate members and the hospital board should appoint them for a minimum of two years. The committee should elect one of its members to be chairperson; he or she should serve for a maximum of two consecutive years. If necessary, the committee should co-opt additional members of the particular discipline under consideration to ensure that at least two members of the particular discipline are present when making credentialling recommendations. For this purpose, general practice is regarded as a discipline. However, at no time should the committee comprise more than nine members.

When dealing with a practitioner in a subspecialty—where there may be only one or two practitioners engaged in that subspecialty in the hospital—the committee should seek the services of outside medical peers, who usually will practise outside of the hospital's geographic area. The hospital should remunerate such peer practitioners for their time. The selection of practitioners to serve on the credentials committee for this purpose should be a decision of the medical staff in consultation with the administration including, for this purpose, the quality management department.

The hospital may also need to use outside medical peers in other circumstances—for example, when contemplating restriction of privileges of a senior and well-regarded member of the medical staff—to ensure credibility, objectivity and fairness. The most difficult aspect of the committee's work is achieving objectivity and fairness to all members of the medical staff. Accordingly, the committee should document fully all of its decisions, and state the reasons and evidence on which they are based. Careful and precise documentation is essential when the committee faces a decision to reduce or deny privileges that a practitioner has previously enjoyed.

The credentials committee must pay close attention to the preparation of its agenda, scrutinise its minutes for accuracy, and operate with the degree of formality detailed in this chapter. The committee should have ready access to legal advice, if and when members think it is necessary.

Where a member of the committee is the subject of a submission to the committee or is in the position of being an applicant for re-appointment or privileges, or for any other circumstances where there may be—or appear to be—a conflict of interest, he or she must absent himself or herself from the committee's deliberations. Appendix A contains model terms of reference for a credentials committee.

425 | Credentialling procedures

425.1 | Credentialling steps

The credentials committee will consider applications by medical practitioners for privileges in association with the triennial appointments, and annually as a routine.

The credentialling process includes the following steps:

- All medical practitioners wishing to practise in the hospital must make application to the manager setting out their training, qualifications and experience and in addition must define the details of clinical work they wish to perform. All procedures for which privileges are sought will be specifically named or identified.
- With the aid of a list of procedures provided by the hospital, doctors will indicate precisely those procedures they wish to conduct. Any procedures not included on the list should be added by the applicant in a way that ensures the procedure can be clearly identified. If credentialling criteria include specific qualifications, training or numbers of procedures performed, the applicant must attach relevant substantiating documentation to the application.
- The application for privileges must be made on the hospital's 'Application for Privileges' form.
- The application is checked to ensure that it is complete and all items have been answered.
- The application is compared, in the case of an annual review or a reappointment, with the previous application and any changes noted.
- Referees' responses are checked for completeness and relevance.
- The quality management department prepares a report for the credentials committee concerning any quality of care problems that have occurred in respect to the applicant over the previous year.
- Copies of the application are forwarded to each member of the credentials committee.
- The application is placed on the agenda for the next meeting of the credentials committee.
- After the committee has met and considered the applications, the chairperson of the credentials committee returns all copies of the applications to the administration together with a completed form of 'Recommendations Regarding Privileges' for each applicant.
- In the case of a first appointment, the quality management department may see fit to make contact with either referees and/or other hospitals where the applicant works, for the purpose of assisting the credentials committee to satisfy itself about the capacity of the applicant in relation to the privileges sought.
- A medical practitioner may make application at any time for privileges to be upgraded.

425.2 | Methods of delineating privileges

425.21 PREFERRED METHOD

There are a number of methods for delineating a doctor's clinical privileges; however, in the case of procedures, one method has clear advantages over the others. This method consists of the granting of privileges for the precise procedures any doctor wishes to perform, and this process should cover all procedures.

The only effective method of delineating clinical privileges for procedural disciplines—quintessentially for surgeons—and for those procedures carried out by members of cognitive disciplines, requires a detailed listing of the procedures that the practitioner wishes to be permitted to carry out in the hospital. Appendix C refers to the use of domains for identifying procedures.

425.22 CREDENTIALLING PROCEDURALISTS

In Australia, both the Commonwealth Government and the Australian Medical Association (AMA) publish a list of fees that include a description of related services. To minimise the task of identifying clinical privileges, hospitals may use the 'left hand side' of the Commonwealth Government's Medical Benefit Schedule or the AMA's list of fees to identify the many procedures and clinical activities that practitioners may want to perform. The applicant for privileges must indicate those activities he or she wishes to carry out. In practice most specialists and general practitioners undertake a relatively focused range of procedures. Listing them in the suggested manner is relatively easy.

Anaesthetists and other medical staff who desire to undertake any anaesthetic work in the hospital must state the clinical groups of procedures for which they wish to provide anaesthetic services. While by no means restricted to doctors requesting anaesthetic privileges, applicants should be prepared to demonstrate competence to a designated member of the medical staff. Appendix C details matters concerning anaesthetic privileges.

425.23 CREDENTIALLING COGNITIVE DISCIPLINES

To an increasing degree, such cognitive domains as internal medicine, paediatrics, psychiatry and dermatology are carrying out their own range of procedures, thus lending themselves to the system of precise delineation of privileges described above. Nevertheless, much of the work of practitioners in these domains remains cognitive and not procedural, and is thus not amenable to this mechanism of credentialling. But it is possible to define criteria for granting privileges for cognitive disciplines. Well-defined practice policies can assist in the credentialling of such disciplines. In general, such policies might state, for example, when a consultation is required, and how specialty-specific the care of certain clinical conditions should be. The medical staff should formulate practice policies; the board should adopt them as hospital policy binding on all appointed medical practitioners for whom they are relevant.

Medical practitioners should formally decide among themselves about certain specific limitations. For example: should a thoracic physician be permitted to manage a patient with diabetic keto-acidosis? Should a consultation be sought with a cardiologist in every case of myocardial infarction or only in certain circumstances and if so which ones? The medical staff should carefully discuss and formally decide such specific limitations and, when desirable, encode them in formal practice policies. For example, while the hospital medical staff may decide to permit specialists in internal medicine to practise in their own subspecialties, it might mandate in a practice policy that patients without a definitive diagnosis after a specified length of stay be referred for a consultation or second opinion to prevent them from languishing on wards and to promote initiation of appropriate therapy. This approach intends to improve quality of care, and appropriate practice policies can enhance achievement of this objective.

The development of practice policies is an important element in assuring the quality of patient care (see Part II). Practice policies can apply to a range of medical staff activities. One such use is the delineation of ways agreed upon to treat patients; another is who does what under certain circumstances. The judicious use of practice policies is an effective technique for defining areas of practice for cognitive disciplines, and of ensuring that only competent practitioners are caring for patients. Used in this way practice policies become an adjunct to credentialling. Practice policies should be separately documented and terms and conditions for appointment should refer to them explicitly. The need for and the extent and contents of practice policies will obviously vary from hospital to hospital.

425.24 CREDENTIALLING GENERAL PRACTITIONERS

General practitioners should be subjected to exactly the same credentialling provisions as their specialist colleagues. In general, blanket provisions concerning general practitioners are highly discriminatory. Each applicant for privileges should be treated individually with regard to his or her training, experience, and, if need be, demonstrated competence. When matters that may affect general practitioners are under consideration, a general practitioner should be represented in the discussions.

Early efforts to determine what procedures should be undertaken by general practitioners—in the absence of effective credentialling—saw the grouping of clinical activity, particularly procedures, into major and minor groupings. This approach merely begged the question as to the definition of what was major and what was minor. Quite frequently it became merely the perception of the medical practitioner involved. A disputes resolution arrangement becomes necessary to adjudicate the arguments that result from such a system—and it rarely satisfies either party.

The approach whereby general practitioners are permitted to carry out a specified list of procedures while no restriction is placed on specialists does not solve the practical problem that transgressions by medical staff are not limited by specialty. Moreover, specialists' transgressions tend to be more serious because their activity usually involves more complex procedures.

425.25 CLINICAL SUPPORT SERVICES

The types of clinical support services provided by pathologists and radiologists do not lend themselves to credentialling in the same fashion as services provided by practitioners in the clinical domains. Radiologists' and pathologists' performance, for example, relates to their capacity to diagnose correctly. Further, the performance of their units and laboratories depends on organisation and management considerations that are similar to industrial quality management. Of greater concern, perhaps, is radiology involving pregnant women and certain invasive radiological services involving contrast media. However, the training, selection of practitioners, and general procedures that are currently in place relating to these domains are such that they do not warrant the same priority in relation to the delineation of privileges as do the clinical domains.

425.3 │ Criteria for credentialling decisions

In reaching its decision the credentials committee must consider a number of matters to satisfy itself about the applicant's competence. In summary, these matters include training, experience, volume of work and working conditions. The committee must satisfy itself that the applicant has enough experience to be competent. It must also interest itself in the volume of work engaged in by the applicant over a twelve-month period. Particularly in respect of certain selected procedures, the number performed during the course of a year has a direct bearing on the provider's continued competence. The obstetrician who only conducts one or two confinements a year, or the surgeon who only performs one cholecystectomy per year, must raise concerns regarding continuing competence.

In general the committee's decisions should be based on:
- the training, qualifications and experience of the practitioner;
- a report concerning the number of selected procedures performed over a given period by each member of the medical staff;

- advice received from the medical staff council, the management, or the quality management department, concerning the performance of the practitioner and any evidence that it is less than acceptable to his or her peers;
- any evidence of serious behavioural problems that the practitioner, despite repeated warnings, has failed to address.

425.4 | Information for credentialling

The credentials committee will in the course of its activities derive information concerning individual medical practitioner performance from the quality management department, if available, including reports of quality of work derived from the results of 'structured quality review'. Where a medical practitioner applies for privileges and where that practitioner performs only a small amount of his or her total work in the hospital, the committee must formally inquire in writing about the practitioner's quality of care, any malpractice episodes, and other activity at other hospitals where the applicant has an appointment.

425.5 | Routine credentialling decisions

The quality management department (QMD) provides information on performance, the credentials committee decides if that performance warrants continuation of privileges, and the board decides whether or not to accept the recommendation of the credentials committee. There should be a clear separation between findings of inadequate performance or poor quality care and the decision which limits a doctor's right to practise in the hospital. The findings of inadequate performance or poor quality care are the result of structured quality review, or other quality assurance activity conducted by the quality management department. Without an effective quality management program objective evidence about the doctor's performance will be difficult if not impossible to obtain. The credentials committee recommends to the board what action should be taken based on these findings. Any decisions of the committee will be in the form of recommendations that, in the case of appointments, will go to the medical appointments advisory committee, and otherwise to the board of directors through the manager.

The business of the committee should be formally conducted and all decisions properly recorded. Minutes should be kept in the form of decisions and should be formally approved and signed at the subsequent meeting. The committee should ensure that all its decisions are objective, without malice and have constant regard for the law of natural justice.

The credentials committee may grant all of the privileges an applicant requested or, in some circumstances, it may deny all or most of the requested privileges. The committee may temporarily suspend privileges relating to the performance of one or a group of clinical activities, subject to the practitioner obtaining further training or education, or may choose to allow the doctor to perform an activity under some form of supervision. Privileges may also be increased.

The committee must base any denial of privileges—whether that denial relates to one procedure or a total denial of right to practise in the hospital—on sound objective grounds. Sound objective grounds means the objective evaluation of valid documentary evidence such as a carefully structured quality review of the practitioner's medical records or a substantiation of complaints and a sound judgment based fairly on the evidence that, as far as is possible, excludes bias or the appearance of bias. The committee's evaluations must be consistent from practitioner to practitioner. To allow medical staff the luxury of denying privileges to a colleague because he or she is unpopular, because his or her manner and style of practise is somewhat controversial, or even because common wisdom and hearsay may suggest that he or she is not competent, is courting legal retribution and is not in patients' best interests. In the case of initial appointments such evidence of performance may not be available and judgment must be made solely on qualifications, experience and references.

The options open to a credentials committee should be stated and defined in hospital by-laws and in terms of reference, and should include the granting of provisional privileges for a stated period, not to exceed one year, during which the practitioner would be supervised by a nominated colleague. For example: the medical practitioner who has only recently been appointed and whom no one knows, or a practitioner whose work is suspect and who wishes to conduct a particular procedure, may have a senior member of the staff designated with the responsibility to supervise him or her and report back to the credentials committee after a certain period of time. When necessary, structured quality review of the practitioner's medical records can supplement such evaluations.

425.6   Non-routine credentialling decisions

425.61 LOCUMS

In private hospitals in particular it is not uncommon to find that a member of the medical staff will arrange for a locum to do his or her work while he or she is on holiday—and that the locum is totally unknown to the hospital. All locums must be credentialled before working in the hospital and usually the credentialling must be for the current twelve months. However, in the case of most private hospitals, the director of nursing and the chairperson of the credentials committee—and in the public hospital situation, the hospital manager and the chairperson of the credentials committee—may under emergency circumstances authorise temporary privileges for a strictly limited period only. Such authorisation will be valid until such time as the credentials committee has had the opportunity to review the practitioner's qualifications and background. The granting of temporary or emergency privileges should be formally documented by letter.

425.62 UPGRADING PRIVILEGES

The committee should upgrade or extend privileges if and when a medical staff member requests such action and provides documented evidence that he or she has acquired the necessary training and expertise. Policies associated with upgrading privileges should be determined by the credentials committee, endorsed by the quality management committee and adopted by the hospital board.

The credentials committee must establish precise criteria that warrant extending privileges. Such criteria may include, for example:

- detailed documentation of retraining or skills acquisition;
- written testimonials from preceptors;
- statements from referees;
- reports from supervisors that the applicant has met requirements to demonstrate new skills to approved members of the staff, or has completed some form of supervised training.

425.63 DOWNGRADING PRIVILEGES

The process of reducing the privileges of a member of the medical staff is always a serious and potentially legally hazardous step to take. The process may be initiated by a report from the quality management department or the medical staff council, or a complaint from a member of the medical or nursing staff or even from a patient. Regardless of the source of information great care must be taken to ensure that the hospital handles the ensuing investigation along predetermined lines, and that at all times the rights of the doctor under review are respected and that the rules of natural justice are followed.

Temporary suspension or limitation of privileges is also a mechanism for protecting the interests and safety of patients when, in the rare situation, a member of the medical staff is seriously or even dangerously ill or where he or she continues to refuse to meet his or her obligations and responsibilities as a member of the medical staff. The ultimate objective is to ensure a working environment in the hospital that is conducive to high quality patient care. Examples might include a practitioner who:

- is psychotic or abusing drugs or alcohol;
- repeatedly refuses to maintain adequate medical records;
- repeatedly arrives late for theatre bookings;
- repeatedly uses abusive language to nursing or other staff.

The threat of curtailment of clinical privileges is usually sufficient to persuade the most recalcitrant practitioner of the need to observe medical staff by-laws.

425.7 Assuring fair play

425.71 MEDICAL STAFF AND OBJECTIVITY

One of the difficulties encountered commonly in Australia is the small size of hospital medical staffs and the difficulty anticipated in operating a credentialling system free from personalities and local bias. This problem is particularly acute in small public hospitals and the majority of private hospitals.

To overcome this problem, for the purpose of credentialling of medical staff small hospitals should function as a group and establish a single credentialling process that embraces all of the medical staff who wish to work in any one of the group's several hospitals. Such a group might be a private hospital chain of hospitals, an area health service and, most particularly, small country hospitals functioning in one regional area. Even a small solitary hospital should be able to contract with its nearest larger institution to assist in conducting an objective credentialling program.

Use of an area-wide or ownership-wide credentials committee avoids potential inconsistencies that may arise from the different decisions of separate credentials committees for each hospital. This would permit a private hospital group to control the quality of medical staff in all its hospitals and will minimise the time commitment of busy medical staff in prolonged committee activity. Such an area committee would decide in which hospitals to grant what privileges. In most Australian states public hospitals are subjected to a system of 'role delineation' that applies broad restrictions concerning the range of procedures that can be conducted in individual hospitals.

425.72 NATURAL JUSTICE

The concept of natural justice is an ancient common law principle that anyone whose rights would be affected by a decision to be made by third parties should be given the right to a fair hearing. These principles are embodied in two concepts:

- the right to be heard; and
- the right to be heard without bias.

Professionals are often much more critical of their own than are any outsiders. This judgment applies particularly to medical practitioners, who are conditioned by years of professional training to aim for excellence and high standards. In making the sort of judgments about their colleagues that arise in situations such as quality management and credentialling, doctors tend to lose sight of some of the legal constraints in their efforts to deal with unsatisfactory practitioners or with questions of incompetence.

The law leans towards ensuring that any doctor coming under the scrutiny of a credentials committee gets 'a fair go'. When a doctor's privileges are subject to limitation he or she must be advised to that effect as soon as possible. Moreover, he or she must be given the opportunity to present any further evidence in support of the application for a continuance of privileges and to argue his or her case before the committee, particularly if privileges are to be withdrawn or limited from those which he or she already enjoys. Whether the practitioner has an automatic right to legal representation before such committees or not should be a matter of hospital policy (e.g. in medical staff by-laws) and all medical staff should be informed about such policies on appointment. If after reconsideration the committee still rejects the doctor's application for privileges, he or she must have the right to an appeal.

425.73 APPEAL MECHANISM

The hospital must establish a formal appeal procedure long before it is ever likely to be used, and the appeal should be determined by persons who have no other connection with the hospital. The appeal procedure should be structured and include:

- a standard form notifying the appellant of the appeals committee and meeting time;
- a standard form completed by the appellant stating the basis of the appeal;
- a standard form to be completed by the appeals committee that documents the decision and the reasons for it;
- a standard letter advising the appellant of the result of the appeal committee's decision.

The appeals committee has to be a standing committee and should consist of:

- a chairperson, who should be appointed by the hospital;
- a nominee of each of the following colleges who has no other association with the hospital:
  —The Royal Australasian College of Surgeons.
  —The Royal Australian College of Obstetricians and Gynaecologists.
  —The Royal Australasian College of Physicians.
  —If the appellant is a general practitioner, a nominee of the Royal Australian College of General Practitioners.
  —If the appellant is of a specialty that is not represented by any of the above colleges (such as a dental practitioner or an oral surgeon), the appropriate organisation or representative body should be asked to nominate a member of the committee.

The hospital should establish a small panel of alternative members who would serve in the temporary absence of a committee member. As in the case of credentials committees, the establishment of area or regional appeals committees has a good deal of merit especially in light of the small number of appeals that any one hospital might expect to generate. Members serving on an appeals committee should be remunerated at daily or hourly rates consistent with the sessional fees that the hospital pays to its medical staff.

426 | Appointments

426.1 | Context

The process of appointing medical staff to hospitals has been well established in Australia in relation to public hospitals, most of which have a medical appointments advisory committee or its equivalent. While refusal to appoint is rarely challenged, refusal to reappoint under Australian law is extremely difficult to defend if and when it has been challenged. Successful challenges have been based largely on denial of natural justice.

Surprisingly, in the 1990s some private hospitals in Australia still do not have a formal appointment mechanism for medical staff working in the hospital. In such hospitals the director of nursing, acting as a combined one person appointments and credentials committee, is the time-honoured—and only—mechanism for protecting the patients and the hospital. We believe that this is a legally hazardous situation for any hospital in the 1990s, quite apart from the fact that it is hardly a satisfactory state of affairs for patients.

426.2 Purpose of appointments

The purpose of the appointment mechanism is to determine whether by virtue of his or her training, qualifications and experience, and his or her conduct and reputation, the practitioner is a fit and proper person to work in the hospital. The appointment of a doctor to a hospital represents a legal contract between the doctor and the hospital. The doctor wishes to work in the hospital; the hospital, having checked the doctor's qualifications, his or her experience, training and good character, together with any other matters, agrees to him or her working in the hospital under its rules and regulations (by-laws). In Australia public hospital appointments by tradition have tended to be on a triennial basis. The situation in private hospitals is variable and loose; in many private hospitals the first appointment lasts for life.

426.3 The nature of appointments

The process of 'appointment' of a medical practitioner to work in a hospital is one of determining whether by virtue of his or her qualifications and training, and his or her character, conduct and reputation, the practitioner is a fit and proper person to work in the hospital. Other questions may include the match between the practitioner's skills and his or her specialty or subspecialty and the hospital's requirements. While a practitioner's suitability for appointment may remain constant in many respects, obviously his or her competence to undertake certain clinical activity may not. Thus what the hospital permits an appointed practitioner to do in the hospital at any one time—as a result of the credentialling process—may vary.

Appointments can be divided into:

- new (initial) appointments (see Figure IV-2-1 on page 547); and
- reappointments.

426.4 Timing of appointments

In Australia the appointment process is traditionally carried out every three years and there is talk of extending it to every five years. Given the nature of the appointment mechanism, it is simply not necessary to conduct it more often. Credentialling, however, should be annual, and in the third (fifth) years combined with reappointment.

426.5 The medical appointments advisory committee's role and function

A medical appointments advisory committee considers applications from medical practitioners who wish to work in the hospital and makes recommendations on appointments to the hospital's board of directors.

The committee's recommendations depend on the appropriateness of medical practitioners' qualifications, skills, character and good standing within the medical profession, and the hospital's requirements for each type of practitioner. The appointment process aims to ensure the highest possible standard of patient care in the hospital for all patients.

426.6 The medical appointments advisory committee's structure and organisation

The committee should comprise seven medical practitioners appointed by the board of directors from nominations by the medical staff association and the manager or his or her delegate. If need be, the committee will have the power to co-opt additional practitioners from appropriate disciplines or specialties, but at no time should the committee comprise more than nine members. Committee members should hold office for a period of three years. The board should fill any casual vacancies on the advice of the medical staff association. Appendix A provides model terms of reference.

427 | Appointment procedures

427.1 | Initial appointment

Advertisements for appointments should be handled by the quality management department and any correspondence should be signed by the hospital manager. When the hospital receives a request for appointment, a letter of reply should include:

- an application for appointment;
- an application for privileges;
- a copy of the by-laws.

When received, the application is checked by the appropriate processing officer (in the quality management department). The appointments officer contacts cited referees by form letter and, if necessary, promptly follows up to ensure that the hospital receives some references. The administrative officer also sends a form letter to the chairperson of the credentials committee asking him or her to convene a meeting to consider the application if the credentials committee does not hold regular (monthly) meetings.

The complete application package will now consist of: the application itself, references and the credentials committee's report. This complete package goes to the next regularly scheduled meeting of the medical appointments advisory committee. The original application is filed so as to ensure its confidentiality.

427.2 | Application for reappointment

Three months prior to the end of the triennium, the administrative officer sends an 'Application for Reappointment' and an 'Application for Privileges' with a letter listing the requirements for reappointment to all medical practitioners with hospital appointments.

The procedure for all applicants for appointments and reappointments is as follows:

QUALITY MANAGEMENT DEPARTMENT
- The application is checked to ensure that it is complete and all items have been answered.
- Referees' responses are checked for completeness and relevance.

CREDENTIALS COMMITTEEE
- Copies of the application are forwarded to each member of the credentials committee.
- The application is placed on the agenda for the next meeting of the credentials committee.
- After the committee has met and considered the applications, the chairperson of the credentials committee returns all copies of the applications to the administration together with a completed form of 'Recommendations Regarding Privileges' for each applicant.

MEDICAL APPOINTMENTS ADVISORY COMMITTEE (MAAC)
- The complete package, now with the recommendations of the credentials committee, is then forwarded to the members of the medical appointments advisory committee for consideration at the next meeting.

- After the committee has met and considered the applications and recommendations regarding privileges, the chairperson of the MAAC forwards all applications and recommendations to the board through the manager.

Board of directors

- Recommendations for appointment from the MAAC are placed on the agenda of the next board meeting for consideration and, if appropriate, approval.
- When the board has considered the applications, the hospital manager sends a letter conveying the board's decision to each medical practitioner up for (re)appointment.
- Decisions concerning each applicant become part of the minutes of the board meeting.
- Hospital boards should give consideration to an appeal mechanism in the case of (re)appointments that they decline to make.

427.3 Criteria for appointment decisions

The medical appointments advisory committee's decisions should be based on the following:

- the qualifications, training and experience of the practitioner;
- in consultation with the administration, the need or requirement for practitioners of a particular specialty or subspecialty at the hospital for which the appointment is to apply;
- whether or not the hospital has the facilities to meet the practitioner's anticipated resource requirements, for example to conduct procedures for which he or she has applied for privileges;
- the practitioner's capacity to provide an adequate level of service to the hospital given his or her other commitments and his or her places of practice and residence;
- the practitioner's moral, ethical and professional character;
- the practitioner's attitude to the hospital and its medical, nursing and other staff.

427.4 Information for appointment decisions

In deliberations about requests for (re)appointment, the medical appointments advisory committee should review:

- copies of the application and supporting documents, for example references;
- the credentials committee's recommendations;
- interview reports;
- other information concerning an applicant that the committee may have requested or that the manager has provided.

Applicants for appointment must be interviewed by the head of the department in which they will be working and, where appropriate, additional members of that department. The head of the department should provide a written assessment and report to the MAAC.

427.5 Appointment decisions

The committee recommends the period of appointment in accordance with the hospital's by-laws. Currently, appointments are usually for a three-year term, or in the case of practitioners over 65 years of age, for a one-year term. The committee should have the power to recommend a provisional appointment for a period not exceeding twelve months. The committee should formally record its decisions and recommendations for the board.

428 | Evaluating credentialling and appointment efforts

Following the first annual credentialling exercise and the first appointment and reappointment effort, the hospital should carefully evaluate its credentialling and appointment activity. Most Australian hospitals will be unfamiliar with the structured process we have described and will need to carefully review the process to assess its costs, its benefits and, more particularly, where and how the process could be improved. Such an evaluation should be conducted by the quality management department and a report prepared for the board.

Appendix A

Model terms of reference for credentials committees

42A0 | **Contents**

42A1. Purpose of this appendix
42A2. Authorisation of the committee
42A3. Purpose of the committee
42A4. Committee membership
42A5. Meetings
42A6. Applications for privileges
42A7. Process considerations of the committee
42A8. Committee recommendations and reporting

42A1 | Purpose of this appendix

If credentialling is to be effective, it must be structured, precise and annual. Credentials committees are more likely to be exposed to legal challenge than almost any other aspect of quality management; hence, the precise role or terms of reference of this committee is of great importance. This appendix provides model terms of reference for a credentials committee. Hospitals should review the situation as it pertains to their circumstances and either adopt or adapt these terms of reference as appropriate.

42A2 | Authorisation of the committee

1. The credentials committee is authorised by the board of directors of the hospital.
2. The credentials committee is a 'standing' committee.

42A3 | Purpose of the committee

1. The credentials committee is the instrument for delineating the clinical privileges of all doctors working in the hospital. This includes full-time staff specialists, visiting medical practitioners, locum tenens and all junior staff in training.

2. The principal aim is to ensure that all work carried out by medical practitioners is consistent with their qualifications, training and competence and has regard to the available resources.
3. The committee will consider applications by medical practitioners for privileges in association with the triennial appointments and annually as a routine.
4. The committee will evaluate any matter relating to the privileges of a medical practitioner referred to it by the manager, the medical staff association or the quality management committee.
5. The committee shall develop policies and procedures for credentialling for recommendation to the board and shall implement such procedures as the board approves.

42A4 | Committee membership

1. The committee will consist solely of registered medical practitioners. The committee comprises five (5) medical practitioners.
2. Members are appointed by the hospital board from among candidates presented by the medical staff association and the manager. The medical staff nominates five candidates and the manager nominates two. The manager's nominees may be the same as or different from those of the medical staff.
3. Members of the committee will serve for two years and will be eligible for reappointment.
4. A member of the committee can be removed from membership of the committee on the vote of two-thirds of the membership of the committee when he or she fails to attend three consecutive meetings without adequate reason, or when the member's behaviour has been such as to be inconsistent with the aims and objectives of the quality management committee. Such removal must be endorsed by the board.
5. In the case of a vacancy on the committee due to death, resignation or otherwise, the medical staff and the manager will each nominate one candidate to the board who will appoint one to serve the remainder of the two-year term. The manager's nominee may be the same as or different from the nominee of the medical staff.
6. The chairperson of the committee is elected annually from among the members of the committee.
7. The committee has the power to co-opt other medical practitioners from appropriate disciplines and specialties, but at no time will the committee have more than nine (9) members. Any additional co-opted members will sit on the committee only until the task for which they were co-opted has been completed and will discuss and vote only on the task for which they were co-opted.

42A5 | Meetings

1. A quorum for the committee to begin and to continue to transact business is three (3) members.
2. Where the physical presence of members is not possible, they may 'attend' by telephone hook-up.
3. Where a member of the committee is the subject of a submission to the committee or is in the position of being an applicant for reappointment or privileges or for any other circumstances where there may be a conflict of interest, real or apparent, he or she must absent himself or herself from the deliberations of the committee.
4. The business of the committee shall be formally conducted and all decisions properly recorded.

5. An agenda shall accompany a notice of regularly scheduled meetings and it shall be distributed not less than ten (10) days prior to the meeting.
6. Minutes will be distributed with the agenda.
7. The committee shall meet monthly or at such other frequency as decided by the committee. However, the chairperson, or in his or her absence any two members, may call for an emergency meeting of the committee without notice or agenda being distributed prior to the meeting.
8. Matters coming before the committee shall be decided by a simple majority vote of those members present and voting in favour of the motion. The chairperson has a casting vote in the case of a tied vote. Proxy voting is not permitted.

42A6 │ Applications for privileges

1. All medical practitioners wishing to practise in the hospital must make application to the manager setting out their training, qualifications and experience and, in addition, must define the details of clinical work they wish to perform.
2. The application for privileges must be made on the hospital's 'Application for Clinical Privileges' form.
3. The committee shall consider applications by medical practitioners for privileges in association with the triennial appointments, and annually as a routine.
4. The manager, the medical staff council, or the QM committee may request changes to a practitioner's privileges at any time. Similarly, an individual practitioner may request changes to his or her own privileges if circumstances warrant. Such requests must be acted upon promptly by the credentials committee.

42A7 │ Process considerations of the committee

1. The committee will in the course of its activities derive information concerning individual medical practitioners' qualifications and performance, if available, from the quality management department and any other appropriate source.
2. The committee will ensure that all its decisions are objective, without malice and have constant regard for the law of natural justice.
3. The credentials committee works in close association with the medical appointments advisory committee, the quality management committee and other committees according to hospital policy and practice.
4. Where a medical practitioner applies for privileges and where that practitioner performs only a small amount of his or her total work in the hospital, or in the case of an initial application, the committee must formally inquire in writing about the practitioner's quality of care, any malpractice episodes, and other activity at all other hospitals where the applicant works.
5. The criteria to be used by the committee shall be solely the competence of the medical practitioner under consideration to provide high quality care given the resources and services that the hospital can make available for such care.
6. The decisions and actions of the committee will at all times have regard to the hospital by-laws and policies, and relevant state regulations and legislation.
7. Confidentiality of the business of the committee shall at all times be paramount. Members will only discuss the committee's business with other members and such other persons who are authorised to provide or receive such information.

42A8 │ Committee recommendations and reporting

1. The committee reports through the manager to the hospital board. Reports will be the minutes of the meeting or such other form as the manager requires.

2. Decisions of the committee shall be in the form of recommendations to the board.
3. Under ordinary routine circumstances, in the case of appointments, recommendations shall go to the medical appointments advisory committee or, in the case of annual privileges, to the board of directors through the manager.
4. Under emergency situations, such as the need to limit a practitioner's privileges immediately, the committee shall make such recommendations for action to the manager who shall act according to the powers delegated to him or her by the board.
5. The committee may recommend modifications to terms of reference to be endorsed by the board prior to taking effect.

Appendix B

DOMAINS FOR CREDENTIALLING

42B0	**Contents**
	42B1. Purpose of this appendix
	42B2. Domains
	42B3. Anaesthesia and credentialling
	42B4. General practitioners and anaesthetics
	42B5. Medical specialty domains

42B1 | Purpose of this appendix

The process of delineating clinical privileges involves a request by medical practitioners of precisely those clinical activities they wish to undertake in the hospital.

This appendix describes:

- the domains or categories of medical disciplines that may be helpful divisions of practice for purposes of delineating clinical privileges;
- the process of credentialling as it applies to the cognitive disciplines;
- the position of general practitioners who wish to apply for hospital privileges;
- credentialling for anaesthetic services, which are not only high-risk procedures but which do not lend themselves readily to defining precise procedures for the purpose of credentialling.

42B2 | Domains

Medical staff of Australian hospitals are quite familiar with the concept of categorising specialties and subspecialties. In larger public hospitals medical staff are also used to restricting their activities to such domains as, for example, gynaecologists limiting themselves to the diseases of the female reproductive organs and cardiologists limiting their activities to diseases of the heart and circulation. Within these two broad groupings, however, considerable subspecialisation occurs. Outside these larger public facilities such demarcations are not quite so rigid. Even within these larger public facilities, while there is a list of procedures which is usually associated solely with a particular domain, not uncommonly one or more domains will perform the same procedure.

For the credentialling of medical staff, it might seem more logical and rather simpler to have a single form listing the procedures for each domain. However, because of the factors mentioned above, this approach would mean that a number of procedures would have to appear in multiple domains, introducing redundancy but still not ensuring completeness.

The recommended approach is to specify the domains that comprise medical practice, and to compile a separate list of procedures for each one. Procedures should be assigned to the domain in which they occur most often. There is no implication that because a procedure was assigned to one domain rather than another that it cannot be performed competently by practitioners in other domains. Procedures listed under domains can be adapted from the Commonwealth government's Medical Benefit Schedule or the AMA's list of fees. These lists, familiar to Australian doctors, attempt to group procedures more or less into the domains of the major specialties and subspecialties.

The domains listed in this appendix include only the common subspecialties. A large tertiary referral hospital will have medical staff working in a number of additional domains; the list can be changed to suit the local circumstances.

The position of general practitioners (GPs) in hospitals has been a matter of some contention for several decades. Like any other practitioners, general practitioners must be able to demonstrate their experience, training and competence when applying for hospital privileges. Indeed, for continuation of privileges, a quality management program should be able to demonstrate that the outcomes of care rendered by general practitioners are the same or better than that provided by specialists to equivalent types of patients. In most hospitals where GPs apply for privileges they will need to apply to work in several domains.

42B3 | Anaesthesia and credentialling

There is no doubt that delineating privileges for anaesthesia by means of identifying individual anaesthetic procedures carries inbuilt anomalies and difficulties. The practice of anaesthesia is itself branching off into a number of specialty areas. Applicants for anaesthetic privileges must be able to indicate their experience and competence in those areas in which they wish to practise.

The following areas of anaesthetic activity provide groups or categories of anaesthetic services for the purpose of credentialling:[1]

- local anaesthesia and minor nerve blocks without intravenous sedatives or narcotics;
- management of problems of pain relief;
- management of cardio/pulmonary resuscitation;
- management of critically ill patients in intensive care units;
- the use of invasive anaesthetic procedures;
- the use of invasive techniques for monitoring;
- paediatrics/neonatal anaesthesia;
- obstetrics anaesthesia;
- neurosurgery anaesthesia;
- ear nose and throat anaesthesia;
- cardiothoracic anaesthesia.

42B4 | General practitioners and anaesthetics

In a country the size of Australia, with its thinly spread rural population, general practitioners will be required to provide anaesthetic services for some time to come. The Faculty of Anaesthetists of the Royal Australasian College of Surgeons has issued the following statement in relation to this matter.[2]

1. A minimum period of experience in anaesthesia under instruction is required. This experience should be:
   1.1 In a department of anaesthetics where a graded program can be arranged.
   1.2 Under the instruction of persons who are competent to teach the trainee. That is, they themselves are qualified in anaesthesia.
   1.3 Full time and with a significant case load.
   1.4 Of at least twelve months duration, which need not necessarily be continuous, and may include three months experience in intensive care.
2. At the conclusion of this time, the practitioner must have acquired the following technical skills:
   2.1 Intubate with confidence over the full age range from neonate to elderly.
   2.2 Cannulate both the peripheral and central venous system.
   2.3 Perform simple regional blocks of the upper limb.
   2.4 Maintain intermittent positive pressure ventilation safely over a period in the intubated and non-intubated patient.
   2.5 Closed chest cardiac compression and defibrillation in simulated circumstances if necessary.
3. The practitioner must possess clinical knowledge sufficient to:
   3.1 Understand the pharmacological and physiological effects of the commonly used anaesthetic agents.
   3.2 Appreciate the additional risk of anaesthesia in the presence of pre-existing disease or injury.
   3.3 Resuscitate patients suffering from fluid and electrolyte depletion, acid-base disturbances and hypoxia with or without hypercarbia.
   3.4 Choose the anaesthetic method most appropriate to a particular patient and procedure.
4. The provision of anaesthetic services implies maintenance and updating of the above skills and knowledge. This implies both continuing education and continuity and adequacy of clinical experience. The latter demands at least weekly involvement and/or 250 procedures per year.

42B5 | Medical specialty domains

For credentialling purposes, we suggest dividing medical practice into the following domains (listed alphabetically for convenience). Miscellaneous procedures, i.e. those that cannot be assigned to a domain of medical practice, can be handled separately.

1. Allergy and Immunology
2. Anaesthesia
3. Cardiology (cardiothoracic surgery)
4. Cardiothoracic surgery
5. Dental surgery
6. Dermatology
7. Ear, nose and throat surgery
8. General surgery (including all subspecialties not listed)
9. Gynaecology
10. Internal medicine (including all subspecialties not listed)
11. Neurosurgery
12. Obstetrics
13. Ophthalmology
14. Orthopaedic surgery
15. Paediatrics (both medical and surgical)
16. Peripheral vascular surgery

17. Plastic and reconstructive surgery
18. Psychiatry
19. Radiology
20. Urology

References

1. This material is based on discussions with Dr Patricia Mackey of the Department of Anaesthesia, Royal Melbourne Hospital, Victoria and material from the American Society of Anaesthesiologists.
2. Essential Training for General Practitioners Proposing to Administer Anaesthetics. Faculty of Anaesthetists, Royal Australasian College of Surgeons 1986.

MODEL TERMS OF REFERENCE FOR MEDICAL APPOINTMENTS ADVISORY COMMITTEES

42C0	Contents

42C1. Purpose of this appendix
42C2. Authorisation of the committee
42C3. Purpose of the committee
42C4. Committee membership
42C5. Meetings
42C6. Applications for appointment
42C7. Process considerations of the committee
42C8. Committee recommendations and reporting

42C1	**Purpose of this appendix**

This appendix provides a model terms of reference for a medical appointments advisory committee. Many public hospitals in Australia have well-structured and developed mechanisms for appointing medical staff. For those that do not and for a significant number of private hospitals, this appendix suggests the terms of reference for such a committee.

42C2	**Authorisation of the committee**

1. The committee is an authorised committee of the board of directors.
2. The medical appointments advisory committee is a 'standing' committee.

42C3	**Purpose of the committee**

1. This committee advises the board of directors concerning the appropriateness of medical practitioners to be appointed to work in the hospital, having regard to

their qualifications, skill, character and good standing within the medical profession. In conducting this function the ultimate aim is to ensure the highest possible standard of patient care in all areas of the hospital for all patients.

2. The committee shall develop policies and procedures for appointments for recommendation to the board and shall implement such procedures as the board approves.

3. The committee recommends both appointments and reappointments, and reappointment is implied whenever appointment is mentioned.

42C4 | Committee membership

1. The committee will consist solely of medical practitioners. The committee consists of a core group of a minimum of five (5) and a maximum of seven (7) medical practitioners.

2. Members are appointed by the hospital board from among candidates presented by the medical staff association and the manager. The medical staff nominates seven (7) candidates and the manager nominates three (3). The manager's nominees may be the same as or different from those of the medical staff.

3. Members of the committee will serve for three (3) years and will be eligible for reappointment.

4. A member of the committee can be removed from membership of the committee on the vote of two-thirds of the membership of the committee should he or she fail to attend three consecutive meetings without providing an adequate reason. Such an expulsion must be ratified by the board.

5. In the case of a vacancy on the committee due to death, resignation or otherwise, the medical staff and the manager will each nominate one candidate to the board who will appoint one of the candidates to serve the remainder of the two-year term. The manager's nominee may be the same as or different from the nominee of the medical staff.

6. The chairman of the committee is elected annually from among the members of the committee.

7. The committee has the power to co-opt other medical practitioners from appropriate disciplines and specialties, but at no time will the committee have more than nine (9) members. Any additional co-opted members will sit on the committee only until the task for which they have been co-opted has been completed and they will not have the right to vote.

42C5 | Meetings

1. A quorum for the committee to begin and to continue to transact business is a majority or five (5) members, whichever is the less.

2. The medical appointments advisory committee receives recommendations from the credentials committee.

3. Where a member of the committee is the subject of a submission to the committee or is in the position of being an applicant for reappointment or privileges, or for any other circumstances where there may be a conflict of interest, real or apparent, he or she must absent himself or herself from the deliberations of the committee.

4. The business of the committee is formally conducted and all decisions properly recorded.

5. An agenda accompanies a notice of regularly scheduled meetings, which is distributed not less than ten (10) days prior to the meeting.

6. Minutes are properly kept and are distributed with the agenda.

7. The committee meets monthly or at such other frequency as will be decided by the committee.

8. Matters coming before the committee shall be decided by a simple majority vote of those members present and voting in favour of the motion. The chairperson has a casting vote in the case of a tied vote.

42C6 | Applications for appointment

1. All medical practitioners wishing to practise in the hospital must make application to the manager setting out his or her training, qualifications and experience.

2. The application for appointment must be made on the hospital's 'Application for Appointment' form.

42C7 | Process considerations of the committee

1. The committee will in the course of its activities derive information concerning an individual medical practitioner's qualifications and performance, including the potential to give high quality care given the hospital's resources, from the credentials committee or any other appropriate source.

2. The committee will ensure that all its decisions are objective, without malice and have constant regard for the law of natural justice.

3. The criteria to be used by the committee in making appointments shall be as follows:

   —in consultation with the administration, the need or requirement for an alteration in the number of practitioners of a particular specialty at the hospital for which the appointment is to apply;

   —the capacity of the practitioner, given his or her other commitments and his or her place of practice and residence, to provide an adequate level of service to the hospital;

   —the moral, ethical and professional character of the practitioner;

   —whether the hospital has the facilities, including equipment and staff, to meet the anticipated requirements of the practitioner;

   —the practitioner's attitude and behaviour towards nursing, medical and other hospital staff;

   —the credentials of the practitioner, that is, training, experience and competence as advised by the credentials committee. If the credentials committee recommends no privileges, the only permitted decision is not to appoint.

4. In consideration of an application from a medical practitioner, the committee will be provided with the following documentation:

   —copies of the application and any supporting documents;

   —the recommendations of the credentials committee;

   —other information concerning an applicant provided by the manager, or that may have been requested by the committee.

5. The committee will arrange to have each new applicant interviewed, and the head of the department in which the applicant would be working and two members of the committee will conduct the interviews. These interviews should be conducted independently, and each of the three interviewers should write a brief report for the committee.

   Alternatively, the committee may ask the applicant to appear before it. The head of the department in which the appointee will be working may be invited to attend the committee for this purpose.

6. The decisions and actions of the committee will at all times have regard to the hospital by-laws and policies, and relevant state regulations and legislation.

7. Confidentiality of the business of the committee shall at all times be paramount. Members will only discuss the committee's business with other members and such other persons who are authorised to provide or receive such information.

42C8 | Committee recommendations and reporting

1. The committee will report through the manager to the hospital board.
2. Decisions of the committee shall be in the form of recommendations which shall go to the board of directors through the manager.
3. The committee will recommend the period of appointment for a one- or three-year term or such other term permitted by the hospital's by-laws.
4. The committee will have the power to recommend a provisional appointment for a period not exceeding twelve months if the credentials committee considers such actions desirable and if the by-laws permit it.
5. The committee may recommend modifications to these terms of reference to be endorsed by the board prior to taking effect.

Chapter 3

PATIENT SATISFACTION SURVEYS

---

430 | Contents

This chapter describes patient satisfaction surveys—the most practical way of assessing the interpersonal aspects of the quality of care—and how to conduct them. It deals with:

431 | Purpose of this chapter

Patients, who are the primary focus of a hospital's activities, are a critical source of information. Doctors, nurses and other providers are well aware that the patient's symptoms are the starting point for all care and that they focus diagnostic interventions. Moreover, the patients' wishes determine the chosen therapy. However, most providers are less aware of the value of patients' opinions about the quality of care. Obtaining such opinions is the function of patient satisfaction surveys. Such surveys, especially when conducted or specified and audited by an external or coordinating body, may form the basis for 'report cards' that consumers can use to compare hospitals' performance. In the US, publication of such report cards is becoming commonplace for such managed care plans as HMOs, and may become mandatory in the years ahead. Patients' reports would encompass their experience with hospitalisation, and they may influence a managed care plan's contracting decisions for enrollees' hospital care, providing contracted hospitals with an incentive to improve at least the interpersonal aspects of the quality of their care.

In principle one must distinguish between patient satisfaction surveys and patient outcome surveys—both of which may involve postdischarge interviews or self-administered questionnaires—although in practice the two types of survey may overlap by design or default. Patient satisfaction surveys gather patients' evaluation and opinions, and are instrumental in assessing the interpersonal aspects of the quality of care. Patient outcome surveys gather patients' reports of symptoms, treatment regimens and health status, and are the key to judging a hospital's technical quality of care and to providing clues about interventions' effectiveness. A single questionnaire can gather both types of information—patients' opinions and reports—but designers must be mindful of their different purposes to avoid potential bias. While the principles of survey research hold equally for both types of surveys, their purposes and hence principles' application differ.

This chapter deals exclusively with patient satisfaction surveys. It covers the various aspects of conducting a survey: purpose, design, data collection (sometimes referred to as questionnaire administration), and analysis and reporting. However, it does not intend to substitute for a text on social survey research and cannot encompass all of the nuances that quality managers are likely to encounter in practice. Quality managers who are contemplating the conduct of a patient satisfaction survey would be well advised to consult with a recognised expert in social survey research or public opinion polling, unless an expert himself or herself. Hospitals may also want to contract for these services.

432 | Prerequisites for success

Hospitals' goals in conducting patient satisfaction surveys should be to:
- produce usable information, which requires competence in survey design, administration, and analysis and reporting;
- use results to improve patient care, which requires the will to act and requisite mechanisms to implement improvement actions.

Hospitals not willing to invest the necessary resources to produce usable information or lacking the will to act on survey results are wasting their efforts in conducting patient satisfaction surveys or, at best, achieving marginal public relations benefits by appearing to care about patients' perceptions and the quality of their care.

The quality management department should be responsible for conducting patient satisfaction surveys and its existence, with appropriate staff, will help ensure their success. Prior to conducting patient satisfaction surveys, the hospital should have put in place an effective quality management organisation (see Part III, Chapter 1) and mechanisms to resolve quality problems (see Part II, Chapter 8). Because patient satisfaction surveys are relatively simple and self-contained activities, hospitals may want to institute them early in the development of their quality management programs (see Part III, Chapter 6) to demonstrate that they are doing something. Demonstrating action is one thing, achieving improvement, another. At all stages of quality maturity, hospitals must match the focus of their patient satisfaction surveys with their ability to act on their results, lest they waste money identifying problems that they will not or cannot remedy.

433 | Managing patient satisfaction surveys

433.1 | Purpose of patient satisfaction surveys

Patient satisfaction surveys intend to systematically collect patients' opinions (evaluations or ratings) about the quality of care they received. Patients are the only valid source of information on the interpersonal aspects of care and patient satisfaction surveys are a practical way to gather it. Patient satisfaction surveys complement, and provide a counterweight to, unsolicited complaints and compliments. They can reveal deficiencies in care that can become the focus of improvement strategies. In this respect they are another problem identification technique (cf. structured quality review) and also offer a means of evaluating certain types of potential improvement strategies prior to their implementation.

By conducting a patient satisfaction survey a hospital is committing itself to remedy any serious deficiencies the survey identifies. There is little point in undertaking a patient satisfaction survey unless one is prepared to act on its findings. While patients may be flattered that the hospital cares about their opinions, their illusions will be replaced by cynicism if any problems they identify persist.

For best results, patient satisfaction surveys should be conducted continuously, with quarterly and annual reports. Continuous sampling of opinion permits trend analysis and monitoring patient satisfaction. Hospitals can supplement this ongoing effort with special surveys targeted to specific issues. Special surveys may require expanding existing or drawing entirely different samples, and supplementing existing or developing separate survey instruments. Patient satisfaction surveys may be divided into two types: point of service and follow-up surveys.

433.2 Point of service surveys

Point of service surveys, as their name implies, are done in the hospital before the patient leaves. An interviewer may record the patient's opinions, the patient may interact directly with a computer program for this purpose, or may simply be given a self-administered form to be left behind or sent in later.

Point of service surveys have several advantages. They are low cost. Questions can be asked of every patient without the cost of finding the patient postdischarge. The patient's experiences are fresh, aiding recall of feelings and thus promoting the survey's relevance. This immediacy may also be a disadvantage. The patient's feelings may be too intense and unconsidered. Further, the patient may be reluctant to discuss care openly with someone whom he or she associates with the care that he or she received. While the goal may be to survey every patient, biases may exist which result in some patients being missed or not filling in the questionnaire, especially if they can take it away. This mix of immediate and delayed completions may also be a biasing factor. Further, it may not be necessary to obtain opinions from every patient. Sampling may be more efficient and, of course, can be done for point of service as well as follow-up surveys.

433.3 Follow-up surveys

As their name implies, follow-up surveys are done some time after the patient has been discharged. Follow-up should occur shortly after discharge so that the survey seems relevant to the patient and the experience is still relatively fresh. The rest of this chapter focuses on follow-up surveys, including those designed to test proposed changes to hospital operations, although the principles apply equally to both point of service and follow-up surveys.

433.4 Contracting out

The quality management department should be responsible for patient satisfaction surveys; however, this does not mean that the department must conduct them. The hospital may find it very advantageous to contract out the design, conduct and tabulation of surveys to a firm specialising in public opinion or social survey research. Nevertheless, hospital management should not abdicate the survey's contents to either an outside firm or to a consultant working in isolation.

A contract with an expert firm avoids the need to hire staff and train people such as survey experts and interviewers. Further, the firm may have sophisticated survey-taking software or other computerised aids that permit it to conduct surveys cost-effectively. A hospital may want to hire a firm based on competitive bids. Hospitals not experienced in developing requests for proposals for surveys may want to retain a consultant to assist them write the request for proposals and evaluate responses.

If a contract is let, the survey manager (the quality management department staff member responsible for the patient satisfaction survey) should keep in close contact and meet periodically with the contractor to review progress and problems. The hospital should evaluate both the survey and the firm's work. It may be advisable to obtain another bid for the survey if the hospital is dissatisfied with the firm's quality, service or price. Working closely with a contractor for an extended period permits one to build a productive relationship. There is no value (and often considerable expense and risk) in obtaining fresh bids for work without the expectation of significant benefits in quality, service or price. Nevertheless, all contracts should be job or time limited to permit the possibility of renegotiation or to obtain another bid for the work, and to alert the contractor that the hospital cares about quality, service and price—which it can reinforce by constant contract monitoring.

433.5 Survey design group

The hospital should appoint a survey design group to assist the quality manager to design patient satisfaction surveys and to interpret resultant data. The group could be a subcommittee of the quality management committee and include an outside social survey expert. Its primary purpose is to assure the survey's relevance to improving the quality of care. The group can, for example:

- adopt and adapt off-the-shelf questionnaires or select among standard questions;
- set priorities among questions;
- review and approve protocols;
- assist in the interpretation of survey data;
- identify problems and improvements to be referred to the hospital's problem resolution mechanism (see Part II, Chapter 8).

433.6 Protocol

The quality management department should develop a protocol (proposal) for each and every patient satisfaction survey it proposes to conduct. The protocol sets out details of:

- the survey's purpose, including intended use of results;
- questionnaire design;
- data collection and processing, including the assessment and assurance of data integrity;
- analysis and reporting;
- how designers and users will evaluate its technical adequacy and utility.

For example, the protocol will specify the intended use of each survey question, the analyses to be performed and the statistical reports to be produced. Often such specifications take the form of tables, graphs and so on to be filled in with survey results. Careful protocol preparation permits all of the many choices involved in conducting a patient satisfaction survey to be considered, set out coherently, and reviewed by those who will use the results. Protocol review permits any design issues that surface in the protocol to be resolved prior to conducting the survey. Time spent planning pays off in terms of the relevance and validity of survey results. Money spent asking the wrong questions or in obtaining invalid answers to the right questions cannot be recouped.

The protocol provides the blueprint or plan (policies and procedures) for conducting the survey. For ongoing patient satisfaction surveys, the protocol should be reviewed annually and, if warranted, revised in the light of experience and changed information needs. A key issue in the revised protocol will be mapping old questions to new ones to permit database continuity. If the survey is contracted out, the 'request for proposal' serves as the outline for the protocol, to be elaborated by the contractor. The protocol should be complete but need not be exhaustive or exhausting. Everything in the protocol must be decided or done at some time during the survey. Doing it at the beginning will help assure the survey's quality.

434 | Sampling

434.1 | Purpose of sampling

While every patient can be surveyed, sampling may, and usually is, more efficient. Sampling must be differentiated from targeting. Sampling refers to selecting subjects from a defined universe (population); targeting, on the other hand, refers to selecting the universe of interest. For example, the hospital may have opened a new outpatient clinic and wants to know patients' opinions about such things as the ambience and the service. In this case it would target only patients using the new service. The hospital could still sample such patients, if there were many of them, to give the desired information at least cost.

434.2 | Sampling strategy

Sampling's objective is to be able to make valid inferences from the sample to the population from which the sample was drawn. Clearly, one must first define the population and then decide how best to sample its members. Poor sampling leads to erroneous inferences. Expert advice should be obtained prior to sampling because sampling errors cannot be fixed after data have been collected. Survey results from unconsidered samples may be useless or, even worse, misleading.

Sampling strategy depends on stating clearly the question to which one wants an answer, and the confidence one wants to be able to have in that answer. There are many different types of samples, although the word itself is often used to mean probability sample, which is the sense that applies here. In probability sampling, each member of the population (universe) of interest has a given probability of being sampled. Common ways to sample are drawing numbers randomly, for example balls in a bag, or systematically, for example every tenth name on a list, where the starting point (between one and ten in the case of this example) is decided randomly. Prior to sampling, the population may be stratified. Stratification is especially useful if the population consists of subgroups whose opinions are of interest but whose numbers of members differ substantially. For example if the hospital treats mostly women and few men, patients should be stratified by sex prior to sampling if the hospital wants to know reliably the separate opinions of women and men. The number of patients of each sex sampled will be roughly equal, but the sampling rate will be quite different: a higher proportion of female patients than of male patients will be sampled.

434.3 | Factors affecting sample size

The correct number of patients to be sampled depends on:

- the size of the population (universe);
- the type of question response, for example dichotomous, yes/no versus multiple categories versus continuous variable;
- the expected frequency of response;
- desired confidence limits—the upper and lower values that specify the chance, usually taken to be 95%, that the population mean will fall in the resultant interval;
- desired significance level (if one intends to use sample statistics to test hypotheses about population parameters)—the probability of rejecting the null hypothesis

when it is true (a type I error), typically set at 0.05—and sometimes power—the probability of rejecting a false null hypothesis, one minus the probability of failing to reject the null hypothesis when it is false (a type II error), typically set at 0.8.

435 | Questionnaire design

435.1 | *Questionnaire focus and contents*

Patient satisfaction surveys can be combined with those seeking patients' reports about such matters as symptoms and health status, subject only to the burden they may place on the respondent. Questionnaires designed to elicit such facts may require telephone or personal interviews. In general, short simple questionnaires are preferable to long complex ones. Patient satisfaction surveys can gather opinions about:

- services received; and
- changes in services the hospital is contemplating.

This section describes both of these types of surveys and discusses the following topics:

- what to ask—sources of questions;
- nature of questions;
- types of questions;
- statement of purpose;
- questionnaire reviews and pretests.

435.2 | *Services received*

Generally a small number of trend items form the survey's core and can be supplemented by point-in-time evaluations and opinions about proposed changes. All survey questions must relate to the survey's purpose. The planned use to which the answer to a question will be put must be explicit and part of the survey design. For example, questions may be included as part of a scale (score constructed from answers to several questions), or to check on the survey's reliability, as well as to provide direct answers to questions. Questions may provide trend information, if included continuously, or point-in-time information, if included only in a single survey.

435.3 | *Service changes*

Often several alternatives exist to resolve problems identified by surveys or other means, and the option of choice may depend on patient acceptance. In these cases, patients' preferences can be solicited through an ongoing patient satisfaction survey (or separate survey if none is ongoing). The opinions of patients who were treated recently may be more relevant than, and as likely to be representative as, a sample of people living in the community that the hospital serves. Moreover, using an ongoing patient satisfaction survey for this purpose is far less costly than conducting a separate community opinion poll. Nevertheless, bias may result from using patient satisfaction surveys for this purpose, and hospitals may want to consider conducting periodic public opinion polls to assess their standing in the community, for example.

435.4 | *What to ask—sources of questions*

Constructing survey questionnaires is both a science and an art, and requires considerable skill and experience. Designers must pay attention to the clarity of questions, their order and their layout. Clarity includes making sure that people can understand what is being asked and that the question is unambiguous, that is, it can be reasonably interpreted in only one way (and thus represents the same question to every respondent). The mode of administration, for example in person, by telephone interview or self-administration, affects the appropriate wording of questions and types of responses as well as the questionnaire's layout.

Patient satisfaction survey items may be taken from standard questionnaires or suggested by anyone in the hospital responsible for care who needs information to evaluate services or choose among alternatives. Initially the quality management department will likely be the primary source of items. However, as the program develops, competition for available survey space may intensify. In this case, the survey users group should assist the quality manager select survey items. Questionnaire designers must convert desired questions into questionnaire items that potential respondents can understand unambiguously.

435.5 │ Nature of questions

Questions must not only focus on satisfaction but also on reasons, especially sources of dissatisfaction and what might be done to remedy them. Satisfaction items are useful for keeping score or comparing oneself to others; however, they say nothing about the hospital's activities that may have led to the patient's opinion. Questions that pinpoint reasons are essential to identify actionable antecedents. For example, if patients were not satisfied with the care received they might be asked to list their experience or reasons for feeling that way. Further, if they list several reasons they might be asked to pick the most important or the one that bothered them the most. Whatever the patients' feelings, they may be asked to identify changes that would improve care and, if appropriate, why they mentioned that particular item. Again, they may be asked to rate or rank items and explain why the top-rated or top-ranked improvement suggestion is most important to them. The key is to elicit results useful to improving the quality of care and to prioritise them.

Survey questionnaires contain the following two broad types of questions:

• structured items; and
• open-ended or unstructured items.

435.6 │ Structured items

In structured items, all the possible responses are defined, even if the list of categories includes 'other' and 'don't know' responses. A possible question of this type might be:

• Overall, how satisfied would you say you are with the care you received at Beneficial General Hospital? Would you say you are:
  (a) Very satisfied.
  (b) Somewhat satisfied.
  (c) Neither satisfied nor dissatisfied.
  (d) Somewhat dissatisfied.
  (e) Very dissatisfied.
  (f) No opinion, don't know (volunteered response). A volunteered response is one that the respondent must say (rather than being read or shown a list of responses or being prompted in another way).

Structured items are easy to analyse because all of the responses have already been categorised. The precategorisation is also a disadvantage, however. One has to be certain that almost all responses will fall easily into one of the defined categories. Obviously this situation is easy to effect for the above type of question, but not so easy for questions with infinite response possibilities. For such situations, open-ended items are more appropriate. Nevertheless, with experience, responses to even these questions can be structured, based on the most frequent responses, with the final possibility being 'other, specify'.

435.7 Open-ended items

Open-ended items have the distinct advantage that the respondent's exact opinions can be captured directly, rather than being fitted into a predetermined category (see coding below). However, in surveys with many respondents, coding open-ended items for subsequent analysis is a complex task. The following is an example of an open-ended item.

- Question—What would you say was the single best thing about your stay at Beneficial General Hospital?
- Illustrative response—'The thing that pleased me most was how kind the nurses were, and the young doctor's attention.'

435.8 Statement of purpose

The finished questionnaire consists of two parts:

- a statement of purpose;
- questions to be answered.

The statement of purpose informs the potential respondent about the survey and permits him or her to decide whether or not to consent to participate in it. It should be brief, to the point, and answer at least the following questions, which might arise in a potential respondent's mind:

- Who is doing the survey?
- Why are you doing this survey?
- What good will it do?
- Why (How) was I selected?
- Why should I participate?
- What happens to my answers? Who will see them?
- Will I get a copy of the survey results? When will I get them?
- What happens if I choose not to participate? What do I get for participating?

435.9 Questionnaire reviews and pretests

The quality management department must thoroughly review and test questionnaires prior to use. Once the draft questionnaire has been developed, a small group of people comprising the users of survey results and one or two experts in social survey or opinion research should first review it. The users check that items will meet their information needs and approve the analysis and reporting plan. The experts focus on clarity and flow of questions, the appropriateness of response choices and other survey design issues. Sometimes this step is called a design review.

The quality management department (QMD) should next pretest the revised questionnaire with ten to twenty patients. Expert, specially trained, interviewers should conduct these interviews. They can gauge respondents' reactions and debrief interviewees to learn what changes should be made to the questionnaire, and discuss its length and complexity. For self-administered questionnaires, a postadministration focus group can perform this same function. Sometimes this step is called an alpha test. If warranted, the QMD can next pretest the revised version of the questionnaire using a much larger sample, for example 50–200 patients. Sometimes this step is called a beta test. If all goes well, the questionnaire is ready to go to the field. If pretests reveal continuing or unexpected difficulties, redesign may be required. The testing cycle is then repeated with the new questionnaire. As mentioned previously, time spent designing and testing pays off in terms of collecting useful, relevant and valid data. Use of standard, tried and true, patient satisfaction questionnaires can both avoid the need for review and testing and save time and money.

436 | Questionnaire administration—data collection

436.1 | Data collection methods

How the questionnaire is to be administered to patients is a key aspect of survey design. For follow-up surveys, the following choices are available:

- self-administration;
- telephone;
- personal interview.

436.2 | Self-administered questionnaires

Self-administered questionnaires are clearly the least expensive way to collect data and are often attractive for this reason. But they are not necessarily the best way. To boost response rates they must prominently display who to call for help and, if not completed on site, include a preaddressed, postage-free envelope in which to return the completed questionnaire, or the questionnaire must be printed on a postcard or as a self-mailer. Self-administered questionnaires have a number of drawbacks, including the following:

- Questionnaires must be simple, in terms of:
  —questions;
  —responses;
  —logic (skipping subsequent questions based on the response to the index question).
- They must be very well designed to avoid confusing would-be respondents.
- They preclude the use of flash cards, prompts, and other interviewing aids or devices.

436.3 | Telephone surveys

These days the telephone interview is likely to be the best, even though not all patients may have a telephone and those who do are not always available. With telephone interviews, some professional polling organisations can enter interview responses directly into a computerised database. Telephone interviews are more expensive because they require an interviewer. However, questions can be clarified and responses probed (but rules are needed to avoid biasing respondents) and more complex questions and logic can be used. Flash cards, for example, still cannot be used. For sampled patients without telephones, the QMD can substitute a personal interview or mailed (self-administered) questionnaire. Ignoring such patients may bias survey results. Moreover, the way in which the survey is administered can influence responses. Thus, if a mixed strategy is contemplated, careful consideration of its potentially biasing effect is essential as part of the survey design process.

436.4 | Face-to-face interviews

In many respects, face-to-face (personal) interviews are the ideal but also the most expensive way to administer questionnaires. They permit observing the patient and, with medically trained interviewers, examination also. Personal interviews are excellent for fact-finding, for example gathering data for outcomes studies, as well as opinion taking. Interviewers can use flash cards (to display respondents' choices for example, which is especially helpful if their number is too many to remember easily) and such other interviewing aids as photographs, diagrams and models. To save interviewers' time in fruitless attempts to interview sampled patients, the quality management department can set up appointments to conduct interviews in advance, by mail or by telephone.

437 Questionnaire processing—data entry

437.1 Data entry steps

Data entry's purpose is to produce a database for analysis. Processing completed questionnaires involves:

- logging in returns;
- coding and editing;
- data entry.

Returned questionnaires must be logged in and matched to sampled patients. Responses to open-ended questions must be coded prior to data entry. All questionnaires must be edited to ensure responses to questions are clear and unambiguous for data entry. Survey managers must provide schemes and rules for these purposes. Questionnaires should be designed not only to facilitate interview or self-administration but also data entry. Many choices are available, depending on the equipment accessible by the hospital or organisation conducting the survey. They include, for example, direct entry, database entry, key-to-card/tape and optical scanning. This section elaborates on each of these processing steps and data entry possibilities.

437.2 Logging in returns

The survey manager must match returned questionnaires with lists of sampled patients. These lists may be unit cards or sheets; hand- or computer-compiled databases. Periodically, the quality management department must attempt to follow-up sampled patients who have not yet been interviewed or who have not yet returned a mailed questionnaire. The survey protocol defines the number and timing of follow-ups. When interviewers have made the required number of call backs for interviews, or when the allowed number of mailings and follow-up time has run out for self-administered questionnaires, the survey manager must make out an appropriate data entry form to record the correct disposition of the sampled patient, and, if part of the protocol, to permit subsampling, for example of non-respondents. Uncontrolled samples, for example, handing out surveys and processing returns, are subject to obvious bias, limiting inferences (see sampling above).

437.3 Coding open-ended responses

In the process of coding, coders assign codes to open-ended responses to categorise them and thus permit analysing them statistically. Before coding can be done, an appropriate coding scheme must exist or be developed. Developing such coding schemes as the International Classification of Diseases (ICD-9-CM) can be a difficult and time consuming task. However, schemes for patient satisfaction surveys are usually less complicated. Survey managers can usually develop an appropriate coding scheme based on responses' frequency and similarity. They can also develop rules for using codes to help to assure consistency. The type of scheme one needs depends on how one intends to use the coded response. A simple approach involves reading twenty to fifty responses and assigning them codes. Using this pilot scheme, one can then code 100–200 responses to see how well the scheme works and to modify it to cope with responses not encountered previously. A key part of the scheme will be identifying synonyms: responses similar enough to be considered the same for analytic purposes.

Once one has the scheme, one must recode all of the responses used to develop it in order to ensure consistency of final codes. If one assigns coding to clerical staff one must check their work, especially early on, to make sure they understand the scheme and are coding correctly. Such review may identify the need to elaborate or revise coding rules. It helps to allocate specific questions to be coded to the same coder to improve consistency. If the coder encounters responses apparently not encompassed by the scheme, the coding scheme's developer or manager (sometimes referred to as a vocabulary controller) should decide if it fits an existing code, if a new code is warranted, or if it should be coded 'other'.

437.4 Editing

Editing questionnaires is the process of assuring that all responses are clear and unambiguous for data entry. Entry can be done by the data entry operator, but in high volume situations may be reserved for specially trained staff to facilitate high productivity. Editing specifications must be established for each question and, of course, will depend on type. At the most simple, the specification may say 'one answer required'. In this case, the editor will make sure that one and only one answer is chosen. If two answers have been chosen, the edit specification may call for a random selection of one of them or entry of 'invalid response'; if no response, that 'no response' is indicated clearly as the data entry item.

437.5 Direct database entry

The most sophisticated data entry systems allow the interviewer (or subject) to answer questions posed directly on a computer screen. The answers are entered directly into the computer database. This system minimises data entry errors. It can also generate reports automatically. However, such systems are unlikely to be available to the average hospital.

437.6 Data screen entry

In data screen entry a clerk transfers questionnaire responses to a computerised database by keying them into a data entry screen that corresponds to questionnaire responses. Commercial microframe, miniframe and mainframe computer database management packages are available for this purpose. However, some programming experience is usually required to construct user-friendly data entry screens. Careful sight verification, supplemented by computerised edit checks if key verification is not used, is necessary to avoid data entry or transcription errors.

437.7 Key-to-card/tape data entry

Responses are keyed to punch cards or to magnetic tape and uploaded to a computer, normally a mainframe. This system has been used traditionally, particularly with large volumes of data. Increasingly PC-based data screen entry is supplanting it. Key verification (repeat entry of the same data with automatic matching to identify discrepancies) is used to reduce data entry errors but, of course, requires double the work.

437.8 Optical scanning data entry

Optical character recognition (OCR) systems permit conversion of marks on paper, including handwriting, to electronic form. Special OCR software creates questionnaires that can be scanned and interpreted to create a database. This data entry system is increasing in popularity as the software is becoming increasingly sophisticated. Already OCR software exists for the reliable interpretation of check marks and constrained handwriting, for example numerals written in boxes or defined areas, that for unconstrained handwriting is still not reliable enough to warrant its general use. The necessary OCR equipment may not be available in the average hospital.

437.9 Data cleaning

The last step in preparing data for analysis is often referred to as data cleaning. It should represent the last step to assure data integrity, but regrettably is sometimes the only quality control point. As with all processing activities errors should be prevented if at all possible (e.g. through improved questionnaire design) or, if not, identified (and if possible corrected) as early in the process as possible (which favours direct database data entry for example, as inconsistencies can be identified automatically and corrected at their source). Some errors (e.g. missed questions) cannot be corrected in processing and represent missing data, diminishing statistical inference.

Typically, data cleaning involves running processed survey data against a set of computer programs that check for missing fields, responses out of valid ranges and inconsistencies, for example. The result is a report that identifies errors that the survey manager can track to the source—the completed questionnaire. Sometimes data cleaning identifies processing errors that can be corrected; sometimes problems that are not amenable to correction, resulting in missing data. Even if errors' resolution is to recode responses 'missing data', data cleaning serves the useful function of eliminating from analysis obviously incorrect or invalid responses that might affect results. Once data have been cleaned, survey responses are available for analysis and reporting.

438 | Analysis and reporting

438.1 | Analysing survey results

The survey protocol should describe the analysis plan necessary to achieve the survey's purpose. Nevertheless, results may suggest additional analyses. Most of the time, hospitals will desire only simple analyses such as frequency distributions and cross tabulations. Whenever survey designers compare distributions or proportions, they should use appropriate statistical tests to gauge the probability of any observed differences arising by chance. Selecting a one in twenty chance as the cut-off for statistical significance is customary. Showing results in graphic form—for example time series plots, bar charts and pie charts—may provide additional insights or improve presentation.

438.2 | Reporting survey results

The quality management department should prepare reports for ongoing patient satisfaction surveys quarterly, except in small hospitals in which biannual or annual reports may be more appropriate. The reports should be simple, to the point, and in a form satisfactory to their users. In general, reports should consist of:
- a brief narrative summary identifying key results, especially trends;
- tables, charts, graphs and diagrams.

In the case of surveys that span several quarters, users may welcome quarterly progress reports rather than waiting to the end for a summative report. However, depending on the survey's design, valid inferences may only be possible after all of the data have been collected.

Particularly valuable are comparisons about patient satisfaction and other responses with results obtained by other hospitals, either individually or in the aggregate. These data are usually available only if an outside agency surveys many hospitals or if mechanisms exist for hospitals to co-ordinate survey questionnaire items and share results.

438.3 | Disseminating survey results

Hospital management must decide to whom to release survey results and when to do so. In particular, it must decide whether or not to provide results to staff, publish them, and/or release them to the press. If results are to be disseminated widely, the hospital should prepare a short, simple report suitable for a general audience. Such a report can be prepared or finished by the hospital's public relations department or if it lacks one by an article writer. A professionally prepared media release may also be appropriate.

439 | Evaluating patient satisfaction surveys

As with all quality management activities, the quality management department should assure and improve the quality of their patient satisfaction surveys. The quality management principles established throughout this manual apply. The QMD can assess, assure and improve the following aspects of patient satisfaction surveys:

- design:
  —questionnaire
  —sampling
- Mechanics:
  —response rate
  —item completion rates
  —interviewer/question reliability
  —processing accuracy
- analysis and reporting;
- utility, value to users:
  —problems identified, what was done about them
  —ideas evaluated, resultant actions.

Patient satisfaction surveys' ultimate payoff is their utility to providers—specifically, the information they generate that hospitals can use to improve patient care. If surveys identify problems that are never acted upon, management should examine its willingness to improve care and the effectiveness of those aspects of the quality management program designed to formulate and implement solutions. If surveys reveal no problems, the quality management department should examine the questionnaire's adequacy. If patients truly believe that the hospital is doing an outstanding job in all respects, sample sizes can be reduced to the minimum consistent with monitoring satisfaction to be sure it does not decline over time. The hospital can increase or supplement this monitoring sample when it wants to seek patients' opinions on proposed changes or other focused matters.

Chapter 4

STRUCTURED QUALITY REVIEW

---

441 | **Purpose of this chapter**

Quality assessment is a prerequisite for quality improvement. Only by identifying quality of care problems can hospitals expect to improve systematically the quality of their care. Quality refers to care and its documentation. Care refers to processes and outcomes. Quality assessment refers here to the process of examining retrospectively a patient's medical record to determine if the care a patient received and the outcomes he or she experienced were what he or she should have received and was expected to experience. Structured quality review refers to the process of assessing retrospectively the quality of care provided to an individual patient for an episode or continuum of medical care, based on the documentation in the patient's medical record.

Structured quality review is a tool for comprehensive quality assessment of care and its documentation. It intends to identify all of the important quality of care problems in a case: processes that if improved would increase patients' health status improvement and/or the certainty of its attainment. By aggregating results, hospitals can create a quality score to monitor quality improvement. Because it can be implemented easily, with minimal commitment of resources, structured quality review is likely to be the initial method for, and remain the mainstay of, systematic problem identification in Australian hospitals for some time to come.

If designed and implemented properly, structured quality review is a powerful learning tool as well as a potent way to identify quality problems. Hospitals and doctors should approach and engender an environment for its use in this spirit, rather than as a means to identify 'bad apples' (practitioners who need to but refuse to or are incapable of improving their practices). Most quality problems result from poorly-designed processes, not individuals' malfeasance.

Structured quality review involves the following three steps (see Figure IV-4-1 on page 591):

- Screening—systematic case-by-case assessment using automated outcome/process assessment screens to identify potential quality problems.
- Review—structured medical record review to confirm potential quality problems and to characterise them.
- Analysis—statistical (pattern) analysis of screening information and medical record review results to reveal patterns of care and illuminate quality problems.

Screening's central purpose is to focus expert clinician reviewers' attention on cases likely exhibiting quality problems, thereby reducing their workload to a manageable level and improving their productivity. Outcome/process assessment screens match what was done and achieved with what should have been done and achieved to identify cases with potential quality problems and thus that require further review. Screening by this means offers objectivity (because it uses explicit practice criteria), and economy (because it can be done by specially trained nurses or medical records technicians).

Structured medical record review (SMR) refers to a systematic process in which expert clinicians examine medical records to confirm quality problems identified by outcome/process assessment screens. Pattern analysis refers to the statistical analysis of screening data and/or structured medical record review findings to reveal patterns of care. It may identify trends in, and reveal the distribution of, quality problems, discover additional quality problems, illuminate their causes, and guide subsequent investigations necessary to identify problems' root causes.

This chapter describes the prerequisites for successful structured quality review in hospitals, considerations in managing the effort, and steps necessary to implement structured quality review. Necessarily the chapter provides general guidance, not detailed how-to instructions, because every hospital's needs and circumstances differ. Part II, Chapter 8 describes structured quality review's conceptual bases.

442 | Prerequisites for successful structured quality review

442.1 | *Structured quality review must be part of a complete system*

Hospitals would be well advised to consider implementing structured quality review only as part of a well-articulated quality management plan. Further, they should only institute structured quality review after first providing, as part of their quality management plan, the resources necessary to support it. To do otherwise is to court disaster because medical practitioners' and others' enthusiasm will turn quickly to disappointment and disenchantment, hindering future efforts to (re)introduce quality management efforts. Because structured quality review identifies quality problems, hospitals must have the will and have institutionalised mechanisms to investigate their root causes and to change care systems and practices to eliminate them. Without the commitment and means to correct quality of care problems, hospitals would be wasting their time and effort in implementing structured quality review.

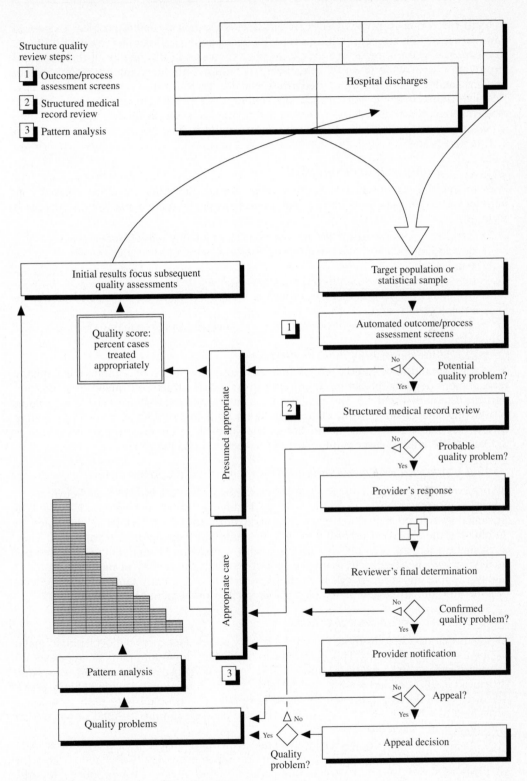

Structure quality
review steps:

1 Outcome/process
assessment screens

2 Structured medical
record review

3 Pattern analysis

Hospital discharges

Initial results focus subsequent
quality assessments

Target population or
statistical sample

Quality score:
percent cases
treated
appropriately

1 Automated outcome/process
assessment screens

No ◁◇ Potential
Yes ▽ quality problem?

Presumed appropriate

2 Structured medical record review

No ◁◇ Probable
Yes ▽ quality problem?

Provider's response

Reviewer's final determination

No ◁◇ Confirmed
Yes ▽ quality problem?

Appropriate care

Provider notification

3

No ◁◇ Appeal?
Yes ▽

Pattern analysis

△ No

Quality problems

Yes ◇ ◀
Quality
problem?

Appeal decision

Figure IV-4-1 *Structured quality review steps*

Structured quality review's conceptual basis is clear: if a quality problem existed in prior care it is likely to recur in future care. By investigating and eliminating the problem's root causes it will not recur in future care, thereby assuring the quality of that care and improving it over what it would otherwise have been. Structured quality review cannot prevent quality problems from occurring initially; only from recurring subsequently. Hospitals must institute intraproduction (rather than postproduction) quality control mechanisms (principally decision support technology) to avert problems and prevent their occurrence initially. Presently such technology is only in its embryonic stages. (See Part II, Chapters 6 and 7.)

442.2 Quality management plan

Prior to introducing structured quality review, the hospital must develop a plan for its introduction. This plan is normally part of the hospital's quality management plan. It includes:

- integrating structured quality review with other quality surveillance systems;
- developing policies and procedures for how structured quality review is to be conducted;
- training doctors in structured quality review;
- installing the management information system for tracking cases and tabulating review results; and
- deciding how results will be reported and used to improve quality of care.

442.3 Quality management department

A hospital should have hired a quality manager and have in place a functioning quality management department before attempting to introduce structured quality review. (See Part III, Chapters 4 and 6.) The quality management department plays a crucial role in conducting and/or supporting clinical divisions in their conduct of structured quality review (see below). Without the quality management department's support, a hospital is unlikely to be able to successfully introduce structured quality review.

442.4 Adequacy of medical records and medical recordkeeping

Before embarking on structured quality review hospitals must ensure that their medical recordkeeping function is up to the task of identifying and tracking medical records. In Australia at the present time many hospitals must invest considerable resources in automating their medical recordkeeping and upgrading their medical record staff. They must make such investments to support quality management generally and structured quality review specifically. In many Australian hospitals the quality of medical records is highly variable and it too needs to be improved. One of the early targets for and effects of structured quality review is to bring about such improvement (see below).

442.5 Make versus buy decisions

Hospitals that decide to institute structured quality review face a crucial decision: to make or buy the requisite system. This decision can be broken down into parts that correspond to structured quality review's three steps: outcome/process assessment screening, structured medical record review, and pattern analysis. A turnkey system will likely prove the most cost-effective approach for most hospitals. The hospital may wish to retain a consultant to advise it on which system to license or to design the hospital's own system if it chooses this alternative.

Presently the only commercially available structured quality review system is QSM (described in Part II, Chapter 8). It provides an outcome/process assessment system for all types of cases, supports structured medical record review and produces reports.

Further, it permits hospitals to tailor these structured quality review aspects to their particular needs and circumstances. A hospital would have to commit tens of millions of dollars over many years to develop a system as good as QSM, which it can license now. Even after making such an investment, it would be a rare hospital that would succeed. Hospitals are simply not in the business of developing such expert systems. Further, using home-grown systems hospitals lose the ability to compare their performance with that of others. Hospitals' ability to benchmark their performance is a distinct advantage of licensing a structured quality review system from a vendor (like QSM) that operates an international database. Alternatively, hospitals can benchmark their performance through co-operative arrangements if they operate a common structured quality review system.

442.6 | Dangers of omitting outcome/process assessment screening

Some hospitals might be tempted to omit the step of automated outcome/process assessment screening, thinking that they could simply use quality assurance nurses to screen records or dispense with screening entirely, and therefore avoid the need to license or develop a complete structured quality review system. Hospitals should resist such temptations because they represent false economies and short-sighted policy.

Available evidence suggests that quality assurance nurses' screening of medical records (without using a valid automated outcome/process assessment screening system) is no better than random selection of cases and therefore of no use in identifying cases that likely contain quality problems. Use of population-based screens—such as clinical indicators to identify providers whose care exhibits a surfeit of quality problems and therefore should be examined closely—is also likely not to prove to be cost-effective. Firstly, these screens' accuracy has never been demonstrated. Secondly, even if accurate they do not specify all of the major quality problems whose existence expert clinicians need to confirm.

Hospitals can use structured medical record (so-called 'peer') review alone to identify quality problems, but for ordinary use it is far less cost-effective than using an outcome/process assessment system to first find the cases on which expert reviewers should focus their attention. Nothing is as deadly to the little enthusiasm that doctors have for reviewing medical records than to search for needles (quality problems) in haystacks (mountains of medical records). With large numbers of medical records and few quality problems, reviewers can easily overlook those that truly exist. Hospitals that opt to use only structured medical record review to identify quality problems will still need to license or develop an information system to track, store, analyse and report review results. Further, screening provides substantial information for pattern analysis.

443 | Managing structured quality review

443.1 | Reasons for implementing structured quality review

Generally, structured quality review will be the basis of hospitals' quality management program. It provides the means to:

- assure the quality of care—by reviewing samples of cases and documenting that patients received care processes that they needed and wanted and that the hospital implemented properly these processes;
- improve the quality of care—by identifying quality of care problems and subsequently eliminating their root causes.

Structured quality review intends to survey care to document its quality and to identify systematically problems in its provision. Using appropriate, statistically significant, samples hospitals can construct quality scores to track the progress of their quality improvement efforts. Early on in their quest for quality, hospitals may use structured quality review to focus on particular areas of care to build their experience while developing their quality management program. However, hospitals' goal must be to institutionalise hospital-wide structured quality review, or some other equally or more cost-effective means of systematic surveillance of the quality of their care.

443.2 Hospital-based versus contracted structured quality review

Generally a hospital's quality management department operationalises its quality management program, including structured quality review. However, the hospital can also contract out this function, in whole or in part, to an organisation specialising in quality assessment (as occurs in the United States, but which is unknown at the present time in Australia). The hospital may want to enter into such a contract for one or more of the following reasons:

- to obtain an 'objective' assessment (one performed by expert clinicians who are not associated with the hospital);
- to avoid the cost of training doctors in or conducting structured quality review (which may be especially attractive to small hospitals);
- to overcome a shortage of expert clinicians to review medical records (because the hospital has only one visiting neurosurgeon for example, who obviously cannot review his or her own work).

Hospitals may contract out all of a quality management department's function (but obviously cannot contract out their responsibility for quality management), the entire quality assessment function, quality assessment of those areas for which it does not have sufficient clinicians to review objectively others' work, or an annual audit to ensure the accuracy and adequacy of its own structured quality review system.

443.3 Quality management department's role

A hospital's quality management department (QMD) is responsible for its quality of care surveillance systems, including structured quality review, even though it may delegate actual reviews to individual clinical departments or divisions. Specifically, the QMD operationalises the hospital's quality management policy and plans, and conducts and/or supports clinical departments in their conduct of structured quality review. The QMD must (assist clinical departments to):

- identify cases for review;
- track review cases;
- ensure that reviews are done in a timely fashion;
- monitor reviewers' performance;
- record, analyse and report review results;
- facilitate use of structured quality review results in practice; and
- evaluate structured quality review efforts.

Generally the quality management department is responsible for abstracting medical records to permit outcome/process assessment screening (especially when it operates the medical record function). However, hospitals can delegate this responsibility to clinical departments. In this case the quality management department is responsible for monitoring abstracters' performance to assure the quality of abstracts (and hence screening). It may also hire and train abstracters or assist clinical departments to perform these tasks. Clinical departments furnish the expert clinicians to review cases failing screens. The QMD trains reviewers or, at least, is a trainer of trainers in the hospital's structured quality review policies and procedures. Individual departments or the QMD may record reviewers' judgments and ask providers whose care reviewers question to respond to their determinations. The QMD is responsible for tracking review cases, ensuring the integrity of structured quality review databases, and for reporting results to the quality manager, hospital manager, quality management committee and the hospital's board of directors.

443.4 | Uniform structured quality review procedures

In collaboration with the medical staff, the hospital's quality manager must develop uniform structured quality review policies and procedures to ensure comparability of results and reports. Such policies and procedures must encompass all of the mechanics covered in this chapter. The hospital may want to retain an expert consultant to facilitate completion of this task. Structured quality review system vendors will likely also be willing to assist hospitals to complete this task.

Hospitals should codify their policies and procedures for structured quality review in writing and distribute them to all visiting medical staff members. They should describe the reasons for and sequence of structured quality review, as well as detail the procedures that the hospital uses to identify potential and confirm genuine quality problems, how the hospital investigates quality problems, and the types of remedies it uses or envisions for resolving particular quality problems.

443.5 | Training in structured quality review

Training doctors in structured quality review is an essential prerequisite for success. To save time and money and ensure a high level of training, the hospital may want to retain an expert consultant to develop training materials, train a core group of staff and doctors in the hospital who can train others, or conduct all of the training. An experienced consultant will already have developed and tested training materials that he or she can adapt to meet the hospital's particular circumstances. Structured quality review system vendors may also offer such training or training materials.

443.6 | Structured quality review management information system

Hospitals must install a quality management information system to track reviews through their various stages, and process, analyse and report quality assessments (reviews)— before they begin structured quality review. Commercially available structured quality review or other quality management information systems can fulfil these functions and some permit hospitals to tailor them to meet their particular requirements. Alternatively, a hospital could develop its own management information system if it has the requisite money and expertise. In any case, hospitals would be well advised to retain an expert consultant to assist them acquire or design and install a structured quality review tracking and reporting system.

Hospitals must incorporate the reports that the system will generate in policies and procedures and in training materials. Doctors and other practitioners engaged in and subject to structured quality review have a right to know how the hospital will process review results, how it intends to use this information and how it will protect confidentiality.

443.7 | Protecting the confidentiality of review information

Quality assessments are always sensitive and the potential for harm (directly to practitioners and indirectly to quality management as a result of practitioners' reactions to breaches of confidentiality) is ever present. Practitioners especially may be harmed unfairly if information is revealed out of the proper context. Hospitals must take appropriate steps to protect the confidentiality of quality assessment information. Their quality management policy must specify that such information is confidential, what steps medical and other staff members are to take to protect its confidentiality, and sanctions for employees who deliberately or carelessly give such information to persons not authorised to receive it.

443.8 | Evaluating structured quality review

Periodically the hospital should review and evaluate its structured quality review efforts to improve their cost-effectiveness. While this function is the quality management department's responsibility, involving an outside expert in this effort is likely to be most worthwhile. Further, the hospital can engage an outside firm to conduct an annual audit of its efforts, to authenticate, and to suggest ways in which it might improve, them.

444 | Deciding which medical records to review

444.1 | Structured quality review's goals in relation to sampling

Structured quality review has two goals:

- quality assurance—confirming that care is delivered to standards, to reassure patients of the hospital's quality of care;
- quality improvement—identifying quality problems so that quality managers can eliminate their root causes and prevent their recurrence, and hence improve the quality of future care.

Hospitals face a knotty question: Which cases to review? There is no one correct answer to this question. *The correct sampling strategy depends entirely on one's purpose and the system's state.* Hospitals can best achieve quality assessment's twin goals by reviewing all of their cases. However, most hospitals lack the resources for 100% review of cases unless they have machine intelligent electronic medical records, which none does now, or a very cost-effective outcome/process assessment screening system, which few have now. Moreover, even if hospitals are willing to review all of their discharges, they must decide which cases they should review first. Finally, 100% review of cases may not be the most cost-effective strategy. Reviewing fewer cases may allow the resources saved to be used elsewhere to improve quality to a greater extent.

Hospitals must avoid following the vaudeville drunk's example of looking for his lost car keys under the street lamp, 'because that is where the light is'. Hospitals need to look for quality problems where they can reasonably expect to find them, not where it is convenient to look for them. In the absence of information about where quality problems may lurk, focusing quality assessment efforts may be difficult. The information available about cases to be assessed influences one's sampling strategy and the extent to which final samples achieve one's intended purpose. The more, and the more accurate, information that is available, the better one can sample. At the start, hospitals may have little information about their cases or quality of care. As they build their experience, initial assessments' results can focus subsequent sampling strategies.

This section reviews briefly the implications for sampling of different levels of quality problems among hospitals' cases and of various sampling strategies. It describes the following sampling strategies:

- 100% review—simple and excellent, but most costly, strategy.
- 1-in-n samples—simple strategy, but not necessarily cost-effective; produces variable confidence intervals, for example for population estimates, test of significance of difference between proportions.
- Probability samples—excellent for quality assurance, but not necessarily best for quality improvement, purposes; requires tracking sampling fractions to produce population estimates.

- Targeted samples—excellent for identifying important quality problems (and hence quality improvement), but precludes quality assurance surveillance; requires targeting mechanism.
- Surveillance system—can achieve cost-effectively both quality assurance and quality improvement purposes; initial quality assessment results determine subsequent sampling strategy.

Sampling involves selecting cases from a population to represent that population in some way. The sampling strategy one chooses and how one implements it affects what one can say about the population based on the resultant data: one cannot make big statements based on small samples. Sampling and resultant analyses and their interpretation are a matter of statistics. Quality managers would be well advised to seek and use competent statistical advice if they decide to sample cases for quality assessment purposes and to make statements about the hospital's—and especially individual providers'—quality of care as a result. While sampling principles are well-established, their correct application can prove tricky. This section intends only to draw readers' attention to sampling's purpose and some general considerations of its application. Specific considerations (which depend on hospitals' purposes and circumstances) are beyond its scope.

444.2 | Quality problems' incidence and its effect on sampling

Reliable estimates of the quality of hospital care are hard to find. A working estimate is that 1–14% of cases exhibit one or more quality problems. For some types of cases the rate may be 30–50%. Including documentation problems could raise this rate to 80% or higher. Before the quality revolution, manufacturers might tolerate defect rates of 2–3%, that is, two or three defects per 100 products. Now manufacturers talk of defects per 1000 and, in some cases, defects per million, products. Toyota, for example, reports a defect rate of one in 100 000 for parts from its Japanese suppliers. At this rate a hospital with 10 000 discharges per year would deviate from practice and documentation standards only once per decade. Today quality problems likely occur in hospitals every day. If a hospital were to reduce the incidence of quality problems to seven cases per 1000 (seventy cases per year would exhibit a quality problem in a hospital with 10 000 discharges), finding those seventy cases, short of reviewing all cases, represents quite a challenge. To fix quality problems, one must first find them.

Ideally, hospitals should assess the care given to every patient. The only barrier is cost; not absolute cost but the value of such expenditures relative to that of other quality improvement activities. The lower the cost of 100% quality assessment, the greater its practicality. The number of cases one assesses and how one assesses them determines the cost of assessment. Structured quality review, which employs automated outcome/ process assessment screens, is the only practical means of assessing the quality of care of large numbers of cases. Mature quality assessment systems tie the assessment rate to the defect (quality problem) rate. As the defect rate rises, the system increases the assessment rate according to an explicit formula. In health care, experience is so limited that such systems have yet to be used routinely.

Hospitals' quality assessment rates are likely to resemble an inverted U. Early on, hospitals can expect cases to exhibit relatively high quality problem rates. They can identify many quality problems from relatively small samples. As they resolve these problems, they will need to assess the quality of a larger proportion of cases to find remaining quality problems. Eventually, hospitals can reduce rates of quality problems to the point where they can employ sophisticated surveillance systems that tie assessment to quality problem rates to both assure and improve quality.

444.3 | Sampling strategies

What is the best sampling strategy? The answer to this deceptively simple question depends on, for example, one's purposes, the information available at the time of the decision, and balancing sampling's costs and benefits. In general, one would expect the most appropriate sampling strategy to vary dynamically, further complicating already complex considerations. Additionally, hospitals may use a mix of strategies. For example, they may review 100% of some cases and samples of others, or may decide to review only high-risk cases and to sample from among them. As circumstances change, hospitals may change their sampling strategies. Over time, they will have populated a database with sampled cases.

The ultimate question for any sample of cases is: What does the sample represent? To answer this question, hospitals must track carefully what cases they reviewed when (and preferably why) they reviewed them. Simply adding cases to a database may jeopardise a hospital's ability to appropriately specify analyses and meaningfully interpret reports. Hospitals should not underestimate the difficulty of sampling, nor that of tracking samples in databases, nor that of using this information to produce meaningful reports. Quality managers would be well advised to think through these issues before embarking on widespread structured quality review, and to retain qualified help to assist them to complete this task.

444.4 | Sampling by time period

Hospitals interested in analysing trends, in types of quality problems among different types of cases for example, must establish statistically significant rates for each year or other appropriate period. If they sample cases, discharge date becomes an important sampling stratification variable. Ideally, one should measure providers' performance for a given type of case over a complete year, for two reasons: seasonality and the temporal distribution of cases. Over a year's course, hospitals' caseload and case mix, and their performance, may vary. For example, one might expect the number of pneumonia cases, and the disease's underlying causes, to vary by time of year. Thus, for example, basing care assessments on one quarter of a year might produce a different picture than basing it on a full year. Further, monitoring trends in quality becomes problematical if one year's data is from one calendar quarter and that for other years from different calendar quarters. Given the availability of complete data for several years, one can examine the potential for such seasonal effects.

Various strategies exist for temporal sampling and hospitals may use them if their circumstances permit. For example, hospitals with substantial numbers of cases might select cases discharged on ten randomly selected days of each month, rather than relying on random samples of cases, to ensure that samples represent the temporal distribution of cases and the quality of care. If the number of certain cases exhibits seasonal variation, hospitals may use admission date as a stratifying variable (one used to control the number and/or proportion of cases sampled in each month, for example). If a hospital infrequently sees certain types of cases, sampling to reduce the number assessed affects its ability to judge quality. If a quality problem in a case is a rare event (no matter how many cases the hospital sees), it must sample all or large samples of cases to find all of its quality problems. If cases or quality problems are rare events scattered throughout the year, one cannot sample by time period.

444.5 | 100% review

Most hospitals will be hard-pressed to start by reviewing 100% of their cases because of start-up and/or resource constraints. Although 100% review is ideal because it assesses quality in all cases (and permits simple construction of a quality score) and can potentially identify all quality problems, it is only practical with machine intelligent medical records or very cost-effective outcome/process screens. Because of the simplicity of its operationalisation, hospitals may want to consider reviewing 100% of cases for documentation adequacy or 100% of certain, high-risk, cases (see targeted samples below).

444.6 | 1-in-n samples

To start, a hospital may decide to assess the quality of a fraction of all or some types of its discharges. Such sampling's goal is to bring review loads into line with available screening and clinician reviewer resources; not to estimate population parameters from sample statistics (see probability sampling below). For example, hospitals may sample every tenth discharge, selected randomly. The number chosen is based solely on resource constraints and has nothing to do with sampling theory. While sample statistics can be taken as population parameters (rates of quality problems, for example), quality managers will need to calculate the estimate's confidence limits. Further, a simple sampling fraction, while easy to operationalise, may neither permit confident estimates of rates of quality problems for different types of cases nor be a particularly efficient sampling strategy.

Random selection of cases for review is necessary to avoid bias or implicit targeting. To improve quality problems' yield relative to quality assessment efforts, a hospital may want to exclude some types of cases (those not expected to exhibit a high rate of quality problems), and take a systematic sample of the remainder. A systematic sample is a convenient way of taking a 1-in-n sample. The hospital can array discharges by date and case number, and select every nth one. The sampling fraction determines the sample's starting point. For example, with a 1-in-10 sample, the hospital selects randomly a number between 1 and 10, starts with that case and then selects every tenth case on the list to create the sample. A systematic random sample of all or certain types of discharges is a useful way to begin because it can both identify quality problems and provide a rough baseline to target cases for review.

444.7 | Probability samples

Probability sampling's primary purpose is to improve the efficiency of data collection. From sample statistics (e.g. rates of quality problems in a given type of case), one can estimate the population parameter (rates of quality problems within the population of cases of interest) within known confidence limits. Given large populations, one can infer their characteristics from relatively small samples of their individual members. For example, from a properly constructed sample of 1600 people, one can estimate how a country's adults view an issue (within a few percentage points)—no matter how large the country's adult population. Simple probability sampling (e.g. 5% of discharges) may not be as efficient or powerful as stratified sampling. If the numbers of different types of cases and the incidence of quality problems in each type varies—which is almost invariably true—one must sample different fractions to maintain constant confidence intervals in resultant population estimates.

For quality assessment purposes, probability samples offer an excellent way of calculating quality scores to monitor the quality of care, but may not be the most efficient way to identify important quality problems (see targeted samples below). Further, sampling efficiency incurs a cost or risk: the confidence that one has in the sample statistic as an estimate of the population parameter. At what point does efficiency balance risk? The confidence that one can place in a sample statistic depends on a number of factors, including one's ability to estimate reliably the size of the population, to estimate reliably quality problems' incidence, and to draw random samples (thereby avoiding bias). Further, the cost of sampling (drawing and administering random samples) must be less than the cost of collecting data on cases not sampled, that is, those cases represented by the difference between the size of the population and of the sample. While one can calculate samples on theoretical grounds, possible interactions among factors make it advisable to model the decision effects of alternative sampling strategies.

444.8 Targeted samples

444.81 PURPOSE AND ADVANTAGES OF TARGETED SAMPLES

Targeting certain types of cases for review makes better use of scarce quality assessment resources than 100% review, simple 1-in-n samples and probability sampling schemes. It is most efficient at identifying important quality problems, but may neither identify them all nor provide reliable estimates of the distribution among different types of cases (see probability sampling above). Given that hospitals are more interested in finding and fixing quality problems than constructing reliable quality scores, targeting is the way to go. By focusing on certain types of cases (those that exhibit most of the important quality problems), a hospital can considerably reduce resource expenditures without losing too much information. The key issue is discerning on which cases to focus.

Targeting refers to reviewing certain types of cases defined by patients' health problems or care processes' characteristics; not cases' outcomes nor their providers (see below). It assumes explicitly that all cases are not equally worthy of review: some are more likely to harbour important quality problems than others and/or it is more important to document the quality of care for some types of cases than others. Stated generally, the goal is to identify those cases that exhibit quality problems whose resolution will yield the greatest increase in patient health status improvement at lowest cost (of identification and resolution) per unit gained. The following questions are relevant in targeting cases for review: What criteria to use to target cases? Where to get the information to operationalise criteria?

444.82 CRITERIA FOR TARGETING CASES

Hospitals can use any number of criteria to target cases for review; however, hospitals may lack the information necessary to operationalise them because of the inadequacies of their current clinical information system, for example. A useful approach is to identify cases with a principal diagnosis or a principal procedure that meets one or more of the following criteria:

- Proper medical care makes a large difference in health status improvement.
- Improper medical care can be very detrimental to the patient.
- There is a significant volume of cases.
- Care is relatively costly (per episode and/or in the aggregate).
- Care is complex, for example defined by the number and nature of interventions and/or of interactions among providers, and may give rise to a substantial number of quality problems.
- Care is of concern, for example people fear it may harbour quality problems because of recent news media revelations.

Using such criteria the hospital can identify which cases to target for review, referred to sometimes as 'high-risk' cases (because of their absolute or relative propensity to exhibit quality problems). For example, based on the above criteria acute myocardial infarction, coronary artery bypass graft and hysterectomy cases may qualify as high-risk cases; tinea pedis, low back pain and Fabry's disease cases may not.

444.83 INFORMATION FOR TARGETING

Hospitals can use one or more of the following three sources of information to focus their quality assessment efforts on cases most likely to exhibit quality problems that if resolved would likely yield the greatest improvement in quality:

- published reports, assuming that if other hospitals experience certain quality problems, one's hospital may have them too (which may or may not be true, and there is no guarantee that the published reports focus on the most important problems);
- structured group judgment methods, for example asking clinicians to identify cases that are common, where medical care makes a difference or is expensive, and whose care could be improved significantly;
- targeting techniques in which early quality assessment results are used to focus subsequent quality problem identification efforts (see below).

Use of published reports is a simple way to start, but they may not address the hospital's most important problems. Structured group judgment methods too are inexpensive but subject to the same types of error, which is inherent in the lack of empirical information to anchor judgments. Targeting techniques can be used to great advantage but require a commitment to structured quality review of statistically significant samples of all types of cases to learn in which types quality problems mostly lurk.

444.84 TARGETING CASES IN PRACTICE

The principal diagnosis* is a useful surrogate of a patient's health problem for quality assessment purposes. Common surgical operations are often targets for structured quality review. All operations must be indicated; operations performed that are not indicated, or that are contraindicated, are serious quality problems. Moreover, surgical operations can and do have untoward outcomes that may result from malprocesses and therefore represent quality problems. Surgical operations are easy to identify and hence to target for review. However, the ease with which hospitals can identify surgical operations, the general acceptance of their review, and their 'clear-cut' nature should not blind hospitals to the need to review other types of cases that may harbour more significant quality problems.

444.85 SAMPLING TARGETED CASES

To reduce further their review loads, hospitals with large numbers of high-risk cases can sample them for quality assessment purposes. Sampling theory is relevant here but not crucial. The primary goal is to identify as many quality problems as exist; not to generalise from the sample to the population. Probability sampling permits such generalisation within pre-established confidence intervals (see above), and is particularly important for pattern analysis. Hospitals have the option of sampling among all cases and/or periods (see above). In general, the best strategy is likely to be 100% review of targeted cases in given periods (e.g. every other month), rather than to draw a random sample of 50% of monthly discharges.

444.86 TARGETING CASES FOR QUALITY ASSESSMENT BASED ON OUTCOME

At first blush, targeting cases with maloutcomes seems a good strategy because their existence represents potentially bad care. However, this strategy poses several difficulties. Firstly, hospitals that do not abstract all cases may have difficulty identifying patients who suffered a maloutcome other than death. Deaths are a natural target for review and many hospitals review these cases routinely. The payoff, however, varies by case type. Patients who die unexpectedly represent a more significant potential quality problem than those

---

* The definition of principal diagnosis varies from country to country and even from state to state within Australia. In Australia, it most commonly refers to that condition which is the main reason for the patient's hospital episode. In the United States, it refers to: after investigation, the condition that resulted in the patient's hospitalisation.

patients whose death is wholly expected. While in principle sophisticated outcome/ process assessment screens can distinguish among deaths for review purposes, in practice they are not yet widely available. Other outcome review targets include nosocomial infections, blood transfusion reactions and adverse drug reactions. However, hospitals might examine many of these types of cases at the expense of examining cases that would reveal more significant quality problems. Moreover, poor quality care does not always result in a detectable maloutcome, even though the potential for one may be ever present. In summary, case type targeting is the best strategy for cost-effective quality problem identification.

444.87 AVOID TARGETING PROVIDERS OR DEPARTMENTS

Hospitals may be tempted to target providers rather than cases for review. This strategy is fraught with difficulties and hospitals would be well advised to avoid it. There is a natural tendency to target for review doctors whom colleagues or managers suspect are less good than others. In principle this is a very logical strategy; in practice it can be disastrous as a starting point. Since systematic quality of care information is lacking, notions of who is a good or a bad doctor may be based on invalid indicators. Given any doctor's quality problem rate, to what is it to be compared? Doctors treat different patient mixes; the normal quality problem rate for each type present in the mix may vary. While the problems identified may be real, they may exist in greater frequency among other doctors' cases. The targeted doctor could rightly complain of being singled out. Moreover, solutions to whatever problems are found may not depend on changing the targeted doctor. Population-based screens (see below) may be an acceptable way of targeting providers for review, but in general such screens' value may not be worth their cost.

Hospitals may wish to start structured quality review in one or two departments, for example, to learn from the experience before spreading it to others. This practice is acceptable provided that the reasons for starting with the designated department are clear and acceptable to their staff, and that the hospital plans to extend structured quality review to other departments in the future. Sometimes certain types of cases are treated mostly in a particular department; thus it becomes easier to target for review all of the cases treated by that department than hunt for the targeted cases throughout the hospital. This approach is practical but not necessarily ideal.

444.88 TARGETING PROVIDERS USING POPULATION-BASED SCREENS

Population-based screens are of unproven value and are likely not cost-effective. (See Part II, Chapter 8.) Population-based screens require: a population parameter, for example principal diagnoses, provider; an indicator, for example death rate; and a criterion, for example upper limit defined by two standard deviations. Thus, for example, using information abstracted from medical records, one could target Dr Smith's cases for review because his patients' death rate lies beyond two standard deviations of all discharges. The sensitivity and specificity of such approaches are largely unknown. A flaw that may be apparent in the example, however, is that Dr Smith may treat only terminal cancer patients. Examples of population-based targeting systems include: so-called severity of illness measurement systems, clinical indicators, and cost or resource utilisation models. Beyond accuracy, the utility of such systems depends on hospitals being able to translate the targeting information into cases pulled for review. The ability to make this translation will depend on the sophistication of the hospital's clinical information system.

To operationalise population-based screens, hospitals have to abstract some information from the medical records of all (or at least all of certain types of) cases. Further, once these screens have identified providers whose cases should be subjected to structured quality review, hospitals must abstract additional medical record information to operationalise case-based outcome/process assessment screens, or proceed directly with medical record review. The totality of this effort may be greater, and the yield less, than assessing directly the quality of high-risk cases for example (with outcome/process assessment screens). Finally, the appearance of targeting certain doctors' cases for review (rather than targeting types of cases, irrespective of provider) may be more trouble than it is worth (see above).

444.9 Surveillance systems

A quality surveillance system's purpose is to achieve as cost-effectively as possible quality assessment's twin goals of reassuring patients of the hospital's quality of care and of finding important quality problems. To accomplish these goals, quality-mature hospitals must have in place a system that:

- targets for review the types of cases that most likely exhibit important quality problems whose resolution will increase the amount of, and/or the certainty of achieving, achievable patient health status improvement;
- surveys appropriate probability samples of all other cases;
- uses information from both types of samples to retarget cases and/or change sampling fractions;
- adjusts outcome/process assessment screens' granularity to reflect the best balance of their sensitivity and specificity relative to identifying important quality problems.

Only hospitals that have instituted hospital-wide structured quality review can implement sampling strategies necessary to operationalise such a systematic surveillance system. Ideally, hospitals should assess periodically the quality of their care for all or statistically significant (probability) samples of discharges for all types of cases. They can then focus their subsequent quality problem identification efforts on those types of cases that exhibit the most important quality problems, to make the best use of their quality assessment resources. Periodic resampling is required to recalibrate this targeting mechanism. Ideally, hospitals should continue to assess the quality of care of some appropriate fraction of non-targeted cases to monitor quality problems' incidence, to permit a change in targets if necessary, and to reassure patients of the quality of their care. Hospitals have a variety of ways to target cases for review and of drawing probability samples (see above).

Structured quality review involves identifying all types of quality problems in a case (rather than a specific type, such as nosocomial infections for example). However, hospitals still have considerable latitude in choosing outcome/process assessment screens' granularity (which determines the fineness of the problems that screens attempt to identify). In general, the finer the screens, the more data—and hence abstracting time— required to operationalise them. Obviously, the finer the screens, the more chance they have of identifying all of the important quality problems in a case. Higher sensitivity rates may come at the expense of lower specificity rates, requiring clinicians to review a greater number of cases that fail screens—increasing quality assessment costs. Based on previous assessments or informed judgments, one might conclude that examining only limited aspects of care might identify most (or the most important) quality problems in a case, and result in greatly reduced assessment costs.

The correct balance between screens' sensitivity and their specificity depends on hospitals' circumstances. In general, early on one might expect hospital managers to be able only to control the types of screens used to review cases (e.g. documentation versus diagnosis-specific screens). Only after many years' experience will they be able to possess the technology and information to fine-tune individual diagnosis-specific screens' granularity to meet quality assessment cost-effectiveness goals. Obviously, the introduction of machine intelligent electronic medical records will obviate the need for such fine-tuning and will also improve immeasurably hospitals' ability to assure and improve the quality of their care. But for most hospitals widespread use of such systems is likely decades away.

445 Screening medical records for quality of care problems

445.1 Purpose of outcome/process assessment screening

The first step in structured quality review is the use of automated outcome/process assessment screens. Screening's central purpose is to focus expert clinician reviewers' attention on cases likely exhibiting quality problems, thereby reducing their workload to a manageable level and improving their productivity. It substitutes less expensive medical abstracter or nurse reviewer personnel for very expensive expert clinician reviewers. While screening is far cheaper per case than unaided medical record review, it can still represent a substantial cost if a hospital abstracts (screens) all of its discharges. Moreover, expert reviewers must examine cases failing screens, adding to the cost. Thus, efficient screening systems must have high sensitivity and specificity (goals which often conflict), and must achieve these goals with the least amount of abstracted medical record information, abstracted as efficiently as possible.

445.2 Nature of outcome/process assessment screens

Outcome/process assessment screens examine care comprehensively (rather than searching for a certain type of quality problem, e.g. nosocomial infections). They match what was done and achieved (processes and outcomes) to what should have been done and achieved for the types of patients whose quality of care they are designed to assess. Because outcome/process assessment screens model the complexities of medical practice, they must be automated (referred to sometimes as computerised) for reasons of reliability and economy. The most accurate outcome/process assessment screens are diagnosis- or procedure-specific and review criteria stem directly from explicit practice policies (or practice criteria) that take into account an individual patient's characteristics and his or her wishes. In the most sophisticated quality assessment systems, users can set screens' scope (the problems for which they search) and granularity (the fineness of the quality problems for which they search). Further, they can modify or add screening criteria, and/or collect other data. Part II, Chapter 8 details the basis for outcome/process assessment screens.

445.3 Availability of outcome/process assessment screening systems

Hospitals would be well advised to license an existing system rather than attempting to develop their own. Development of a valid, practical outcome/process assessment system could be expected to cost many millions of dollars and take several years. The only automated outcome/process assessment system available commercially is QSM (Quality Standards in Medicine, Boston, Massachusetts). (See Part II, Chapter 8.) This system contains diagnosis- and procedure-specific, and specialty, screens, for example those pertaining to obstetrics cases. Hospitals, therefore, can use it to screen all of their discharges. It also supports subsequent further review of cases failing screens. Tools like QSM are both cheap enough to screen all cases (essential for comparing providers who may treat only a small number of cases of any one type during a year) and accurate enough to be useful.

Several vendors license so-called empty-shell systems into which hospitals can enter their own outcome/process assessment screening criteria. They must either develop these criteria de novo or adapt existing criteria from other sources and, of course, keep them current. These efforts may involve considerable cost. Further, empty-shell systems are not as efficient as sophisticated purpose-built systems like QSM. Hospitals may also face such problems as interfacing or integrating the empty-shell system with other licensed systems or its own structured quality review management information system, for example to support structured medical record review, and to analyse and report review results.

445.4 Mechanics of outcome/process assessment screening

Outcome/process assessment screening depends on examining retrospectively individual patients' medical records to identify cases with potential quality of care problems (to be confirmed by subsequent structured medical record review). Hospitals should review designated cases as soon after the patient leaves the hospital as practical. The sooner a hospital identifies its quality problems, the sooner it can address and resolve them. Medical record documentation should be complete within seven days of discharge, including, for example, the doctor's completed discharge summary, principal diagnosis coding, and filed laboratory reports. Indeed, one purpose of a hospital's quality management program is to ensure that this (or a similar) goal is met.

The quality management department may abstract cases or delegate this task to individual clinical departments. For its efficient completion, hospitals must pay attention to the flow of records (for efficient record handling) and track this step in their medical record systems (to control workflow and track records). It is obviously most efficient to handle a patient's medical record only once after discharge. If a hospital finds it impossible to arrange its workflows to accomplish this end, at least it should have well-established workflows to code the principal diagnosis, check the documentation's completeness, and abstract recorded information and so on.

In hospitals with machine intelligent electronic medical records, outcome/process assessment systems can extract automatically the information they need to screen cases. Today hospitals lack such records. In some circumstances they can transfer automatically to the outcome/process assessment system what relevant machine intelligent information they do have—for example patients' demographics—and abstract the remainder. Specially trained medical record technicians or other personnel, for example nurses, must abstract from patients' medical records the information needed to operationalise screens.

Outcome/process assessment screens with smart abstracting systems (like QSM) serve questions to abstracters and limit them to the minimum number needed to assess the particular case, thereby reducing to a minimum the amount of abstracted information. To further improve abstracters' productivity, these abstracting systems can also collect simultaneously all other information that the hospital needs to manage quality and its operations. Presently, in some hospitals medical record personnel handle the patient's medical record multiple times after discharge to abstract from it the information the hospital needs to meet its various purposes. Such multiple handling and abstraction add considerable cost to patient care.

445.5 Data-based strategy for outcome/process assessment screening

Using fine screens at the beginning may result in a very high percentage of cases failing screens (and therefore requiring further review), defeating screening's primary purpose of sparing reviewers' effort (although it does allow reviewers to address the specific quality problems that screens identify). Many cases may fail screens because of documentation deficiencies. To avoid an excessive number of cases requiring further review for this reason, hospitals may wish to start by screening all or selected medical records for documentation adequacy. Such screening can involve not only the presence or absence of required documentation but also its adequacy, for example the recording of specific items in a patient's medical history (see below).

This strategy has the added advantage that it does not require further review of medical records by clinicians because the medical record abstracter can determine the presence or absence in the medical record of the required documentation. The quality manager can report screening results directly. Through this feedback to doctors, nurses and other caregivers, hospitals can improve the adequacy of their medical record documentation. With adequately-documented medical records, hospitals may proceed to screen for substantive quality of care problems at the initial level of granularity, progressing to finer screens as warranted.

445.6 | Documentation review

The oft-mentioned poor quality of medical records is not a barrier to, but rather a target of improvement opportunity for, structured quality review. Outcome/process assessment screens address both patient care and its documentation. Good documentation is essential for good patient care and for quality management. Poorly documented care cannot be of high quality, no matter how adequate the doctor's patient management may have been. For quality assessment and risk management purposes the rule is 'if it isn't in the medical record it wasn't done or observed'. For example if, according to practice policies, a patient should have been given a course of conservative therapy before undergoing lumbar laminectomy, either the surgeon should have documented the conservative regimen employed and noted its failure in terms of the patient's symptoms or he or she should have noted clearly why conservative therapy was not indicated in this case. Failure to document one or the other will cause the case to fail the lumbar laminectomy screen.

If documentation of conservative therapy is missing, the clinician who reviews the case (because it failed the screen) cannot determine whether or not it was tried (or was not indicated in the particular case, unless the patient's medical record documents symptoms, signs or signals indicating this fact). The reviewer must assume that the surgeon did not attempt indicated conservative therapy. The surgeon is then left to respond to the reviewer's determination that 'conservative therapy was indicated but not attempted'. He or she may well be able to state (or preferably document) that conservative therapy was indeed attempted and that it failed, indicating the need to operate. The need to respond, and convince reviewers that the performed surgical operation was indicated, provided an incentive for the surgeon to document adequately in future cases what care was given (and why it was or was not given). Failure to respond automatically results in the hospital considering that the operation was not indicated. If the surgeon convinces reviewers that the surgical operation was indicated, his or her documentation of the case remains noted to have been deficient. This type of information is useful when considering the surgeon's recredentialling or reappointment to the hospital's staff.

Documentation review intends to assess the medical record's completeness and its adequacy. Hospitals may start with this type of review before proceeding to outcome/ process assessment screening of patient care (see above). Automated screens can complete this review, saving both quality management department staff's and expert reviewers' time. Depending on screens' sophistication the review can check only for the presence or absence of required documentation or also its adequacy. Examples of items that screens can check and report include:

- principal diagnosis;
- secondary diagnoses;
- discharge summary;
- admission history;
- admission physical examination;
- report for each surgical operation and other major procedures;
- pathology report, if specimen taken at operation or biopsy;
- imaging reports, if any procedure done;
- progress notes.

445.7 | Building a database for structured outcome measurement

Outcome/process assessment screening can be the first step toward establishing a structured outcome measurement system. The extracted or abstracted information describes the index intervention. The index intervention is the process of care for which one wishes to determine the long-term outcomes. Subsequently, hospitals can follow-up patients, learn of their long-term outcomes and postindex intervention outcome influencing processes or events, and enter this information into the database that contains the initial information on the index intervention. Hospitals can analyse resultant data to validate and improve their practice policies and, to some limited extent, assess interventions' effectiveness.

445.8 | Results of outcome/process assessment screening

Outcome/process assessment screens produce substantial information for pattern analysis (see below) and, if the hospital uses this process to collect additional information, for other purposes as well. Screens divide cases into the following two categories:

- those that do not require further review because they:
  - —met all of the screening criteria for that type of case and, therefore, care can be presumed to have been appropriate (based on the screen's scope and its granularity);
  - —contain quality problems that do not merit further review and that can be analysed statistically, for example absence from the medical record of a pathology report for a specimen taken at surgical operation;
- those that exhibit potential quality of care problems and require further review.

Cases that require further review to confirm or deny quality problems' existence are said to have failed the screen. In cases failing quality screens, there is no implication that care was inadequate; only that a potential quality problem exists and that further review is required to determine whether or not a quality problem does in fact exist. Cases may fail screens because their circumstances are beyond those that the screen was designed to assess. Even the most sophisticated screens have limits because of designers' limited knowledge or cost-effectiveness considerations, and some cases' circumstances may exceed them. Customarily, the term 'potential quality problem' refers to findings of cases failing screens, because expert clinician review of cases failing screens is necessary to confirm a quality problem's existence.

446 | Conducting structured medical record review

446.1 | Purpose of structured medical record review

The second step in structured quality review is structured medical record review of cases failing outcome/process assessment screens. It intends to:

- confirm (or deny) quality problems identified by outcome/process assessment screens (and any others that expert clinician reviewers may also identify);
- determine whether any maloutcomes resulted more likely than not from malprocess and, if so, the putative malprocess involved;
- decide if malprocesses constitute an imminent danger to patients.

Structured medical record review's primary goal is to find facts—to identify genuine quality problems (to avoid chasing quality ghosts); not to find fault with individual providers (even though reviewers may find some providers' performance to have been deficient). Useful pattern analysis, structured quality review's third and final step (see below), depends first upon establishing firm facts. Once reviewers have established the fact of poor quality care, the hospital can then set about determining its root causes and taking steps to eliminate them. Deficient care may have one or more root causes that produce poor provider performance. Eliminating these causes will improve the quality of care. Poor performance may not be the provider's 'fault', but may stem from the system of care.

446.2 | Nature of structured medical record review

Structured medical record review is a systematic process for examining medical records to confirm or identify quality of care problems—care processes that if changed would increase patient health status improvement (and/or the certainty of its attainment), reduce cost or enhance patient satisfaction. It consists of the following five steps (see Figure IV-4-1 on page 591):

- Initial review (involving one or more reviewers) to confirm (or deny) a quality problem.
- If reviewers confirm (or identify) one or more probable quality problems, inviting the doctor who rendered the care (or other person responsible for the care process at issue) to comment on reviewers' determination, in a structured manner.
- Final review (involving the same or different reviewers) to confirm (determine a genuine) quality problem exists in light of providers' comments on reviewers' initial determination.
- Communication of final review results to responsible providers.
- The possibility of providers' appeal of reviewers' final determination, and ultimate adjudication of whether or not care exhibited a quality problem.

Specially trained doctors conduct structured medical record review. They review only those types of cases that they are competent to judge, for example involving the same specialty or subspecialty in which they were trained and practise currently. They review *all* aspects of the quality of an episode or continuum of care; they do not limit their review to a certain aspect of care, for example a surgical operation, or medical care defined narrowly as what doctors do or for what they are responsible. Expert reviewers:

- focus on cases with potential quality problems (cases failing outcome/process assessment screens);
- are trained in and use a structured approach to conducting such reviews;
- look for all quality problems, not just those associated with doctors;
- record findings in a systematic coherent fashion;
- are subjected to rational argument (rebuttal) by the providers of the care they criticise, so that quality problems must be substantiable and substantiated.

Usually, structured medical record review focuses on quality problems that pertain to patients' health status. Additionally, reviewers can identify process problems that increase the cost of, or diminish patient satisfaction with, care (whether or not they affect health status). The principles are the same.

446.3 | Mechanics of structured medical record review

446.31 NEED FOR PROCEDURES AND STRUCTURE

Hospitals must establish a written policy and standardised procedures for conducting structured medical record review, and provide the means to support its conduct and record and report review results. This section covers the following points:

- managing structured medical record review;
- who should review;
- matching cases to reviewers;
- training reviewers;
- conflicts of interest;

- when and where to review;
- how to review;
- tracking reviewers' performance.

446.32 MANAGING STRUCTURED MEDICAL RECORD REVIEW

The hospital's quality manager, in consultation with the heads of clinical departments, must formulate standardised procedures for conducting structured medical record review that pertains to all doctors in all clinical departments. The hospital's board must ratify these procedures and institutionalise them in policy, hospital by-laws and other procedures. These procedures must include reviewer training, recording forms, and all other aspects of conducting structured medical record reviews.

Structured medical record review must follow predetermined steps, with the findings of each step recorded on standardised forms which can be keyed into computer software (or recorded directly into a computerised system) for tabulation and analysis. In principle, expert systems can be easily designed to assist reviewers and record their judgments. In practice, clinicians who are unfamiliar with structured medical record review cannot usually cope with the added unfamiliarity of computer-aided review and are best asked initially to record their judgments using pencil and paper. Subsequently, hospitals can switch to computer-aided, paperless review systems.

In structured medical record review, doctors are the primary measurement system. Unlike machines, they suffer from fatigue and other psychological problems that impair the quality of reviews. Their job is to review medical records to confirm or identify quality problems. This task is a difficult one. The reliability and validity with which doctors confirm or identify quality problems depends on various factors. They include: the state of the records, for example organisation, legibility; the degree of systematisation of the review; experience in structured medical record review; readiness to do review; the number and complexity of prior reviews conducted in the particular review session; and the rate of cases examined that exhibit genuine quality problems.

Asked to review 100 cases, only the 95th of which has a quality problem, the reviewer may miss it. Asked to review 100 cases, 99 of which have a quality problem, will likely result in a higher proportion of existent problems being discovered. Moreover, problem-rich reviews may reduce the discovery rate of non-existent problems because there is no need to find something wrong to justify conducting the reviews. Thus the more likely that whatever medical records are reviewed contain genuine quality problems the better. The ability to concentrate on cases with identified potential problem care is the greatest advantage of outcome/process screening systems—others being improved accuracy and cost savings.

446.33 WHO SHOULD REVIEW CASES

Hospitals should involve all visiting medical practitioners in structured medical record review. Various alternative ways to involve them exist. For example, practitioners could rotate on structured medical record review committees, or each practitioner could be called on to conduct so many reviews per year. The process of structured medical record review is educational. Thus participating in—as well as knowing that one is subject to—structured quality review may be expected to improve care. The educational value of participation favours involving all medical practitioners. However, reviewing medical records for quality of care problems is a learned skill, and requires training and experience. This fact favours limiting reviews to clinician 'peers' expert at and experienced specifically in structured medical record review. One can resolve the apparent dilemma that these seemingly conflicting objectives pose by training everyone in structured medical record review and by reserving the most proficient or experienced reviewers for final response reviews (see below).

There is no implication that only doctors can be reviewers. Since doctors are primarily responsible for ordering or implementing most patient care, most reviewers will need to be medical practitioners. Other health care providers can serve on structured medical record review committees or provide individual reviews to provide additional perspective on the appropriateness of care processes. However, non-medical practitioners can never be the sole reviewers (because it is never appropriate to examine only the nursing or occupational therapy aspects of care, for example) and, for the most part, medical practitioners will constitute all or the majority of reviewers.

446.34 TRAINING REVIEWERS

Most doctors find it difficult to review medical records for quality assessment purposes and training for this task is essential. Clinicians interested in becoming expert reviewers must understand what is expected of them and receive training in the proper way to conduct reviews and record findings. The intent of such training is to make doctors competent reviewers, not experts in quality management. A quality management professional experienced in structured medical record review activities should design training materials. Hospitals may wish to contract for training material, training of trainers, or for all training. Vendors of quality assessment systems may provide such material and/or training. Training is best done in small groups so that trainers can assist doctors conduct them and constructively critique practice review results. Hospitals may want to establish a library of well-assessed test patient medical records to test reviewers' performance and to evaluate training's effectiveness.

Training must cover the hospital's policies and procedures, and the specific steps reviewers must follow and forms they must use, as well as introducing doctors to the concepts of quality management and principles of structured quality review. It is particularly important to train reviewers in what to look for, how to look for it and how to record findings on forms. Obviously, the simpler the procedures and forms, the less training is likely to be required, and the greater the reliability of recorded judgments. If the hospital uses committees to review medical records additional training in committee chairmanship and participation will probably be needed.

446.35 MATCHING CASES TO REVIEWERS

Doctors (and other providers) should review only those cases that they are qualified to review. Hospitals should establish criteria for medical records' reviewers in their quality management policies and procedures. These criteria should parallel their practice policies with respect to who may treat various types of patients, if such have been established. For example, only paediatricians should review paediatric cases. But who should review a case of acute myocardial infarction? Should it only be a cardiologist? What if a family practitioner—or a chest physician on call—treated the patient?

Hospital policy should assign cases for review based on established criteria relating to diagnosis and intervention, not who treated the patient. Quality assessment must always address the key issue of whether or not the right type of practitioner treated the patient given the circumstances. Thus, for example, hospital practice policies may state that it is acceptable for the on-call chest physician to treat the patient in an emergency, provided he or she called in a cardiologist at the earliest practical time. For quality assessment purposes, however, the hospital may insist that a cardiologist review the case. If quality problems exist with the patient's emergency care, it may be the system of care (which allows chest physicians to treat such emergencies) that is the problem rather than the treating physician. If panels or committees review cases, they may consist of eligible practitioners from two or more relevant disciplines, to provide greater perspective.

What type of practitioner should treat certain types of patients is always a sticky question. Cardiologists, for example, may do a better job of treating acute myocardial infarctions (AMIs) than internists or general practitioners. Then again, patient outcomes for certain AMI cases might be no different no matter what type of practitioner treated the patient, and the more specialised medical practitioners may order more tests and other interventions, increasing costs (but not improving outcomes). The answer to who should treat patients—and how they should treat them—is based more on tradition than science. Structured quality review and structured outcomes measurement are useful tools for providing information toward answering these types of questions.

446.36 CONFLICTS OF INTEREST

Reviewers should only review cases for which no real or apparent conflict of interest exists. The hospital's policies and procedures should be clear on this point. Reviewers have an obligation to identify such a conflict when it exists so that the hospital can assign another reviewer to the case. Obviously, a doctor cannot review his or her own care. In some instances, for example a neurosurgeon, the doctor may be the only neurosurgeon on the staff. In other instances only a limited number of doctors are qualified to review care and they work closely together. In such instances the hospital will have to contract for, or make other arrangements to obtain, objective reviews. While this may seem like an added expense or burden, biased reviews are not useful for quality management purposes and represent a waste of time and money. The alternative to objective reviews is to let quality problems remain hidden and unaddressed, which is likely an even more costly strategy.

446.37 WHEN AND WHERE TO REVIEW CASES

Quality management resource personnel should schedule cases for structured medical record review as soon as outcome/process assessment screens have identified those requiring further review. In practice, they may send reviewers weekly lists of cases to be reviewed. Automated quality review systems will perform this task. Reviewers should complete their assigned reviews promptly. The hospital's quality management policies should provide incentives (and, if needed, sanctions) to accomplish this end.

The quality management department should set aside a special area in which clinicians can review medical records. This space should be quiet and comfortable. It may consist of cubicles for individual reviewers, and/or a conference room for committees. The advantage of setting aside such space in the quality management department is that medical records do not have to be carried far, nor released from the confines of the medical records area. If the quality management department releases medical records to reviewers, its quality management personnel must enter such transfers into the hospital's medical records tracking system.

446.38 HOW TO REVIEW CASES

The quality management department (or individual clinical departments delegated to conduct reviews) should employ one or more resource persons trained in the specifics of the hospital's structured quality review process. This person may assist reviewers complete forms, if necessary on a one-to-one basis. This personal approach is very resource intensive, but can overcome any deficiencies in reviewer training. With properly trained reviewers, a resource person need only be on call to answer questions and solve procedural problems. In almost all cases the resource person will be responsible for notifying reviewers that they have cases to review, obtaining the records for review, arranging for reviewers to complete reviews, collecting completed review forms, checking their completeness, entering results into the computerised management information system, and managing the entire structured quality review process. Automated structured quality review systems may perform many of these tasks for the resource person.

449.39 TRACKING REVIEWERS' PERFORMANCE

Given the present state of the art, reviewers' performance is likely to remain an important variable in review results' reliability. Thus, structured medical review systems must analyse reviewers' performance and, if necessary, hospitals must adjust review processes, including the selection and training of reviewers, based on results. Improving the quality of review, like any process, depends on reducing variability.

Quality managers must track reviewers' performance and their quality management information systems must be capable of providing the requisite data. The simplest level of performance evaluation involves tracking the extent to which individual reviewers promptly complete their assignments and record clearly their judgments for all relevant points. Also of interest is reviewers' ability to reliably discern genuine quality problems. Structuring medical record review and training reviewers will help to ensure reliable reviews. The review process provides more or less information for judging reviewers' reliability, depending on how the hospital decides to conduct reviews and whether or not it conducts routine quality assurance or special studies of reviewers' reliability. For example, panel reviews offer a built-in way of assessing reviewers' reliability (see below). Quality managers can track the proportion of a given reviewer's cases in which he or she identifies quality problems that are confirmed by subsequent sequential reviewers (see below). Review quality assurance studies are required to identify reviewers who fail to identify or confirm quality problems that exist (as opposed to those who falsely label a case as containing a quality problem when in fact it does not). Methods for calculating and interpreting accuracy, statistics and intra- and inter-rater reliability scores are beyond this manual's scope.

446.4 | Numbers of reviewers and review structure

446.41 SOME OPTIONS FOR STRUCTURING MEDICAL RECORD REVIEWS

Hospitals have many options in organising the way they conduct initial reviews (of cases failing screens) and final reviews (of providers' responses to initial reviewers' determinations). They relate to the number of reviewers and the review structure. A hospital may choose one option for the initial, and another for the final, review. This section describes the following options:

- single reviewer;
- multiple independent reviewers (panels);
- sequential reviewers;
- committee review.

446.42 SINGLE REVIEWER

Usually a single clinician reviews the medical record of cases failing screens. This approach has the distinct advantage of economy—a single reviewer decides all review questions. However, it has the distinct disadvantage that results of individual reviews are likely to be more variable than those that result from the various forms of multiple reviews (see below).

A single reviewer may make a 'predetermination' before submitting cases with 'confirmed' quality problems to a departmental quality of care committee. This system has the advantage that a single reviewer disposes of cases failing screens that do not exhibit a genuine quality problem (e.g. because the particular case was beyond the screens' scope). It has the disadvantage that the single reviewer's judgment may not be reliable and that different individuals may differ in their judgments. This latter consideration is important because a given individual is likely to perform this review function for a limited time. The net result of such a system may be a large reduction in cases for the committee to review (high specificity) but reduced sensitivity (some cases with genuine quality problems escape the committee's attention).

446.43 MULTIPLE INDEPENDENT REVIEWERS: PANELS

The term 'panels' refers to an ad hoc collection of qualified reviewers each of whom reviews the case independently, with one reviewer acting as co-ordinator. Panels can consist of two to five, or more, reviewers. The co-ordinator is responsible for collecting the independent reviews, reconciling any differences that may exist regarding key findings, and completing the forms that constitute the completed review. Computerised systems exist or can be designed to take multiple individual reviews and produce automatically a co-ordinated review based on pre-established rules. The independent review of each case by multiple clinicians with pooling of or census judgments would likely yield superior assessments. Further, because several individuals each review the same cases quality managers can use panels' results to judge individual reviewers' reliability (performance). However, this approach may be prohibitively expensive for routine use.

446.44 SEQUENTIAL REVIEW

Sequential review, as its name implies, involves multiple reviewers examining the patient's medical record in sequence. The result of one step determines whether or not another reviewer is needed. The most common procedure involves three potential reviewers. If the first reviewer identifies or confirms a probable quality problem, a second qualified reviewer conducts an independent assessment to confirm (or deny) it, to avoid the simple possibility that the initial reviewer overlooked or misread something in the medical record, and to avoid asking providers whose care might have been criticised erroneously from having to respond accordingly. If the two reviewers disagree, a third independent reviewer breaks the tie. The third reviewer's decision is determinant (because it constitutes a 2:1 decision).

This form of review is more efficient than independent panels, and also provides the advantage that at least two experts agree that a quality problem exists before seeking providers' comments. It reduces false positives (cases stated to exhibit a quality problem that in fact do not have one) but, compared to panels, may increase false negatives (cases with missed quality problems) because the first reviewer's judgment of 'no quality problem' completes case review.

446.45 COMMITTEES

Committees are a tried and true method for conducting medical record review. Like panels, they have the advantage that several clinicians can review the same case, and the added advantage that reviewers can discuss the quality of care before deciding whether or not the case exhibits a quality problem. However, committees can only function like panels if committee members independently review the case, which is impossible within the constraints of the meeting without copying the entire medical record. Moreover, committees require all members to be in the same place at the same time, posing scheduling problems. In contrast, members of panels can review cases at their convenience. Committees may be best reserved for response (and appeal) reviews where discussion of practices and evidence may be most fruitful to determining whether or not a case exhibits a genuine quality problem.

446.5 | Initial review of cases failing screens

446.51 REVIEWERS' TASKS

Structured quality review improves the effectiveness and efficiency of medical record review in two ways. It:

- permits expert reviewers to focus on those cases that exhibit potential quality problems and displays those problems to reviewers;
- structures the subsequent review of cases failing screens.

Reviewers' task is to:

- identify (confirm) all quality problems—deviations from appropriate care processes or practices, including care documentation—whether or not they led to a maloutcome;
- determine who was responsible for any deviation—lack of an action or an inappropriate action—that seems to have occurred, so that the person responsible for the process in question (e.g. doctor, chief nurse, head of pharmacy) can comment on reviewers' determination;
- decide if any maloutcome that the patient may have suffered was more likely than not the plausible result of malprocess and, if so, identify the putative process;
- consider whether or not any malprocess represents an imminent danger to patients.

446.52 CORRECT APPROACH TO IDENTIFYING QUALITY PROBLEMS

Reviewers must use implicit criteria when reviewing cases failing outcome/process assessment screens. If objective criteria exist for assessing the quality of care for the type of case being reviewed, they would have been built into screens (assuming that sophisticated screens are in use). Reviewers must determine if a potential quality problem identified by screens is a genuine quality problem in the particular case (which means the reviewer must rule out any circumstances that exist in the case which are beyond screens' ability to assess that would suggest that care was appropriate in the particular case). Reviewers, who are usually medical practitioners, must address all aspects of care and assess all quality problems; not just confine themselves to the 'medical' aspects of care (those for which they believe doctors are responsible)—for example the patient's surgical operation if the reviewer is a surgeon. Structured quality review's goal is to identify *all* quality problems in a case so that the hospital can identify and eliminate their root causes. In structured quality review, the clinician reviewer is the principal instrument for identifying genuine quality problems, no matter who is responsible for them.

Structured quality review intends to identify all of the deficiencies and problems that may have existed in the provision of hospital care. If medical reviewers do not address all aspects of care and attempt to identify all quality problems, they will remain hidden. For example, the reviewer may notice that a patient with pneumonia was not given antibiotics within four hours of admission, the hospital's standard of care. The reviewer noted that the admitting medical officer had written the medication order on admission. Certainly the doctor had acted correctly; equally certainly, care was deficient (assuming no recording error).

The reviewer should clearly note the problem, not ignore it because the doctor acted correctly. In the example's case, he or she should note: 'patient did not receive antibiotics within four hours of admission', and, if discernible, the responsible process and/or entity, for example, 'drug not dispensed (pharmacy responsible)'. Analysis of many cases may reveal this particular problem to be a common one. Subsequent investigation may reveal that all of the patients were admitted at night, when the pharmacy was closed. A solution to the problem would be to keep the pharmacy open twenty-four hours a day; there may, of course, be several other solutions. In this example, reviewers identified a quality of care problem beyond the action or responsibility of any individual medical practitioner; a real problem nonetheless.

The quest for quality improvement is the correct mind-set for reviewing medical records. Reviewers must not only assess care based on what was known or done, or could have been known or done, at the time of care provision, but also be mindful of—and note—any shortcomings of existing limitations or problems in existing care processes. For example, one could criticise a doctor for admitting a patient to the hospital whose condition did not warrant admission. However, it would be unreasonable to do so if this criticism is based entirely on information that came to light and could only have been known after the patient had been admitted. Nevertheless, an inappropriate admission to the hospital does constitute a quality problem. However, the correct mind-set must be to determine what, if anything, could be done to provide the admitting doctor with the information to judge better whether or not admission is needed at the time that he or she must make this decision; not to criticise him or her for making a decision that was reasonable given all of the information that was available at the time, even though, in retrospect, it turned out to be a wrong decision. The right question is: How can we improve a process that led to a maloutcome (an inappropriate admission in the example's case)?

446.53 MECHANICS OF CONFIRMING (OR DENYING) QUALITY PROBLEMS

For each review case, the individual clinician who (or the committee that) will conduct the review should have screening results and the patient's medical record. Screening results should list screens used and should also list (and describe in relevant detail) quality problems that they identified. Reviewers should have immediate access to screening criteria and other reference documentation, if they need to refer to them. To speed the review, a quality management resource person can flag the places in the medical record relevant to each of the reasons that the case failed screens. Figure IV-4-2 on page 616 shows a QSM case summary that indicates the reasons a case failed quality assessment screens and requires further review. Chapter 8 in Part II describes QSM.

The screening printout may suggest that the surgical operation the patient received was not indicated, for example—a potential serious quality of care problem. The reviewer must examine the patient's medical record to see if the surgeon stated why he or she operated on the patient, that is, recorded an indication for the operation. If not, the reviewer should note the quality problem 'no indication documented'. It is the surgeon's responsibility to document the indication, not the reviewer's to discern it. If the surgeon documented the indication, the reviewer must determine whether or not the screen encompassed it (rare indications may be beyond its scope) and, in either case, determine whether or not the clinical findings in the medical record substantiated it.

In the case that the indication was beyond the screen's scope, the reviewer might note that the operation was indicated and state what was the indication (and possibly note that the particular indication was beyond the screen's scope). In the case that the indication was within the screen's scope, the reviewer may find that the patient's clinical findings do not support the documented indication, and (barring the case in which the surgeon omitted relevant findings from the patient's medical record) the surgeon would seem to have no grounds for having performed it. In this latter case, the surgeon should have the opportunity to mention relevant findings that he or she did not record (a documentation problem at the very least) and/or explain why he or she performed the operation (see below, 'Provider's response to reviewers' determination').

The reviewer must address each reason that the case failed screens that requires confirmation of a quality problem's existence and record results on standardised forms. Some reasons, for example 'no pathology report for a specimen taken at operation', may not need confirmation, but would, nevertheless, appear on the screening report. Which

```
Printout: 01/01/95        QSM Case Summary              Page: 1


QSM Screen(s): Hernia repair, medical, surgical, anesthesia

M R Number: 005412                              LOS: 9 days
Discharge Date: 12/12/94                        Sex: F
Admission Time: 12:12                           Age: 72 years
Disposition: Home or self care
Principal Diagnosis: 552.01 REC UNIL FEM HERN W OBST
Provider: 412
Principal Procedure: P53.29 UNIL FEMOR HERN REP NEC
Surgeon: 201
Anesthesiologist: 165
_____

REASONS FOR PEER REVIEW
Treatment Selection
     Hernia repair
         No bowel resection performed: gangrene present
Outcomes to be reviewed
     Hernia repair
         LOS > 5 days: incarceration or strangulation managed
         without bowel resection
     Surgical
         Unscheduled return to operating room for a further procedure
_____

OTHER REASONS
Diagnostic workup
     Hernia repair
         No pelvic exam
         No rectal exam
Outcomes to be monitored
     Medical
         Positive urine culture > 24 hrs after admission; not positive
         or can't tell on admission; Rxed or negative by discharge
     Anesthesia
         Can't tell about oxygen saturation during operation
Discharge Status
     Medical
         Temperature >= 37.8°C (100°F) p.o. in 24 hrs prior to discharge
     Surgical
         No, or can't tell about, instructions for wound dressing:
         healed or healing wound at discharge not established
         Can't tell about surgical wound complications
```

Figure IV-4-2 *Quality Standards in Medicine case summary*

failure reasons require confirmation is a policy decision. Ideally, for a potential quality problem that requires confirmation, the reviewer should state whether or not it is a quality problem, for example by marking the appropriate box on the form. If a reason that the case failed the screen is not a quality problem, the reviewer should state briefly why it is not. If it is a quality problem, he or she should state what exactly is the problem, which may simply be confirmation of the screening report reason (e.g. by checking a box) or a modification of it (e.g. by penning an elaboration of the printed reason).

The reviewer may also want to review the chart to identify quality problems beyond those identified by outcome/process assessment screening. Sophisticated diagnosis- or procedure-specific screens are likely to be quite sensitive and hence identify all or almost all important quality problems in a case. With their use, reviewers are likely wasting their time hunting for additional quality problems because the yield is unlikely to be commensurate with the additional effort. If outcome/process assessment screens have low sensitivity, they may lull reviewers into a false sense of security, and they may not look for quality problems that screens fail to identify, and these problems will remain hidden. For this reason, quality managers must know screens' sensitivity. If a reviewer does spot an additional quality problem (especially of a type that screens do not encompass), he or she should note it on the review findings form. This information (and reasons cases failed screens but do not exhibit a quality problem) is useful not only for disposing of the case in question, but also in screens' further development.

The types of potential quality problems reviewers must confirm (listed on the screening report) depend obviously on the specific outcome/process assessment screens used. For readers' information, we list below the essential types of questions that screens (and hence reviewers) might address. They are illustrative, not exhaustive.

Intervention planning
- For non-emergency admission, was each phase of the treatment planned appropriately?
  —Were tests performed prior to admission when appropriate?
  —Before or on admission was the patient's expected discharged status determined and appropriate plans made? For example, if the patient was expected to require discharge to professional home care or to a nursing home, were such arrangements made on admission, to permit the shortest possible hospital stay and to prevent patients languishing on wards?

Diagnostic workup, including inferences based on test results and other diagnostic information, for example consultations
- Was the patient investigated adequately? If not:
  —What tests should have been, but were not, done?
- Was the patient diagnosed correctly (e.g. right tests, wrong inference)? If not:
  —What was the correct diagnosis?
- Was the patient's problem investigated promptly (or was there delay in diagnosis)? If so:
  —What interventions were delayed?
- Were any non-indicated tests done? If so:
  —Which tests were non-indicated?
  —Why were they non-indicated?
- Were indicated tests done too often? If so:
  —Which ones?
- Were any tests done in the hospital that could have been done prior to admission? If so:
  —Which ones?
- Were necessary consultations obtained in a timely manner? If not:
  —What consultations were not obtained that should have been obtained?
  —Which needed consultations were delayed?
  —Which consultations were unnecessary?

Treatment selection, including informed consent

- Was hospital admission indicated? If not:
  —Why not?
- Was treatment (including surgical operations) indicated and in accordance with the patient's wishes? If not:
  —Which treatments should have been selected?
  —Why should these treatments have been selected?
- Was treatment initiated promptly (or was there delay in treatment)? If so:
  —What interventions were delayed?
- Were any non-indicated treatments given? If so:
  —Which ones?
  —Why were they non-indicated?
- Were indicated treatments given in the appropriate amounts or intensity? If not:
  —Which ones?
- Were treatments carried out in the right place? If not:
  —Which ones were carried out in which wrong places?
- Was the patient informed properly of interventions' expected benefits and risks? If not:
  —What was done improperly, or not done at all?
- Was the patient's consent documented properly? If not:
  —What was done improperly, or not done at all?

Treatment implementation, including management of complications

- Were treatments implemented properly? If not:
  —What was done incorrectly?
- Were all abnormal findings investigated (e.g. elevated serum potassium) and explained (e.g. did the doctor document the actions he or she took consequently)? If not:
  —What was not followed-up or explained satisfactorily?
- If maloutcomes ('complications') occurred, were they more likely than not the result of malprocess (error of omission or commission)? If they are the result of malprocess:
  —Which process(es) was (were) implemented improperly?
  —What should have been done differently?
- If maloutcomes occurred, were they managed properly? If not:
  —What should have been done differently?
- Was the patient's length of stay appropriate? If not:
  —What should have been done differently?

Patient instructions and follow-up

- Was the patient instructed properly at separation, for example about risk factors, medications, follow-up? If not:
  —What was missed?
  —What was done incorrectly?
- At separation, had appropriate follow-up arrangements been made? If not:
  —What was not done that should have been done?

Preventive interventions to reduce the risk of, or the severity of disease if, recurrence of the health problem

- Did the patient receive, or was he or she scheduled to receive needed preventive interventions? If not:
  —Which interventions should have been, but were not, given or scheduled?

446.54 DETERMINING WHO SHOULD RESPOND TO REVIEWERS' DETERMINATIONS

Reviewers must identify who is or might reasonably be expected to be responsible for the process that gave rise to an identified quality problem. Reviewers (or alternatively quality management department staff) can complete this task simply by classifying the type of quality problem, for example medical care, nursing care, housekeeping. The hospital's structured quality review management information system can then send the responsible person—for example patient's doctor, chief nurse or head of housekeeping— a copy of the reviewers' determination and invite his or her comments (see below). The system automatically links the type of problem with the person the hospital has decided is responsible for the processes or practices that produced it (which does not imply that the so-called responsible entity can necessarily determine the problem's root causes nor resolve them even if known—see Part II, Chapter 8). As a rule, only one entity is usually responsible for commenting on a particular quality problem.

Take the case of a sponge left in the patient's abdomen during a surgical operation. If Dr Smith failed to order a sponge count, Dr Smith is the responsible entity. If he ordered the count but Nurse Jones failed to do it and Dr Smith failed to check, two problems exist. Nurse Jones did not do the count and Dr Smith failed to check that it was actually done. Even though Nurse Jones failed to count the swabs it may not be appropriate to blame her for the deficiency. For example, subsequent pattern analysis may reveal this or related problems are common. Further investigation may reveal that operations are scheduled too tightly. Better scheduling would likely reduce the problem. Nurse Jones could not do her job properly because she was not allowed to, not because she was incapable of doing it under proper circumstances.

446.55 LINKAGE OF MALOUTCOME WITH MALPROCESS

For each maloutcome—for example, death, inadvertent laceration of an organ, nosocomial infection or fall from bed—reviewers should decide if it resulted more likely than not from malprocess (as opposed to being an inevitable consequence of the patient's disease and/or inherent in its treatment). The implication of a 'more likely than not' finding is that the maloutcome was potentially preventable and that some change in care processes will likely reduce the chances for its future recurrence. Reviewers should also identify the process or processes they believe led or contributed to the maloutcome.

Sometimes reasons for maloutcomes are unclear. Reviewers should only attribute them to malprocess if a plausible, preferably scientifically substantiated, connection exists between it and the maloutcome. Reviewers' findings can be subjected to pattern analysis (see below). Such analysis can examine the relationship between maloutcomes' occurrence and reviewers' findings about their association with malprocess to permit quality managers to determine if a genuine quality problem exists whose root causes they should investigate, if not obvious. Maloutcomes attributable to supposed malprocesses will decline if hospitals rectify such malprocesses and eliminate their root causes.

446.56 IMMINENT DANGERS TO PATIENTS

Based on their assessment of review findings, reviewers should indicate whether or not imminent danger to patients or a potentially serious quality problem exists. The implication of such determinations is that the hospital must have in place the machinery— authority and mechanisms—to quickly judge their merits and, if warranted, to act immediately.

Hospitals must have the ability to act decisively to remove an imminent danger created, for example, by an impaired doctor who may expose a patient to avoidable serious harm. For example, a surgeon who caused a patient's death and whom reviewers believe acted negligently may represent an imminent danger to other patients. An imminent danger suggests the need for immediate action, based on a single case, for example immediate suspension of privileges in the case of the surgeon. However, the hospital manager cannot act decisively without having in place the machinery to confirm imminent dangers and the authority to take necessary steps to eliminate them. Recklessly suspending a surgeon's privileges because of a disgruntled colleague's biased opinion is an obvious danger to the surgeon's reputation and the hospital's quality management program. But allowing impaired surgeons to continue to operate is a danger to patients and the hospital's financial wellbeing and reputation.

A finding of a potentially serious quality problem is less urgent than an imminent danger, but draws the quality manager's attention to the need for prompt action. It suggests that the quality manager decide immediately the need to complete promptly a focused investigation to determine if a serious problem exists or not. Delay, as might occur through the normal course of the hospital's structured quality improvement process, would expose patients to avoidable serious harm if a genuine and serious quality problem exists. Again, if investigation confirms the existence of a serious quality problem, the hospital manager must have in place the machinery to take swift action to resolve it.

446.57 RISK MANAGEMENT ISSUES

For risk management purposes, the hospital may ask reviewers to estimate the risk to which any malprocess may have exposed the patient, even if he or she did not suffer a maloutcome, and to grade its seriousness. For example, a serious breach of theatre protocol could have led to the patient's death, but luckily the patient neither died nor suffered any discernible harm. Nevertheless, risk managers are interested in knowing that the situation that occurred represents a serious risk to patients' (and potentially the hospital's financial) health. Reviewers may grade the extent of (actual or potential) harm in terms of its duration (e.g. temporary or permanent) and seriousness (e.g. amount of health status loss). More simply, reviewers may grade quality problems as major or minor (based on their implicit assessment of its potential to reduce patients' health status). These classifications may be useful for analytic purposes but can be omitted, since they are not central to structured quality review's purpose (identifying quality problems to permit their resolution) and are often unreliable.

446.58 ABSTRACTION ACCURACY

Sometimes abstracters will make errors that result in cases failing screens inappropriately, for example because of a simple keystroke error, misinterpreting something in the medical record, or conflicting documentation. Reviewers should be alert to this possibility and check that the reason the case failed the screen is in fact valid. If reviewers discover abstracters' errors, they should note the true situation on the review form and describe the type of apparent error. This correction permits the quality manager to update the case file so that it truly reflects the care provided, to monitor documentation issues, and to track abstracters' performance, with a view to improving the abstracting process (which may involve changing medical record policies, retraining abstracters, improving abstracting software, for example).

446.59 RECORDING REVIEW RESULTS

Reviewers should be responsible for recording review results on standardised forms designed for this purpose, or entering them directly into a computerised system if the hospital uses one to support structured medical record review. The quality management department should make available a quality management resource person to facilitate forms' proper completion. If the hospital does not use a computerised system to support structured medical record review, this person should enter review results recorded on forms into its structured quality review management information system immediately after the reviewer completes them. The system should be capable of accepting both structured items, for example quality problem confirmed, yes/no; and unstructured items, for example a description of the problem's exact nature.

446.6 | *Providers' response to reviewers' determinations*

Hospitals should give providers or others responsible for care processes that reviewers criticise (i.e. draw attention to probable malprocess or maldocumentation) the chance to respond to such criticisms. The opportunity to provide feedback is vital to establish facts. Reviewers can overlook or misread, misinterpret or misunderstand something in the medical record, which may be a documentation deficiency or lack of diligence on reviewers' part. Providers or other responsible persons may offer reasoned and reasonable explanations as to why what was done was appropriate (which may shed new light on care processes, thereby affecting reviewers' judgments). The structured medical record review process should encourage doctors and others responsible for care processes to cite literature or research reports in support of their responses, since reviewers rarely know everything. The goal is a rational exchange of views of the evidence regarding care's appropriateness, rather than adamant statements based on no rational evidence; light rather than heat.

For example, reviewers may determine that a doctor failed to obtain a needed imaging study and that a nurse gave the wrong dose of a drug. The structured quality review process should transmit reviewers' determinations to the responsible entity: the patient's doctor (the lack of the needed test) and the chief nurse (the wrong dose). The hospital's structured quality review management information system should be able to send these notices automatically (to save costly clerical time). The process should give each party a fixed time to respond (e.g. thirty days), with the possibility of seeking extensions (e.g. for vacations, need to obtain additional information to respond). The doctor's response may reveal that the test was done prior to the admission, but that he or she failed to document this fact in the patient's hospital record (a documentation problem), or that he or she does not consider the test necessary for the particular type of patient involved, or that he or she agrees that the test should have been done. The chief nurse, having checked the situation, may concede that the nurse gave the wrong dose because he or she misread the doctor's writing, and that so would anyone else.

Hospitals should provide a structured format to respond to reviewers' determinations—either a printed form or instructions about how to respond and what items to cover in the response. At the end of the allowed period, for example thirty days, if a provider has not responded he or she should be reminded about the chance to respond and a new date for the response should be set. If the provider fails to respond after being reminded of the chance to do so, reviewers' initial determinations become final. In this case the quality manager should notify the provider or other responsible person of the determinations' finality. Hospitals with completely automated structured quality review systems and local area computer networks can accomplish this exchange of information in a paperless fashion.

Providers may occasionally claim they never received the request to comment (including reminders) or were away for several months (and failed to mention this fact to anyone). In such cases the hospital must decide whether or not to reopen the case. The possibility exists for truly extenuating circumstances, but such option should be exercised infrequently to avoid taking away the incentive to respond in a timely manner and to provide a complete picture of the quality of care being delivered. Failure to respond to quality assessment findings is itself a quality problem because without the ability to establish facts in a timely fashion, hospitals cannot improve the quality of their care.

446.7 Review of providers' responses: final determinations

The final review's purpose is to confirm the facts about patient care processes; to determine whether or not a genuine quality problem exists in light of providers' and others' responses to reviewers' initial determinations. The same or different reviewers can perform this final review (referred to sometimes as the response review). Hospitals may want senior reviewers (e.g. department heads) to perform this function, or may assign it to the departmental quality improvement committee. If more than one responsible party was asked to comment on reviewers' initial determinations, for efficiency purposes hospitals should collect all of them (or wait until the period allowed for response has elapsed) before conducting the final review. The hospital's policies and procedures should specify who reviews providers' responses.

Reviewers should consider separately each provider's response (if multiple). They should use a structured format to consider and record their opinions. Reviewers should answer the following types of questions, for example. They are illustrative, not exhaustive.

Care and its documentation

- In light of providers' responses to reviewers' initial determination, were care processes appropriate? If yes:
  —What new information changed reviewers' initial determination, for example:
  · Reviewer misread something in the medical record. (A reviewer performance problem that the quality manager must track.)
  · Provider obtained the test, but did not record this fact, and the findings, in the patient's hospital record. (A documentation, but not a care, process problem, that the quality manager must track.)
  · Provider supplied a journal article that indicated the test was not needed for the type of patient involved. (The quality manager must track the need to change the hospital's practice policies and/or educate reviewers.)
- If care processes were not appropriate (a genuine quality problem exists):
  —What exactly was the quality problem and who is (or ought to be) responsible for the malprocess that gave rise to it, for example:
  · The nurse misread the doctor's order and gave the wrong dose. (The quality manager must track such errors with the view of finding some way to reduce their frequency of occurrence.)
  · The doctor's orders were illegible and this fact should be brought to his or her attention. (The quality manager should track this problem with the view of drawing reviewers' attention to the need to delve behind the obvious when identifying initially quality problems—e.g. the initial reviewer should have seen that the doctor's order was illegible and included this fact as a quality problem in his or her initial determination—and of finding some way of avoiding bad penmanship—e.g. computerised order entry, if it turns out to be a common and serious problem.)
- For risk management purposes an assessment of the extent to which the malprocess (including maldocumentation) affected (could have affected) the patient's health status.

Evidence
- What types of evidence did the respondent (provider or other responsible entity) supply in support of his or her responses? (Useful to track the basis of responses, and how often each type influenced reviewers, to improve the structured quality review process.)
- Did the initial reviewers misread, misunderstand or misinterpret the medical record? If so:
  —What was misread? (Useful for educating reviewers and, possibly, revising medical record policies.)
- Did the provider or other respondent give new information (not in the medical record originally)? If so:
  —What was this new information? (Useful for revising medical record policies.)
- Did the provider forward documented evidence that care was acceptable, for example a journal article? If so:
  —What was the journal article and its essential points? (Useful information for considering changes to practice policies or educating initial reviewers.)
- Did the provider make a compelling argument that care was acceptable? If so:
  —What were the essential points of the argument? (Useful information for considering changes to practice policies or educating initial reviewers.)

If a provider cites studies in support of his or her patient care, reviewers must assess their relevance and validity, preferably using structured protocols designed for this purpose. Such assessment might necessitate obtaining the opinion of an expert in research methods. Providers can sometimes misunderstand results or rely mistakenly on conclusions from inadequate studies.

If response reviewers find one or more quality problems, despite or in light of the provider's response, they give a reasoned explanation for this determination. The quality manager should forward reviewers' final determinations to each provider who responded to reviewers' initial determinations and any other that these responses revealed were responsible for malprocesses (e.g. in the above example's case, the doctor whose illegible handwriting led to a nurse giving the patient a wrong dose of medication). Unless the hospital permits the provider to appeal, these determinations are final. The hospital should enter reviewers' final (like their initial) determinations into the hospital's structured quality review management information system to permit case tracking, and data analysis and reporting.

446.8 | Appeals of reviewers' final determinations

Hospitals would be well advised to include an appeals procedure as part of their structured quality review process, to handle those cases in which reviewers say a genuine quality problem exists but the responsible provider is adamant that one does not exist. With a well-designed structured quality review process, one would expect less than 1% of cases reviewed initially to merit appeal.

If the hospital permits an appeal of final (response) reviewers' determinations, it should establish policies and procedures for such an appeal. They should specify a maximum period in which a provider can lodge an appeal and, in general, parallel those for responding to reviewers' initial determinations. In particular, providers or other individuals responsible for processes that gave rise to a quality problem must spell out the bases for their appeal. For example, the provider must argue the specifics of the case in terms of the interpretation of facts and inferences based on them.

Appeals' reviewers should be different persons than those who conducted initial or response reviews. A hospital-wide committee or an expert outside of the hospital (if it conducts its own structured quality reviews) may decide appeals. Appeals' reviewers should complete a structured review (appeal) format designed to answer the same types of questions considered in a final (response) review. Appeals reviewers will likely emphasise the relevance and validity of any scientific evidence that the provider gave in support of the appropriateness of care. A hospital must promptly notify the appellant of an appeal's outcome, and update its structured quality review management information system accordingly. Fully-automated structured quality review systems will perform these functions based on entering the appeal's results.

446.9 | Quality assessment (structured quality review) results

Quality assessment's (structured quality review's) purpose is to establish facts: to identify genuine quality problems. It is not to condemn doctors or anyone else. Separate procedures must exist to discipline doctors, for example for misconduct or other breaches of duty. Quality assessment provides the starting point for quality improvement (and the means to know that action intended to improve quality did in fact result in its improvement). An effective structured quality review process will establish the following facts:

- Care, including its documentation, given to an individual case was appropriate, because:
  —it met all outcome/process assessment screening criteria (the majority of cases);
  —initial reviewers determined care was appropriate, even though the case failed screens (many cases, because their circumstances were beyond screens' scope);
  —final reviewers determined care was appropriate, based on providers' responses to initial reviewers' determination (some cases);
  —appeals' reviewers determined care was appropriate, based on providers' appeal of final reviewers' determinations (very few cases).
- After considering providers' responses to initial reviewers' determination, final (appeals') reviewers determined that care or its documentation exhibited a genuine quality problem (that stemmed from malprocess), described its exact nature, and identified the malprocess involved.

At each stage in the review process, reviewers must follow structured procedures and record findings in a structured way to ensure their comparability. The quality manager must enter review results into a computerised database to permit subsequent pattern analysis and reporting. If a hospital reviews all or properly drawn samples of cases it can use structured quality review results to construct a quality score (percentage of cases meeting standards, i.e. without quality problems) with which to quantify and track the effectiveness of its quality improvement efforts.

447 | Analysing patterns of care

The third and final step in structured quality review is statistical analysis of review findings—the results of both outcome/process assessment screening and structured medical record review—often referred to as pattern analysis and sometimes as provider profiling. It intends principally to describe quality problems' distribution in space (distribution analysis) or time (trends analysis), may identify additional potential or actual quality problems to be investigated consequently, and may guide such investigations. Key analysis variables may relate to person, time and place, among other factors. Part II, Chapter 8 details appropriate types of pattern analyses. If the hospital licenses a structured quality review system it will likely perform automatically a number of relevant analyses, for example trends in types of quality problems for given types of cases, and may contain expert systems to monitor them. Generally the cost of developing expert systems to track structured quality review results and support quality managers' decisions is beyond most hospitals' current capabilities.

Hospitals will likely be most interested in quality problems' distribution and their trends. Distribution refers generally to where quality problems occur, for example in certain types of cases, with certain providers, in certain departments. Automated structured quality review systems, for example, can profile providers' performance (e.g. track the completeness of their medical records) and draw the quality manager's attention to providers whose performance is exemplary and those whose performance is exceptionally poor, either based on a threshold (hospital standard) or cut-off (e.g. exceeding the norm or average by two standard deviations).

Virtually any process or outcome variable is grist for various pattern analyses. Quality managers must think about the analysis' purpose, the appropriateness of the analytic model, the quality (integrity) of data, and the intended use of results. They must always exercise caution in interpreting results. Poorly specified analyses may produce misleading results, that is leading one to conclude a quality problem exists when in fact it does not exist. If hospitals review samples of cases, analyses must adjust for this fact in producing population estimates and/or interpreting differences between rates, for example. Moreover, patterns exist in the mind of the beholder (who may see them where none exist) and even statistically significant results may be artefacts or lack decision relevance. Hospitals wanting to undertake pattern analyses would be well advised to retain qualified biostatisticians, epidemiologists, and health systems researchers, who are experienced in analysing quality of care data, to assist in specifying analyses and interpreting their results.

448 | Reporting and using structured quality review results

448.1 | Structured quality review data

Structured quality review produces the following types of data:

- Structured quality review:
  —inputs, for example aggregate abstracter time;
  —processes, for example average time to abstract cases, reviewers' performance;
  —outcomes, for example proportion of cases treated to standards, types of quality problems.
- Patient care provision:
  —inputs, for example patient demographics or case characteristics;
  —processes, for example lengths of stay, durations of surgical operations;
  —outcomes, for example death, nosocomial infection, 'complications' rates.

This information-rich database can be supplemented further with patient follow-up data to permit measurement of long-term outcomes to determine their relationship to care processes in order to validate and improve practice policies and to assess interventions' effectiveness. This section deals only with some structured quality review management reports (useful to monitor and improve the hospital's SQR process) and some reports useful to quality managers and providers in their quest to improve quality.

448.2 | Type of reports

Quality managers need two types of reports: standard reports (those produced periodically) and ad hoc reports (those produced when needed to address a particular issue). Licensed structured quality review systems should contain a number of useful standard reports and provide ad hoc reporting capability. Hospitals that develop their own structured quality review management information system must develop the standard and ad hoc reporting capabilities that they need.

Standard reports are those that quality managers (including heads of clinical departments, providers and others responsible for quality) have decided are necessary to structured quality review and to monitor and improve the quality of care. A critical part of the hospital's quality management plan involves defining these standard reports. This section provides some general suggestions for the following broad types of reports:

- activity;
- action;
- feedback;
- quality of care.

448.3 | Activity reports

These reports are of primary interest to the quality manager. They inform him or her of structured quality review process' performance. For example, one report may describe the time needed to abstract medical records; another, to complete structured medical record reviews. By examining variances in abstracting times for comparable populations of records, for example, the quality manager can monitor abstracter productivity and spot those abstracters requiring additional training.

448.4 | Action reports

These reports are of primary interest to the quality manager, and through him or her the hospital manager. They describe actions to be considered or taken that stem from structured quality review results. For example, if a structured quality reviewer suggests that an imminent danger or a potentially serious problem exists, this fact must be brought immediately to the quality manager's attention. He or she must decide what, if any, action to take. The hospital must have in place the machinery to effect whatever actions are required (see above).

448.5 | Feedback to doctors

A hospital's quality management policy should require that periodically (e.g. quarterly) each visiting medical practitioner receive a report showing which of his or her cases were reviewed and the results of those reviews. This feedback provides vital information to stimulate change: to improve one must first know how one is performing. Comparison of the individual practitioner's performance with that of colleagues enhances this feedback. If the hospital provides such comparisons, they must be valid lest they produce misleading information. For example, if a practitioner's death rates are compared with others, the patients and their conditions must be similar enough with respect to characteristics affecting patient outcomes to permit valid comparisons. Generally, comparison data fits on a spectrum ranging from useless (grist for legal action), to potentially interesting (grist for research), to signal for action (grist for quality improvement), as comparability increases. Part II, Chapter 8 discusses issues relevant to comparing providers' performance.

448.6 | Quality of care reports

The quality manager, heads of clinical departments, the hospital manager, and members of the board of directors must receive periodic quality of care reports. The reports that each person receives, and how often he or she receives them, will be different of course, depending on their exact information needs. At the board level, reports must be simple and show, for example, trends in the hospital's quality of care. Graphic presentations, for example time series, may be most appropriate. Other reports may focus on specific problems and their incidence over time. Hospital managers and others will be interested in these same reports but in greater detail and more often. The quality manager must review relevant reports at least weekly.

Hospitals can construct and report a simple but meaningful quality score from quality assessment (review) results (if they review all or statistically significant samples of cases):

percentage of cases managed appropriately (i.e. not exhibiting a quality problem). For example, if a hospital treated all of its cases to quality standards, its score would be 100%. If the hospital deviated from its quality standards in five cases out of 100, its score would be 95%. Hospitals can construct such scores for each type of case they treat and use them to monitor the effectiveness of their quality improvement efforts. They can also construct quality scores for individual doctors. However, they are less useful than hospital-wide quality scores because individual doctors can be criticised only if reviewers said they (rather than the nursing service for example) were responsible for a quality problem, and most problems stem from poor care systems.

448.7 Ad hoc reports

Routine review of standard reports may suggest avenues worthy of investigation. Investigating quality problems' root causes, for example, may require analyses of existing structured quality review results, and care process and outcome data. To facilitate these types of analyses and reports, the quality management department should have access to statistical software packages and ad hoc reporting capabilities, and the expertise needed to use them correctly. Stated simply, an ad hoc report is any report other than a standard report. The quality manager will be a major user of ad hoc reports, and any number of other people may demand ad hoc reports.

The quality manager, as part of the hospital's quality management plan, should establish policies and procedures for requesting and generating ad hoc reports. If possible, the hospital should make the contents of the structured quality review database available to authorised users so that they can generate their own analyses and reports. This strategy has two distinct advantages: the quality management department does not have to generate reports for others (who may become frustrated if their requests go unfulfilled or if their completion is delayed); and the availability of data may encourage their use. A properly constructed structured quality review database may be a goldmine for research purposes, especially if mechanisms exist to collect patient follow-up data to measure long-term patient outcomes. The hospital should encourage its doctors to use the database to explore clinical issues of interest to them. With widespread access to data, the quality manager and his or her staff must be prepared to assist users specify, produce and interpret analyses and reports.

448.8 Interpreting and the interpretability of reports

To the extent possible, all reports should be self-explanatory, especially at the board level. However, useful information may inherently be contained in reports that are not familiar to managers. Most managers would have little difficulty reading statements of accounts. They are familiar with these reports and their meaning. They have been trained or have acquired the experience to interpret them. The uninitiated, which includes most doctors, would have difficulty reading statements of accounts, and the information they contain would be lost. Clinical and administrative managers need to be initiated into the world of quantitative quality management. They will need training in reading reports and support in interpreting them until they have become thoroughly familiar with their contents and meaning. Even the most sophisticated manager must rely on the quality management department to produce interpretable, useable reports.

When managers read statements of accounts for example, they assume that all transactions conform to certain standard accounting practices, that cash figures correspond to deposits in banks etc. Similarly, the quality manager is responsible for evaluating data's integrity, defining for users all of the concepts used in reports, describing all of the transactions involved and, most importantly, stating what inferences can (and cannot) be drawn validly from the report.

Quality management reports' interpretability depends largely on the samples of cases underlying their compilation. For quality of care reports for example, results from samples must be extrapolated properly to the population they intend to represent. Reports based directly on results of sampled cases may be misleading, because of variation in sampling rates occasioned by stratification for example. In drawing samples one must be ever mindful of the use to which results will be put, that is, the reports users want and how they will be generated.

Other factors may affect reports' interpretability. For example, presentation of hospital nosocomial infection rates means virtually nothing. Quality managers must display them by site and patient type, for example. Control charts (a type of quality report—see Part II, Chapter 2), for example, must show confidence limits (see above) so that rates tending out of control or that have crossed a predetermined limit become a signal for action. Valid comparisons to regional or national averages provide additional anchor points to establish limits for quality control purposes. While, ideally, nosocomial infection rates should be zero, money spent reducing a rate on a par with all hospitals may be better spent on other quality improvement activities because they would yield a higher pay-off for patients.

448.9 Use of quality assessment results in practice

Hospitals can use structured quality review results to monitor and to improve the quality of their care. The quality problems that structured quality review identifies are the grist for the hospital's mechanisms to investigate and eliminate their root causes. Structured quality assessment results are also useful in the revision of practice criteria (used for outcome/process assessment screening) and, if existent, practice policies. Structured quality review, because it involves outcome/process assessment screens based on explicit practice criteria, provides a first step toward the establishment of practice policies. Institutionalisation of structured medical record review (with or without case-based screening) provides a possible point of entry for the subsequent development of practice policies. They arise from review results, to communicate to everyone in the hospital how each type of patient should be managed.

449 Evaluating structured quality review results and efforts

449.1 Need to evaluate structured quality review

Structured quality review involves a substantial resource commitment. Hospitals should make every reasonable effort to ensure that the process is as cost-effective as possible. All of the principles that this manual enumerates for assuring and improving the quality of patient care apply also to assuring and improving the quality of a hospital's structured quality review process. Part II, Chapter 9 reviews basic principles of program evaluation, Chapter 8, principles that underpin structured quality review, and Chapters 3 and 8, concepts of sensitivity and specificity. This section describes how hospitals can judge the performance of their structured quality review process. It focuses first on impact, then on outcome, process and structure.

Obviously impact is the most important level of evaluation, but also the most difficult to determine. Structure is the easiest level of evaluation, but also the one that provides the least amount of information that matters the most: the process' effectiveness toward improving the quality of care. As part of the structured quality review process, hospitals must put in place information systems to collect the information they need to evaluate, and to know that any changes they make improve, the process' performance.

449.2 | Impact of structured quality review

A principal prerequisite for successful structured quality review is hospitals' willingness (and concomitant means) to resolve quality problems that structured quality review identifies. If the hospital is unwilling to make this commitment to change and improve, structured quality review—and all other quality management activities—are a waste of time and money. A corollary of this view is that any hospital lacking such programs has not yet committed itself to delivering high quality health care.

To evaluate their structured quality review efforts, hospitals can monitor the proportion of quality problems identified by all means and those identified by structured quality review that they resolve successfully, and that they address (whether or not resolved successfully). For purposes of evaluating structured quality review efforts the percentage of quality problems addressed is the most important information. If this percentage is low, the hospital is obviously wasting its resources by identifying, but not addressing, quality problems. If a hospital resolves only a small fraction of those problems it addresses, it obviously has a problem in some other component of its quality management machinery. Addressing a high proportion of identified quality problems (by structured quality review or other means) begs the following question: What fraction of its quality problems is the hospital identifying?

449.3 | Types of structured quality review outcomes to evaluate

Structured quality review is primarily a system for identifying quality of care problems that consists of three principal parts (see above). Hospitals can evaluate this system's ability to identify quality problems in the following two ways:
- its accuracy in identifying quality problems among cases subjected to structured quality review;
- the proportion of a hospital's quality problems that its structured quality review efforts identify.

449.4 | Sensitivity and specificity

Accuracy refers to the system's sensitivity and specificity. Sensitivity is the extent to which the hospital's structured quality review system identifies quality problems that exist in assessed cases. Specificity is the extent to which its structured quality review system rejects cases that do not exhibit a quality problem. Hospitals face great difficulty in measuring their SQR system's accuracy. However, the following approaches are useful.

A hospital can conduct, or preferably contract for, an annual audit of samples of cases that it reviewed, and compare the audit's results with its own to identify discrepancies and understand why they occurred. Describing methods for conducting such an audit is beyond this manual's scope. In general, the accuracy of both outcome/process assessment screening and structured medical record review mostly determine structured quality review systems' sensitivity; outcome/process assessment screening, their specificity. The audit will shed light on which parts of the hospital's SQR process need to be reviewed and revised to improve their performance. Part II, Chapter 8 discusses the evaluation of outcome/process assessment screens' sensitivity and specificity.

Quality managers can derive useful information on their structured quality review process' performance from the rates at which quality problems are identified and confirmed at each stage of review. For example, for a given health problem quality managers can compare the rate of cases failing screens with that for cases with reviewer-identified quality problems; the rate of cases with reviewer-identified quality problems with that for cases with confirmed quality problems after review of providers' feedback of initial reviewers' determinations. Individual reviewer performance data may also be instructive. For example, one reviewer may habitually initially identify quality problems that are not confirmed subsequently.

Quality managers can change their structured quality review process based on the results of these types of analyses. The appropriate changes to make depend on their exact findings. For example, redesign of outcome/process assessment screens may improve their accuracy. Reviewers who constantly identify problems that are not genuine problems or those who often fail to identify important quality problems may benefit from additional training or, if they do not, may be replaced with more accurate reviewers.

449.5 Proportion of quality problems identified

Structured quality review's goal is to identify all of the important quality problems in a case and, by extension, all of the cases with important quality problems. The SQR process' sensitivity speaks to the first consideration (see above); its targeting and SQR's inherent ability to pick up all important quality problems, to the latter consideration. If the hospital reviews routinely all of its cases, targeting is not an issue. The extent to which structured quality review can identify all of a hospital's important quality problems is an open question.

Hospitals can gauge their targeting system's (or sampling approach's) effectiveness by comparing the proportion of cases with confirmed quality problems in a statistically significant random sample of cases and that in its targeted sample. Clearly, the proportion of confirmed quality problems in the targeted sample should be higher, and preferably much higher, than that in the random sample of cases. The ratio of rates of confirmed quality problems is a measure of the targeting system's effectiveness. If a hospital reviews random samples of cases for surveillance purposes, it can use the rate of confirmed quality problems in these samples as the point of comparison for its targeted samples. Obviously it should not include these surveillance samples among its 'targeted' cases. Hospitals can adjust their targeting systems based on these types of analyses' results.

Determining the fraction of all quality problems that structured quality review can identify is quite difficult. Firstly, one must define in measurable terms what is a quality problem and then determine which of these problems one can expect structured quality review to identify. For example, one could reasonably expect structured quality review to identify cases with unindicated diagnostic tests, and even to determine whether or not an indicated test was done with the right frequency (an issue which current outcome/process assessment screens rarely address now). However, SQR cannot identify whether or not the hospital's clinical laboratory is performing the test in question with maximum efficiency. If a hospital has multiple problem identification mechanisms (as all should, if only SQR, incident and complaint tracking and reporting systems, and patient satisfaction surveys), the quality manager can compare quality problems identified by the hospital's SQR process with those identified by all other means. Key questions here are: What problems that SQR did not identify should it have identified? What problems that SQR identified were also identified by other means? Based on answers to these questions a hospital might change its mix of quality problem identification strategies and improve accordingly the cost-effectiveness of its structured quality review process.

449.6 Processes of structured quality review

Quality managers can evaluate the processes in place to perform the various parts of structured quality review. For example, they can examine the cost of screening and determine whether or not alternative arrangements would reduce screening costs. An efficient abstracting system that can gather essential information in half the time needed for the one in use now would obviously permit the hospital to abstract more cases or to reduce its abstracting costs if abstracting more cases would not bring a worthwhile addition to the number of quality problems identified. Similarly, quality managers can examine the ways in which reviewers examine cases failing screens to see if there are more efficient ways of performing these tasks. Whatever changes they make, quality managers must be mindful of their effect on the SQR process' performance. Trade-offs between effectiveness (the proportion of important quality problems identified) and efficiency (the cost of their identification) are inevitable, and the quality manager must strike the right balance, which is likely to change as the hospital's quality management program evolves.

449.7 | Structures of structured quality review

The simplest evaluation is to compare the structured quality review process that the hospital has in place with what experts might recommend. Quality managers can compare their structured quality review process with that described in this manual, for example, or ask an expert consultant for his or her opinion. This type of evaluation may be sufficient early on, but once a hospital has accumulated data on the time needed to abstract medical record, rates of quality problems and so on, it should begin to evaluate processes, outcomes and impacts.

449.8 | Need to collect information on costs and effects routinely

To assess the cost-effectiveness of their quality improvement efforts, hospitals must routinely collect, for example, the cost of identifying quality problems through screening and structured medical record review, and of corresponding effectiveness, for example the proportion of quality problems these efforts identify in comparison to the costs and effects of alternative means of identifying them. Hospitals must design and deploy mechanisms to collect cost and effectiveness data as part of their quality management plans and structured quality review management information systems. They must also implement the routine collection of such data and assess periodically their accuracy. The quality manager must measure the cost of abstracting, for example, by monitoring the number of cases abstracted per hour, determining the number of minutes needed to abstract each case, and converting this time to a cost by multiplying by the average abstracter's salary loaded for on-costs, supervision and other overhead items. The same technique can be used to monitor the cost of expert clinician reviewers. However, if they are not paid (but volunteer their time), shadow price or nominal costs may be substituted for doctors' sessional fees.

PART V

RISK MANAGEMENT

SUMMARY

This part of the manual focuses on risk management, which as a discrete function is almost unknown in Australian hospitals. Certainly the concept of minimising risk to either the hospital or its staff, in the form of legal liability for malpractice or for the consequences of inadequate occupational health and safety, is not a high profile activity in the minds of most hospital staff. In the US, there is much greater concern for risk management, especially with respect to patient care activities. Hospitals throughout the world would do well to follow the principles expressed here, even though they may have to adapt practices to local circumstances. The material is presented as follows:

Chapter 1   *Introduction to and purpose of Part V*—provides a general background to the concept of risk.

Chapter 2   *Professional liability*—focuses on the risks inherent in the provision of patient care and provides an insight into professional liability.

Chapter 3   *Occupational health and safety*—deals with occupational health and safety as an important element of quality management. The authors have attempted to recognise the practical difficulties of the average hospital manager trying to cope with the occupational health and safety of his or her staff.

Chapter 1

INTRODUCTION TO AND PURPOSE OF PART V

---

510 | Contents

This chapter considers the issue of risk management under the following headings:

511. Purpose of this part
512. Contents of this part
513. Purpose of this chapter
514. Risk concepts
515. Types of risks
516. Planning ahead

---

511 | Purpose of this part

Risk management is an important part of an overall hospital quality management program. Hospital professionals in general rarely think about risk management and such risk management as does exist in Australian hospitals is rarely directed at the two areas of highest risk—professional liability and occupational health and safety. This part attempts to redress this situation and to describe how risk management fits into a quality management program. The chapters intend to fulfil the needs of hospital professionals involved in quality management; they are not detailed texts on managing professional liability nor on implementing occupational health and safety programs.

512 | Contents of this part

This part consists of three chapters. The first chapter explores the concept of risk. The second chapter describes professional liability from the hospital's perspective. Chapter 3 discusses occupational health and safety and how and why that activity fits into a quality management program.

513 | Purpose of this chapter

This chapter introduces Part V and exposes readers to the concept of risk management as it impinges on quality management. It outlines the concepts of risk, describes the types of risks that hospitals face, and serves to lead readers into greater detail regarding professional liability and occupational health and safety. Environmental hazards (such as the environmental aftermath of a chemical factory explosion), disaster preparedness (such as the familiar disaster plan already existing with most hospitals), and what we refer to as commercial risks (such as malfeasance, embezzlement, property theft, fire, violence in the workplace, sexual harrassment, and other risks inherent in organisations), while properly included under the umbrella of risk management, are beyond this manual's scope.

514 | Risk concepts

Everyone, and every enterprise, faces many types of risk. Risks, like opportunities, lurk everywhere. Risk is the dark side of opportunity and is inherently part of life. In a business or commercial context, risk is often expressed as the chance of suffering a financial loss or other injury that damages the organisation's profitability.

The objective of risk management is to reduce such risk to the lowest level commensurate with achieving the organisation's purpose. Essentially, three strategies exist for managing risk:

- risk avoidance, preventing or reducing the possibility of a loss occurring;
- damage control or loss prevention, minimising the magnitude of a loss should one occur;
- risk transfer or insurance, in which all or part of the loss is transferred to someone else in exchange for a premium.

A prudent home-owner, for example, might remove fire hazards from his or her house and take other steps to reduce the chance that it will catch fire (a preventive strategy). He or she might install fire extinguishers or build it near a fire brigade so that if the house did catch fire it could be dealt with quickly (loss prevention or minimisation). Finally, he or she might insure the house so that in the event of a partial or total loss, he or she could rebuild the house and pay for temporary accommodation while doing so (risk transfer).

Clearly, rational analysis could be applied to the chances of loss, the probability and cost of preventing losses, and the cost of losses that might occur to yield the best mix of strategies. However, particularly in the situation of hospitals, estimates are often difficult to make and may be shaky, involving a wide range of factors that could materially influence the result. For example, a spectacular or well published failure may damage one's reputation or credibility leading to immediate embarrassment or loss of one's job and result in lost revenues or patient referrals for years to come. Moreover, such calculations inevitably value human life and limb in monetary terms, and create other ethical dilemmas. The greater the value placed on human life and limb, the more emphasis must be placed on prevention rather than accepting that losses will be made good through insurance or the hospital's budget.

Not all risks are insurable. For those that are insurable, it may not always be prudent to buy insurance, because of premium costs for example, especially if avoidance or prevention strategies are less expensive. Even in the case of an insured risk (e.g. defending an allegation of malpractice), secondary consequences (e.g. loss of reputation and future income) are not insurable.

515 | Types of risks

The manager of any hospital faces many risks. They can be arranged into the following four categories:

- professional liability and losses resulting from injuries to patients and visitors; injuries to visitors being seen here as a commercial risk;
- occupational health and safety, resulting from injuries to staff and employees;
- environmental hazards—resulting from injuries to persons in the community—that are the consequence of the organisation's action or inaction or those of its staff, employees or patients;
- commercial risks, resulting from injuries to the organisation such as fire, theft, sabotage of computers, assassination of the chief executive, malfeasance; all of which are beyond this manual's scope.

516 | Planning ahead

While most hospitals do not face the risk of such catastrophes as Chernobyl, the Challenger space-shuttle disaster, Hubble trouble, the Piper alpha oilrig explosion in the North Sea, or the bombing of Pan Am 103 over Lockerbie, Scotland, lesser disasters can be equally damaging within the community in which the hospital operates. Every hospital should periodically evaluate the risks it faces and plan accordingly. This plan must include prevention, damage control, and insurance strategies for all types of relevant risks. Such a plan must include very infrequent risks that, if they occurred, would be disastrous or materially affect operations. For example, a hospital's operations would be disrupted if it had to receive the victims of a major plane crash. The chances of effective damage control or coping with a crisis improve if the appropriate responses have been thought through in advance and established mechanisms exist to invoke and implement them when needed. Such mechanisms must include public relations and identification of a spokesperson to liaise with the media.

Chapter 2

PROFESSIONAL LIABILITY

---

520 | Contents

This chapter focuses on the risks which represent professional liability and explores the following:

521. Purpose of this chapter
522. Risk avoidance
523. Damage control
524. Risk transfer
525. When malpractice is alleged

521 | Purpose of this chapter

This chapter summarises ways in which hospitals can manage the risks inherent in delivering patient care. It focuses on those risks that arise to patients, and adopts the hospital's perspective. For the practitioner these risks represent professional liability and their consequences become manifest in the form of malpractice suits. An effective quality management program reduces the hospital's risk of being sued for malpractice and of the probability of suits being successful. Since this manual's primary focus is quality management, this chapter serves simply to bring together those aspects of such a program that relate to risk management. Risk management involves:

- risk avoidance;
- damage control;
- risk transfer.

It also considers the handling of malpractice allegations.

522 | Risk avoidance

522.1 | *Ways to minimise risk*

Successful malpractice suits can be reduced by eliminating malpractice. Bad or poor outcomes can give rise to suits, but not all bad outcomes result from malpractice. Medical care by its very nature involves inherent risks that cannot always be foreseen or prevented. These outcomes were once seen as acts of God, but increasingly people believe that if something went wrong someone was at fault and in some cases, it is true, such blame may be justified. Suits based on maloutcomes without malpractice may still succeed because of the imperfections of the legal system. Nevertheless, an effective quality management program can reduce the risk of a suit and improve the chances for defending oneself against allegations of malpractice if one is brought. Risk avoidance— preventive measures—may be divided into three classes based on: structure, process and outcome.

522.2 │ Structural risk avoidance

Proper planning is essential for crisis and risk management. Lack of a well-articulated plan about what to do in the event of a serious maloutcome can turn an already serious situation into a disaster. Structural interventions may relate to patients, practitioners, or to the hospital/patient care environment. Hospitals can reduce risk by:

- providing only services for which the hospital has proper facilities, equipment and staff (appropriate service or products policy);
- accepting only patients that it can treat properly (appropriate admissions policy);
- ensuring visiting medical practitioners are competent to treat patients (appropriate appointments and credentialling procedures, and mechanisms to ensure practitioners limit their practices to those activities for which they have been granted privileges and follow adopted practice policies);
- employing appropriately qualified, trained, and experienced nursing and other staff in sufficient numbers appropriately deployed and supervised to meet service objectives and implement policies;
- acquiring and maintaining in proper operational condition sufficient equipment to meet service objectives and implement policies;
- insisting on proper medical records (and conducting regular reviews to ensure their accuracy, objectivity, legibility, timeliness, comprehensiveness, and completeness including alterations), and recordkeeping practices (security and maintenance of confidentiality etc.);
- requiring adequate informed consent policies, for example for surgical operations and practices, such as clear documentation in the medical record that the doctor explained the consequences of alternative therapies for the patient's condition;
- protecting research subjects with proper review of research protocols prior to the implementation of the study, and monitoring of ongoing research projects;
- adopting proper practice policies regarding consultations and other matters germane to proper patient care, including who is responsible for the patient's care and an adequate nominee system for holiday periods;
- paying proper attention to the scheduling of staff and their workloads to avoid hazardous or overload situations that may facilitate errors, including practitioners managing too many patients or being given insufficient time to manage a patient properly;
- adopting and implementing proper management policies and practices to meet service objectives, including an effective quality management program to assess and assure the quality of patient care, and periodic review and evaluation of this quality assurance system including risk management;
- stressing risk management by educating staff about its importance and that of quality management; effective dissemination of policies and their adoption in practice, including proper incentives to adopt them.

522.3 │ Process risk avoidance

Quality controls placed on the process of medical care, including its documentation, can play an important part in risk avoidance. Such controls include well-accepted measures, such as specific crossmatching of blood before it is administered, as well as those that are less widely implemented. Included in the latter category is a mechanism to ensure that procedures are carried out only by practitioners with the requisite privileges, and procedures exist to pick up untoward outcomes quickly and sufficiently early to enable prompt action to minimise any damage. We could also include in this group computer programs to check on medications, including interactions, before they are dispensed. Early intervention, such as an inadvertent drug overdose detected promptly and managed appropriately, may result in little residual injury. The same overdose left undetected could result in the patient's death.

Accurate and timely information flow is the key to process risk avoidance. Efficient, well-articulated systems should be in place to process clinical information. Such systems should be under constant surveillance to avoid lost laboratory slips and radiology reports, and other deficiencies, and to ensure that practitioners see and act on information pertinent to the patient's proper care.

522.4 | Outcome risk avoidance

Strictly speaking, outcome risk avoidance is a contradiction. Maloutcomes that have occurred cannot be prevented; however, recurrences can be. Quality assessment, infection control and other outcome surveillance systems can identify problems early so that remedial interventions can be instituted promptly. In some instances they can detect processes in danger of going out of control before serious maloutcomes occur.

Pattern analysis of practitioner performance, for example, may identify a practitioner in need of continuing medical education or whose privileges should be limited. In such cases avoidance of serious outcomes—disasters waiting to happen—can be a real possibility. Routine analysis of incident reports and patient complaints by the hospital's quality management department are other important sources of risk management information.

523 | Damage control

Inevitably, serious maloutcomes may occur to patients and some may have involved malpractice. The hospital can control losses resulting from such outcomes in a number of ways. The key is a well-formulated management strategy, prepared well in advance, for handling such incidents when they occur. Such a plan includes:
- a senior person to co-ordinate damage control activities;
- a spokesperson to represent the hospital (and practitioners) to the media;
- liaison with the patient and family members to explain the untoward event and help cope with its consequences;
- completion of an incident report, and interviewing everyone with any knowledge of events and the circumstances leading up to the event;
- proper documentation of the medical record;
- notification of the hospital's liability insurer and the practitioner's medical defence organisation;
- inquiring into the matter to determine why the serious event took place and how it might have been prevented, in order that steps may be taken to prevent its recurrence.

An important aspect of damage control policy is delineating criteria for judging which patient maloutcomes are serious enough to warrant damage control and which may be graded into levels of response depending on the seriousness of the maloutcome. A massacre on Ward 10 or an amputation of the wrong leg need no contemplation. However, deaths, for example, occur regularly and hospitals need clear policies to indicate when incident reports must be made out and when damage control measures must be set in motion. Usually the hospital's insurer will decide, in the light of inquiries which demonstrate that the hospital was at fault, whether an out-of-court negotiated settlement is the appropriate course to take.

524 | Risk transfer

Prudent risk management requires assessment of risks that cannot be prevented entirely and the purchase of appropriate insurance. Insurable risks include those resulting from patient care (suits by patients) and from quality management activities (suits by doctors). Medical practitioners are expected to be members of a medical defence organisation and it is the hospital's responsibility to check that they are.

Medical staff involved in quality management activities on the hospital's behalf should be indemnified against law suits resulting from their participation in such activities. In the case of public hospitals such indemnity is automatically achieved by quality management committees being authorised committees of the board of the hospital. Private hospitals will have to purchase insurance, to protect their medical staffs.

Some residual risk may be retained (self-insurance), and some transferred by insurance purchase. The balance depends on many factors, including the absence of statutory or regulatory requirements, the hospital's financial resources and the cost of premiums. The insurance aspects of risk management are beyond this manual's scope. Similarly, we do not intend dealing with legal actions against third parties, such as equipment manufacturers, to recoup losses that hospitals may have suffered, from successful malpractice claims involving defective equipment. In such situations hospitals are well advised to seek competent legal advice.

525 | When malpractice is alleged

If legal action occurs in the form of a writ or if it is merely threatened, the practitioner should notify the hospital immediately (if the incident involved the hospital) and his or her medical defence organisation. The hospital should notify its insurer and both parties should obtain competent legal advice.

The incident may have already been the subject of damage control activity or an inquiry. If not, other relevant aspects of damage control policies should be pressed into service at this point and an inquiry held. Patient complaints, while not as serious as allegations of malpractice, may foretell more serious problems. Their routine analysis by the hospital's quality management department is an important source of outcome risk avoidance information.

Chapter 3

OCCUPATIONAL HEALTH AND SAFETY

---

530 | Contents

This chapter manifests our view that occupational health and safety is an integral part of risk management and hence quality management. It is not intended to be a textbook on occupational health and safety, but rather an account of how to minimise workplace hazards and to bring their consideration within the ambit of a quality management program. This chapter deals with:

531 | Purpose of this chapter

This chapter describes generally the manner in which occupational health and safety (OH&S) is currently organised in most Australian hospitals, and examines risks to hospital staff and how to detect, prevent and mitigate them.

Hospitals are potentially dangerous places in which to work and staff must be constantly alert to those dangers. Management, through its quality management program, has an obligation to conduct occupational health and safety programs towards minimising these dangers and diminishing the risks that employees face.

The purpose of an occupational health and safety program is to ensure employees' well-being. Employers have a duty to protect their employees, and in so doing reduce the hospital's liability for employee injury or illness resulting from employment. Incidental to this responsibility, the manager will find that his or her staff will be contributing maximally to the hospital's task. An OH&S program contributes to product (health care) quality in several ways. It can:

- prevent injury to patients, for example the transmission of HIV infection from staff member to patient, or injury of a patient by an impaired provider;
- prevent direct injury to staff, for example the transmission of HIV infection from patient to staff, or the injury of a staff member in the course of lifting a patient;
- improve the work environment and worker morale, thereby contributing to improvements in both health care quality and productivity.

Hazards in hospitals that present an immediate risk of injury and disease are usually well known and readily identifiable. They include, for example, manual handling, slips and falls, electricity, sharp instruments and hot surfaces. Long-term consequences of hospital hazards may be far less evident. Thus, clinically manifest hepatitis B may not be revealed for three months after contact; and repeated heavy lifting of patients may have long-term degenerative consequences in the spine of lifters. An effective OH&S program also addresses these less obvious hazards.

An effective OH&S program requires:

- knowledge about hazards (what to look for);
- information on how well you are doing (current risk);
- knowledge about what and how to improve (potential risk reduction);
- a mechanism and the will to implement change (reduced risk).

In the broadest sense, an OH&S program can be viewed as encompassing the following functions:

- hazard control;
- health promotion;
- stress management (employee assistance, counselling);
- employee health services;
- employee management.

532 | Hazards and risks

The terms 'hazard' and 'risk' tend to be used interchangeably in common parlance. We use them as follows:

- Hazard: object or situation that is potentially harmful.
- Risk: or the 'chance of harm' is a measure of the extent to which a person is exposed to harm, for example reduced health status. Risk is influenced by, for example, the probability, severity, intensity and length of exposure to hazards, the precautions taken, and training etc.

533 | Background to occupational health and safety in hospitals

533.1 | *Occupational health and safety is important; often neglected*

Occupational health and safety in Australian hospitals has been developed largely as a product of industrial legislation. Frequently, as an activity it has been driven by industrial awards, and in most hospitals it is seen as the personnel department's responsibility. If the product of a hospital is patient care, the hospital staff are an important element in that production process. Managing the quality of the product, therefore, also involves caring for the occupational health and safety of its producers. This line of reasoning places occupational health and safety within the ambit of a quality management program.

Under most state legislation, risk containment is a responsibility of the hospital's management. This requirement is manifest in the provision of a healthy, safe workplace and compliance with regulations, standards and codes of practice. Other obligations come under compensation, rehabilitation and prevention legislation. Mostly, legislation does not require specific programs, but the programs provide the means of compliance with regulatory requirements. Even hospital committees and their composition are defined within the contents of such legislation as *OH&S Committees in the Workplace Act 1984* in New South Wales, and are matched more or less in the other Australian states. One experienced fire and safety officer emphasised this industrial background as follows: 'Occupational health and safety on many occasions has been used (by unions) to beat management over the head.' In an environment where management has not been particularly attentive to occupational health and safety, unions have used the issue for industrial confrontation.

While a small number of major hospitals have an association with a university department of occupational medicine and the expert resources which that may contain, most hospitals in Australia do not. For example, at one large metropolitan hospital which has over 2000 staff, the occupational health and safety staff consists of one fire and safety officer. This level of staffing is the rule rather than the exception.

While there is a climate in industry generally, particularly among large, responsible employers, to seek to achieve the optimum standard of worker, bystander and environmental safety realistically possible, hospital priorities and budgetary restraints mean that in reality hospitals still have a long way to go before the ideal and the practical can approximate. Unfortunately, the very industrial nature of occupational health and safety and its separate development from the culture of clinical services results in an even lower priority being attached to it than should be the case. It is doubtful whether clinical staff are even aware of many of the occupational risks to which they and other staff are exposed, and are probably not even aware of the fact that their hospital has an occupational health and safety program.

533.2 | Hospitals are hazardous workplaces

Hospitals constitute a very large industry. For example, in 1990–91 health care accounted for 8.1% of Australia's gross domestic product.[1] In 1989–90, Australian hospitals accounted for 51.6% of recurrent expenditures.[2] In 1986 the Australian health sector employed approximately 500 000 people or 7% of the workforce, and 70% of all health workers worked in hospitals and nursing homes. In common with all developed countries, health industry employment is growing faster than employment generally. In their structure, large hospitals resemble small cities and are more complex than almost any other kind of workplace. They embody facilities not only for their prime function of caring for the sick and injured but also for research and teaching. They employ a remarkable diversity of professionals, technicians, tradespeople, administrators and servicepeople, who are exposed to a remarkable range of hazards. Although this chapter deals with hazards and their control in hospitals, its content applies broadly to all types of health care settings. As in any other industry, the protection of hospital workers from harm and the promotion of their health is the product of occupational health and safety programs.

The hospital can be a hazardous place in which to work. The range of hazards encountered is greater than that of almost any other type of workplace. Incidence rates for compensatable injury and illness are about double the average rates of all combined service industries and equal to those of the manufacturing industry. The rates in certain classes of hospital workers exceed those of some occupations generally regarded as dangerous. Compared to the total workforce, hospital workers are more likely to record compensatable sprains and strains, dermatitis, hepatitis, other infections, mental disorders and eye injuries. No other industry presents such a high risk of exposure to infection, ionising radiation and toxic hazards. Mental distress and substance abuse are more prevalent in hospital workers. Furthermore, hospital workers suffer more episodes of acute illness than other workers.[2]

533.3 Availability and reliability of data

Existing comparisons are unlikely to represent the true state of harm to hospital workers because of the usual shortcomings of epidemiological studies. On the one hand, hospital workers may tend to reveal more illness and injury than their counterparts in other industries as they work in a medical setting and might be expected more often to report their complaints because sick bay facilities are to hand. On the other hand, many unskilled hospital workers who are exposed to hazards may not comprehend the risk. Further, they may be unwilling to report for a variety of reasons. Also, sense of duty and commitment may encourage workers to soldier on and not report; or they may undertake 'corridor consultations' with physicians, nurses and therapists with whom they work, which are not reported. Drug and alcohol dependency tends to be hidden whenever it occurs, but compared with industry generally, fewer statistics seem to be available in hospitals on overall morbidity among their workers and on general health status. Moreover, what statistics there are may be unreliable. Finally, as in industry generally, the usual morbidity statistics do not reveal the prevalence and incidence of minor and chronic complaints, nor much mental distress, disaffection, unfitness and fatigue, all of which hinder productivity.

The availability of accurate data about the incidence of accidents, injuries and illnesses coming under the category of occupational health and safety in Australian hospitals was, until relatively recently, limited. Not only was there reason to believe that many episodes of injury and illness were not reported, but also the breakdown of figures was not sufficiently detailed to enable an accurate assessment of the real situation in acute care hospitals to be made. In New South Wales there were 5747 workplace injuries in one year, 1986–87, or an incidence of 55.1 per 1000 workers, and 534 cases of occupational diseases or an incidence of 5.1 per 1000 workers.[3] How reliable such data were when applied to hospitals and whether or not these numbers could be extrapolated reliably to other states was uncertain. Certainly, when compared with data in reports of the US National Institute of Occupational Safety and Health (NIOSH) the incidence of illness and injury would appear to have been far below what might have been expected.[4]

With the advent of Worksafe Australia more accurate national data is becoming available. Its overview for 1991–92 indicates that the OH&S performance of the Hospitals and Nursing Homes industry group is significantly below that of Australian industry standards in general. As a whole it experiences 25% more injuries per 1000 employed than the incidence rate for Australian industries overall.[5] The overview went on to comment: 'The incident rates for the industry are of even more concern when it is remembered that approximately 370 000 persons are employed within this industry group. Further, nearly one-fifth of injury/illness occurrences result in severe conditions (i.e. entailing more than 60 days of lost time).' (See Figure V-3-1 and Figure V-3-2 on pages 644 and 645.)

A recent press release from the National Occupational Health and Safety Commission referred to the 100 000 cases of occupational back disorders that occur each year in Australia.[6] The health industry experienced some 12% of this number (while employing 4% of the workforce). The Commission's statement went on to say: 'Back disorders account for a startling 52% of all injuries suffered by nurses making it the single most serious occupational health and safety problem facing the nursing profession.'

While all types of information systems in Australian hospitals are far from adequate, existing data relating to occupational health and safety in acute care hospitals evoke even less interest among hospital managers and doctors than data relating to patient care. Bringing occupational health and safety closer to the clinical mainstream through a quality management program that recognises its impact on the quality of care is one mechanism which could eliminate this deficiency.

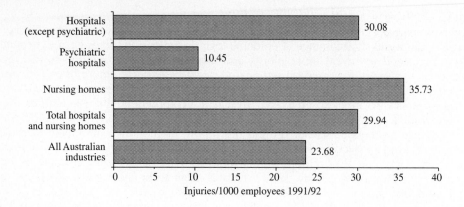

Figure V-3-1 *Injury incidence in Australian hospitals and nursing homes. Source: Hospitals and Nursing Homes Industry,* Occupational Health and Safety Performance Overview. *Worksafe Australia, 1991/92*

533.4 Present state of OH&S in hospitals

Despite high incidence rates of work-related disease and injury, most hospital workers are poorly served by health and safety programs. In a survey of 2600 hospitals in 1972 in the United States (a country more advanced than most others in this regard), only half had employee health services, and only 8% of the hospitals were regarded as having met the nationally recommended minimum criteria for an adequate service. The same report, however, indicates that since the survey of 1972, 'Many hospitals have since taken steps to initiate or improve worker health services'.[7] Data for Australian hospitals do not exist, but there is no reason to believe that the situation is any better, only that it is worse.

Hospitals mostly do not meet industrial safety criteria and standards laid down by regulation. What little is done is usually assigned to security personnel or administrative sections, whose officers lack sufficient training in work health and safety. The safety standards in most hospitals would appal a safety officer in industry. Such occupational health and safety programs that do exist seem to be focused mainly on the containment of hazards, particularly safety hazards, with little if any attention to health promotion, employee assistance, employee health services, or employee management in such areas as workloads. Individual hospitals' situations vary widely; these and the following comments accordingly apply to the average hospital.

It is an ironic paradox that hospitals bristling with health professionals whose whole ethic is caring for patients on many occasions give the appearance of either failing to recognise worker health and safety as deserving attention or, at the very least, give it a much lower priority. No one reason for the paradox is dominant; rather a variety of reasons has been advanced, all hypothetical, even if plausible, and none having been subjected to statistical and epidemiological proof. The reasons may be listed as:

- government role;
- hospital management's role;
- sickness not health.

533.5 Government role

No single set of laws, regulations, standards, codes of practice or industrial agreements applies to the health and safety of hospital workers or to all aspects of hospital work generally, though codes have been developed for particular hazards, for example radiation and the manual handling of patients. Further, governments, having introduced

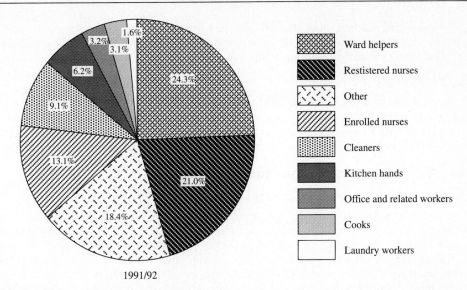

1991/92

Figure V-3-2 *Distribution of injuries in Australian hospitals and nursing homes by occupation, 1991/92. Source: Hospitals and Nursing Homes Industry,* Occupational Health and Safety Performance Overview. *Worksafe Australia, 1991/92*

modern occupational health and safety legislation in recent years, have in general failed to provide the resources needed to support its application and policing, even in hospitals for which they are responsible. Deficiencies in this area, of course, are not confined to the Australian scene but appear to be universal. Even so, hospitals appear not to attract anything like the attention given by regulatory authorities to manufacturing industry, despite being as dangerous. A 1982 study noted that in Florida the annual rate of illness and injury reported for hospital workers was 100 per 1000 workers—about the same as that recorded for sheet metal workers, auto mechanics and paper-mill workers.[4] Recent workers' compensation legislation in New South Wales, which applies to all industry including hospitals, tends to incorporate strong provisions also for prevention of work-related injury and disease, and for rehabilitation, though once again inadequate support is given to train the people needed to implement the provisions.

533.6 | Hospital management's role

While a considerable amount of information exists about certain hospital hazards, there is no doubt that information on this aspect of hospital activity in Australia is no better than most other hospital data. Consequently, hospitals may be unaware of all of their hazards. Equally important, however, is hospital managers' failure to recognise problems or to be aware of generally applicable industrial standards, and of the means used to control hazards in industries other than hospitals. The need for management to engage outside consultant help in this area is, it would seem, rarely acknowledged.

Few hospitals employ in their worker health services professionals trained in occupational health, and therefore capable of advising on modern concepts of hazard control and health promotion. While occupational health and safety in industry generally is seen as saving costs in the long run, even if incurring cost in the short run, most hospitals, operating as they do within the public sector, have not had the same financial incentives to introduce these programs. Probably due to the prevailing hospital culture, there has also been little visible action by hospital employee unions to press for better health and safety rather than just for better wages and fringe benefits. Lastly, if public hospital operating budgets are slashed, the first services to go are those not seen to contribute directly to acute patient care, including what few employee occupational health and safety programs may have been in place.

533.7   Sickness not health

Hospitals and their workers are geared towards the cure and care of sick and injured patients, and more focused on crisis intervention rather than prevention. It is therefore not surprising that workers may neglect their own health and safety and be less than mindful of their obligation to safeguard that of others under their supervision or influence.

534   Types of hazards and their consequences

534.1   Hospital specific and general occupational hazards

Hazards in hospitals can usefully but broadly be subdivided into those specific to or especially common in hospitals and those which may occur equally commonly in any industrial setting. The latter, such as lifting loads, slipping and falling, being struck by and striking against objects, lead to far more injuries than do the more hospital-specific hazards such as infective and anti-neoplastic agents. This situation is understandable because most employees are exposed to the general industry type of risk and relatively few to the hospital type. Moreover, the hospital type is often recognised to be dangerous and possibly life threatening, whereas the general risk is usually regarded as everyday and marked by lack of instruction, protection and care, if not indifference.

Table V-3-1 on page 647 lists some pre-eminent hospital hazards. Many of them encompass a great range of substances. For example, in 1985 the National Institute of Occupational Safety and Health found some 159 primary skin and eye irritants and 135 potential carcinogens, mutagens or teratogens to which individuals could be exposed in hospitals.[4] The field of occupational health and safety hazard knowledge and its discovery is large and complex. The following text intends only to give the reader an appreciation of hazards and their consequences and not to be a comprehensive text on this subject.

The potential disease and injury consequences of exposure to some hazards are mostly inherent in the nature of the hazard. Some pre-eminent hospital hazards are highly specific, that is, electricity to electrocution, and rubella to teratogenesis. Exposure to the HIV virus may lead to HIV positivity and ultimately AIDS. However, many hazards have multiple and various effects. For example, asbestos causes a range of cancerous and degenerative diseases; and particular solvents may have irritant, allergic, degenerative and cancerous effects. Conversely, a disease may result from many different hazards: lung cancer, bronchial asthma and contact eczema each present the same clinical and pathological picture regardless of the cause or trigger mechanism in any particular instance.

Some hazards may have only short-term effects, which may be reversible, for example eye irritants; some have long-term effects, which may be irreversible, for example asbestos-induced mesothelioma; others again have both short- and long-term consequences, for example mercury and ionising radiation. The complexity of the situation and the difficulty of tracking and identifying hazards and their effects can be emphasised by acknowledging that there are both general and specific work environments either of which or both may contribute to work-related conditions. The elucidation of such situations is often complex and requires special skills and knowledge. For purposes of description, hospital hazards can be categorised as:
- physical;
- chemical;
- biological;
- psychological.

Table V-3-1 *Selected pre-eminent hospital hazards, by type of hazard*

Physical	Chemical	Biological	Psychological

Fire	Disinfectants	Bacteria
		  staphylococcus
		  streptococcus
		  n. meningitidis
		  m. tuberculosis
		  h. pertussis
			Overload
			stress
			
			  Physical
			  Mental

Patient handling	Antiseptics	Viruses
		  HIV
		  Hep A, B, C
		  Rubella
		  CMV
		  Zoster
		  H Simplex
		  Influenza
			Hours of work

Sharps	Sterilisants	Parasites	Exposure to death
Falls, injuries	Pharmaceuticals	Scabies	Fear of harm
Electricity	Anti-neoplastics	Fungi	Technological change
Explosion	Substances of abuse (narcotics)	Organic dusts	Access to drugs
Heat, steam	Irritants		Insecurity

Radiation
  Ionising
  Non-ionising
	Carcinogens		Role ambiguity

Radionucleotide	Teratogens		Job mismatch
Assaults	Mutagens		
	Lab. chemicals		

534.2 | Physical hazards

534.21 FIRE

Hospitals are potent sources of fire hazards because of the large number of diverse flammable and combustible materials that must be stored and used in widespread parts of the hospital in various types of use. About a third of hospital fires originate in wards or employee quarters, mostly from smoking. In other areas, linens, equipment, solvents, gases, welding, heaters, waste, oily rags, cleaning materials, lubricating oils and oil-based paints are potential sources of fire.

The morbid consequences of involvement in fire and explosion are obvious. Hospital fires are particularly dangerous because employees must evacuate patients as well as protect themselves. Deaths are due mostly to suffocation rather than to direct exposure to the fire. Most public hospitals in Australia stress fire prevention, although persuading health professionals to attend fire drills is not always easy. Other steps, if not already taken, include prohibition of smoking on hospital premises.

534.22 PATIENT HANDLING

Patients present a unique type of manual handling problem which is responsible for much loss attributable to back, shoulder, arm and leg strains and sprains, and to hernias. Back injuries constitute by far the largest single source of compensatable injury loss in hospitals and occur most commonly in nurses' aides, orderlies, nurses' and others who regularly lift patients.

534.23 NEEDLE STICK INJURY (SHARPS)

Cuts, lacerations and puncture wounds are common among hospital workers because of the many opportunities for contact with needles, sharp instruments, glass equipment and sharp edges.

534.24 FALLS AND INJURIES

The next greatest source of compensatable loss in hospitals results from injuries, including back strains, occasioned by trips, slips and falls on the same level, owing to wet, polished, uneven, greasy or cluttered floor surfaces, to unsafe footwear, and to the moving of carts, beds and other heavy objects.

534.25 ELECTRICITY

Electrical hazards also abound in hospitals, particularly where there is electricity in wet areas. Apart from the risk of electrocution, electrical malfunction is the next most common cause, after smoking, of fires in hospitals, due to defective equipment, ungrounded appliances (including some beds), damaged cords, lasers, and energising of exposed non-current-carrying metal parts of equipment.

534.26 EXPLOSION

Compressed gases are often flammable, all are explosible, and some are toxic in various ways. They include the anaesthetic gases cyclopropane, diethyl ether, ethyl chloride, ethylene, oxygen and nitrous oxide, and such others as acetylene, ammonia, argon, chlorine, ethylene oxide, helium, hydrogen, methyl chloride, nitrogen and sulphur dioxide.

534.27 HOT AND COLD MATERIALS

Hot and cold materials, including steam and cryogens such as liquid nitrogen and dry ice, are again omnipresent in hospitals, and present risk of burns.

534.28 RADIATION

Ionising radiation is produced in hospitals from diagnostic X-ray, fluoroscopy, angiography and computerised tomography; from X-ray therapy; from radioisotopes used in diagnostic and therapeutic procedures; from linear accelerators; from radiopharmaceuticals; and from stored or discarded radioactive materials. The types of hazard presented by exposure to radiation external to the body are entirely different from those presented by radioactive sources in the body. The latter may enter the body by inhalation, injection through punctures, absorption from intact or damaged skin, or accidental ingestion (e.g. from contaminated hands). The consequences may be short or long term, local or disseminated through the body, depending on the type of source and mode of exposure.

The types of non-ionising radiation encountered in hospitals include ultraviolet (UV), visible (including laser), and infrared (IR) light, radiofrequency (RF) microwave, and ultrasound. Effects of exposure to UV radiation include burns of the skin, conjunctivitis, loss of sight and skin cancer; to lasers, concentrated burns of the skin and the retina; to IR radiation, skin burns and pigmentation and possible eye damage; to RF/microwave radiation, heating of deep body tissues and (possibly) other changes; and to ultrasound radiation, possible temporary hearing loss and local effects on parts contacted.

534.29 ASSAULTS

Anecdotal accounts suggest, although once again documented evidence is poor, that assaults on staff by patients are common, particularly in reception, emergency rooms and psychiatric wards. Visitors may also assault staff and assaults also occur elsewhere in and around hospitals, in shrubbery, parking lots, tunnels and footpaths, particularly where visibility is limited and others are not present.

534.3 Chemical hazards

It is not possible here to describe the remarkable diversity of chemicals and pharmaceuticals encountered in hospitals and their manifold effects. Certain chemicals worthy of mention because of their potential for harm include asbestos (now being replaced or sealed), formaldehyde, glutaraldehyde, anti-neoplastic drugs, ethylene oxide, methyl methacrylate, anaesthetic gases, ammonia, mercury, and various carcinogens, mainly in laboratories, such as benzene, benzidine and carbon tetrachloride.

Hospital workers encounter a large number of chemicals. Some are pre-eminently or almost exclusively used in hospitals, others are common to various industries. Some are in widespread use throughout hospitals; use of many others is confined to particular areas and categories of staff. Each of the broad categories of chemical hazards listed in Table V-3-1 on page 647 covers a wide range of individual chemical substances.

Each of these substances has its own particular toxic effects depending on the concentration and duration of exposure, the route of exposure (through the skin, by inhalation, by ingestion), and the form of the substance (liquid, solid, gas, fume, vapour, dust etc.). Many of the chemicals are mixtures of substances having diverse potential for harm, the effects being possibly influenced also by the individual's use of alcohol, tobacco and drugs. The effects may be topical, on exposed surfaces such as skin, eyes, nose, throat, bronchial passages and gut; or systemic, after absorption into the body. The effects may be acute, immediate, delayed, chronic or long term, and may take the form of irritation, inflammation, burns, suffocation, degeneration, metabolic change, allergic or other immunological disorder, cancer, genetic mutation, deformity or other change. Some substances have multiple effects.

534.4 Biological hazards

Hospitals may bring together many of the serious diseases consequent on infection by biological agents. The potential for transmission of infective agents to employees and others is greater in hospitals than in almost any other workplace. The potential exists not only in the obvious areas of patient care and laboratory but also in sterilisation, laundry, waste disposal and elsewhere.

The infective agents listed in Table V-3-1 on page 647 represent only a sample of the innumerable biological hazards that workers may encounter in hospitals. The HIV-positive provider, or patient, is a potential biological hazard and of increasing concern. Spread of infection in a hospital requires a source of infecting organisms, a susceptible host and a means of transmission. The sources may include patients, staff and visitors, in whom the associated infective disease may not be evident or who may be unaffected carriers of the organism. Secondary sources include contaminated objects such as linen, utensils, equipment and medications.

Susceptibility to infection, always variable in 'normal' people, is greatly enhanced in patients (and perhaps in some staff members) who are weakened by age or disease or whose immunity is compromised by corticosteroids, irradiation, immunosuppression or other therapy. Non-infective biological agents of disease, including a large range of organic dusts, cause bronchial asthma and allergic alveolitis (hypersensitivity pneumonia). Hospital laboratory personnel handling animals are exposed to risk of inhalation of fur, droppings, feed and other detritus and possible consequent sensitisation. Humidifier fever may result from faulty airconditioning.

534.5 | Psychological hazards

Mental disorders are far more common than are the more widely publicised consequences of infective and toxic hazards. Job stress contributes to anxiety and depression, to maladaptive behaviour and lifestyle, and to alcohol and other substance abuse. Hospital employees are exposed to some of the most stressful job situations found anywhere. They deal with distressing life-threatening injuries and illnesses in a situation often compounded with job overload, long hours, understaffing, deadlines, responsibility, shift work, complex and malfunctioning equipment, fear of infection and toxic substances, dependent and demanding patients, and death. Moreover, hospital employees work in one of the most complex organisational structures in our modern society, often with divided professional and organisational loyalties, and value conflicts.

These job factors may lead to worker frustration and job dissatisfaction, a state which, coupled with fatigue, may be visited on patients, other employees and family. It may lead further to withdrawal, expressed as apathy, mental illness, disaffection, absenteeism, workers compensation for minor disorders, and staff turnover. Hospital workers, particularly in nursing, medical and technical areas, consistently show up in studies of mental ill health by occupational categories as being among the most highly affected. Rates of suicide and substance abuse are particularly high. Psychological hazards and their consequences therefore constitute a source not only of much distress in hospital workers but also of great economic loss. Their impact on the quality of patient care can only be guessed, but is likely considerable.

534.6 | Distribution of hazards

Australian hospitals have a very diverse workforce. Registered nurses comprise 35% of the total workforce, while doctors and other health professionals account for approximately 10%. Non-professional staff, including tradespersons, clerks, laundry workers, plant operators and so on, comprise almost 50% of the total workforce.[3] (See Table V-3-2 below.)

These main groups conceal a further wide diversity of occupations and tasks. Within major occupational groups, each subgroup confers its own characteristic pattern of hazards and risks. For example, oncology physicians and nurses are exposed to quite different risks than doctors and nurses in infectious disease departments. Nevertheless, in broad terms of nature of risk, hospital populations can be subdivided into professional, technical, service and administrative/clerical groups. To all these employees at risk must be added the patients and the many friends, relatives, other visitors, and perhaps students, who for varied reasons attend nearly all parts of the hospital each day, and whom the hospital has a responsibility to protect from risk of injury and disease while on its premises.

Table V-3-2 *Persons employed in hospital and nursing homes, 1986*

Occupation	No.	No. in group	Percent
Managers and Administrators: Group 1	8 096	8 096	2.5
Professionals: Group 2			
General medical practitioners	7 164		
Specialist medical practitioners	2 722		

continues

Table V-3-2 *continued*

Occupation	No.	No. in group	Percent
Dental practitioners	241		
Pharmacists	1 412		
Occupational therapists	1 638		
Optometrists	11		
Physiotherapists	2 673		
Chiropractors and osteopaths	3		
Speech pathologists	503		
Radiographers	2 488		
Podiatrists	154		
Other professionals	14 244		
Total Group 2		33 253	10.4
Para-professionals: Group 3			
Registered nurses	111 912		
Other para-professionals	6 504		
Total Group 3		118 416	37
Tradespersons: Group 4			
Food tradespersons	7 426		
Other tradespersons	8 466		
Total Group 4		15 892	4.9
Clerks: Group 5	27 808	27 808	8.7
Salespersons and personal service workers: Group 6			
Enrolled nurses	30 183		
Dental nurses	306		
Others	4 495		
Total Group 6		34 984	10.9
Plant/machine operators and drivers: Group 7	2 638	2 638	0.8
Labourers and related workers: Group 8			
Cleaners	18 617		
Laundry workers	4 242		
Kitchen hands	13 456		
Ward helpers	31 678		
Other labourers and related workers	7 558		
Total Group 8		75 551	23.6
Inadequately described/not stated	2 932	2 932	0.9
Total	319 570	319 570	100.0

Source: Modified from C. Grant and H. M. Lapsley, 'The Australian Health Care System 1992'.

Table V-3-3 *Extent of some hazards in selected hospital departments*

Hazard	Patient care	Operating theatres	Offices	Laboratory	Food service	Laundry	Main- tenance
Physical:							
Patient lifting	++	+					
Other manual handling	+	+	+	+	++	++	++
Slips, falls	+	+	+	+	++	++	++
Tools, machinery				+	+	+	++
Repetition work			++				+
Assaults	++	+					+
Ionising radiation	+	+		+			
Electricity	+	++		++	+	+	++
Noise					+	+	++
Heat, cold				+	++	++	+
Flammables, explosives	+	+		++	+		++
Chemical:							
Toxic substances	+	+	+	++	+	+	++
Therapeutic substances	++	+		+			
Biological:							
Infective agents	++	++		++		+	
Air quality	+	+	+	++	++	+	++
Psychological:							
Psychosocial	++	++	+	+			

Key: Exposure to risk: + some; ++ considerable

The exposure to hazards and the risk therefrom is clearly not evenly distributed among the various occupational categories in hospitals, and it will clearly vary from hospital to hospital depending on the type and range of services provided. Thus sprains and strains, particularly low back injuries, which constitute by far the largest single source of injury and economic loss in hospitals as in most other industries, are commonest among nurses, nursing aides, orderlies and other staff who regularly lift patients, and in other sections of hospitals where much heavy manual handling is undertaken, such as laundries and stores. The risk for infections such as hepatitis B is greatest in doctors and nurses. Medical practitioners also have high rates of drug dependence and suicide. Table V-3-3 above categorises hospitals' various departments by the pattern of hazards to which employees in those areas are particularly exposed.

The matrix of hazards and areas displayed in Table V-3-3 is not exhaustive but rather illustrates the diversity of hazards that may be encountered in various parts of the hospital environment. The absence of data relating to occupational health and safety in Australia makes it impossible to quantify the degree of risk afforded by the presence of a hazard either in the hospital industry as a whole or in an individual department. Any work environment will probably consist of a complex mix of hazards. These can be categorised as:

- general hazards present in the hospital, such as falls and sharps, and those present in its environment, for example distributed through the airconditioning system;
- specific hazards, such as those encountered in certain places or circumstances, for example from equipment in theatres or laboratories.

The total number of hazards present should be enumerated rather than assumed, so as to measure the total risk. Of course, certain hazards, such as massive radiation leaks, represent such a high risk that where they occur the contribution of other risks may be insignificant.

535 | An effective occupational health and safety program

535.1 | Elements of an OH&S program

An OH&S program comprises a number of functional elements. They include:

- occupational health and safety hazard control, which is the core business. Most hospitals will struggle to succeed even confining their efforts to this core element;
- health promotion or wellness programs;
- stress management (encompassing all types of employee assistance programs);
- employee health services;
- employee management.

In addition the OH&S service, the department or division whose job it is to implement the program, may engage in consulting, teaching and research.

535.2 | OH&S risk management

Occupational health and safety risk management encompasses:

- risk avoidance (hazard control);
- damage control;
- risk transfer.

The main role and function of the OH&S service is to control hazards and minimise risk. It is the main core business of occupational health and safety. Involvement of the service in hazard control, in collaboration with other hospital professional services, may call for simple common sense management intervention. On the other hand, from time to time there may be a need for expertise in the areas of occupational hygiene, safety engineering, ergonomics, toxicology or occupational health psychology. Evaluating the effectiveness of hazard containment measures may involve environmental and biomedical surveillance and monitoring.

Generally, safety and medical services in hospitals are separated organisationally, but it is now essential that they be combined so that control of physical hazards is not artificially isolated from that of other types of hazards. In addition, by bringing the OH&S service within the organisational framework of quality management, its activities can be supplemented with the analytical resources of the quality management department. One illustration of the common ground that should exist between medical and safety services is the identification and prevention of nosocomial infections.

535.3 | Risk avoidance

Occupational injuries and diseases should be prevented and risks avoided, if at all possible, as in many cases there are no satisfactory treatments for, by way of example, degenerative back disease (from inadvisable patient lifting), AIDS (from needle sticks), or mesothelioma (from exposure to asbestos). Risk avoidance is achieved through hazard control and results in risk reduction. Preventive, risk avoidance strategies can be classified under structure, process and outcome. Necessarily, examples are illustrative. Specific hazards require specific control strategies, and readers responsible for OH&S risk management would do well to obtain expert advice. Just as for quality management in general, it is essential that management has the right attitude, sees to it that right policies are developed and that correct practices are implemented. Policies and practices for which management should have regard can be categorised by structure, process and outcome as follows:

- Structure:
  —employ people who are capable of doing the job (physically fit, properly trained etc.);
  —educate all staff concerning the occupational hazards they may face;
  —train and educate line managers concerning OH&S awareness;
  —substitute safe materials for dangerous ones, if at all possible;
  —engineer out hazards where appropriate; for example, alter processes to minimise worker contact with hazards and progressively install fail-safe systems;
  —vaccinate at-risk employees with, for example, hepatitis B vaccine and TB vaccine;
  —limit worker exposure to unavoidable hazards, for example by job rotation;
  —devise proper training and incentives for staff and supervisors in relation to safety consciousness and incident reporting etc.;
  —consider money incentives for safety.
- Process:
  —design safe work practices, for example for infectious waste disposal;
  —provide and train staff in correct use of personal protective devices, clothing, safety gear etc.;
  —insist that good housekeeping practices be followed;
  —insist that such safe work practices be carried out and devise incentives to that end.
- Outcome—set up appropriate surveillance, monitoring and information systems encompassing for example:
  —radiation exposure monitoring;
  —physiological markers, such as blood lead levels;
  —outcomes, such as accidents and injuries;
  —absenteeism and employee sickness including such conditions as spontaneous abortion, congenital anomalies/genetic defects in offspring and infertility; and
  —other relevant indicators of potential workplace hazards.

535.4 | Damage control

Although the OH&S service should stress prevention, it should be available or make arrangements to handle medical emergencies to the extent of resuscitation and urgent treatment where no other facility is available. The use of a sick bay or the accident and emergency department will vary according to circumstances from hospital to hospital. The service must also be able to cope with the need to deal with a range of outside agencies and organisations which may become involved in a variety of ways with work-related episodes. Hospitals should prepare relevant plans including, for example, to:

- identify and assist the individual (e.g. QM manager or hospital manager) who deals with press and family where this is necessary;
- investigate and report on incidents depending on their nature and magnitude;
- notify and liaise with insurer when appropriate;
- liaise with emergency services when and if necessary.

535.5   *Risk transfer*

All hospitals currently engage in a range of risk transfer mechanisms, various types of insurance, including the following for example. We mention them merely for completeness:

- workers compensation insurance;
- fire insurance;
- liability insurance.

536 | Additional occupational health and safety activities

536.1   *Health promotion*

While hospital health and safety programs' first priority must always be for the protection of employees, patients and visitors from harm in the hospital environment, so-called non-occupational disorders occasion far more employee morbidity than work-related disease and injury. The associated financial loss, in sickness absence, turnover, premature death and retirement, and ineffective work, warrants a major improvement effort. Health promotion is not then a matter of hospitals merely being caring employers or of their usurping a community health role; rather it is a matter of diminishing the risk of ill health. Health promotion or disease prevention is now commonly the subject of special programs in industry, within the general health and safety program, though they may be conducted separately. Hospital work sites present a particularly fertile ground for such programs. Canteens, for example, can serve healthy, nutritious meals, or label foods to inform consumers which are healthy or which pose risks, and smoking may be prohibited throughout the hospital. As with hospital hazard programs, health promotion may be the subject of specific programs that may cover the following:

- anti-smoking, smoking cessation;
- hypertension and coronary heart disease;
- cancer, glaucoma and diabetes;
- mental health;
- physical fitness, nutrition.

Limitations of staff and budgets will dictate that most hospitals will have limited opportunity to engage in this type of health promotion. Larger hospitals, particularly with the help of outside agencies, will see these programs as benefiting staff morale and enhancing their risk reduction initiatives. It is important that decisions on such programs should be authorised by the QM committee on the recommendation of the OH&S committee.

536.2   *Stress management—employee assistance programs*

Many industries combine, under the heading of employee assistance programs, such aspects of health promotion as the management of emotional distress, maladaptive behaviour and drug and alcohol dependence. Though these aspects may rightly be viewed as extensions of occupational health and safety, employee assistance programs may also provide counselling for gambling, financial difficulty and other 'non-health' problems, often under the auspices of the personnel management and human resources department. External sources usually provide stress management programs, but they are likely to be more successful if integrated with management activities designed to counteract causes of distress outlined above. Thus, regular staff meetings, adequate staffing, flexible and efficient job design and work organisation, education, skills enhancement, action on legitimate complaints, availability of non-judgmental counselling, and group therapy on dealing with disease and death are some measures open to hospitals that may prevent or mitigate distress. They also represent good management practice.

536.3 Employee health services

Employee health services comprise:

- clinical services related to occupational health and safety, such as pre-employment examinations and clinical surveillance. Some services such as pre-employment examinations may be delegated to the employee's own general practitioner, while others may require specialist occupational health practitioners;
- general medical services which actually substitute for the employee's general practitioner. In general, except in isolated situations where general practitioner services may not be available, such service may be neither desirable nor in the employee's best interests;
- the tracking and monitoring of sickness reports from the employee's general practitioner, to determine if patterns exist and to explore their relationship to possible occupational hazards.

536.4 Health assessment, employment examinations

Health assessment includes information and judgments on health status of employees derived from many sources such as self-administered questionnaires, preplacement, periodic and special medical examinations, and various records of illness, absence and work-related injury and disease. The preplacement examination is intended to ensure that a new employee is not adversely placed, and to provide a baseline health record for ongoing health surveillance, often over a working lifetime. Opportunity is taken to record a full occupational history.

The question of the desirability of pre-employment examination for all workers, as against certain target staff, is far from unanimous. In addition, hospitals employ large numbers of staff, among whom there is often a rapid turnover. The sheer physical and economic task of such routine examinations will prevent many hospitals entertaining the idea. Periodic health appraisals may be made for workers exposed to risk of harm, or on return from sickness or injury absence, or who are on transfer to another job, or who are retiring or leaving. Biological monitoring may be part of periodic surveillance and, together with information on environmental exposure to certain hazards, may constitute an ongoing cumulative record of exposure.

Health assessments provide the opportunity to explain to work applicants and employees the hospital's health and safety program, to educate them in the particular risks of their job, and to advise where appropriate on aspects of lifestyle and general health. The employees should be given assurance on their rights to privacy and to access to their own personal records.

536.5 Medical services

It may or may not be a function of the OH&S service to provide a sick bay or medical service for staff. Nevertheless, a close liaison with any staff treatment service and with external practitioners is necessary to ensure speedy and effective rehabilitation to work and for feedback as to the possible work-relatedness of morbidity or mortality. It also may afford continuity of care on return to work, in collaboration with private practitioners.

Any employee consultation facility should afford medical, psychological and social counselling, particularly in the areas of substance abuse and of HIV and hepatitis B infection, with appropriate consideration of confidentiality. The occupational health service may give this assistance if no other is available. In any case, the service needs to be aware of the extent of such problems because its role includes containing any risks that may exist.

536.6 | Health records

The occupational health service should maintain a health record of all hospital employees including such relevant source documents as general practitioners' sickness certificates. The records should include results of surveillance examinations, reports of incidents and accidents, biological and environmental monitoring data, and sickness data generally. Records must be confidential and available only to accredited people within the service. The usual professional ethical obligations attach to all of the service's activities. Periodically the service, with proper biostatistical or epidemiological assistance, should report on the data it collects. Reports should focus on identifying potential preventive actions. Analysis of record data may be descriptive, on the distribution of health, injury and disease by occupational, environmental, organisational, personal and social variables in order to identify or monitor problems and the effectiveness of solutions. The service should investigate apparent epidemics (unusual occurrences of morbidity and disability) to confirm their existence and if possible identify and eliminate their causes.

The vexed question of who is entitled to what information is beyond the scope of this manual. Suffice to say, diagnoses must not be reported to hospital management, although management does have a right and need to know certain information for administrative purposes, for example on ability to work and on work restrictions. The only exceptions relate to aggregate data, legal requirements, subpoena, workers compensation, written authorisation by the employee, or in certain cases of contagious disease. All potentially work-related illnesses and injuries among staff should be the subject of reporting to employers and insurers in conformity with workers compensation legislation. Policies on the disclosure of privileged information should be explicit and widely disseminated throughout the hospital, and management should enforce sanctions if employees breach these policies.

536.7 | Employee management

Employee management consists of advising management and employees about schedules, workloads and the wide range of personnel management issues which affect worker performance and job satisfaction.

The health and safety service touches upon employee relations in a number of ways, for example in stress management (employee assistance) programs. Other relevant aspects of employee management include scheduling (particularly of nurses), workload (particularly of doctors) and shift work (which may disturb circadian rhythms). These and other aspects of work discussed elsewhere can cause distress and fatigue and thus can affect performance and ultimately the quality of patient care. Employee management concerns are properly part of the occupational health service's responsibility to advise hospital management, including the personnel department.

536.8 | Consultancy teaching and research

Consulting, teaching and research of necessity will be activities undertaken only in large teaching hospitals that have a full-blown OH&S service, usually in association with a university department. The service's occupational physician acts as a consultant to others in the hospital on matters related to the health and safety programs; but is also available to provide consultancy to colleagues within and outside the hospital on patients (not necessarily hospital employees) with potentially work-related illness and injury. In this way, small hospitals in regions or area health services can make use of the expertise in the central base or teaching hospital.

537 | Establishing and improving an effective OH&S program

537.1 | Setting priorities

An effective occupational health and safety program requires a number of key elements, the absence of any one of which will like as not spell failure for the undertaking. They include the following:

- knowledge from in-house experts and/or outside consultants;
- information from outside surveys and/or in-house data systems;
- resources from the board and management;
- organisation to get the job done;
- commitment and the will to succeed.

Keys to improving hospital occupational health and safety can be summarised as follows:

- select measures by which to evaluate progress, and set priorities;
- progress measures should be specific to the problem, for example reduction in injury rates;
- priority setting measures must be commensurable across all problems. Priority setting as a rational exercise is quite complex and requires data and knowledge likely beyond most hospitals' present capabilities. The best approach is to select the obvious and the big problems (which initially might have to be identified from industry-wide rather than from hospital-specific sources);
- some useful measures (criteria) include:
  —health status loss to employees;
  —productivity losses;
  —other costs, such as insurance premiums and legal suits;
  —employee morale, for example judged from surveys or absenteeism rates.

537.2 | Relation to quality management

If care is about quality, employees who provide the care are surely critical to the successful implementation of quality. Work health and safety promotes quality patient care. A cared for employee is a caring and productive employee. Thus effective and efficient management of a health and safety program can be expected to result in:

- enhanced recruitment and retention of good workers;
- improved morale and hence productivity;
- safer conditions, which in turn lead to fewer legal suits and lower workers compensation costs;
- better patient care as a result.

Management cannot assume that individual health professionals automatically understand and act to control risks to their wellbeing and the hospital's benefit. In any case, solutions should not and often cannot rest with individual employees, whatever their knowledge of prevention. Obviously, individuals need to understand the hazards of their workplace and should act responsibly. However, many preventive activities are beyond an individual's capacity to implement. Employee health and safety is a management responsibility. Hospital managements also have a legislated responsibility and increasingly will be under pressure from unions, from media publicity on particular issues such as the transmission of HIV and reproductive risks to their employees, and from general community expectations on workplace standards and accountability for the cost of carelessness. There is an increasing awareness in the community and in industry generally about health and safety programs, though there are still major deficiencies in most hospitals.

The occupational health and safety program is also responsible for impaired providers. The quality management committee is responsible for developing policies to deal with situations where a provider, a medical practitioner in particular, is, or is suspected of being, impaired. One such situation might be a surgeon who is HIV positive. The QM committee needs to consider such questions as: Should the hospital have a policy for testing all or certain providers for HIV or drugs? Should patients be told prospectively that their doctor is HIV positive or has AIDS? If a surgeon, for example, is discovered to be HIV positive, or to have died of AIDS, should the hospital notify all of his or her patients so that they can be tested?

537.3 Management commitment

An effective occupational health and safety program should be part of a comprehensive quality management structure. In this fashion, the traditional attitude that occupational health and safety is a benefit bestowed by an industrial award, and that it should therefore be separate from the health culture of hospitals, may need to be corrected. The correct attitude will produce a better awareness by all concerned of the importance of OH&S to the hospital generally. If an influential committee such as the quality management committee were made aware of some of the effects of employee injury on hospital performance, for example, greater resources and influence would inevitably be brought to bear on the issue.

Hospital managements have an economic obligation to provide effective and efficient programs and services, partly because of the need to cut costs and the risk of litigation. They also have a community obligation in that their hospital operations may constitute a threat to employees and others, and hospital employment affects general health (or ill health) status.

No health and safety program can succeed without the hospital board's and management's unequivocal commitment. Such a commitment is usually expressed in a written policy that states the commitment in a sentence or two, and summarises the hospital's strategy for operationalising that commitment. The statement may cover the establishment of a program and of a health and safety committee; the goals of the program; responsibilities of the OH&S committee, line management and staff; and procedural policies. Policies should be set in consultation with employees, who will be represented on the OH&S committee. Most important is the commitment of resources to implement policies and to get the job done.

537.4 Getting started

The hospital should proceed to:

- appoint a health and safety committee (such committees are now required by legislation in all Australian states) that would be a subcommittee of the hospital QM committee;
- determine the OH&S committee's reporting arrangements and frequency of its reports;
- determine the functional relationship of the occupational health and safety service to the personnel department;
- appoint its occupational health and safety officer and other personnel;
- budget and allocate funds for the elements of the OH&S program and OH&S service;

- ensure that the organisational structure is in place;
- ensure that the hospital has at least the minimum number of staff for the role;
- if the hospital does not have them, hire consultants and experts to provide essential advice and guidance;
- develop an OH&S plan, which ultimately will have quantitative targets; for example a reduction in injuries from 200 per 1000 employees per year to 100 per 1000 employees. The plan should also contain specific implementation steps and identify people who are to be held accountable for the implementation;
- establish or augment data collection and reporting systems for appropriate monitoring;
- convert data to information, set priorities, and update the OH&S plan, including resource requirements;
- match progress to plans and, if progress falls short, analyse the reasons why.

537.5 The occupational health and safety committee

537.51 REGULATORY REQUIREMENTS

Australian states generally now require the establishment of health and safety committees in places of work beyond a certain (low) minimum size, and specify the general aims, composition, functions and responsibilities of such committees. The legislation may, for example, require the committee to have equal management and employee representation, with employee chairmanship. Thus, at the present time the committee is bipartite, with advisory attendance by an in-house health professional such as the safety engineer or occupational physician or nurse, if any of these professionals is available. However, in the majority of Australian hospitals they are not.

537.52 THE OCCUPATIONAL HEALTH AND SAFETY COMMITTEE'S PURPOSE

The role of the OH&S committee is to:

- develop an OH&S plan;
- monitor progress of OH&S activity in the hospital;
- determine priorities and set strategies;
- draw up detailed procedures for hazard identification and control;
- develop training and education and motivation programs for employees;
- maintain appropriate records in accordance with regulations and for effective control of hazards;
- institute mechanisms for ongoing OH&S program review and quality management;
- provide an information base, including library of material safety data sheets;
- develop policies on health promotion programs;
- conduct regular workplace inspections;
- provide input to new construction, renovation, work systems and equipment;
- investigate accidents, unusual occurrence of disease etc.

Most hospitals may well lack the necessary expertise to accomplish all of these tasks and will require the assistance of outside consultant advice. However, it is the committee which must carry the ultimate responsibility for the recommendations that are developed for management's consideration.

537.53 OH&S COMMITTEE MEMBERSHIP

The committee should consist of from seven to thirteen members.[8] Regard needs to be paid to statutory provisions, which stipulate that these committees must represent both management and workers, and that the number of worker representatives must always exceed that of management. The hospital board appoints members who should serve for a minimum of two years. Membership of this committee would include the OH&S officer (who ideally should be a suitably qualified medical practitioner or registered nurse but who at the present time is more commonly the fire and safety officer—a non-health professional), the QM manager, the personnel officer, and the in-house health professional such as the safety engineer or occupational physician or nurse, if any of these professionals is available.

The committee may co-opt additional expertise if and where the need arises. Such experts would be advisory and would not have a vote. Ideally, the occupational physician should chair this committee, if legislation does not require the chairperson to be a rank-and-file employee. Unfortunately, at the present time few hospitals have an occupational physician. The chairperson of the OH&S committee should be a member of the QM committee.

537.54 AUTHORISATION OF THE COMMITTEE

The OH&S committee should be a standing committee authorised by the board of directors of the hospital.

537.55 COMMITTEE MEETINGS

The committee should meet monthly or at such other frequency as the committee decides. An agenda should accompany a notice of regularly scheduled meetings and it should be distributed not less than ten days prior to the meeting. The business of the committee should be formally conducted and all decisions properly recorded.

537.56 REPORTING RELATIONSHIPS

As an integral component of quality management, the occupational health and safety committee in the hospital should be a subcommittee of the hospital QM committee. Part of the business of the QM committee should be a regular review and report on the incidence of employee illness and injury, and the occupational health and safety officer should personally present this report and answer questions on it.

537.6 Specialised subcommittees

The occupational health and safety committee must be prepared to address the whole gamut of hazards that hospitals may present. Hazard analysis and control and review of control measures' effectiveness constitute the program's prime justification. Nevertheless, certain hazards are so common or so potentially serious as to warrant special control programs within the overall program. Some of these special programs have long attracted the formation of special committees within hospitals, which, in the past, often but undesirably functioned in isolation from each other. Such subcommittees must have access to expert advice and data, and must be action driven. Moreover, because of the traditional lack of integration of these activities in many hospitals, the co-ordinating role of the OH&S committee, with the support of the quality management department, needs continual emphasis. Any specialty OH&S subcommittees should report to the statutory OH&S committee. Examples of such independent functions often resulting in subcommittees include the following:

- back injuries, strain injuries generally, or manual handling of patients and other loads;
- noise;
- radiation and radionucleotide safety;
- infections, possibly subdivisible also into nosocomial, MRSA, hepatitis B, AIDS and other infectious diseases;
- laboratory safety;
- anti-neoplastic (cytotoxic) drugs;

- waste disposal and public and environmental hygiene;
- fire and explosion risk.

Such specific programs may demand greater resources than most hospitals can muster. Certainly, in larger teaching hospitals many of these programs will be indicated. Small hospitals will tailor programs to suit what they assess as their greatest risks, and they will inevitably be on a much smaller scale. Smaller hospitals may also find it beneficial to group themselves on some mutually satisfactory arrangement to gain access to some of these specialised services.

One of the OH&S committee's important responsibilities is product safety, including such matters as recalls on supplies and machines, and equipment generally. Functionally, the OH&S committee may assign this responsibility to a QM subcommittee whose remit would also include implant registries and manufacturers' recalls of patient supplies and equipment, such as cardiac pacemakers.

538 | The occupational health and safety plan

538.1 | Aspects of an occupational health and safety plan

The OH&S director's central responsibility is to produce a realistic OH&S plan in collaboration with the OH&S committee. While such a plan would have many aspects, those of particular importance include:

- analysing risks and setting priorities for their reduction;
- establishing program objectives and setting strategies to achieve them;
- selecting key measures of success and developing information systems to track progress.

538.2 | Priority setting

Priority setting in OH&S is a difficult task, as it is in other complex areas. The objective is to implement strategies that will produce the greatest reduction in risk given the resources available, within policy constraints. Rational priority setting depends heavily on the availability of information and appropriate analytical models. Essentially, it is necessary to:

- identify hazards and existing risks, and the extent to which existing regulations are being met and good practices are being implemented;
- assess the consequences of existing risks, in such terms as health status loss and financial loss;
- for significant existing risks, analyse their major underlying causes and formulate preventive or remedial strategies;
- estimate the extent to which any set of strategies will reduce the risk and the initial and recurrent cost of implementing these strategies;
- select and implement the most cost-effective strategies;
- monitor the extent to which risks are reduced, and reassess priorities and revise the plan.

538.3 | Risk analysis

Risk analysis has two components:

- risk assessment;
- risk evaluation.

Risk assessment measures risk. Risk evaluation is a judgment about the acceptability of any risk, and consequently about the value of its reduction. While it is incumbent on hospital managers to assess risk, judgments about their acceptability may have been pre-empted by social custom, regulation or legislation.

For example, assessing risk implies prior identification of particular hazards such as patient lifting, and then determination of consequences. In this case consequences may be back or other strain injury, and the level of its severity in the nursing and other patient handling staff, and injury to patients. Thus, with a given hazard in a given situation, one attempts to establish the number of persons potentially at risk, the probability that exposure to risk will occur and, if exposure occurs, the probability, nature and severity of harm over time, including costs.

On the other hand, risk evaluation is a social, industrial, political and psychological judgment of the acceptability of risks. In the back injury example, it could be argued that the high rate of hospital employee morbidity and cost from injuries incurred in lifting patients and other loads is presently accepted by employees, managements and governments (and taxpayers) who foot the bill.

538.4   Information on hazards

Information on hazards and risks can be drawn from two sources: published reports and hospital information (incident reporting) systems. The basis of successful risk reduction is reliable, relevant and useable data. Unfortunately, such data have not been available at the national level in Australia, nor in many cases in a useful form at the individual hospital level.

Injuries, especially falls and strains, are known to be major problems in hospitals and serve as a good example of hospital hazards. More specifically, back injuries in nursing staff represent a particular hazard.

At the hospital level, accident reports, illnesses and absences should be part of the incident recording and tracking component of a quality management program. The reporting and tracking of all incidents, whether related to staff, patients or visitors, should be part of one integrated system and as such form a vital component of the total quality management program. Risk from injuries/accidents can be assessed from good hospital information systems. Risk from diseases in the workplace for some time to come will be calculated from published material. Nevertheless, one should remember that published data must either originate in special studies or information systems.

The following example of data assembly illustrates what we believe every hospital should be doing on a routine and regular basis, even though this collection of data relates only to a narrow range of physical hazards and should ideally include all types of hazards. While larger hospitals using more sophisticated technology will have more complex hazards, most hospitals will find that collecting data on accidents and injuries will provide at least one fruitful way of identifying problems.

One major metropolitan hospital in Australia provided data on staff accidents for the calendar year 1990 and the financial year 1993/94. In 1990 the hospital employed 2000 staff and reported 301 work site accidents involving staff during that calendar year (about 151 per 1000 employees). In 1993/94 the staff employed had risen to about 2500 and reported accidents to 405 (about 162 per 1000 employees).

In 1990 the hospital's rate of injuries (151 per 1000 workers) was 6.4 times the 1991/92 national average for industry generally and 5 times that for hospitals. By 1993/94 the rate had risen to 162 per 1000 workers. Figure V-3-3(a) on page 664 shows the hospital's distribution of accidents per 1000 employees by type for 1990 and 1993/94. The three most common types of accidents in 1990—sharps (needle sticks), manual handling (lifting), and slips and falls—were still the three most common types in 1993/94. The rate of reported sharp injuries fell almost 40%, from 51 per 1000 workers in 1990 to 37 per 1000 in 1993/94. Accidents involving objects striking workers, and vice versa, also fell

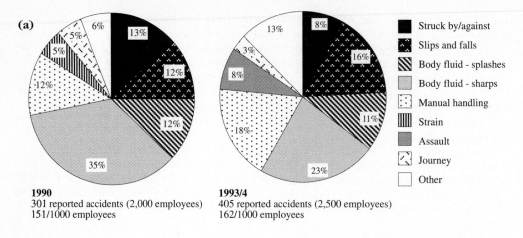

(a)

Legend:
- ■ Struck by/against
- Slips and falls
- Body fluid - splashes
- Body fluid - sharps
- Manual handling
- Strain
- Assault
- Journey
- Other

1990
301 reported accidents (2,000 employees)
151/1000 employees

1993/4
405 reported accidents (2,500 employees)
162/1000 employees

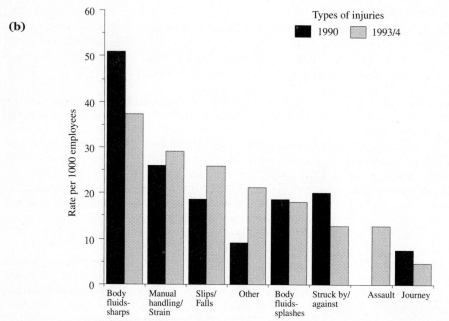

(b)

Figure V-3-3(a) and (b) *Distribution of reported staff accidents at a 500-bed metropolitan hospital, 1990 and 1993/94*

appreciably, from 20 per 1000 to 13 per 1000 workers. However, overall, other types of accidents—most notably slips and falls, assaults and others—more than made up for these improvements.

Over the three to four year period the number and rate of staff accidents have increased. However, the hospital is unable to determine whether this result merely reflects an improvement in the reporting of accidents or a real increase in accidents. Better reporting can make it appear that the situation is deteriorating when in reality it may be improving. Accurate reporting is necessary to measure progress in quality management. Most importantly, to realise quality improvement, management must provide the incentives and resources to investigate accidents' root causes and to change procedures and practices to prevent or reduce their occurrence. Whether there has been improved reporting or not, the occupational health and safety officer believes that a significant number of accidents are still not being reported. In commenting on these data, he was critical of a continuing failure to report incidents, and when reported, the poor standard of the reports by departmental heads and the absence of corrective action taken to prevent problems even when the problem was clearly identified. He views these deficiencies as a reflection of the staff's indifference to accidents. Most likely this situation stems from management's lack of interest in and commitment to reporting and resolving these problems.

538.5 From information to action

The hospital's rate of recorded injuries, 143 per 1000 workers in 1990 and 162 per 1000 workers in 1993/94 is many times the national average, and the multiple is increasing. The higher incidence of injuries may be real or it may be due to better than average reporting. The better a hospital's reporting system the worse it may look, rendering comparisons with other hospitals (with less good systems) misleading. However, the better the system, the more information is available to reduce the risk. Clearly, reducing strains—the most common problem—would reduce total injuries. On the other hand, maybe it would be easier to reduce contact injuries by greater attention to good housekeeping practices. Based on careful analysis of what is possible, the hospital might set an objective of reducing its injury rate by half, for example to 75 per 1000, for the next year and implement what it concluded were the most cost-effective strategies to achieve this end.

In this particular hospital, the figures show that on average about one in six members of the hospital staff suffered an accidental injury over the course of the year. However, the focus in this hospital, as in most, is simple accidents and injuries. It is hard to believe that drug abuse, psychological stress or diseases relating to the workplace would surface in a program where a fire and safety officer was the sole responsible individual. No recorded incidents relating to chemical or biological hazards in a hospital of over 2000 staff reinforces this view. Should this suggested under-reporting exist, the OH&S incident rate would be even higher.

While a fire and safety officer is quite capable of managing accident and injury identification, without appropriate medical practitioner input into the OH&S committee, it is highly unlikely that workplace diseases and other incidents will either be thought of or identified. The noted failure to report OH&S incidents, while consistent with our remarks about hospital incident reporting in general, emphasises the overall attitude of hospital staff and management to occupational health and safety. By integrating the reporting of OH&S incidents within the framework of quality management, we would hope to see a more realistic attitude on behalf of hospital staff over the course of time.

539 The occupational health and safety service

539.1 Functions of services

The OH&S service is the operational arm of the health and safety program. In line with our view that OH&S is properly part of quality management, the service should be part of the quality management department. In large hospitals it may be a freestanding department or division. The OH&S service provides the professional staff for the hospital's OH&S program. It advises and co-operates with the health and safety committee on which its director sits, but is responsible to the quality manager (or hospital manager, if a separate department). Its role is predicated on the hospital's health and safety policy, its program's goals, and the service's terms of reference and rules of procedure. In Australia, when even large hospitals employ one, usually non-medical, fire and safety officer, its capabilities are likely to fall far short of the ideal. As with all aspects of quality management it is necessary for the hospital, specifically the OH&S committee, to assess the OH&S service's performance with a view to continual improvement.

539.2 | Organisation

The OH&S service's organisation will depend very much on the size of the hospital, program responsibilities and to some extent management preferences. Nevertheless, it is important to stipulate a number of requirements including the following:

- there must be a director of the OH&S service who is responsible for implementing the OH&S program;
- there must be a mechanism for obtaining expert outside assistance when needed;
- the OH&S director should chair the OH&S committee and be on the QM committee.

The line management configuration will vary from hospital to hospital. Although we prefer the first one in most circumstances, the following three models are possible:

- the director of OH&S reports to the manager through the QM manager;
- the director of OH&S reports directly to the manager, in parallel with the QM manager;
- the director of OH&S is separate from QM and reports to the manager through the personnel manager.

539.3 | Occupational health and safety service director

Legislation usually does not specify the numbers and make-up of work health and safety services or staff. In large hospitals the director of the service is usually a full-time occupational physician. In hospitals where a physician attends part time, the director is usually the chief occupational nurse but may be an occupational health and safety manager from a diversity of backgrounds who has a postgraduate qualification in the field. The director must:

- have entry, and make regular and ad hoc visits, to all parts of the hospital;
- establish liaison with all hospital departments and services and with relevant external agencies;
- ensure the collection, keeping and confidentiality of appropriate records; and
- generally advise management on the hospital's health and safety program.

539.4 | Occupational health and safety service staff

The staff of the health and safety service may be employed or contracted. The numbers and diversity of staff of a hospital employee health service vary with the size of the hospital, although as already mentioned a fire and safety officer is frequently the only staff available. In a small hospital of up to 100 bed capacity the only professional staffing feasible may be that of a part-time occupational nurse with a visiting occupational physician. Hospitals of up to 300 bed capacity may rate one or two full-time occupational nurses and a physician shared half time with another hospital. Larger hospitals rate not only full-time occupational physician(s) and nurses but also, depending on size, an occupational hygienist, occupational psychologist or psychiatrist, safety engineer and possibly ergonomist and toxicologist.

The reality, of course, is that these benchmarks for staff fall far short of what exists in most hospitals today. The average hospital, almost regardless of size, has one non-medical safety officer with a variable degree of knowledge and experience, and an occupational health and safety committee on which experts may or may not be represented. It is possible, however, to obtain outside expert advice in a part-time or ad hoc consultative capacity, which can be shared by smaller hospitals on a regional or group basis. Twenty-four hour coverage in smaller hospitals may be arranged by a telephone roster service.

539.5 | Qualified and trained staff

As for any hospital service, the key to an effective OH&S service is the training, experience and qualifications of the staff involved in the provision of that service. The service will not be effective and efficient unless each of its professional staff is properly trained and qualified in the respective occupational health and safety discipline. Hospitals must provide opportunities for continuing education of their services' professional staff by sending them to professional meetings, courses and seminars. Attendance at such meetings is good for morale and allows development of networks of potentially helpful contacts as well as exchange of experience on hospital problems.

539.6 | Service facilities

The rooms, equipment, furniture and other facilities provided for the hospital's health and safety services will vary with the size and type of hospital and the extent to which other facilities obviate the need for duplication. Usually, regulations or codes of practice governing services in industry generally do not provide firm standards for facilities. The space provided may range from a single clinic room in a small hospital to a suite of rooms, including occupational hygiene laboratories, in large hospitals. Even in small hospitals the premises of the service should be a space identifiable and dedicated as such. Clearly, however, there is no need for hospitals to duplicate such facilities as pathology laboratories or other resources. The guiding rule should be that the facilities must be commensurate with the tasks to be undertaken by the OH&S service. All records, whether computerised or not, must be in a secure area to guarantee confidentiality.

References

1 Health expenditure bulletin, No 7. July 1992. Australian Institute of Health & Welfare.
2 Health expenditure bulletin, No 8. April 1993. Australian Institute of Health & Welfare.
3 Grant C, Lapsley HM. The Australian health care system; 1992. (Australian studies in health service administration, No.75). Sydney, Australia: School of Health Services Management, University of New South Wales.
4 National Institute for Occupational Safety and Health: Guidelines for protecting the safety and health of health care workers. Washington, DC: U.S. Government Printing Office, 1988, (Publication No:88–119), p 1–2.
5 Hospitals and Nursing Homes Industry. Occupational Health and Safety Performance Overview. Australia, 1991–92. Worksafe Australia. National Occupational Health and Safety Commission.
6 Employment injuries New South Wales hospitals and nursing homes; 1986–87.
7 National Institute for Occupational Safety and Health: Guidelines for protecting the safety and health of health care workers. Washington, DC: U.S. Government Printing Office, 1988, (Publication No:88–119), p 1–2.
8 National Occupational Health and Safety Commission. Media release; August 9, 1989.
9 National Institute for Occupational Safety and Health; Guidelines for health care workers, op.cit. p 1–8.

PART VI

QUALITY MANAGEMENT AND THE LAW

SUMMARY

This part intends to introduce some legal facts into an environment which has been characterised by much speculation, very little understanding of the law, and not a little anxiety on the part of hospital medical staff. While there is little doubt that some activity necessary for quality management in a hospital does pose potential exposure to legal action, such a threat certainly does not exist with the current level of quality management activity commonly seen in Australia.

This part's contents apply strictly to Australia, and in some cases only to the State of New South Wales. This latter material intends to illustrate situations that may, but do not necessarily, exist in other Australian states and territories. Clearly laws, and the customs on which they are based, vary from State to State, as well as from country to country. Nevertheless, we believe that such principles as respect for individuals and their privacy, rules of natural justice or due process, and truth-telling and striving for objectivity ought to apply everywhere.

This part describes the various aspects of the law that impinge on quality management activity. The avoidance of risk of legal consequences hangs heavily on the appropriate structures and processes, matters discussed in Part III. Chapters in this part are:

Chapter 1   *Introduction to and purpose of Part VI*—provides perspective concerning legal aspects of quality management activity.

Chapter 2   *Liability of hospitals and medical practitioners*—deals with such matters as negligence, duty of care, hospital liability, visiting medical officers and quality assurance.

Chapter 3   *Natural justice*—describes the legal concept of natural justice and the important part it plays when there are disputes between doctors and their colleagues or hospitals.

Chapter 4 *Defamation*—explores the subject under a number of headings including what is the meaning of defamation, popular misconceptions and quality management and defamation.

Chapter 1

INTRODUCTION TO AND PURPOSE OF PART VI

| 610 | **Contents** |

This chapter provides some perspective concerning the legal consequences of quality management activity and examines the current state of confusion which is in evidence. It describes:

- **611.** Purpose of this part
- **612.** Contents of this part
- **613.** Purpose of this chapter
- **614.** Current concerns
- **615.** Indemnity
- **616.** Risks in perspective
- **617.** Risk minimisation

| 611 | **Purpose of this part** |

Part VI aims to provide readers with a straightforward account of the legal situation with particular reference to doctors when they are engaged in hospital quality management and quality assurance activities. Myth and rumour abound among medical staff concerning their liability in relation to quality management activities in hospitals. This part provides basic and factual information to assist hospitals and their medical staff better understand the legal environment in which they find themselves when engaged in quality management. However, this material cannot substitute for good experienced legal advice and guidance should hospitals or their medical staff find themselves in any doubt.

612 | Contents of this part

This part contains four chapters that cover the critical areas of medical staffs' legal concerns regarding hospital quality management. The first chapter provides the context for the material in subsequent chapters dealing with liability of doctors and hospitals, the law of natural justice and the issue that worries doctors more than anything else—defamation.

613 | Purpose of this chapter

There is, at the present time, widespread concern among certain groups within the medical profession regarding their legal exposure if and when they involve themselves in quality management activity. These concerns have, in reality, a somewhat flimsy basis, but the fact that they are genuinely held has significant consequences on the participation by some medical staff in quality management and quality assurance activity. Surgeons—and obstetricians in particular—seem to believe that they are unreasonably exposed to risk of legal actions against them if they engage in any quality management activity whatsoever.

This chapter explores the reasons for this belief and hopefully provides some reassurance to them and to others that their concerns are largely unfounded. We also describe the methods by which medical staff and hospitals can minimise risks inherent in quality management.

614 | Current concerns

It is coincidental that the move to introduce formal systems of quality management into Australian hospitals parallels a significant rise in medical and hospital malpractice litigation. As a result there has been a heightened awareness in the minds of many hospital doctors of the legal hazards of their daily activities.

Unfortunately they have sometimes translated this coincidental chain of circumstances into a totally uninformed concern about their legal exposure while involved in legitimate quality assurance activity. The risk inherent in daily hospital duties far exceeds any risk of engaging in legitimate quality management including quality assurance.

While, initially at least, some medical staff have used the concern about legal risk more as an excuse to avoid any involvement with quality management, the situation has reached the stage where many hospital staff genuinely believe that they are at risk. This concern has now escalated to a point where medical staff in some hospitals have refused to participate in 'quality assurance' until they have been provided with some 'protection'.

The 'protection' sought quite often is a guarantee that no one in any circumstances will be able to initiate legal action against them. This desire, while understandable, is of course unrealistic. Such 'protection' is enjoyed by very few individuals or groups of individuals in our society and is granted very rarely. Parliamentarians while in parliament are almost the only example of such 'protection'. Further, adequate protection for medical staff currently exists—provided proper process is observed. Recent Commonwealth and state legislation provides additional safeguards for medical practitioners who engage in quality management activities.

615 | Indemnity

Doctors can reasonably expect to be indemnified against the costs of any legal action against them while engaged in quality assurance on behalf of the hospital. Doctors working in public hospitals on committees authorised by the board of the hospital or area health service should be entitled to the same indemnity as the board itself. In most states the indemnity is provided by the Department of Health itself. However, doctors would be well advised to seek clarification of the question of their indemnity from the hospital manager, and preferably in writing. Doctors in a private hospital should also be protected against the costs of any legal actions and the hospital should negotiate such indemnity with its insurer. Such arrangements should specifically mention the committees whose members are to be indemnified.

616 | Risks in perspective

How real are the legal risks about which so many hospital medical staff are concerned? What do these risks entail?

The risk to hospitals and medical staff from medical and hospital malpractice litigation is far greater than any risk incurred by doctors participating in properly conducted quality management activity. 'Properly conducted' quality management activity is a crucial qualification because much of what we see in hospitals presently is either ineffective quality management or it is conducted in such a way as to risk exposing medical staff unnecessarily.

Medical staff's greatest concern seems to relate to possible action for defamation initiated against them by one of their colleagues. While this concern would be understandable in the environment of a credentialling committee which had the task of denying or limiting individual doctors' privileges, we have yet to see such a committee functioning in this fashion anywhere in Australia. Similar risks could exist with the process of structured quality review to which we refer in Part IV. This concern about defamation seems to us to represent a misunderstanding concerning the major aspects of quality management. Quality management is rarely about dangerous and negligent doctors. In more instances than not it is about system defects or failures rather than people failures. However, even where an aberrant medical practitioner is the issue, if a committee functions correctly and follows proper procedures, the risks to medical staff are small.

Obstetricians are very concerned about their risk of malpractice legal suits and with good reason. However, we have talked to obstetricians who have refused to keep any records of what they claimed to be quality assurance activity because of fear of defamation from colleagues, and fear of documents being subpoenaed and subsequently used in action for malpractice. In addition, in spite of their exposure to malpractice litigation, some obstetricians have great difficulty disciplining themselves to maintain adequate medical records. Good medical records and an effective quality management program properly documented would do more to reduce the current wave of malpractice actions against obstetricians than any other action they might take.

617 | Risk minimisation

Rigid adherence to principles and procedures is necessary to minimise the risk of any legal action as a result of quality management activities. Part III establishes these principles and describes procedures necessary for effective committees. Nevertheless, documentation prepared even by a properly constituted and effectively run quality assurance committee may still be subpoenaed in any proceedings concerning an incident that such a committee reviewed. Such legal action, of course, does not expose committee members to any liability. However, such documentation may well be used against the hospital or doctors involved in the incident that the committee reviewed. There is no means to prevent such use, other than legislation.

A number of principles must be observed if members of committees dealing with matters such as quality assurance or the credentialling of medical staff can enjoy reasonable protection from the risks of legal actions. These elements are:

- A properly constituted committee: the authority for the establishment of the committee must be in written form and should clearly state under what authority the committee functions and to whom it reports.
- Carefully drafted terms of reference: not only should a committee's terms of reference be carefully drafted but the chairperson's responsibility to strictly adhere to them.
- Confidentiality: one would think that doctors concerned about defamation would not have to be told about confidentiality. Unfortunately, however, a failure to observe strict confidentiality is a common problem. Minutes of meetings are left in public places; a problem concerning a colleague is discussed in the surgeons' room or over the dinner table; particularly in country towns it is not uncommon to find an unwelcome colleague to have been defamed by rumour and innuendo.
- Carefully prepared and checked minutes: as we have discussed in a previous chapter (Part III, Chapter 3), minute preparation is far from satisfactory in many hospitals. When legal issues are at stake, it is crucial that the minutes be prepared as if they were to be read in court. Wherever possible, individual names should not appear and resolutions should be carefully and accurately recorded. The minutes should be checked by two people before distribution. Until and unless committees become privileged by legislation, their minutes are subject to subpoena.
- Strict observance of the rules of natural justice: while doctors, when dealing with colleagues usually have the interests of the hospital and high quality care uppermost in their minds, the law says that everyone, even a doctor suspected of poor practice, must be given a 'fair go'. It is surprising how often this is forgotten and doctors find themselves in legal actions as a result. The next chapter deals with the concept and the law pertaining to natural justice.
- A carefully designed formality: one cannot overemphasise the importance of formality for effective committee functioning. Of even greater importance, lack of formality may increase committee members' exposure to legal hazards. Examples of the failure to follow established procedures for committee functioning include the following: failure to adhere to terms of reference; unstructured discussion; failure to insist on properly worded motions, seconded and voted upon.
- All medical staff subjected to the same process: when it comes to credentialling of medical staff presently one may find that the only person subjected to detailed review is the person whose activities are to be curtailed. Credentialling must apply to all medical staff, and it is the credentials committee's task to see that all medical staff are subjected to the same process.
- Recommendations to the board: when decisions of a committee relate to medical staff, all such decisions should be in the form of recommendations to the board of the hospital. In this way the board of directors takes the responsibility for a decision that it is empowered to make.

An effective quality management program, including a process of delineation of clinical privileges, is the greatest safeguard any hospital or its medical staff can have against the risk of legal action against them. Such a program of course will not eliminate all such legal suits. However, the existence of such programs will enable both hospitals and doctors to better defend themselves in such circumstances.

Chapter 2

LIABILITY OF HOSPITALS AND MEDICAL PRACTITIONERS

---

620 Contents

This chapter looks at the legal liability that hospitals and doctors may incur in the course of quality management. It deals with the material under the following headings:

621. Purpose of this chapter
622. Civil damages
623. Hospital liability

621 Purpose of this chapter

This chapter's main purpose is to set out the law as it relates to the liability of hospitals and doctors as simply and in as easily understandable fashion as possible. It deals only with civil actions and excludes criminal liability. Legal issues and the consequences of legal liability play an important part in the process of quality management generally and risk management specifically. Failure to observe minimal rules and to comprehend the demands made by the law inevitably leads to even greater liability.

622 Civil damages

622.1 Causes of action

A civil case for damages against a hospital and/or medical practitioner is usually based upon the following causes of action:

- breach of contract;
- negligence;
- assault and battery;
- false imprisonment.

Cases involving assault and battery and false imprisonment are rare and deal mainly with situations where consent has not been obtained for treatment (assault and battery), or hospitalisation (false imprisonment). On the other hand, it has become more common for claims alleging a breach of a duty of care to be pleaded both in contract and tort. In most cases the duty will be the same and the cases determined pursuant to the principles of negligence.

622.2 | Negligence

The following elements must be established in order for a plaintiff to succeed in a negligence action:
1. the existence of a duty of care;
2. breach of that duty;
3. damage to the plaintiff;
4. a causative link between the breach of a duty and the damage suffered.

622.3 | Duty of care

When a hospital accepts a patient or a medical practitioner undertakes to diagnose, advise or treat a patient, each comes under a duty to that patient to exercise reasonable care. This duty applies to each person involved in the care of a patient including, for example, a nurse, the assisting surgeon, the pathologist and the anaesthetist. The relationship which is established as a result of the act of undertaking the care of the patient results in a duty of care which is recognised by law.

622.4 | Breach of duty

The standard of care usually applied is that set out in the often quoted English case of *Bolam v Friern Hospital Committee* in which McNair J summed up to the jury as follows:

> ... I must explain what in law we mean by negligence. In the ordinary case which does not involve any special skill, negligence in law means this: Some failure to do some act which a reasonable man in the circumstances would do, or doing some act which a reasonable man in the circumstances would not do; and if that failure or doing of that act results in injury then there is a cause of action. How do you test whether this act or failure is negligent? In an ordinary case it is generally said, that you judge that by the action of the man in the street. He is the ordinary man. In one case it is said that you judge it by the conduct of the man on the top of the Clapham omnibus. He is the ordinary man but when you get a situation in which it involves the use of some special skill or competence, then the test whether there has been negligence is not the test of the man on top of a Clapham omnibus, because he has not got this special skill. *The test is the standard of the ordinary skilled man exercising and professing to have that special skill. A man need not possess the highest expert skill at the risk of being found negligent. It is well established law that it is sufficient if he is exercising the ordinary skill of an ordinary competent man exercising that particular art* ... (emphasis added)

This standard is applied to both a hospital and a medical practitioner.

McNair also noted that a doctor 'is not guilty of negligence if he has acted in accordance with a practice accepted as proper by a responsible body of medical men skilled in that particular art ... putting it the other way round, a man is not negligent if he is acting in accordance with such a practice, merely because there is a body of opinion who would take a contrary view'.

However, this does not mean that if a hospital and its medical staff (the relevant medical community) totally failed to keep up with developments in medical science that they could escape liability.

In the New South Wales Court of Appeal's decision in *Albrighton v Royal Prince Alfred Hospital* (1980) 2 NSWLR 542 at page 563 His Honour Mr Justice Reynolds said:

> It also, in my view, is based on a wrong assumption that a jury should be directed that, if what is charged as negligence is shown to have been done in accordance with the usual and customary practice and procedure then prevailing in what was called a

particular 'medical community' they cannot find negligence. This, in my opinion, is plainly wrong, because it is not the law that, if all or most of the medical practitioners in Sydney have habitually failed to take an available precaution to avoid foreseeable risk or injury to their patients, then none can be found guilty of negligence. Medicine is, of course, a science, and the totality of human knowledge increases day by day. Generally, it may be thought the progress is gradual; but at times there are dramatic breakthroughs such as the discovery of antibiotics and the developments of organ transplants.

Each case depends upon its own circumstances. It is the function of the court to ultimately decide whether a practice is negligent or not, although in most cases it can be said that compliance with accepted practice (even though a minority practice) undertaken by responsible practitioners in the field in question is generally an answer to a negligence claim.

622.5 | Causation and damages

It is an essential link in the negligence claim to show that the alleged breach of duty has caused damage suffered by the plaintiff. For example, a nurse or medical practitioner may well have been negligent in misreading a monitor in circumstances where the patient suffered complications following a procedure. However, the incorrect monitor reading may not have had anything to do with the complication which the patient suffered. If that is the case the error did not 'cause the damage' and therefore the tort of negligence has not been established. Only harm suffered that was caused by a hospital's or medical practitioner's breach of duty of care to the plaintiff will be compensated by the law of negligence.

623 | Hospital liability

623.1 | Organisation's liability

A hospital is under an obligation to take reasonable care in relation to the provision of staff, equipment, nursing care and other functions. A departure from reasonable standards will leave the hospital liable in negligence.

This extends to the hospital organisation itself as was set out in the English Court of Appeal decision of *Wilsher v Essex Area Health Authority* [1981] WN302:

> A health authority which so conducts its hospital that it fails to provide doctors of sufficient skill and experience to give treatment offered at the hospital may be directly liable in negligence to the patient. There is no reason why, in principle, the health authority should not be liable if its organisation is at fault.

It is also well established that a hospital is liable for the negligence of all members of its staff, including nurses and employed doctors ('vicarious liability').

623.2 | Total care

Quite apart from vicarious liability there is another basis upon which hospitals can be liable for the negligence of doctors. This involves the *'total care'* concept and is more applicable to a public than to a private hospital. In cases where a hospital undertakes to a patient to render complete medical services through its staff, it comes under a duty of care in respect of the totality of those services. This concept was developed in England and found approval with J. A. Reynolds in *Albrighton v Royal Prince Alfred Hospital:*

> The hospital, by admitting the Appellant, could be regarded as undertaking that it would take reasonable care to provide for all her medical needs, and whatever legal duties were enforced upon those who treated, diagnosed, or cared for her needs from this time, there was an overriding and continuing duty upon the hospital as an organisation.

623.3 | Visiting medical officers

A vexed issue in the area of hospital liability is the responsibility of the hospital for the actions of a visiting medical officer. In the recent decision of the New South Wales Court of Appeal in *Ellis v Wallsend District Hospital* the court held in the circumstances of that case that the visiting medical officer in treating a private patient was not an employee of the hospital and accordingly the hospital was not vicariously liable for his acts or omissions. The issue as to the responsibility of a hospital where a visiting medical officer is treating a public patient has not yet been finally decided.

623.4 | Quality management

As indicated above, a hospital is under a duty to take reasonable care in the provision of its services to patients and in its organisation of such services. If a particular hospital employee is at fault or the hospital system is at fault, the responsibility and therefore liability will lie with the hospital. From a legal point of view, it is therefore important that loss prevention and risk minimisation measures be put into place in all hospitals by means of effective quality management programs.

Not only does a quality management program provide for loss prevention and risk minimisation, the absence of such a program may, in fact, lead to a greater apportionment of liability to a hospital in certain circumstances. They may include for example:

- the repetition of similar errors prior to a particular incident without detection;
- the continued employment of a doctor the hospital knows, or should know, is deficient in certain respects.

A quality management program also provides a forum for discussion of the advice and warnings which acceplable practice dictates should be given to a patient. This is a 'growth area' in civil litigation against hospitals and medical practitioners, and should be regularly discussed. Hospitals should be aware that, in Australia, while there has not yet been a recorded action against a hospital for failing to undertake quality management activities, including credentialling, they can no longer dismiss this possibility.

Chapter 3

NATURAL JUSTICE

---

630 | Contents

This chapter deals with the legal concept of natural justice, which not infrequently becomes an issue when doctors deal with their colleagues or when a hospital attempts to deal with an aberrant medical practitioner. It discusses the matter under the following headings:

631. Meaning of natural justice
632. Natural justice protection
633. Rules of natural justice
634. Quality management committees

631 | Meaning of natural justice

Rules have been developed over time to ensure that the rights and interests of individuals are protected in decision-making processes. These two basic rules are the principle that a decision maker must:

1. afford an opportunity to be heard by a person whose interests will be adversely affected by the decision (the 'right to be heard rule');
2. be disinterested or unbiased in the matter to be decided (the 'bias rule').

Legislation often provides that an official or other authority must observe a prescribed hearing procedure when exercising its statutory powers. More commonly, however, no such procedure is enacted but judicial-type procedures are still followed. The courts will imply a duty on the part of the decision-making authority to observe the principles of natural justice.

632 | Natural justice protection

In *Ridge v Baldwin* [1964] AC 40 Lord Reid identified three main categories of legal rights attracting the protection of natural justice. These were:

- property rights (for example, an order made controlling and regulating the use of, or the keeping of, animals on premises);
- membership of professional, social and other non-statutory bodies (for example expulsion from a professional association, trade union etc.);
- the holding of a public office (for example the dismissal of a police officer on the ground that he or she had been found guilty of a criminal offence).

Other categories of rights protected by natural justice have also developed:

- trading, commercial or occupational licences (for example the right to hold a licence as a taxicab driver);
- 'legitimate expectations' (for example renewal of a licence, or a reappointment to a position);
- other interests which have been held as attracting the protection of natural justice include: reputation; the interests of university students facing disciplinary or exclusion proceedings; and the interests of prisoners facing disciplinary proceedings within prison.

634 Rules of natural justice

No strict guidelines have been developed with respect to operationalising rules of natural justice. Basically, a procedure which is adopted in determining the rights and interests of individuals must be 'fair'. What is 'fair' depends on the unique circumstances of each case. A host of factors will be taken into consideration in this regard including administrative frameworks, nature and importance of the subject matter, and the relative seriousness of the consequences in the exercise of power.

634 Quality management committees

It is of the utmost importance that quality management committees observe rules of natural justice when arriving at their recommendations or decisions. For example, credentials committees and medical appointments advisory committees should afford medical practitioners and others the opportunity of being heard by the committee with respect to recommendations or decisions affecting their particular rights and interests.

It is also important for hospitals to adhere strictly to their own rules and procedures once they have developed them. These rules and procedures are best specified in committee's terms of reference (see Chapter 3 in Part III, which includes model terms of reference for credentialling and medical advisory committees). In disputes involving persons affected by committee decisions, the issue may hinge on whether or not the committee followed its own rules and whether or not they were appropriate (that is, on procedural matters); not on the actual merits of the case, nor the correctness of the decision.

Chapter 4

DEFAMATION

---

640 | Contents

Nothing seems to worry medical staff more than the perceived risk of defamation. This chapter explores the subject under the following headings:

641 | Purpose of this chapter

For some reason the risk of legal action against them for defamation seems to occupy an abnormal amount of nervous energy on the part of many hospital medical staff. Whether this is due to the embellished stories of circumstances in the United States or not, we are not sure. One thing, however, is certain, and that is that the understanding of the average hospital doctor about the law of defamation is far from complete. This chapter is an attempt to inform without becoming too legally complex.

642 | What is defamation?

> A man who wants to talk about smoke may have to pick his words very carefully if he wants to exclude the suggestion that there is also a fire . . . but it can be done. (Lord Devlin: *Lewis v Daily Telegraph*)

The law of defamation within Australia varies between each state and territory. Some states apply the common law, others apply a mix of both the common law and statute, while some states are governed solely by statutory provisions. The following material does not pretend to be comprehensive but is intended to be a general guide.

A defamatory statement is one that holds a person up to hatred, ridicule or contempt or tends to lower the person in the estimation of a right thinking ordinary decent Australian. The intention of the writer or the publisher is irrelevant in determining whether or not a statement is defamatory.

To be defamatory an imputation needs to have no actual effect on a person's reputation; the law only looks to its tendency. Further, public opinion has to be measured from time to time, and the place of publication is also considered in measuring how defamatory an imputation is.

A defamatory statement may be conveyed by words or visual images, either singularly or in conjunction. An imputation may be conveyed even though it is not apparent on the face of the words alone. However, there may be a certain class of person who is aware of some additional fact which makes the statement defamatory. Accordingly, defamation does not need to be direct and can be conveyed by inference.

A person will establish a cause of action in defamation if all of the following elements exist:

- the meaning of the words carry a defamatory imputation (meaning);
- the matter is capable of identifying the person (identification);
- the matter has been communicated to at least one other person (publication).

643 Popular misconceptions

The matter of defamation abounds with misconceptions among non-lawyers and nowhere is this more so than among medical staff of hospitals. Below, we provide the correct situation for some popular misconceptions:

- That a dead person cannot sue is true. However, what is said about a deceased person may defame someone who is living, such as a family member, and such a person can sue.
- A person who is not named can sue. Such a person need only be able to be identified by people as being referred to in the defamatory matter.
- Not only can the person you intend to refer to sue you, but others to whom you did not intend to refer can also sue you. You may intend to refer to Dr Joe Smith as being a murderer, when there are in fact several doctors called Joe Smith. All of them would be entitled to commence proceedings.
- Companies can sue for statements relating to their trading or business reputation and equally, a trade union or local council can sue for statements adversely reflecting on their reputations.
- You can be sued for an honest mistake or misprint. A misprint or honest mistake does not protect a publication, as defamation liability is particularly strict.
- You can be sued for quoting another person's statements. By republishing other persons' statements you assume the liability for those statements unless they are completely refuted.
- The publication of a denial of the defamatory imputation may not protect you from liability. This protection will occur only if the denial goes exactly to the imputation that is conveyed and outweighs it. This is known as bane and antidote. It should be noted that this is particularly difficult to establish.

644 Defences against defamation

644.1 Types of defences

There are a number of defences against an action for defamation that have particular relevance to hospital quality management situations. The following defences are described below.

- Truth
- Contextual truth
- Fair comment
- Fair report

- Qualified privilege
- Absolute privilege
- Privilege under special legislation (next section).

644.2 Truth

Truth (sometimes referred to as justification) is the best defence to an action for defamation. However, in the state of New South Wales for example, the material published must be a matter of public interest. The criterion for public interest varies from state to state. However, for practical purposes most material published by the media relates to matters of public interest, apart from such matters as the private lives of individuals. Proving the truth of something in a court may be extremely difficult. Remember, it is not unusual for witnesses to an event to each provide a different description of that event.

644.3 Contextual truth

In circumstances where material published may convey a variety of defamatory meanings and only some of them may be true, it is a defence that the defamatory meanings that are true produce such an effect on the reputation of the person referred to that other meanings conveyed by the material, that are not true, do not cause any additional injury to their reputation. For example, if a man is described as a liar, bank robber and an illegal immigrant, the defence of contextual truth would succeed as the untrue assertion that he was an illegal immigrant does not cause any additional injury to his reputation, if indeed he was a proven liar and bank robber.

644.4 Fair comment

Material which is a statement of opinion that contains within it a reference to the basis upon which the opinion is formed may be defensible as comment. The opinion must be honestly held and must be based on proper material for comment, that is, accurately states facts and relates to matters of public interest. If the author of the material is malicious, or if the comment is based on untrue facts, the defence will fail. It is often difficult to distinguish between a statement of fact and a comment. Therefore care should be taken in ensuring a comment is expressed to be such and based on clearly defined facts.

644.5 Fair report

Everyone is entitled to publish fair and balanced reports of proceedings of various bodies, for example those specified in Schedule 2 of the *New South Wales Defamation Act*, including:

- court proceedings;
- parliamentary proceedings;
- parliamentary inquiries or royal commissions;
- proceedings of various bodies such as the Medical Tribunal and Equal Opportunity Tribunal.

The defence of fair report also applies to reports of official and public documents and records such as judgments of the court, reports of a professional standards committee and government records or documents which are open to inspection by the public. Similar defences are available in most jurisdictions.

644.6 Qualified privilege

The defence of qualified privilege is also available at common law and its essential elements are as follows:

- The publisher must have a duty (legal, social or moral) to publish the material.
- The person to whom the publication is made has a reciprocal duty to receive the information.
- The publisher must have an honest belief in the truth of the material.
- The publication is made without malice.

The occasion on which the communication is made must be one where the person making the communication has a legal, social or moral duty to publish it to the person to whom it is made, who must have the reciprocal legal, social or moral duty to receive the information. For example, the distribution of a report and minutes of a conference of a professional body such as a college of practitioners to the members of that college, would be privileged even if they contained a defamatory statement. However, if it could be shown that they were published to persons outside the college without any duty to receive the information, the common law of qualified privilege would be lost. Any person who 'leaks' material to the media will be responsible for that republication. If the author of such material was unaware of the 'leak', or otherwise did not authorise the republication he or she will not be held liable. It is therefore important to examine the nature of the communication and the person receiving it and the likely distribution of the material to assess whether this defence is available.

A defence of qualified privilege is available under Section 22 of the *New South Wales Defamation Act* in circumstances where a report is on a matter of public interest, published to people who have an interest in knowing about the matter, and the conduct of the publisher in publishing the material is reasonable. However, the defence is difficult to establish and the author of a report should:

- contact or attempt to contact the person or company referred to in any report and put any allegation to be made to them;
- if that person comments on those allegations, his or her comments should be published;
- take care to use reliable sources and each available source of information; and
- check the accuracy and authenticity of any material contained in any report.

644.7 *Absolute privilege*

Section 17 of the *New South Wales Defamation Act* provides absolute privilege in a number of different situations. These include:

- publication to or by the New South Wales Medical Board, a professional standards committee, a medical tribunal or a member of any of those bodies as such a member for the purpose of any procedure under the *Medical Practitioners Act 1938*;
- publication of a report made under Section 100(6) of the *Children (Care & Protection) Act 1987*;
- publication made under Section 33H of the *Public Hospitals Act* of a decision and the reasons for the decision.

645 Privilege under special legislation

645.1 *State and Commonwealth privileges*

In recent years, in response to the concerns of medical practitioners, legislation has been enacted to provide specific protection to doctors and others engaged in quality management. Next sections describe such:

- state legislation;
- Commonwealth legislation.

645.2 | State legislation

Specific state statutes are (by year of enactment):

- *South Australian Health Commission Act 1976*
- *Health Administration (Quality Assurance Committees) Amendment 1989 (New South Wales)*
- *Health Services Act 1986 (Victoria)*
- *Health Services Act 1990 (Australian Commonwealth Territory)*
- *Health Services Act 1991 (Queensland)*
- *Health Regional Boards Act 1991 (Tasmania)*

Provisions under these recent additions to state (and also federal) legislation are cumbersome and, inevitably, limiting. Once again, we emphasise that doctors' greatest protection is 'properly conducted' quality management and quality assurance activity. Given those circumstances, doctors and hospitals should have few concerns, and the number of hospitals that need to avail themselves of protection under these special provisions is likely to be small.

New South Wales, Victoria, Queensland, South Australia, Tasmania and the Australian Capital Territory (ACT) have a basic framework which generally includes the following elements:

- committees are authorised formally by the relevant minister or governor;
- the public interest must be seen to be served by granting protections;
- information gathered cannot be divulged to any person, including courts and tribunals;
- procedural fairness and good faith are central to the committees' functioning.

The New South Wales legislation provides for specific protections for an approved quality assurance committee. Other state, and federal, legislation has similar provisions relating to quality assurance committees. Jurisdictions, such as the ACT, extend the functions of a quality assurance committee to the evaluation of clinical privileges. However, generally, the activities that fall within statutory protections are the assessment and evaluation of the quality of health services as distinct from credentialling and disciplinary processes.

Section 20J of the New South Wales Act provides as follows:

1. Anything done by a committee, a member of a committee or any person acting under the direction of a committee in good faith for the purposes of the excercise of the committee's functions does not subject such a member or person personally to any action, liability, claim or demand.
2. Without limiting sub-section 1 a member of a committee has qualified privilege in proceedings for defamation in respect of:
   a. any statement made orally or in writing in exercise of the function of a member; or
   b. the contents of any report or other information published by the committee.
3. The members of a committee are entitled to be indemnified by the prescribed establishment that established the committee in respect of any loss incurred in defending proceedings in respect of liability against which they are protected by this section.

The above legislation provides for members of a quality assurance committee (approved under Section 20E of the legislation) a defence of qualified privilege to any claim made against them and also an indemnity for the costs incurred in defending proceedings. Approval for a committee in New South Wales is by the Minister for Health. This Act provides the members of a quality assurance committee operating under the Act considerable protection against claims for defamation so long as the members of the committee are acting in good faith or in other words without malice. Proving lack of good faith or malice is difficult, provided the committee acts fairly.

Section 20I provides that a finding of a committee as to the need for changes or improvements in a practice or procedure is not admissible as evidence in proceedings that the procedure or practice was careless or inadequate. Section 20H(1) provides that information generated for the committee cannot be released to courts, nor can the courts request the information. However, section 20H(2) reflects the importance of observing rules of natural justice. It provides an exception to the protection relating to non-disclosure. Moreover, section 20H(1) does *not* apply 'to a requirement made in proceedings in respect of any act or omission by a committee or by a member of a committee as such a member'. Committees which exercise their functions fairly in accordance with the rules of natural justice and the provisions of the legislation should not fear this exception.

645.3 COMMONWEALTH LEGISLATION

An argument was raised that the statutory protections that exist in a number of states and territories would not protect information in actions taken in federal courts or under Commonwealth legislation such as the *Trade Practices Act*.

To remedy this problem the Commonwealth enacted its own legislation in 1992 as part of the *Health Insurance Act 1973*. The amendments provide a statutory protection in the form of confidentiality and immunity provisions for quality assurance committees that are 'declared' by the relevant minister. The protections are only to be conferred where the interest in the quality of health care clearly outweighs the right of the public to freedom of information and legal action. Principles of procedural fairness and good faith underpin the ability to rely on the protections.

Information created solely for the purpose of the committee cannot be disclosed to the courts; however, this does not extend to information such as medical records that are created in the ordinary course of health care. Where information concerns a serious criminal matter, the minister may authorise its disclosure for the purpose of law enforcement, royal commissions etc. There is no power to compel the quality assurance committee members to disclose information.

Importantly, where the Commonwealth and state legislation apply to the same activity, the state Act prevails. This reverses the usual position under Section 109 of the Constitution whereby the Commonwealth legislation would take precedence. In addition, the Act is designed only to operate in areas where the Commonwealth has an interest; for example, activities carried out across state borders and those which have an Australia-wide significance.

646 | Quality management and defamation

646.1 | 'Be accurate, fair and objective'

A quality management program that intends to prevent loss and minimise risk may sometimes involve the examination by committees and/or boards of the various practices of medical practitioners, nurses and other health professionals within a hospital. Government has recognised the importance of these programs by introducing the Health Administration (Quality Assurance Committees) legislation in New South Wales and similar legislation in the other states and at the Commonwealth level.

There is also no doubt that any full and frank discussions by such a committee will involve making statements that (even if they are true) are prima facie defamatory of any of the persons under consideration. Therefore such a committee will have to ensure that its procedures enable it to rely on legislation or any other defence (including the truth of statements) to any action taken for defamation that may arise.

While a committee is afforded considerable protection under legislation (see previous section), not all committees will necessarily be approved under the legislation nor will they wish to seek approval. In any event, if the following matters are taken into consideration any committee should have considerable protection from legal action for defamation.

The best method of ensuring a defence available is to ensure that committee discussions and any report or determination are '*accurate, fair and objective*'. You cannot achieve one of these criteria without having achieved the others. Further, any committee that reports its findings to another person or body should ensure that person or body has the same legal, social and moral duty to receive the information as the committee does in providing it. The committee must also have an honest belief as to the truth of the material and must not be actuated in publishing the material by any wrong or improper motive, otherwise known as 'malice'. Therefore the publication of information to another responsible body is usually protected by qualified privilege. However, care should be taken to ensure that publication does not spread beyond any person to whom the committee has a duty to publish the material and who may not have a duty to receive it.

For example, either a quality assurance committee or a committee involved in the assessment of the quality of clinical care may conduct its own inquiry into the procedures followed by a doctor within a hospital. It may then report on its findings to the board of the hospital and make certain recommendations. Generally such a report would attract qualified privilege. The provision of such a report to a specialist college of which the practitioner was also a member is also likely to attract the defence of qualified privilege, depending on the circumstances. However, the provision of a report to another specialist college may not necessarily be protected. It is clear that the provision of such a report to a journalist or a member of the public who has no duty to receive the information would not attract a defence of qualified privilege. A member of the medical staff who is the subject of such a report should be given the right to respond at an early stage. However, providing nothing affects 'honest belief', the position of the committee is unchanged. Therefore, it is clear that such a report referred to above should be carefully handled and clearly marked as to its distribution. This consideration may involve marking it 'strictly private and confidential' and arranging some security of any copies.

Committees should also consider the following when preparing a report or determination:

- An accurate and fair report requires time and considerable care.
- Always assume that the assertions in the report may have to be subjected to questioning in court, therefore be prepared to establish those matters asserted as fact, to the high standard required. It is not sufficient to rely on one person's version of events if other versions or corroborative evidence can be obtained.
- Gather the facts carefully. While certain facts may be sought, it is always possible that they may not be available. Nevertheless, there is a need to document the fact that the search has been fruitless. It is important to adopt a slightly cynical approach and to question the veracity of all material submitted or gathered.
- Having obtained all the information reasonably possible, it then requires careful assessment.
- Once satisfied that sufficient and coherent information has been obtained, the report may then be prepared. Reporting should be objective, balanced and supported by the evidence. Inferences must be supported by reasoning as well as facts. Avoid all extraneous matter, especially irrelevant personal opinions. If one member of the committee prepared the report, others should review it with the above-mentioned points in mind.

646.2 Check list for reports

The following check list we believe will be helpful for anyone preparing a report. If the answer to all of the following questions is in the affirmative, considerable protection will follow, and possibly a legal defence should that ever become necessary.

REPORT CONTENTS

- Is it accurate?
- Have you relied on several and reasonable sources of information? (Many people will have their own motives in supplying information.)
- Have you considered the veracity of sources and facts?
- Have you checked the accuracy of reported facts and documented their source, in working papers if not in the report itself?
- If relevant, did you attempt to contact the person or persons referred to in the report and put any allegation to them and include their comments?

IS IT FAIR?

- Have you clearly distinguished between facts and your comments or opinions? If you express your own opinion have you clearly stated the facts on which it is based? Is it your honest opinion? (You should not express an opinion for an improper or malicious purpose.)
- Have you chosen your words carefully to avoid such things as ambiguity, misconstruction and inadvertent implications?

IS IT OBJECTIVE?

- Does the report state only what the facts support?
- If contradictory facts exist are they weighed and evaluated in an even-handed manner?
- Does the report contain only material relevant to its purpose (and no ad hominem or other extraneous remarks)?

PURPOSE AND AUDIENCE

- Is the report's purpose clear?
- Is the report addressed (or being published to) the appropriate person?
- If appropriate, has the report been marked 'confidential', and have steps been taken to control circulation of copies?

REVIEW

- Have all members of the committee been given the opportunity to review the draft?
- Has the report been reviewed specifically with the above points in mind, preferably by a committee member who did not draft the document or by someone with experience in preparation of such reports who is not a member of the committee (except if the latter would jeopardise confidentiality)?

646.3 Obtaining advice

Like all matters of the law most people other than lawyers find themselves caught in a confusing web of ideas and words. Hospital medical staff should not allow themselves to be stampeded into panic, which is often made worse by the endless supply of 'bush lawyers' to be found around every hospital corner.

Where questions arise bearing on legal matters related to quality management, the quality management department should know where to obtain competent legal advice that is specific to the peculiar environment of hospital practice, so as to provide doctors and others with authoritative answers.

PART VII

QUALITY MANAGEMENT RESOURCES

SUMMARY

Part VII explores the problems of finding resources to support the design and implementation of quality management programs in hospitals and other health care facilities. Specifically, it outlines the difficulty of keeping up to date with developments in, and of accessing the world's literature on, health care quality management. To assist quality managers, health care administrators, providers and others keep current, this part provides a directory of the world's English-language newsletters, journals and other periodicals—all of which may be of assistance in one way or another to someone engaged in the difficult task of quality management implementation.

Outside of the United States especially there are few quality management resources and there is only limited access to journals and newsletters dealing with the spectrum of quality management issues. Most peer-reviewed scientific medical journals, for example, carry only occasional articles on the subject and, subsequently, for workers in the field such articles are very difficult to find—despite their total number.

This part consists of the following two chapters:

Chapter 1   *Introduction to and purpose of Part VII*—describes this part's purpose and reasons for its inclusion in the manual, some organisational resources for quality management, and the world's literature on this subject.

Chapter 2   *Quality management periodicals*—describes the methods used to identify the world's English-language periodicals that focus exclusively or principally on one or more aspects of quality management, lists these publications alphabetically, chronologically, and by country, and provides a short, structured description of each publication.

Chapter 1

INTRODUCTION TO AND PURPOSE OF PART VII

---

710 | Contents

This chapter explores problems in identifying resources to support or assist with the introduction and implementation of quality management programs in hospitals and other health care facilities under the following headings:

711. Purpose of this part
712. Contents of this part
713. Purpose of this chapter
714. Organisations
715. Books and monographs
716. Articles in journals

711 | Purpose of this part

Part VII intends to provide readers with an appreciation of:

- the (paucity of) resources available to assist quality managers and others to design and implement quality management programs;
- the volume of material relating to health care quality management that has been published in the last 20–30 years;
- the newsletters, journals and other periodicals available to help quality managers, health care professionals, and other interested individuals keep current with developments in health care quality management.

712 | Contents of this part

This part consists of two chapters, including this one.

- This chapter, *Introduction to and purpose of Part VII*, describes this part's purpose and reasons for its inclusion in the manual, some organisational resources for quality management, and the world's literature on this subject.

• Chapter 2, *Quality management periodicals*, describes the methods used to identify the world's English-language periodicals that focus exclusively or principally on one or more aspects of quality management, lists these publications alphabetically, chronologically, and by country, and provides a short, structured description of each publication.

713 | Purpose of this chapter

This chapter intends to give readers an overview of the resources available to assist them introduce quality management programs into hospitals, and facilitate programs' further development. Such resources consist principally of organisations and published materials. Specifically, it alerts readers to the paucity of relevant organisations and other resources available in Australia—and elsewhere—to assist quality managers in the difficult dual tasks of developing a quality-focused organisation and implementing an effective quality management program to achieve quality maturity and substantial and sustained quality improvement. This chapter also describes the growth in the health care quality management literature in the past 20–30 years and some ways to access it.

714 | Organisations

We considered providing a list of organisations that could be of practical, hands-on help to hospitals in Australia. Unfortunately, however, too few experienced organisations exist in Australia to bear listing. The Australian Council on Healthcare Standards remains, with the exception of organisations associated with the authors, the only resource available. Perhaps the next step in quality management implementation in Australia is the development of additional resource centres and organisations to help the Australian hospital industry. We have in mind, particularly, Interwest Quality of Care in the United States, which provides assistance to several hospitals in Utah under a grant from the Robert Wood Johnson Foundation, and CBO, the Netherlands organisation which assists hospitals to improve the quality of care.

Table VII-1-1 on page 693 lists organisations in principal industrialised English-speaking countries that perform functions similar to those of the Australian Council on Healthcare Standards or that act as a clearing house for quality management information. By contacting these organisations, readers may be able to secure leads to organisations that, or individual consultants who, could assist them to implement an effective quality management program.

715 | Books and monographs

The authors gave careful consideration to providing a list of books and monographs on quality management. However, while there are many useful books and monographs, none offers the kind of practical guidance needed to improve the quality of care in Australian hospitals. Indeed, this lack provoked the production of this manual. Moreover, existing books and monographs are of uneven quality and relevance to Australian hospitals.

716 | Articles in journals

The number of articles on quality management and related topics is large and growing rapidly in health (medical) journals. Moreover, most of the material that has been published over the past 20–30 years has emanated from the United States. Because of the subject's breadth and diffuseness, academics and clinicians in Australia—and elsewhere—have expressed difficulty in easily accessing it. The volume of material involved is far too extensive to index in this manual. We did consider including a select bibliography of journal articles for readers' reference. However, the topics that they covered were either very broad (philosophy) or very narrow (dealing with specific techniques), and we did not consider them to be of immediate interest to a wide audience. Finally, we decided to compile a comprehensive list of English-language periodicals as being the most practical and useful approach to help readers learn about, and keep current with developments in, health care quality management (see next chapter).

The medical literature is truly vast—and one must add to it the general literature on (industrial) quality management. This vastness compounds the problem of accessing relevant articles. There is virtually no way to access graded information—for example only articles meeting certain criteria of soundness or utility for a particular purpose. Everyone is essentially on his or her own with respect to evaluating research reports' scientific supportability, for example.

MEDLARS is the world's principal index of medical literature. MEDLARS (MEDical Literature Analysis and Retrieval System) is the computerised system of databases and databanks offered by the US National Library of Medicine (NLM). MEDLARS comprises 40 online databases containing over 18 million references. MEDLINE (MEDlars on LINE) contained about eight million articles at the end of 1994 from more than 3700 biomedical journals, beginning in 1966. The National Library of Medicine adds about 31 000 citations each month.[1]

The National Library of Medicine produces HEALTH (HEALTH planning and administration), one of the MEDLARS databases, in consultation with the American Hospital Association (AHA). It contained about 800 000 articles at the end of 1994 on the non-clinical aspects of health care delivery, beginning in 1975. The American Hospital Association adds about 5000 citations each month. HEALTH draws citations from the following three sources:

• journals with a special emphasis on health administration (not indexed in MEDLINE);
• articles on health care delivery from journals indexed in MEDLINE;
• a collection of over 9000 monographs, technical reports, and theses with a health planning orientation inherited in 1983 from the (US) National Health Planning Information Center.

In addition to being on-line through MEDLARS, HEALTH is available on CD-ROM for use on personal computers from NLM-licensed vendors. The American Hospital Association produces the *Hospital and Health Administration Index* (from 1945 until 1995, the *Hospital Literature Index*), the most comprehensive printed bibliography on health care administration. Other services based on HEALTH include vendors' *Selective Dissemination of Information* services (which provide monthly printouts of relevant citations according to requested search parameters), NLM's *Current Bibliographies in Medicine* (extensive bibliographies on selected medical and health care topics), and the AHA's Resource Center's *Selected Resources* (short bibliographies on selected health care delivery subjects).[2]

Table VII-1-2 on page 694 shows that there was a steady growth in the number of articles in HEALTH classified under the term 'Quality Assurance Health Care' added each year between 1985 and 1990, and a surge in articles added in 1991. The largest number of articles was added in 1993, although the proportion was greatest in 1992. In total, HEALTH contains almost 10 000 articles classified under the term 'Quality Assurance Health Care', and over 40 000 with descriptors that fall under 'quality assurance' in the hierarchy of Medical Subject Headings (the NLM article indexing scheme). The broader term 'quality assurance' includes, for example, practice guidelines and total quality management. One must interpret trends somewhat cautiously because the classification scheme and individual clarifications are revised from time to time.

References

1 Fact sheet: NLM online databases and databanks. Bethesda, MD: US National Library of Medicine, 1994.
2 Fact sheet from the AHA Resource Center: Health planning and administration database (HEALTH). Chicago: American Hospital Association, undated.

Table VII-1-1 *Hospital accreditation and similar quality management organisations*

Australia
Peter Blythe
Executive Director
Australian Council on Healthcare Standards
Level 1, 7-9A Joynton Avenue
Zetland, NSW 2017
Australia
Tel: 61-2-662-2311
Fax: 61-2-662-6370

Canada
Elma Heidemann
Executive Director
Canadian Council on Health Facilities Accreditation
1730 St Laurent Boulevard, Suite 430
Ottawa, Ontario KIG-5LI
Canada
Tel: 1-613-738-7800
Fax: 1-613-523-2820

New Zealand
Peter O'Connor
Executive Director
New Zealand Council on Healthcare Standards
Level 6, Molesworth House
101 Molesworth Street
Wellington
New Zealand
Tel: 64-4-499-0367
Fax: 64-4-499-0368

United Kingdom
Tessa Brooks
Director
The King's Fund
2 Palace Court
London, W2-4HS
United Kingdom
Tel: 44171-221-7141
Fax: 44171-221-1266

United States of America
Dennis O'Leary
President
Joint Commission on Accreditation of Healthcare Organizations
One Renaissance Boulevard
Oakbrook Terrace, Illinois 60181
United States of America
Tel: 1-708-916-5600
Fax: 1-708-916-5644

Margaret O'Kane
Executive Director
National Committee on Quality Assurance
1350 New York Avenue, NW, Suite 700
Washington, DC 20005
United States of America
Tel: 1-202-628-5788
Fax: 1-202-628-0344

World Health Organization Collaborating Center

Evert Reerink, Director
CBO (Centraal Begeleidingsorgaan voor de Intercollegiale Toetsing)
Postbus 20064
3502 LB Utrecht
Netherlands
Tel: 31-30-96-06-47
Fax: 31-30-94-36-44

Table VII-1-2 *Growth in HEALTH citations, 1974–94*[a]

Year	HEALTH Articles	Quality assurance, health care[b]		Quality assurance, extended term[c]	
		QAHC Articles	Rate/1000	QA Articles	Rate/1000
1974	11 050	0	0.00		
1975	26 737	20	0.75		
1976	26 038	23	0.88		
1977	26 420	10	0.38		
1978	31 219	21	0.67		
1979	32 550	56	1.72		
1980	29 457	168	5.70		
1981	28 484	204	7.16		
1982	29 849	189	6.33		
1983	32 983	183	5.55		
1984	33 199	225	6.78		
1985	34 289	241	7.03		
1986	34 839	273	7.84		
1987	36 199	356	9.83		
1988	40 061	430	10.73		
1989	43 614	549	12.59		
1990	49 870	667	13.37		
1991	55 608	1150	20.68	2 570	46.22
1992	61 747	1292	20.92	2 963	47.99
1993	68 369	1362	19.92	3 767	55.10
1994	68 103	666	9.78	2 934	43.08
Total	779 490[d]	9758	12.94	42 776	56.74

Footnotes

[a] HEALTH (HEALTH planning and administration) is produced by the US National Library of Medicine in consultation with the American Hospital Association. It is one of 40 MEDLARS databases and databanks.

[b] QAHC = Quality assurance   health care (a MeSH indexing term). MeSH = Medical Subject Headings (the US National Library of Medicine article indexing scheme).

[c] QA = All descriptors that fall under quality assurance in the hierarchy of MeSH terms: quality assurance health care, plus guidelines, practice guidelines, and total quality management. The number of articles classified under QAHC and QA depends on: the number of journal indexed, number of articles in these journals on these topics in indexed journals, and indexing rules used.

[d] Total is current as of the end of 1994. Because of on-going adjustments, yearly figures in columns do not sum to totals.

Source: American Hospital Association Resource Center, Chicago, Illinois, 1995.

Chapter 2

QUALITY MANAGEMENT PERIODICALS

| 720 | **Contents**

This chapter provides a directory of the world's English-language newsletters, journals and other periodicals dealing with one or other aspect of health care quality management under the following headings:

721. Purpose of this chapter
722. Criteria for identifying quality management periodicals
723. Search methods
724. Search results
725. Accuracy of directory information
726. Directory format
727. Directory of quality management periodicals

| 721 | **Purpose of this chapter**

This chapter describes the scope of the search for the world's English-language health care quality management (QM) periodicals, the methods used to conduct the search, and its results, in the form of a directory of such publications. In this chapter the term 'quality management' refers specifically to health care quality management.

| 722 | **Criteria for identifying quality management periodicals**

The search's objective was to identify all English-language newsletters, journals and other periodicals that focus exclusively or principally on one or more facets of health care quality management. This concept encompasses all aspects of the following subjects:

- outcomes and/or effectiveness research, including technology assessment;
- practice guidelines (practice policies and criteria);
- quality assurance, encompassing both quality assessment and quality improvement;
- utilisation review;
- risk management.

The search's scope was limited to periodicals—publications that are published at least annually. The most common periodicals are newsletters (which are often published weekly, fortnightly, or monthly) and journals (which are usually published monthly or quarterly). Increasingly, publishers in the United Stated are producing annual publications (sometimes referred to as source books) relevant to quality management. We decided to include them because publishers have made a commitment to revise them annually. We decided to exclude program newsletters—those devoted to a single quality management program—such as the *CDAC Newsletter, CEPRP Bulletin*, and *HEDIS Bulletin*—as well as special issues of non-QM journals devoted to quality management.

723 | Search methods

In 1990 the authors compiled an initial list of the English-language newsletters and journals known to them, and others obtained from reference works available at the US National Library of Medicine (NLM). Sources of additional titles were serendipity and those listed in compilations of other quality management periodicals.

In the fourth quarter of 1990, the authors designed a questionnaire to elicit information to compile the directory, and sent it to publishers of seemingly relevant newsletters, journals or other periodicals. They prepared standard descriptions of relevant publications based on the resultant information. In the first quarter of 1991, in 1993 and again in 1994 the authors asked publishers to verify or amend descriptions. For example, in 1994 the authors asked publishers to indicate whether or not the publication was available in an electronic medium. Finally, the authors compiled a directory of all publications that they deemed relevant.

724 | Search results

The authors identified 80 English-language quality management periodicals meeting criteria for inclusion. During the four-year search period, 1991–94, eleven of the periodicals ceased publication. Figure VII-2-1 on page 697 shows the growth of quality management periodicals. Their rate of introduction increased in every quinquennium since 1971. The majority of existing periodicals are published in the United States, and four publishers account for about one half of current US publications.

During the search period a number of other trends was also evident. First, many periodicals changed their name to reflect a broader or more current focus, for example, changing from a title that mentioned quality assurance to one that included quality improvement or quality management. Second, for most periodicals the number of subscribers that publishers claimed increased substantially. Third, prices have edged upwards. Fourth, at least one item of information in every description changed annually.

Table VII-2-1 on page 698 lists periodicals in publication as of the first quarter of 1995 in alphabetical order. Table VII-2-2 on page 700 lists them according to the year that they were first published. Table VII-2-3 on page 701 lists periodicals by country of publication.

725 | Accuracy of directory information

The authors have taken care to verify information. However, they cannot vouch for its accuracy. A particular publication may be sold, change its name or cease publishing. Further, frequency of publication, contents and prices are all subject to change with time. Currency equivalents are also liable to fluctuate.

726 | Directory format

The remainder of this chapter lists quality management newsletters, journals and other periodicals in alphabetical order following bibliographical convention. (Table VII-2-1 provides a listing.) Abbreviations are treated as words. For each publication, the directory provides the following information:

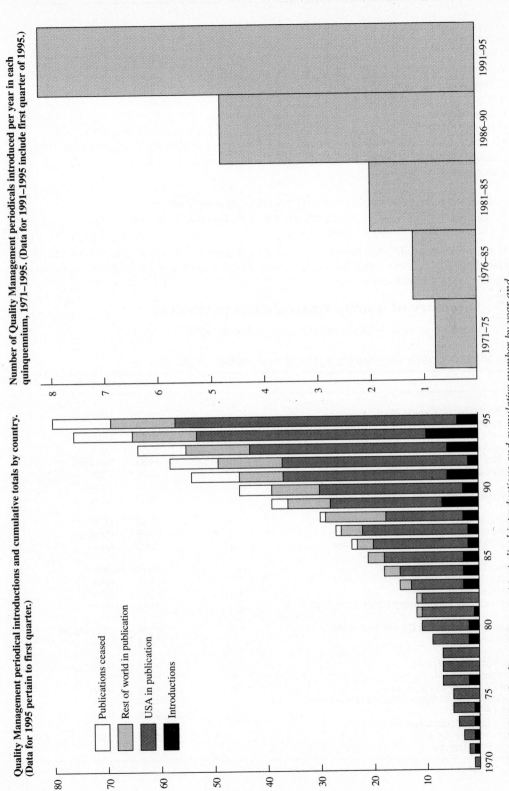

**Quality Management periodical introductions and cumulative totals by country.
(Data for 1995 pertain to first quarter.)**

Number of Quality Management periodicals introduced per year in each quinquennium, 1971–1995. (Data for 1991–1995 include first quarter of 1995.)

Publications ceased

Rest of world in publication

USA in publication

Introductions

Figure VII-2-1 *Quality management periodical introductions and cumulative number by year and country*

- Type of publisher
- Publisher's name, address, telephone and fax numbers, and email address, if any
- Editor
- Circulation (and the basis of the estimate)
- Year first published
- Number of issues per annum
- Subscription address
- Subscription rate per annum (in local currency and US dollar equivalent)
- Membership requirements (if published by a membership organisation and subscription is a benefit of membership)
- Purpose
- Focus
- Whether or not the publication accepts editorial contributions
- The electronic media in which the publication is available, if any
- The publication's ISSN or ISSB, if any

If the publisher failed to provide or to verify information by press time, we included at least the name of the publication and the publisher, and the annotation 'publisher declined to provide information'.

727 | Directory of quality management periodicals

[Directory entries in alphabetical order, based on the periodical's title.]

Table VII-2-1 *Quality management periodicals, alphabetically by title*

Title	Year	Country
A		
AMCRA's Managed Care Monitor	1971	USA
AQH Journal	1988	UK
Abstracts Of Clinical Care Guidelines	1989	USA
Accountability News For Health Care Managers	1994	USA
Accreditor	1983	Australia
American Journal Of Medical Quality	1986	USA
B		
Behavioral Outcomes and Guidelines Sourcebook	1995	USA
C		
CQI Quality Chronicle	1992	USA
Canadian Journal Of Quality In Health Care	1988	Canada
Clinical Performance & Quality Health Care	1993	USA
D		
Directory Of Practice Parameters	1989	USA
Drug Outcomes Sourcebook	1995	USA
Drug Utilization Review	1985	USA
Dynamic Quality Improvement Network Newsletter	1991	UK
E		
European Newsletter On Quality Assurance	1984	Netherlands
Eye On Improvement	1994	USA
H		
Health Technology Trends	1987	USA
Healthcare Quality Abstracts	1993	USA
Homecare Quality Management	1995	USA
Hospital And Health System Quality Management	1989	USA
Hospital Benchmarks	1994	USA
Hospital Case Management	1993	USA
Hospital Infection Control	1973	USA
Hospital Peer Review	1976	USA

continues

Table VII-2-1 *continued*

Title	Year	Country
Hospital Risk Management	1979	USA
Hospital Risk Management Forms, Checklists & Guidelines	1989	USA
Hospital's Critical Path Manual	1994	USA
I		
ISTAAC Newsletter	1989	Netherlands
International Journal Of Technology Assessment In Health Care	1984	USA
International Journal For Quality In Health Care	1989	UK
International Journal Of Health Care Quality Assurance	1987	UK
International Journal Of Risk & Safety In Medicine	1990	Netherlands
Interwest Quality Catalyst	1992	USA
J		
Joint Commission Journal On Quality Improvement	1974	USA
Joint Commission Perspectives	1952	USA
Journal For Healthcare Quality	1979	USA
Journal Of Clinical Outcomes Management	1994	USA
Journal Of Healthcare Risk Management	1980	USA
Journal Of Nursing Care Quality	1986	USA
Journal Of Quality In Clinical Practice	1981	Australia
M		
MEDTEP Update	1994	USA
Managed Care Quality	1995	USA
Medical Outcomes & Guidelines Alert	1993	USA
Medical Outcomes & Guidelines Sourcebook	1993	USA
Medical Quality Management Sourcebook	1994	USA
Medical Utilization Management	1972	USA
N		
Nursing Quality Connection	1991	USA
O		
Outcomes Measurement & Management	1990	USA
Outcomes Research Digest	1994	USA
P		
Patient-Focused Care	1993	USA
Plant, Technology, And Safety Management	1985	USA
Q		
QI/TQM	1991	USA
QRC Advisor	1984	USA
Quality Advocate	1983	USA
Quality Connection	1991	USA
Quality Evaluation News	1985	USA
Quality In Health Care	1992	UK
Quality Letter For Healthcare Leaders	1989	USA
Quality Management In Health Care	1992	USA
Quality Management Update	1991	USA
Quality Matters	1994	USA
Quality Of Care	1980	USA
Quality Resource	1983	USA
Quality Times	1991	UK
R		
Report On Medical Guidelines & Outcomes Research	1990	USA
Research Activities	1976	USA
S		
Strategies For Healthcare Excellence	1988	USA
T		
Technology News	1987	USA
U		
Update	1994	USA

Table VII-2-2 *Quality management periodicals, by when introduced, alphabetically by quinquennium*

Title	Year	Country
1970 and earlier		
Joint Commission Perspectives	1952	USA
1971–75		
AMCRA's Managed Care Monitor	1971	USA
Medical Utilization Management	1972	USA
Hospital Infection Control	1973	USA
Joint Commission Journal On Quality Improvement	1974	USA
1976–80		
Hospital Peer Review	1975	USA
Research Activities	1976	USA
Hospital Risk Management	1979	USA
Journal For Healthcare Quality	1979	USA
Journal Of Healthcare Risk Management	1980	USA
Quality Of Care	1980	USA
1981–85		
Journal Of Quality In Clinical Practice	1981	Australia
Accreditor	1983	Australia
Quality Advocate	1983	USA
Quality Resource	1983	USA
European Newsletter On Quality Assurance	1984	Netherlands
International Journal Of Technology Assessment In Health Care	1984	USA
QRC Advisor	1984	USA
Drug Utilization Review	1985	USA
Plant, Technology, And Safety Management	1985	USA
Quality Evaluation News	1985	USA
1986–90		
American Journal Of Medical Quality	1986	USA
Journal Of Nursing Care Quality	1986	USA
Health Technology Trends	1987	USA
International Journal Of Health Care Quality Assurance	1987	UK
Technology News	1987	USA
Canadian Journal Of Quality In Health Care	1988	Canada
AQH Journal	1988	UK
Strategies For Healthcare Excellence	1988	USA
Abstracts Of Clinical Care Guidelines	1989	USA
Directory Of Practice Parameters	1989	USA
Hospital And Health System Quality Management	1989	USA
Hospital Risk Management Forms, Checklists & Guidelines	1989	USA
ISTAAC Newsletter	1989	Netherlands
International Journal For Quality In Health Care	1989	UK
Quality Letter For Healthcare Leaders	1989	USA
International Journal Of Risk & Safety In Medicine	1990	Netherlands
Outcomes Measurement & Management	1990	USA
Report On Medical Guidelines & Outcomes Research	1990	USA
1991–95		
Nursing Quality Connection	1991	USA
QI/TQM	1991	USA
Dynamic Quality Improvement Network Newsletter	1991	UK
Quality Connection	1991	USA
Quality Management Update	1991	USA

continues

Table VII-2-2 *continued*

Title	Year	Country
Quality Times	1991	UK
CQI Quality Chronicle	1992	USA
Interwest Quality Catalyst	1992	USA
Quality In Health Care	1992	UK
Quality Management In Health Care	1992	USA
Clinical Performance & Quality Health Care	1993	USA
Healthcare Quality Abstracts	1993	USA
Hospital Case Management	1993	USA
Medical Outcomes & Guidelines Alert	1993	USA
Medical Outcomes & Guidelines Sourcebook	1993	USA
Patient-Focused Care	1993	USA
Accountability News For Health Care Managers	1994	USA
Eye On Improvement	1994	USA
Hospital Benchmarks	1994	USA
Hospital's Critical Path Manual	1994	USA
Journal Of Clinical Outcomes Management	1994	USA
MEDTEP Update	1994	USA
Medical Quality Management Sourcebook	1994	USA
Outcomes Research Digest	1994	USA
Quality Matters	1994	USA
Update	1994	USA
Behavioral Outcomes and Guidelines Sourcebook	1995	USA
Drug Outcomes Sourcebook	1995	USA
Homecare Quality Management	1995	USA
Managed Care Quality	1995	USA

Table VII-2-3 *Quality management periodicals, by country, alphabetically by country*

Title	Year
Australia	
Accreditor	1983
Journal Of Quality In Clinical Practice	1981
Canada	
Canadian Journal Of Quality In Health Care	1988
The Netherlands	
European Newsletter On Quality Assurance	1984
ISTAAC Newsletter	1989
International Journal Of Risk & Safety In Medicine	1990
UK	
International Journal For Quality In Health Care	1989
International Journal Of Health Care Quality Assurance	1987
AQH Journal	1988
Dynamic Quality Improvement Network Newsletter	1991
Quality In Health Care	1992
Quality Times	1991
USA	
AMCRA's Managed Care Monitor	1971
Abstracts Of Clinical Care Guidelines	1989
Accountability News For Health Care Managers	1994
American Journal Of Medical Quality	1986
Behavioral Outcomes and Guidelines Sourcebook	1995

continues

Table VII-2-3 *continued*

Title	Year
CQI Quality Chronicle	1992
Clinical Performance & Quality Health Care	1993
Directory Of Practice Parameters	1989
Drug Outcomes Sourcebook	1995
Drug Utilization Review	1985
Eye On Improvement	1994
Health Technology Trends	1987
Healthcare Quality Abstracts	1993
Homecare Quality Management	1995
Hospital And Health System Quality Management	1989
Hospital Benchmarks	1994
Hospital Case Management	1993
Hospital Infection Control	1973
Hospital Peer Review	1976
Hospital Risk Management	1979
Hospital Risk Management Forms, Checklists & Guidelines	1989
Hospital's Critical Path Manual	1994
International Journal Of Technology Assessment In Health Care	1984
Interwest Quality Catalyst	1992
Joint Commission Journal On Quality Improvement	1974
Joint Commission Perspectives	1952
Journal For Healthcare Quality	1979
Journal Of Clinical Outcomes Management	1994
Journal Of Healthcare Risk Management	1980
Journal Of Nursing Care Quality	1986
Journal Of Clinical Outcomes Management	1994
MEDTEP Update	1994
Managed Care Quality	1995
Medical Outcomes & Guidelines Alert	1993
Medical Outcomes & Guidelines Sourcebook	1993
Medical Quality Management Sourcebook	1994
Medical Utilization Management	1972
Nursing Quality Connection	1991
Outcomes Measurement & Management	1990
Outcomes Research Digest	1995
Patient-Focused Care	1993
Plant, Technology, And Safety Management	1985
QI/TQM	1991
QRC Advisor	1984
Quality Advocate	1983
Quality Connection	1991
Quality Evaluation News	1985
Quality Letter For Healthcare Leaders	1989
Quality Management In Health Care	1992
Quality Management Update	1991
Quality Matters	1994
Quality Of Care	1980
Quality Resource	1983
Report On Medical Guidelines & Outcomes Research	1990
Research Activities	1976
Strategies For Healthcare Excellence	1988
Technology News	1987
Update	1994

Abstracts of Clinical Care Guidelines

Publisher: public company
Mosby-Year Book, Inc
11830 Westline Indus-
trial Drive
St Louis, MO 63146-
3241
USA
Tel: 1-314-872-8370
Fax: 1-314-453-7005

Editor: Louise Kaegi

Circulation: 2000 (publisher's
estimate)

First published: 1989

Issues per year: 10

Subscription address: same as publisher

Subscription rate: US$95.00 in USA;
US$112.35 in Canada;
US$105.00 elsewhere;
single issue, US$15.00

Purpose: to disseminate illustrated summaries of and
expert commentaries on
clinical practice guide-
lines and to report on
developments in prac-
tice guideline develop-
ment, dissemination and
use

Focus: practice guidelines

Contributions: accepts practice guidelines and comprehen-
sive review articles that
offer recommendations
to guide clinicians' and
patients' decisions; news
and commentaries;
books and newsletters
and journals for review
or notice

ISSN: 1042-4423

Accountability News for Health Care Managers

Publisher: private corporation
Atlantic Information
Services, Inc
1050 17th Street, NW,
Suite 480
Washington, DC 20036
USA
Tel: 1-202-775-9008
Fax: 1-202-331-9542

Editor: Dorya Currie

Circulation: not available

First published: 1994

Issues per year: 24

Subscription address: same as publisher

Subscription rate: US$295.00 (if prepaid),
US$315.00 (if invoiced)
in USA and elsewhere

Purpose: to provide reliable man-
agement-focused news
on quality-based
accountability standards,
performance measures,
and reporting require-
ments for health plans
and providers

Focus: quality-based performance measures and
standards

Contributions: does not accept

ISSN: 1076-8432

Accreditor

Publisher: non-profit educational/
research (accrediting)
organisation
Australian Council on
Healthcare Standards
(ACHS)
Level 1,
7–9A Joynton Avenue
Zetland, NSW 2017
AUSTRALIA
Tel: 61-2-662-2311
Fax: 61-2-662-6370
Email: theachs @
slim.sinsw.gov.qv

Editor: Wendy Rotem

Circulation: 5300 (publisher's
estimate)

First published: 1983

Issues per year: 3

Subscription address: same as publisher

Subscription rate: free in Australia;
A$15.00 (about
US$11.00) elsewhere to
cover postage; single
issue, free

Purpose: to update health care
professionals on ACHS
accreditation and quality
assurance issues

Focus: accreditation, standards
development, quality
assurance

Contributions: accepts health care statistics, articles

AMCRA's Managed Care Monitor

Publisher:	trade association American Managed Care and Review Association (AMCRA) 1200 19th Street, NW, Suite 200 Washington, DC 20036 USA Tel: 1-202-728-0506 Fax: 1-202-728-0609
Editor:	Amanda Orr
Circulation:	1500 (publisher's estimate)
First published:	1971, as AAFMC (American Association of Foundations for Medical Care) Newsletter; name changed in 1983 to AMCRA Newsletter; in 1991 to present name
Issues per annum:	6
Subscription address:	same as publisher
Subscription rate:	free to AMCRA members; US$125.00 in USA and elsewhere; single issue not available; free sample issue on request
Membership:	open to any organisation associated with the managed health care industry, including, but not exclusively, HMOs, PPOs, VROs, IPAs, FMCs, and PHOs. Annual dues vary by membership category
Purpose:	to provide information about the managed health care industry to AMCRA members
Focus:	managed health care at the state and national levels
Contributions:	accepts unsolicited manuscripts on topics of interest to the managed care industry, such as technology assessment, quality assurance, utilisation review

American Journal of Medical Quality

Publisher:	professional association American College of
	Medical Quality (ACMQ) 9005 Congressional Court Potomac, MD 20854 USA Tel: 1-301-365-3570 Fax: 1-301-365-3202
Editor:	David Jones, MD
Circulation:	3400 (publisher's estimate)
First published:	1986 as Quality Assurance and Utilization Review; name changed in 1992
Issues per year:	4
Subscription address:	Williams & Wilkins 428 East Preston Street Baltimore, MD 21202-3993 USA
Subscription rate:	free to ACMQ members; US$70.00 in USA; US$84.00 in Japan; US$80 elsewhere; institutions add US$5.00; single issue, US$18.00 in USA, US$20.00 elsewhere
Membership:	open to anyone interested in quality assurance or utilisation review. Annual dues: US$295.00, fellow/member (restricted to medical doctors); US$80.00, affiliate
Purpose:	to provide a forum to exchange ideas, strategies, and methods
Focus:	quality assurance, utilisation review, cost containment
Contributions:	accepts

Best Practices in Hospital Quality: The Resource Manual

Publisher:	private corporation American Health Consultants PO Box 740056 Atlanta, GA 30374 USA Tel: 1-404-262-7436 Fax: 1-404-262-7837
Editor:	Allyson Harris
Circulation:	not available

First published: 1994
Issues per year: manual plus quarterly updates
Subscription address: same as publisher
Subscription rate: US$319.00 in USA and elsewhere; single issue not available
Purpose: to provide tools for quality management
Focus: quality management
Contributions: does not accept

Canadian Journal of Quality In Health Care

Publisher: professional association
Canadian Association for Quality in Health Care (CAQHC)
1 Eva Road, Suite 409
Etobicoke, Ontario
M9C-4Z5
CANADA
Tel: 1-416-626-0102
Fax: 1-416-620-5392
Editor: Irene Petersen, RN, BN, MBA
Circulation: 700 (publisher's estimate)
First published: 1988 as Canadian Journal of Quality Assurance; name changed in 1993
Subscription address: same as publisher
Subscription rate: free to CAQHC members; C$101.65, including 7% GST (about US$73.00) in Canada and elsewhere
Membership: open to health care professionals, and others, engaged in quality management, quality assurance, utilisation review, risk management. Annual dues: C$160.50 (about US$115.00)
Purpose: improve patient care through information dissemination
Contributions: accepts

Clinical Performance & Quality Health Care

Publisher: private corporation

Slack, Inc
6900 Grove Road
Thorofare, NJ 08086
USA
Tel: 1-609-848-1000
Fax: 1-609-853-5991
Editor: Richard P Wenzel, MD, MSc
Circulation: 2000 (publisher's estimate)
First published: 1993
Issues per year: 4
Subscription address: same as publisher
Subscription rate: US$96.00 in USA; US$120.00 (surface), US$150.00 (airmail) elsewhere; single issue, US$30.00; institutions, add US$10.00; discounts for multiple year subscriptions
Purpose: to publish original research, commentaries, and reviews that examine critically the structures, processes, and outcomes of health care
Focus: clinical performance in relation to quality of care
Contributions: accepts
ISSN: 1063-0279

CQI Quality Chronicle

Publisher: type not specified
SSM Health Care System
477 North Lindbergh Boulevard
St Louis, MO 63141
USA
Tel: 1-314-994-7800
Fax: 1-314-994-7900
Editor: Carol A. Bales
Circulation: 20 000 (publisher's estimate)
First published: 1992
Issues per year: 4
Subscription address: same as publisher
Subscription rate: free
Purpose: to provide information about continuous quality improvement
Focus: SSM Health Care System activities

Contributions: does not accept

Directory of Practice Parameters

Publisher:	professional association American Medical Association (AMA) 515 North State Street Chicago, IL 60610 USA Tel: 1-312-464-5000 Fax: 1-312-464-4184
Editor:	Margaret C Toepp, PhD; Naomi Kuznets, PhD
Circulation:	3100
First published:	1989 as Practice Parameters Update; name changed in 1990
Issues per year:	directory, plus 3 Practice Parameters Updates
Subscription address:	Order Department (publication number OP270395) American Medical Association PO Box 109050 Chicago, IL 60610-9050 USA
Subscription rate:	US$99.00 for AMA members; US$149.00 for non-members in USA and elsewhere; single issue not available
Membership:	open to medical doctors. Annual dues vary by membership category
Purpose:	to provide an index of information on practice parameters (guidelines) from physician and other organisations to health care and quality professionals
Focus:	practice parameters (guidelines); strategies for patient care management to assist clinical decision-making
Contributions:	accepts from national physician and other organisations
Electronic media:	Practice Parameters on CD-ROM (since 1993), includes a text search capability: US$995.00 single user version

(publication number OP270495), US$1,495.00, network version (OP270695) in USA and elsewhere

Drug Outcomes Sourcebook

Publisher:	public company Faulkner & Gray 11 Penn Plaza, 17th floor New York, NY 10001-0373 USA Tel: 1-212-967-7000 Fax: 1-212-967-7180
Editor:	Alicia Ault Burnett
Circulation:	not available
First published:	1995
Issues per year:	1
Subscription address:	same as publisher
Subscription rate:	US$235.00 in USA and elsewhere
Purpose:	not specified
Focus:	drug outcomes
Contributions:	not specified

Drug Utilization Review

Publisher:	private corporation American Health Consultants PO Box 740056 Atlanta, GA 30374 USA Tel: 1-404-262-7436 Fax: 1-404-262-7837
Editor:	Theresa Waldron
Circulation:	not available
First published:	1985
Issues per year:	12
Subscription address:	same as publisher
Subscription rate:	US$349.00 in USA, US$369.00 elsewhere; single issue not available
Purpose:	to guide subscribers in the cost-effective use of pharmaceuticals
Focus:	utilisation review
Contributions:	accepts

European Newsletter on Quality Assurance

Publisher:	non-profit educational/ research organisation CBO (Centraal Begeleidings Orgaan Voor de

Intercollegiale Toetsing—the National Organization for Quality Assurance in Hospitals)
PO Box 20064
3502 LB Utrecht
NETHERLANDS
Tel: 31-30-96-06-47
Fax: 31-30-94-36-44
Email: cbo @ erc.eur.nl

Editor: Evert Reerink, MD, PhD; Nick Klazinga, MD; Strasimir Cucic, MD

Circulation: 5000 (publisher's estimate)

First published: 1984

Issues per year: 4

Subscription address: same as publisher

Subscription rate: free

Purpose: to disseminate facts and news about quality assurance in health care to interested parties

Focus: quality assurance in health care

Contributions: accepts reports of studies, announcements of meetings, new books, etc; sometimes personalised articles

ISSN: 0920-2153

Eye on Improvement

Publisher: non-profit educational/ research organisation
Institute for Healthcare Improvement
1 Exeter Plaza, 9th floor
Boston, MA 02116
USA
Tel: 1-617-424-4800
Fax: 1-617-424-4848

Editor: Connie Koran

Circulation: 1000 (publisher's estimate)

First published: 1994

Issues per year: 24

Subscription address: Eye on Improvement
PO Box 38100
Cleveland, OH 44138-0100
USA
Tel: 1-216-235-8580
Fax: 1-216-235-2714
Email: CompuServe 75032,345

Subscription fee: US$90.00 in the USA and Canada; US$110.00 elsewhere

Purpose: to provide health care leaders with comprehensive, convenient, timely information about continual improvement gleaned from the published literature and unpublished reports

Focus: health care quality and improvement

Contributions: accepts

Healthcare Quality Abstracts

Publisher: private corporation
COR Healthcare Resources
PO Box 40959
Santa Barbara, CA 93140
USA
Tel: 1-805-564-2177
Fax: 1-805-564-2177

Editor: Dean Anderson

Circulation: not available

First published: 1993

Issues per year: 11

Subscription address: same as publisher

Subscription rate: US$98.00 in USA and Canada, US$110.00 elsewhere; single issue, US$10.00

Purpose: to summarise selected articles on health care quality improvement

Focus: continuous quality improvement, total quality management, critical pathways, practice guidelines, data management, and outcomes measurement

Contributions: does not accept

ISSN: 1073-0303

Health Technology Trends

Publisher: non-profit educational/ research organisation
ECRI
5200 Butler Pike
Plymouth Meeting, PA 19462
USA
Tel: 1-610-825-6000

Fax: 1-610-834-1275
Email: ecri @ hslc.org

Editor:	Cynthia Wallace
Circulation:	2000 (publisher's estimate)
First published:	1987, as Health Technology Critical Issues for Decision Makers; name changed in 1989
Issues per year:	12
Subscription address:	same as publisher
Subscription rate:	US$295.00 for the first year, US$245.00 thereafter, in USA and Canada; US$295.00 each year elsewhere; single issue, US$40.00
Purpose:	to inform health care executives about health care technologies
Focus:	health care technologies
Contributions:	does not accept
ISSN:	1041-6072

Homecare Quality Management

Publisher:	private corporation American Health Consultants PO Box 740056 Atlanta, GA 30374 USA Tel: 1-404-262-7436 Fax: 1-404-262-7837
Editor:	Cheli Brown
Circulation:	not available
First published:	1995
Issues per year:	12
Subscription address:	same as publisher
Subscription rate:	US$187.00 in USA; US$207.00 in US possessions and Canada; US$227.00 elsewhere; single issue not available
Purpose:	to help quality managers maximise quality improvement through practical, real world, hands-on information
Focus:	risk management, outcomes, benchmarking
Contributions:	accepts guest columns

Hospital and Health System Quality Management

Publisher:	public company Aspen Publishers, Inc.

200 Orchard Ridge
Drive, Suite 200
Gaithersburg, MD 20878
USA
Tel: 1-301-417-7500
Fax: 1-301-417-7550

Editor:	Howard S Rowland; Beatrice L Rowland
Circulation:	1300 (publisher's estimate)
First published:	1989 as Hospital Quality Assurance Manual; named changed in 1994
Issues per year:	two base volumes, plus 2 supplements per year. Supplements revise and update existing material and add new material
Subscription address:	same as publisher
Subscription rate:	US$275.00 in USA; US$369.00 elsewhere; plus US$65–$95 for each supplement (price depends on size of supplement)
Purpose:	to inform hospitals how to set up all aspects of a quality assurance program
Focus:	hospital quality assurance
Contributions:	does not accept
ISSB:	0-834-0072-4

Hospital Benchmarks

Publisher:	private corporation American Health Consultants PO Box 740056 Atlanta, GA 30374 USA Tel: 1-404-262-7436 Fax: 1-404-262-7837
Editor:	Allyson Harris
Circulation:	not available
First published:	1994
Issues per year:	12
Subscription address:	same as publisher
Subscription rate:	US$349.00 in USA and elsewhere; single issue not available
Purpose:	to communicate best practices and processes
Focus:	hospital benchmarking case studies, both clinical and operational
Contributions:	does not accept

Hospital Case Management

Publisher:	private corporation American Health Consultants PO Box 740056 Atlanta, GA 30374 USA Tel: 1-404-262-7436 Fax: 1-404-262-7837
Editor:	Kevin New
Circulation:	not available
First published:	1993
Issues per year:	12
Subscription address:	same as publisher
Subscription rate:	US$269.00 in USA; US$279.00 in US possessions and Canada; US$289.00 elsewhere; single issue not available
Purpose:	to provide clinicians and quality professionals with information on hospital case management, critical paths, and related subjects to manage length of stay
Focus:	length of stay
Contributions:	accepts guest columns

Hospital Infection Control

Publisher:	private corporation American Health Consultants PO Box 740056 Atlanta, GA 30374 USA Tel: 1-404-262-7436 Fax: 1-404-262-7837
Editor:	Garry Evans
Circulation:	not available
First published:	1973
Issues per year:	12
Subscription address:	same as publisher
Subscription rate:	US$299.00 in USA; US$309.00 in US possessions and Canada, US$319.00 elsewhere; single issue not available
Purpose:	to provide news and advice on preventing nosocomial infections in hospital employees and patients

Focus:	infection control
Contributions:	accepts guest columns

Hospital Outcomes Management

Publisher:	private corporation American Health Care Consultants PO Box 740060 Atlanta, GA 30374 USA Tel: 1-404-262-7436 Fax: 1-404-262-7837
Editor:	Kevin New
Circulation:	not available
First published:	1994
Issues per year:	12
Subscription address:	same as publisher
Subscription rate:	US$299.00 in USA; $309.00 in US possessions and Canada; US$319.00 elsewhere; single issue not available
Purpose:	to report on how hospitals are tracking medical outcomes
Focus:	health care outcomes
Contributions:	accepts guest columns

Hospital Peer Review

Publisher:	private corporation American Health Consultants PO Box 740056 Atlanta, GA 30374 USA Tel: 1-404-262-7436 Fax: 1-404-262-7837
Editor:	Jan Dale-Nichols
Circulation:	not available
First published:	1976
Issues per year:	12
Subscription address:	same as publisher
Subscription rate:	US$279.00 in USA; US$289.00, in US possessions and Canada; US$299.00, elsewhere; single issue, US$30.00
Purpose:	to provide quality management professionals with practical strategies
Focus:	quality assurance, quality improvement, utilisation review, discharge planning, Joint Commission on Accreditation of Healthcare

Organizations' standards, the Medicare program and its Peer Review Organizations' requirements

Contributions: does not accept
ISSN: 0149-2632

Hospital Risk Management

Publisher:	private corporation American Health Consultants PO Box 740056 Atlanta, GA 30374 USA Tel: 1-404-262-7436 Fax: 1-404-262-7837
Editor:	Cheli Brown
Circulation:	not available
First published:	1979
Issues per year:	12
Subscription address:	same as publisher
Subscription rate:	US$257.00 in USA, US$267 in Canada, US$277.00 elsewhere; single issue, US$22.00
Purpose:	to help hospital-based risk managers reduce the risks to their hospitals, and to improve risk managers' professional standing
Focus:	hospital-based risk management
Contributions:	accepts guest columns from experts

Hospital Risk Management Forms, Checklists & Guidelines

Publisher:	public company Aspen Publishers, Inc. 200 Orchard Ridge Drive, Suite 200 Gaithersburg, MD 20878 USA Tel: 1-301-417-7500 Fax: 1-301-417-7550
Editor:	Howard S Rowland; Beatrice L Rowland
Circulation:	800 (publisher's estimate)
First published:	1989

Issues per year:	base volume, plus 1 supplement per year. Supplement revises and updates existing material and adds new material
Subscription address:	same as publisher
Subscription rate:	US$210.00 in USA; US$286.00 elsewhere, plus US$65–$95 for the supplement (price depends on size of supplement)
Purpose:	to provide up-to-date information on risk management approaches
Focus:	hospital risk management
Contributions:	does not accept
ISSB:	0-8342-0131-6

Hospital's Critical Path Manual

Publisher:	private corporation American Health Consultants PO Box 740056 Atlanta, GA 30374 USA Tel: 1-404-262-7436 Fax: 1-404-262-7837
Editor:	Kathy Cline
Circulation:	not available
First published:	1994
Issues per year:	manual plus quarterly updates
Subscription address:	same as publisher
Subscription rate:	US$495.00 in USA and elsewhere; single issue not available
Purpose:	to provide hospital-based case managers with critical paths, variance tracking tools, outcomes measurement guidance, and other case management resources
Focus:	critical pathways, outcomes measurement
Contributions:	accepts guest columns

International Journal for Quality in Health Care

Publisher:	public company Elsevier Science Ltd The Boulevard, Langford Lane Kidlington, Oxford OX5-1GB, England, UK Tel: 44-1865-843-479 Fax: 44-1865-843-952
Editor:	R Heather Palmer, MB, BCh, SM
Circulation:	1500 (publisher's estimate)
First published:	1989 as Quality Assurance in Health Care; name changed in 1994
Issues per year:	4
Subscription address:	North America: Elsevier Science Inc 660 White Plains Road Tarrytown, NY 0591-5153, USA Australasia: DA Information Services 648 Whitehorse Road Mitcham, Victoria 3132, AUSTRALIA Rest of the world: same as publisher
Subscription rate:	free to ISQua members; US$224.00 in the USA or equivalent elsewhere in the Americas; £150.00 in the UK (plus VAT) or equivalent elsewhere in the world; negotiable discounts for multiple copies delivered to the same address; single issue, £40.00 (US$64.00)
Membership:	membership in the International Society for Quality in Health Care (ISQua) is open to anyone who is working or interested in the field of health care quality improvement. Institutional membership is also available. Annual dues for individual members are US$35.00; for institutional members, determined by the ISQua board
Purpose:	to publish original

articles describing empirical research, or demonstrations, or programs in all disciplines related to the quality of health care, including health services research, health economics, and clinical and nursing care relating to quality of care

Focus:	quality of health care
Contributions:	accepts articles, editorial letters, book reviews, etc.
ISSN:	1353-4505

International Journal of Health Care Quality Assurance

Publisher:	private corporation MCB University Press Ltd 60-62 Toller Lane Bradford, West Yorkshire BD8-9BY UK Tel: 44-1274-499-832 Fax: 44-1274-547-142
Editor:	Professor Robin Gourlay
Circulation:	1000 (publisher's estimate)
First published:	1987
Issues per year:	7
Subscription address:	same as publisher
Subscription rate:	£249.00 (about US$395.00) in UK and elsewhere
Purpose:	to provide a forum for the international exchange of theoretical and practical aspects of quality assurance and quality management in health care
Focus:	health care quality assurance
Contributions:	accepts
ISSN:	0952-6862

International Journal of Risk & Safety in Medicine

Publisher:	public company Elsevier Science BV PO Box 181 1000 AD Amsterdam NETHERLANDS

Tel: 31-20-485-3911
Fax: 31-20-485-3249
Editor: M N G Dukes
Circulation: 260
First published: 1990
Issues per year: 6 (in 2 volumes)
Subscription address: same as publisher
Subscription rate: DFL980 for both volumes (about US$592.00), including shipping and postage in the Netherlands and elsewhere; bulk subscription negotiable; single issue not available
Purpose: inform readers about the management and containment of risk in health care
Focus: risk/benefit ratio in medicine
Contributions: accepts reviews, primary research articles, short communications
ISSN: 0924-6479

International Journal of Technology Assessment in Health Care

Publisher: public company
Cambridge University Press
40 West 20th Street
New York, NY 10011
USA
Tel: 1-212-924-3900
Fax: 1-212-691-3239
Editor: Egon Jonsson, PhD; Stanley J Reiser, MD, PhD
Circulation: 1500 (publisher's estimate)
First published: 1984
Issues per year: 4
Subscription address: USA and Canada: same as publisher
Elsewhere:
Cambridge University Press
The Edinburgh Building
Shaftesbury Road
Cambridge CB2-2RU
England, UK
Subscription rate: free to ISTAHC (International Society of Technology Assessment in

Health Care) members; US$134.00 for institutions, US$92.00 for individuals in USA; £86.00 (about US$137.00) elsewhere
Membership: Open to anyone. Annual dues: US$95.00
Norman W Weissman, PhD
ISTAHC
2121 Wisconsin Avenue, NW, Suite 220
Washington, DC 20007
USA
Tel: 1-202-333-5637
Fax: 1-202-333-5586
Purpose: to provide scholarly articles
Focus: technology assessment
Contributions: accepts
ISSN: 0266-4623

Interwest Quality Catalyst

Publisher: non-profit educational/research organisation
Interwest Quality of Care, Inc
455 East 400 South, Suite 200
Salt Lake City, UT 84111
USA
Tel: 1-801-359-1390
Fax: 1-801-359-1392
Editor: Lori Wingeleth
Circulation: 450 (publisher's estimate)
First published: 1992
Issues per year: 4
Subscription address: same as publisher
Subscription rate: free
Purpose: to inform consortium members and interested parties of resource centre activities
Focus: quality management
Contributions: accepts

ISTAHC Newsletter

Publisher: professional association
International Society of Technology Assessment in Health Care (ISTAHC)
TNO Prevention and Health Sector Medical Technology Assessment

PO Box 2215
2301 CE Leiden
NETHERLANDS
Tel: 31-71-181-483
Fax: 31-71-181-906

Editor: H David Banta, MD, MPH

Circulation: 1440 (publisher's estimate)

First published: 1989

Issues per year: 4

Subscription address: same as membership

Subscription rate: restricted to ISTAHC members

Membership: Open to anyone. Annual dues: US$95.00. Norman W Weissman, PhD ISTAHC 2121 Wisconsin Avenue, NW, Suite 220 Washington, DC 20007 USA Tel: 1-202-333-5637 Fax: 1-202-333-5586

Purpose: to provide a worldwide overview of current technology assessment activities

Focus: technology assessment

Contributions: accepts news items

Joint Commission Journal On Quality Improvement

Publisher: public company Mosby-Year Book, Inc 11830 Westline Industrial Drive St Louis, MO 63146-3241 USA Tel: 1-314-872-8370 Fax: 1-314-453-7005

Editor: G. Jake Jaquet

Circulation: 8000 (publisher's estimate)

First published: 1974 as QRB (Quality Review Bulletin); name changed in 1993

Issues per year: 12

Subscription address: same as publisher

Subscription rate: US$115.00 in USA, US$139.10 in Canada; US$130.00 elsewhere; single issue, US$15.00 (special, theme issue US$25.00)

Purpose: to serve as a forum for practical approaches to improving quality and value in health care

Focus: innovative thinking, strategies, and practices in improving health care quality

Contributions: accepts

ISSN: 1070-3241

Joint Commission Perspectives

Publisher: public company Mosby-Year Book, Inc 11830 Westline Industrial Drive St Louis, MO 63146-3241 USA Tel: 1-314-872-8370 Fax: 1-314-453-7005

Editor: Bruce H. Ente

Circulation: 27 000 (publisher's estimate)

First published: 1952, as Perspectives on Accreditation; name changed in 1979 to JCAH Perspectives; in 1988 to present name

Issues per year: 6

Subscription address: same as publisher

Subscription rate: US$80.00 in USA; US$90.00 elsewhere; single issue, US$15.00

Purpose: to improve quality by helping health care organisations understand and comply with Joint Commission standards, participate in the Indicator Measurement System, and utilise quality improvement tools

Focus: accreditation standard, policies, and procedures; survey process; performance measurement; improving organisational performance

Contributions: accepts

Electronic media: online through MEDIS, Mead Data Central

ISSN: 0277-8327

Journal for Healthcare Quality

Publisher:	professional association National Association for Healthcare Quality (NAHQ) 5700 Old Orchard Road, 1st floor Skokie, IL 60077-1057 USA Tel: 1-708-966-9392 Fax: 1-708-966-9418
Editor:	Mary Marta, MSN, RN, CPHQ
Circulation:	7000 (publisher's estimate)
First published:	1979 as Journal of Quality Assurance; name changed in 1992
Issues per year:	6
Subscription address:	same as publisher
Subscription rate:	free to NAHQ members; US$110.00 in USA and elsewhere; single issue, US$20.00
Membership:	open to all organisations and persons in health care organisations involved in the management of health care quality. Annual dues: US$325.00 for institutions; US$100.00, for individuals
Purpose:	to educate members
Focus:	all aspects of health care quality management
Contributions:	accepts
ISSN:	1062-2551

Journal of Clinical Outcomes Management

Publisher:	private company Turner White Communications 125 Stafford Avenue, Suite 220 Wayne, PA 19087-3391 USA Tel: 1-610-975-4541 Fax: 1-620-975-4564
Editor:	Debra Dreger
Circulation:	80 300
First published:	1994
Issues per year:	6
Subscription address:	same as publisher

Subscription rate:	US$65.00 in USA; US$85.00 in Canada; US$150 elsewhere; US$10.00 discount for two-year subscription; single issue, US$15.00.
Purpose:	to translate outcomes and policy for, and to demonstrate their relevance to, clinicians
Focus:	health care outcomes
Contributions:	accepts
ISSN:	1079-6533

Journal of Healthcare Risk Management

Publisher:	trade association American Hospital Association 1 North Franklin Chicago, IL 60606 USA Tel: 1-312-422-3980 Fax: 1-312-422-4580
Editor:	Margaret Veach
Circulation:	2900 (publisher's estimate)
First published:	1980 as Perspectives in Healthcare Risk Management; name changed in 1992
Issues per year:	4
Subscription address:	same as publisher
Subscription rate:	available only to members of the American Society for Health-care Risk Management
Membership:	limited to health care risk managers. Annual dues: US$90.00
Purpose:	to inform members
Focus:	health care quality and risk management
Contributions:	accepts
ISSN:	1074-4797

Journal of Nursing Care Quality

Publisher:	public company Aspen Publishers, Inc. 200 Orchard Ridge Drive, Suite 200 Gaithersburg, MD 20878 USA Tel: 1-301-417-7500 Fax: 1-301-417-7550
Editor:	Patricia Schroeder, MSN, RN

Circulation:	7000 (publisher's estimate)
First published:	1986 as Journal of Nursing Quality Assurance; name changed in 1991
Issues per year:	4
Subscription address:	USA, Canada, Japan: Aspen Publishers, Inc 7201 McKinney Circle Frederick, MD 21701 USA Elsewhere: Swets Publishing Service PO Box 825 2160 SZ Lisse NETHERLANDS
Subscription rate:	US$86.00 in USA and Canada, US$92.00 elsewhere; discounts for bulk purchases; single issue, US$25.00
Purpose:	to provide practising and quality assurance nurses with useful information on the application of quality assurance principles and concepts to practice
Focus:	health care quality assurance
Contributions:	accepts
ISSN:	1057-3631

Journal of Quality in Clinical Practice

Publisher:	public company Blackwell Science Pty Ltd on behalf of ACHS and AMA 54 University Street PO Box 378 Carlton, Victoria 3053 AUSTRALIA Tel: 61-39347-0300 Fax: 61-39347-5001
Editor:	Professor John Duggan
Circulation:	2800 (publisher's estimate)
First published:	1981 as Australian Clinical Review; name changed in 1994
Issues per year:	4
Subscription address:	same as publisher

Subscription rate:	A$199 US$199 for overseas; single issue not available
Purpose:	to communicate information about the evaluation of clinical practice, quality studies, in healthcare and technology assessment
Focus:	clinical practice
Contributions:	accepts
ISSN:	1320-5455

Managed Care Quality

Publisher:	private corporation American Health Consultants PO Box 740056 Atlanta, GA 30374 USA Tel: 1-404-262-7436 Fax: 1-404-262-7837
Editor:	Allyson Harris
Circulation:	not available
First published:	1995
Issues per year:	12
Subscription address:	same as publisher
Subscription rate:	US$279.00 in USA; US$289.00 in US possessions and Canada; US$299.00 elsewhere; single issue not available
Purpose:	to inform and assist quality management professionals in managed care organisations
Focus:	accreditation, credentialling, practice guidelines, quality improvement programs, report cards
Contributions:	accepts guest columns

Medical Outcomes & Guidelines Alert

Publisher:	public company Faulkner & Gray, Inc. 11 Penn Plaza New York, NY 10001-0373 USA Tel: 1-212-631-1406 Fax: 1-212-695-8172
Editor:	Louis Wingerson

Circulation:	not available
First published:	1993
Issues per year:	24
Subscription address:	same as publisher
Subscription rate:	US$365.00 in USA and elsewhere
Purpose:	not specified
Focus:	health care outcomes and practice guidelines
Contributions:	not specified

Medical Outcomes and Guidelines Sourcebook

Publisher:	public company Faulkner & Gray 11 Penn Plaza, 17th floor New York, NY 10001-0373 USA Tel: 1-212-967-7000 Fax: 1-212-967-7180
Editor:	Spencer Vibbert
Circulation:	not available
First published:	1993
Issues per year:	1
Subscription address:	same as publisher
Subscription rate:	US$265.00 in USA and elsewhere
Purpose:	not specified
Focus:	health care outcomes
Contributions:	not specified

Medical Quality Management Sourcebook

Publisher:	public company Faulkner & Gray 11 Penn Plaza, 17th floor New York, NY 10001-0373 USA Tel: 1-212-967-7000 Fax: 1-212-967-7180
Editor:	Spencer Vibbert
Circulation:	not available
First published:	1994
Issues per year:	1
Subscription address:	same as publisher
Subscription rate:	US$365.00 in USA and elsewhere
Purpose:	not specified
Focus:	health care outcomes
Contributions:	not specified

Medical Utilization Management

Publisher:	public company Faulkner & Gray's Healthcare Information Center 11 Penn Plaza, 17th floor New York, NY 10001-0373 USA Tel: 1-212-967-7000 Fax: 1-212-967-7180
Editor:	Lisa Bender
Circulation:	not available
First published:	1972 as PSRO letter; named changed in 1981 to Medical Utilization Review; in 1994 to present name
Issues per year:	24
Subscription address:	same as publisher
Subscription rate:	US$385.00 in USA and elsewhere; US$100.00 for each additional copy mailed in the same envelope; single issue not available
Purpose:	to inform subscribers about health care cost containment, PROs, private review, and quality assurance
Focus:	public- and private-sector cost containment and quality assurance/ utilisation review
Contributions:	does not accept

MEDTEP Update

Publisher:	national government US Agency for Health Care Policy and Research 2101 East Jefferson Street, Suite 501 Rockville, MD 20852 USA Tel: 1-301-594-1364 extension 162 Fax: 1-301-594-2283
Editor:	William N. LeVee
Circulation:	5000 (publisher's estimate)
First published:	1994
Issues per year:	4
Subscription address:	same as publisher
Subscription rate:	free

Purpose: to provide information on the findings, dissemination and implications of the Medical Treatment Effectiveness Program (MEDTEP). MEDTEP activities are undertaken to determine the most effective and appropriate strategies for diagnosis and prevention, treatment and management of clinical conditions

Focus: health services research, clinical practice guidelines development, database development, and related dissemination and evaluation activities

Contributions: does not accept

NAQA Journal

Publisher: professional association
Association for Quality in Healthcare
9 Chesil Street
Winchester, Hants,
SO23-0HU
England, UK
Tel: 44-1962-877-700
Fax: 44-1962-877-701

Editor: Nancy Dixon

Circulation: 2000 (publisher's estimate)

First published: 1988; relaunched in 1993

Issues per year: 4

Subscription address: same as publisher

Subscription rate: free to members; £65.00 (about US$103.00) in UK and elsewhere; single issue, £9.00 (US$14.00)

Membership: open to all individuals who have a specific interest in or responsibility for the standard of health care provision. Annual dues: £45.00 (about US$238.00) individual; £150.00 (US$72.00) group; £250.00 (US$397.00) corporate

Purpose: to disseminate information

Focus: health care quality

Contributions: accepts

ISSN: 1351-5969

Nursing Quality Connection

Publisher: public company
Mosby-Year Book, Inc.
11830 Westline Industrial Drive
St Louis, MO 63146-9934
USA
Tel: 1-314-872-8370;
1-800-325-4177 (in USA)
Fax: 1-314-432-1380

Editor: Patricia Schroeder, MSN, RN

Circulation: not available

First published: 1991

Issues per year: 6

Subscription address: same as publisher

Subscription rate: US$65.00 for institutions, US$49.95 for individuals, US$32.50 if ordering five or more copies for the same address in the USA; US$70.00 for institutions, US$54.94 for individuals elsewhere; single issue, US$8.00

Purpose: to provide timely and practical information about approaches to improving quality in health care, including standards and guidelines and clear example of how to apply the newest approaches in clinical settings

Focus: nursing-specific health care quality

Contributions: accepts

Outcomes Measurement and Management

Publisher: private corporation
The Zitter Group
90 New Montgomery,
Suite 820
San Francisco, CA 94105
USA
Tel: 1-415-495-2450
Fax: 1-415-495-2453

Editor: Karl A. Thiel

Circulation:	4200 (publisher's estimate)
First published:	1990
Issues per year:	12
Subscription address:	same as publisher
Subscription rate:	US$249.00, in USA and elsewhere; less 20% for more than 10 copies to the same organisation; single issue, US$25.00
Purpose:	to inform subscribers
Focus:	health care outcomes measurement and management
Contributions:	does not accept

Patient-Focused Care

Publisher:	private corporation American Health Consultants PO Box 740056 Atlanta, GA 30374 USA Tel: 1-404-262-7436 Fax: 1-404-262-7837
Editor:	Deborah Goldman
Circulation:	not available
First published:	1993
Issues per year:	12
Subscription address:	same as publisher
Subscription rate:	US$249.00 in USA; US$259.00 in US possessions and Canada; US$269.00 elsewhere; single issue not available
Purpose:	to help hospitals navigate patient-focused care and other forms of organisational restructuring designed to bring care closer to patients and make it more efficient
Focus:	patient care
Contributions:	accepts guest columns

Plant, Technology, and Safety Management

Publisher:	public company Mosby-Year Book, Inc 11830 Westline Industrial Drive St Louis, MO 63146-3241 USA Tel: 1-314-872-8370 Fax: 1-314-453-7005
Editor:	Kristine M Tomasik
Circulation:	3000 (publisher's estimate)
First published:	1985
Issues per year:	base volume, plus 4 theme monographs
Subscription address:	same as publisher
Subscription rate:	US$140.00 in USA, US$190.00 elsewhere, for first year; US$95.00 for each subsequent year in USA, US$135.00 elsewhere; single issue, US$40.00 in USA, US$50.00 elsewhere
Purpose:	to inform professionals responsible for a facility's environmental systems and safety
Focus:	plant and equipment management and safety
Contributions:	accepts

QI/TQM

Publisher:	private corporation American Health Consultants PO Box 740056 Atlanta, GA 30374 USA Tel: 1-404-262-7436 Fax: 1-404-262-7837
Editor:	Jennifer Allen
Circulation:	not available
First published:	1991
Issues per year:	12
Subscription address:	same as publisher
Subscription rate:	US$339.00 in USA, US$359.00 elsewhere; single issue not available
Purpose:	to guide quality improvement through quality management
Focus:	total quality management, quality improvement
Contributions:	accepts guest columns

QRC Advisor

Publisher:	public company Aspen Publishers, Inc. 200 Orchard Ridge Drive, Suite 200 Gaithersburg, MD 20878 USA

Tel: 1-301-417-7500
Fax: 1-301-417-7550

Editor: Barbara J Youngsberg, RN, MSW, JD

Circulation: 2000 (publisher's estimate)

First published: 1984

Issues per year: 12

Subscription address: PO Box 990
7801 McKinney Circle
Frederick, MD 21701-9788
USA

Subscription rate: US$199.00 in USA;
US$239.00 elsewhere;
single issue, US$25.00

Purpose: to provide practical, vital information to quality assurance, risk management, and cost control personnel on strategies and techniques, news and developments that will help them perform their jobs more effectively

Focus: health care quality and risk management

Contributions: does not accept

ISSN: 0747-7384

Quality Advocate

Publisher: trade association
American Medical Peer Review Association (AMPRA)
1140 Connecticut Avenue, NW, Suite 1050
Washington, DC 20036
USA
Tel: 1-202-331-5790
Fax: 1-202-833-2047

Editor: Patricia Madigan

Circulation: 1300 (publisher's estimate)

First published: 1983 as AMPRA Review; name changed in 1994

Issues per year: 6

Subscription address: same as publisher

Subscription rate: free to AMPRA members; US$100.00 in USA and elsewhere; single issue, US$25.00

Membership: open to individuals and institutions dedicated to health care quality through community-based independent quality improvement and evaluation. Annual dues: variable for institution; US$2,000.00, associate; US$75.00, individual

Purpose: to update members and others on latest strides in community-based quality improvement in health care delivery

Focus: community-based quality improvement in health care

Contributions: accept articles and job bank service for members

Quality Assurance Network Newsletter

Publisher: professional society
Royal College of Nursing
Dynamic Quality Improvement Programme
National Institute for Nursing
Radcliffe Infirmary
Oxford, OX2-6HE
England, UK
Tel: 44-1865-224-667
Fax: 44-1865-246-787

Editor: Gill Harvey

Circulation: 8000 (publisher's estimate)

First published: 1991

Issues per year: 2

Subscription address: same as publisher

Subscription rate: free to Royal College of Nursing members; £30.00 (about US$48.00) in UK and elsewhere

Purpose: to guide quality improvement, clinical audit, and clinical guidelines

Focus: health care quality improvement

Contributions: accepts articles on all aspects of quality assurance initiatives in health care

Quality Connection

Publisher: non-profit educational/research organisation

Institute for Healthcare Improvement (IHI) (formerly National Demonstration Project on Quality Improvement in Health Care)
1 Exeter Plaza, 9th floor
Boston, MA 02116
USA
Tel: 1-617-424-4800
Fax: 1-617-424-4848

Editor: Valerie Weber
Circulation: 25 000 (publisher's estimate)
First published: 1991
Issues per year: 4
Subscription address: same as publisher
Subscription rate: free
Purpose: to offer support to leaders in all health care settings who are involved in improving quality and value through the application of continuous improvement principles, through the exchange of information about relevant initiatives, innovative uses of methods and tools, new concepts and their applications, and 'lessons learned'
Focus: health care quality
Contributions: accepts

Quality Evaluation News
Publisher: non-profit educational/research organisation
Center for Clinical Quality Evaluation (CCQE)
1140 Connecticut Avenue, NW, Suite 1010
Washington, DC 20036
USA
Tel: 1-202-833-3045
Fax: 1-202-833-2047
Editor: Carole J Magoffin, MS
Circulation: 1000
First published: 1985 as Quality Review News; name changed in 1995
Issues per year: 4
Subscription address: same as publisher
Subscription rate: restricted to CCQE members

Membership: open to organisations and individuals concerned with change and innovation in medical quality evaluation and research. Annual dues: US$3,000.00 for institution; US$1,000.00, associate organisation; US$100.00, individual, US$35.00, student
Purpose: to inform and be a resource for members
Focus: medical quality evaluation, treatment effectiveness, practice guideline and development of performance measurement systems, outcomes measurement, shared patient–physician decision-making
Contributions: accepts

Quality in Health Care
Publisher: professional association
BMJ Publishing Group
British Medical Association
BMA House
Tavistock Square
London, WC1H-9JR
England, UK
Tel: 44171-383-6241
Fax: 44171-1383-6661
Editor: Fiona Moss
Circulation: 1500 (publisher's estimate)
First published: 1992
Issues per year: 4
Subscription address: same as publisher
Subscription rate: £97.00 (about US$154.00) for institutions, £59.00 (US$94.00) for individuals in UK and elsewhere
Purpose: to explore all aspects of quality in health care, including the issues associated with developing a multiprofessional approach to quality assurance, and to build the academic base for quality improvement
Focus: quality in health care

Contributions:	accepts
ISSN:	0963-8172

Quality Letter for Healthcare Leaders

Publisher:	private corporation Bader & Associates Inc. 5640 Nicholson Lane, Suite 226 Rockville, MD 20852 USA Tel: 1-301-468-1610 Fax: 1-301-770-4919
Editor:	Reggi Veatch
Circulation:	2500 (publisher's estimate)
First published:	1989
Issues per year:	10
Subscription address:	PO Box 2106 Rockville, MD 20847-2106 USA
Subscription rate:	US$279.00 in USA and Canada, US$325.00 elsewhere; US$75.00 for each additional subscription up to 9, and US$52.00 thereafter, mailed to the same address in the USA and Canada; US$99.00 each additional subscription up to 9 and US$69.00 thereafter, mailed to the same address elsewhere; single issue, $23.00
Purpose:	to provide health care executives, physician leaders, and governing board members timely, thought-provoking, and practical articles related to their quality-related responsibilities
Focus:	health care quality and quality management
Contributions:	does not accept
ISSN:	1047-5311

Quality Management in Health Care

Publisher:	public company Aspen Publishers, Inc. 200 Orchard Ridge Drive, Suite 200 Gaithersburg, MD 20878 USA

	Tel: 1-301-417-7500 Fax: 1-301-417-7550
Editor:	Glenn Laffel, MD, PhD
Circulation:	2000 (publisher's estimate)
First published:	1992
Issues per year:	4
Subscription address:	USA, Canada, Japan: Aspen Publishers, Inc 7201 McKinney Circle Frederick, MD 21701 USA Elsewhere: Swets Publishing Service PO Box 825 2160 SZ Lisse NETHERLANDS
Subscription rate:	US$134.00 in USA and Canada; US$155.00 elsewhere; single issue, US$40.00
Purpose:	to provide a forum to explore theoretical, technical, and strategic elements of quality management, and to assist those who wish to implement this discipline in health care
Focus:	health care quality
Contributions:	accepts
ISSN:	1063-8628.

Quality Management Update

Publisher:	public company Faulkner & Gray Information Center 11 Penn Plaza, 17th floor New York, NY 10001-0373 USA Tel: 1-212-967-1000 Fax: 1-212-967-7155
Editor:	Joseph Mangano
Circulation:	not available
First published:	1991
Issues per year:	24
Subscription address:	same as publisher
Subscription rate:	US$275.00 in USA and elsewhere; single issue not available
Purpose:	to provide health care professionals with current, practical information on techniques of, and developments

Focus: in, health care quality management applications of total quality management techniques, and information on activities of external surveying agencies, and on management areas relating to quality management, including utilisation review and risk management

Contributions: accepts occasionally

Quality Matters

Publisher: non-profit educational/research (accrediting) organisation National Committee for Quality Assurance 1350 New York Avenue, NW, Suite 700 Washington, DC 2005 USA Tel: 1-202-628-5788 Fax: 1-202-628-0344

Editor: Ann Greiner

Circulation: not available

First published: 1994

Publisher declined to provide information.

Quality of Care

Publisher: state government New York State Commission on Quality of Care for the Mentally Disabled (NYSCQC) 99 Washington Avenue, Suite 1002 Albany, NY 12210-2895 USA Tel: 1-518-473-4057 Fax: 1-518-473-6296

Editor: Marcus A Gigliotti

Circulation: 14 000 (publisher's estimate)

First published: 1980

Issues per year: 4 to 6

Subscription address: same as publisher

Subscription rate: free

Purpose: to inform professionals, service recipients, family members, and advocacy groups about the activities, actions, and

Focus: concerns of NYSCQC and its programs monitoring quality of care and advocating quality care and treatment for people with mental disabilities

Contributions: accepts articles related to focus

Electronic media: free bulletin board service at 1-518-486-7711

Quality Resource

Publisher: professional association Quality Assurance Section American Health Information Management Association (AHIMA) 919 North Michigan Avenue, Suite 1400 Chicago, IL 60611 USA Tel: 1-312-787-2672 Fax: 1-312-787-9793

Editor: Patrice Spath, ART

Circulation: 3000 (publisher's estimate)

First published: 1983 as QA Section Connection; name changed in 1993

Issues per year: 6

Subscription address: same as publisher

Subscription rate: restricted to members of the quality assurance section of AHIMA

Membership: open to anyone. Annual dues are US$35.00 in addition to AHIMA dues

Purpose: to inform members about important contemporary issues

Focus: quality management, quality assurance and quality improvement; contents are articles and literature reviews

Contributions: accepts articles on quality management, quality assurance or quality improvement

ISSN: 1040-2950

Quality Times

Publisher: professional association Association for Quality

in Healthcare
9 Chesil Street
Winchester, Hants,
SO23-0HU
England, UK
Tel: 44-1962-877-700
Fax: 44-1962-877-701

Editor: Michael Pryce Jones

Circulation: 2000 (publisher's estimate)

First published: 1991 as NAQA Newsletter; name changed in 1992

Issues per year: 4

Subscription address: same as publisher

Subscription rate: free to members; £20.00 (about US$32.00) in UK and elsewhere

Membership: open to all individuals who have a specific interest in or responsibility for the standard of health care provision. Annual dues: £45.00 (about US$238.00) individual; £150.00 (US$72.00) group; £250.00 (US$397.00) corporate

Purpose: to promote quality in health care

Focus: quality assurance, quality improvement, quality management

Contributions: accepts

Report on Medical Guidelines & Outcomes Research

Publisher: private corporation Capitol Publications Inc 1101 King Street, Suite 444 Alexandria, VA 22314 USA Tel: 1-703-683-4100 Fax: 1-703-739-6517

Editor: Kathryn DeMott

Circulation: not available

First published: 1990

Issues per year: 24

Subscription address: same as publisher

Subscription rate: US$495.00 in USA and elsewhere; discounts for multiple copies sent to the same address; single issue, US$25.00

Purpose: to provide news and analysis of issues, legislation, developments, etc., related to medical practice guidelines, their use and development, and how outcomes data can be collected and applied to guidelines use, and quality improvement

Focus: medical practice guidelines, health care outcomes, quality improvement, report cards and other performance measures

Contributions: does not accept

ISSN: 0896-6567

Research Activities

Publisher: national government US Agency for Health Care Policy and Research 2102 East Jefferson Street, Suite 501 Rockville, MD 20852 USA Tel: 1-301-594-1364 Fax: 1-301-594-2283

Editor: Mary Grady

Circulation: 40 000 (publisher's estimate)

First published: 1976

Issues per year: 12

Subscription address: AHCPR Publications PO Box 8547 Silver Spring, MD 20907 USA

Subscription rate: free

Purpose: to disseminate findings of research supported by the Agency for Health Care Policy and Research

Focus: research related to quality management, clinical practice guidelines, patient outcomes research, and other health care issues

Contributions: does not accept

Strategies for Healthcare Excellence

Publisher:	for profit corporation COR Healthcare Resources PO Box 40959 Santa Barbara, CA 93140 USA Tel: 1-805-564-2177 Fax: 1-805-564-2177
Editor:	Susan J Anthony
Circulation:	not available
First published:	1988
Issues per year:	12
Subscription address:	same as publisher
Subscription rate:	US$197.00 in USA; US$199.00 elsewhere; single issue, US$20.00
Purpose:	to provide information on innovative approaches to quality and effectiveness in health care delivery
Focus:	organisational restructuring to boost quality, productivity, responsiveness and effectiveness
Contibutions:	accepts
ISSN:	1058-7829

Technology News

Publisher:	professional association American Medical Association (AMA) Department of Technology Assessment 515 North State Street Chicago, IL 60610-4377 USA Tel: 1-312-464-5000 Fax: 1-312-464-5841
Editor:	Sona Kalousdian, MD, MPH; Michael J Glade, PhD
Circulation:	not available
First published:	1987
Issues per year:	10
Subscription address:	same as publisher
Subscription rate:	US$325.00 for the first year in USA and elsewhere; US$485.00 for two years
Membership:	open to medical doctors. Annual dues vary by membership category
Purpose:	to cover clinical issues and health policy related to technology assessment
Focus:	medical technology assessment
Contributions:	accepts only on a case-by-case basis

Update

Publisher:	non-profit educational/research organisation Health Outcomes Institute 2001 Killebrew Drive, Suite 122 Bloomington, MN 55425 USA Tel: 1-612-858-9188 Fax: 1-612-858-9189
Editor:	open
Circulation:	9000 (publisher's estimate)
First published:	1994
Issues per year:	4
Subscription address:	same as publisher
Subscription rate:	free
Purpose:	to inform interested parties about the Health Outcome Institute's work
Focus:	health outcomes
Contributions:	accepts

INDEX